Irritable Bowel Syndrome: Diagnosis and Treatment

Irritable Bowel Syndrome: Diagnosis and Treatment

Editor: Boden Collins

AMERICAN
MEDICAL PUBLISHERS
www.americanmedicalpublishers.com

AMERICAN
MEDICAL PUBLISHERS
www.americanmedicalpublishers.com

Cataloging-in-publication Data

Irritable bowel syndrome: diagnosis and treatment / edited by Boden Collins.
p. cm.
Includes bibliographical references and index.
ISBN 979-8-88740-645-9
1. Inflammatory bowel diseases. 2. Irritable colon.
3. Intestines--Diseases. 4. Gastroenteritis. I. Collins, Boden.
RC862.I53 I54 2023
616.344--dc23

American Medical Publishers,
41 Flatbush Avenue,
1st Floor, New York,
NY 11217, USA

ISBN 979-8-88740-645-9 (Hardback)

Contents

Preface

Irritable bowel syndrome (IBS) refers to a condition that causes abdominal pain and bowel changes. The common symptoms of IBS include changes in bowel movements, bloating, stomach cramps, and frequent diarrhea or constipation. In menstruating women, IBS symptoms may be even worsen. People with IBS usually have a lower pain tolerance. The precise cause of IBS is unknown. Some of the factors that seem to play a role include severe infections, intestine muscle spasms, changes in gut microbiota, and early life stress. IBS can be diagnosed by performing a physical examination along with a review of the symptoms, family history, and medical history. The IBS treatment aims to alleviate the symptoms with the help of probiotics, dietary changes, counseling, and medicine. This book contains a detailed explanation of the various diagnostic and therapeutic techniques associated with irritable bowel syndrome. It aims to shed light on some of the unexplored aspects of this condition. A number of latest researches have been included to keep the readers up-to-date with the latest concepts with respect to this medical condition.

This book unites the global concepts and researches in an organized manner for a comprehensive understanding of the subject. It is a ripe text for all researchers, students, scientists or anyone else who is interested in acquiring a better knowledge of this dynamic field.

I extend my sincere thanks to the contributors for such eloquent research chapters. Finally, I thank my family for being a source of support and help.

Editor

1

Effect of librax (chlordiazepoxide and clidinium) in the treatment of irritable bowel syndrome

Hassan KH. Rajab

Abstract

Irritable bowel syndrome (IBS) is one of the commonest disorder of the gastrointestinal tract, IBS is long standing dysfunction associated with abdominal pain for which no organic cause can be found. a fifty three patients were included in this study all of them diagnosed as irritable bowel syndrome clinically after excluding organic causes. The patients receive a treatment with "librax "(chlordiazepoxide 5 mg & clidinium 2.5 mg) before meal twice daily plus "spasmopan"(hyoscine N- butylbromide 10 mg) after meal three times daily. The treatment continue for 1.5 -2 month.The results showed an improvement in 68% of the patients. No significant differences observe except in female, age group of 20-30 years old, patients with positive family history of the disease & patients with psychotic disorders (stress, worried & anxiety). Initiation of combine drugs therapy plus psychotherapy a good approach in treatment of irritable bowel syndrome.

Introduction

Irritable bowel syndrome (IBS) is one of the commonest disorder of the gastrointestinal tract, IBS is long standing dysfunction associated with abdominal pain for which no organic cause can be found. Bowel habit is disturbed by diarrhea or constipation occurring alone or alternatively (1) The prevalence of irritable bowel syndrome is 10-20% of population (2), (15-20)% (3) & 7.26% (4)

Irritable bowel syndrome caused by [1, 5, 6, 7, 8]:

1. psycholgical disturbance especially anxiety, stress individual & worried person
2. some relate the onset of symptoms to an attack of infectious diarrhea.
3. in other, food may precipitate the symptoms

The syndrome more frequent in women than men between age(20-40) years old. the commonest symptoms are: 1-abdomial pain relief by defecation, refered to right or left iliac fossa or to hypogastrium. 2-bowel habit variable. 3-painless morning diarrhea. 4-abdomial distension due to excessive flatus. 5-sensation of incomplete emptying of the rectum. 6-audible borborygmi. 7-nausea, headache, tiredness, dyspepsia, atypical chest pain. 8-palpable tender distended bowel. 9-mucus in stool(1, 13).

The diagnostic evaluation of IBS comprises a limited routine laboratory investigation, and endoscopic exploration to exclude organic disease of the gastrointestinal tract & to look for what we called it a red flags as shown in table -1- (1, 6, 9).

Table-1-(6) Red Flags in Evaluating for Irritable Bowel Syndrome

Anemia
Family history of colon cancer or inflammatory bowel disease
Fever
Heme-positive stools
New or recent onset in patient older than 50 years Nocturnal symptoms
Palpable abdominal or rectal mass
Persistent diarrhea or severe constipation Recent antibiotic use
Rectal bleeding
Weight loss

After exclusion of the organic bowel disease the diagnosis based on Rome I Criteria & Rome II Criteria as shown in table 2[6, 10, 11, 12].

Table -2- Criteria of diagnosis of IBS.

Rome I Criteria	Rome II Criteria
At least three months of continuous or recurrent symptoms of abdominal pain that is: Relieved by defecation and/or Associated with a change in stool consistency and/or Associated with a change in frequency of stool Plus two or more of the following greater than 25 percent of the time: Altered stool frequency (more than three per day or less than three per week) Altered stool form (lumpy, hard or watery, loose) Altered stool passage (straining, urgency, or incomplete evacuation) Passage of mucus Bloating or feeling of abdominal distention	12 or more weeks of continuous or recurrent abdominal pain or discomfort Plus at least two of the following: Relieved by defecation and/or Associated with change in frequency of stool and/or Associated with a change in form (appearance) of stool

Current pharmacological treatment option of irritable bowel syndrome are limited and lack specificity (1, 2). Table 4 show many medication used in treatment of irritable bowel syndrome (6, 7, 9) :

Table -3- Medications Used in the Management of Irritable Bowel Syndrome

Predominant symptom	Medications	Dosage	Comment
Diarrhea	Loperamide (Imodium)	2 to 4 mg up to four times a day	Use as needed or prophylactically in times of anticipated stress
	Cholestyramine (Questran)	4 g one to six times a day	Second-line agent
	Alosetron	1 mg per day titrated to two times a day if tolerated	Restricted use in female patients only
Constipation	Fiber	Start low and titrate up to 20 to 30 g a day	May worsen bloating
	Osmotic laxative	Magnesium citrate, lactulose, or polyethylene glycol dosed as appropriate	
Abdominal pain	Antispasmodics and anticholinergics (e.g., dicyclomine [Bentyl], hyoscyamine [Levsin])	Dicyclomine, 10 to 20 mg, two to four times a day	Used as needed only
	Tricyclic antidepressant (e.g., amitriptyline [Elavil])	Start amitriptyline, 10 to 25 mg at bedtime or twice daily, or desipramine (Norpramin), 50 mg three times a day	Needs to be given daily, not as needed, therefore generally reserved for patients with more severe pain
	Tegaserod (Zelnorm)		FDA approved for short- term treatment of women
Gas or bloating	Simethicone (Mylanta)	40 to 125 mg up to four times a day as needed	Anecdotal evidence only
Comorbid depression or anxiety	Antidepressants or anxiolytics as indicated	Dose as appropriate	Treating depression has been shown to improve bowel symptoms

The aim of the study is to evaluate the efficacy of librax & spasmopan in treatment of IBS

Patients and methods

During a 10-month period, 53 out patients with IBS, after exclusion of organic bowel pathology and meeting Rome I Criteria & Rome II Criteria for the diagnosis of irritable bowel syndrome were included in this study. They were assessed using the Personality Questionnaire [including age, sex, psychological state (stress, anxiety & worried), family history of the disease, social habits (drinking & smoker) & history of antibiotic intake within the last six month prior development of the disease]. The diagnosis (was done by physician) is established on the basis of typical symptoms and specific exclusion of relevant differential diagnoses. The heart of the diagnostic evaluation comprises a limited routine laboratory investigation, and endoscopic exploration to exclude organic disease of the gastrointestinal tract. All the patient receive a treatment regimen with "librax "(chlordiazepoxide 5 mg & clidinium 2.5 mg) before meal twice daily plus "spasmopan"(hyoscine N-butylbromide 10 mg) after meal three times daily. The treatment continue for 1.5-2 month.

Statistical analysis was done by using Chi square.

Results

This study included a fifty three patients their ages range between 18-55 years old (mean = 34.35 years of old), 21(39.6%) of them were Male & 32 (60.4%) of them Female, 28 of them were under stress, 31 of them were anxious, 17 of them were worried, 2 of them were drinker, 20 of them were smoker, 6 of them of positive antibiotic intake in the last 6 months & 13 of them had positive family history of the disease(IBS).

The efficacy of the treatment was positive in 36 patients (68%) & negative in 17 patients (32%). The efficacy of the treatment according to the age group were 3 out of 3, 9 out of 18, 18 out of 25 & 6 out of 7 respectively, there is a statistical significant difference in age group rang 20-30 as showed in table -4-.

The efficacy among male was 10 (48%) & 26 (81%) was the efficacy among female, there is a statistical significant difference between male and female as showed in table -5-.

The efficacy among smokers and non smokers was 35% & 30.3% respectively, there is no statistical significant difference between them as shown in table -6-.

The efficacy among patients with positive & negative family history of irritable bowel syndrome was 61.5% & 22.5% respectively, there is a statistical significant difference between them as shown in table -7-.

The efficacy among patients under stress/not under stress 43% &94% respectively, there is a statistical significant difference between them as showed in table -8-.

The efficacy among patients under anxiety/non anxiety patients 55% & 86.4% respectively, there is a statistical significant difference between them as showed in table -9-.

The efficacy among patients under anxiety/non anxiety patients 65% & 69.4% respectively, there is a statistical significant difference between them as showed in table -10-

Table-4- The efficacy of treatment & age of patients:

Age range	Total No.	Positive results %		Negative results %		Significance
Less than 20 years	3	3	100%	0	0%	N.S*
20-30 years	18	9	50%	9	50%	S**
30-40 years	25	18	72%	7	28%	N.S*
More than 40 years	7	6	86%	1	14%	N.S*
Total	53	36		17		

*N.S : statistically not significant / **S : statistically significant

Table-5- The efficacy of treatment & sex of patients :

sex	Total No.	Positive results & %		Negative results & %		Significance
male	21	10	48%	11	52%	S**
Female	32	26	81%	6	19%	
Total	53	36		17		

****S : statistically significant**

Table-6-The efficacy among the smoker & non-smoker patients

Smoker state	Total No.	Positive response &%		Negative response &%		Significance
Smoker	20	7	35%	13	65%	N.S*
Non-smoker	33	10	30.3%	23	69.7%	

N.*S : statistically not significant

Table-7- The efficacy among positive & negative family history of the disease patients

family history	Total No.	Positive response &%		Negative response&%		Significance
Positive history	13	8	61.5%	5	38.5%	S**
Negative history	40	9	22.5%	31	77.5%	

**S : statistically significant

Table-8- The efficacy according to stress state of the patients

State of stress	Total No.	Positive response &%		Negative response	&%	Significance
Under stress	28	12	43%	16	57%	S**
Not under stress	25	24	96%	1	4%	

**S : statistically significant

Table-9- The efficacy according to anxiety state of the patients

Anxiety state	Total No.	Positive response & %		Negative response & %		Significance
positive	31	17	55%	14	45%	S**
negative	22	19	86.4%	3	13.6%	

**S : statistically significant

Table -10- The efficacy according to the worried state of the patients

Worried state	Total No.	Positive response & %		Negative response &%		Significance
positive	17	11	65%	6	35%	S**
negative	36	25	69.4%	11	30.6%	

*S : statistically significant

Discussion

This study was demonstrated that irritable bowel syndrome is more common in female than in male [60.4% & 39.6%] respectively. This is in agreement with irritable bowel syndrome more common in female aged 20-40 years[1], women are affected more often than men[13] & female to male ratio 1.5:1[11, 14].

This study was demonstrate that the etiology of irritable bowel syndrome as follow psychiatric causes (anxiety, stress & worried), positive famil history of the disease, positive history of taken antibiotic in the last 6 months & those with social habits (especially smoker), this in agreement with[1, 15, 5, 6, 7, 13, 16].

The diagnosis of irritable bowel syndrome was done depending on clinical features and Rome (τ& π) criteria after excluding of organic causes be cretin investigational methods and this in agreement with[4, 10, 11, 16, 17].

The efficacy of our treatment in this study was 68% by using combination of librax (consist of chlordizepoxide & clidinium bromide) plus spasmopan" (hyoscine N-butylbromide). Librax of both anxiolytic & sedative effects while spasmopan anticholinergic of both decreasing gastrointestinal motility & anti-secretary effects, both drug may be use in treatment of irritable bowel syndrome alone or in combination, although there is no specific treatment of irritable bowel syndrome the present treatment is symptomatic treatment only. This in agreement with previous findings[18, 19]. While other studies use each element alone in treatment of irritable bowel syndrome as with[16, 20].

The deference among age groups not significant with exception of 20-30 years age range which shows a significant deference. This may contribute to the fact that these female group is a group of sensitive & more liable to follow physician opinion than male.

The deference among sex was significant deference. This mat contribute to the fact that these age group is a group of activity & working which could be consider as psychotherapy in one hand & in the other hand such job providing a body tiredness with their worried about their job to get no problems in it all contribute to a high efficacy & response to treatment.

No significant deference found among smoker patients so smoking no affecting treatment results in irritable bowel syndrome.

A significant deference found in the patients of psychiatric disorders & those of positive family history of the disease, this could be contribute to the environmental causes of illness. sometimes a hereditary & social factors to be consider[21].

Conclusion

1. irritable bowel syndrome a Multi- component disorder.
2. no specific treatment found but symptomatic treatment consider.
3. psychiatric disorder play a role in the results of treatment.
4. younger age group 20-30 years old identical to initiate both medical & psychiatric therapy to over come the disorder.

Recommendation

1. start both medical & psychiatric therapy at the same time on management of irritable bowel syndrome.
2. 2-using of single therapy consider in chronic disorder to be symptomatic therapy according to patient complaining

Author details
Hassan KH. Rajab
University of Tikrit, college of medicine, Department of clinical pharmacology.

References

1. Christopher. R.W.Edwards and Ian.A.D.Bouchier. 1991.Davidsons principle and practice of medicine. Churchill Livingstone Educational Low- priced Books scheme funded by the British Government, U.K. p. p 447-478.
2. Pattee PL, Thompson WG. Drug treatment of the irritable bowel syndrome Journal: Drugs. Augus1992 ; 44:200-6, 1992.
3. Foxx-Orenstein, -A-E; Clarida, -J-C. Irritable bowel syndrome in women: the physician patient relationship evolving. J- Am-Osteopath-Assoc. 2001 Dec; 101(12 Suppl Pt 2): S12-6.
4. Thompson WG. Irritable bowel syndrome: pathogenesis and management Journal: Lancet. 19June 1993 ;341:1569-72,.
5. Drossman DA. Do psychosocial factors define symptom severity and patient status in irritable bowel syndrome? Am J Med 1999;107:41S-50S.
6. Drossman DA, Corazziari E, Talley NJ, Thompson WG, Whitehead WE. Rome II: the functional gastrointestinal disorders: diagnosis, pathophysiology, and treatment: a multinational consensus. Gut 1999;45(suppl 2):1-81.
7. Monnikes, -H; Tebbe, -J-J; Hildebrandt, -M; Arck, -P; Osmanoglou, -E; Rose, -M; Klapp, B; Wiedenmann, -B; Heymann-Monnikes, -I. Role of stress in functional gastrointestinal disorders. Evidence for stress-induced alterations in gastrointestinal motility and sensitivity. Dig-Dis. 2001; 19(3): 201-11.
8. Drossman DA. Irritable bowel syndrome and sexual/physical abuse history. Eur J Gastroenterol Hepatol 1997;9:327-30.
9. Paterson WG, Thompson WG, Vanner SJ, Faloon TR, Rosser WW, Birtwhistle RW, et al. Recommendations for the management of irritable bowel syndrome in family practice. CMAJ 1999;161:154-60.
10. Tovey, -Philip. A single-blind trial of reflexology for irritable bowel syndrome. Br-J Gen-Pract. 2002 Jan; 52(474): 19-23.
11. Pan, -G; Lu, -S; Ke, -M; Han, -S; Guo, -H; Fang, -X. Epidemiologic study of the irritable bowel syndrome in Beijing: stratified randomized study by cluster sampling. Chin-Med-J (Engl). 2000 Jan; 113(1): 35-9.
12. Vanner SJ, Depew WT, Paterson WG, DaCosta LR, Groll AG, Simon JB, et al. Predictive value of the Rome criteria for diagnosing the irritable bowel syndrome. Am J Gastroenterol 1999;94:2912-7.
13. Maxwell, -P-R; Rink, -E; Kumar, -D; Mendall, -M-A. Antibiotics increase functional abdominal symptoms. Am-J- Gastroenterol. 2002 Jan; 97(1): 104-8:
14. Fock, -K-M; Chew, -C-N; Tay, -L-K; Peh, -L-H; Chan, -S; Pang, -E-P. Psychiatric illness, personality traits and the irritable bowel syndrome. Ann-Acad-Med- Singapore. 2001 Nov; 30(6): 611-4.
15. Mayer EA. Emerging disease model for functional gastrointestinal disorders. Am J Med 1999;107: 12S-19S.
16. Farhadi, -A; Bruninga, -K; Fields, -J; Keshavarzian, -A. Irritable bowel syndrome: an update on therapeutic modalities. Expert-Opin-Investig-Drugs. 2001 Jul; 10(7): 1211-22.
17. Ragnarsson, -G; Hallbook, -O; Bodemar, -G. Abdominal symptoms and anorectal function in health and irritable bowel syndrome. Scand-J-Gastroenterol. 2001 Aug; 36(8): 833-42.
18. Iraqi Drugs Guide. 1990. National Board for the selection of drugs and the central drug information Bureau, Baghdad, Iraq. First edition. p.p 38-39.
19. Tougas, -G. Irritable bowel syndrome: new approaches to its pharmacological management. Can-J-Gastroenterol. 2001 Oct; 15 Suppl B: 12B-13B.
20. David F.Altman. Drugs used in Gastroentistinal Diseases. In the Basic and clinical pharmacology, edited by Bertram G.Katzun. MeCraw-Hill. New-York, 8th U.S.A. 2001 p.p 385 and 1064-1068.
21. Levy, -R-L; Jones, -K-R; Whitehead, -W-E; Feld, -S-I; Talley, -N-J; Corey, -L-A. Irritable bowel syndrome in twins: heredity and social learning both contribute to etiology. Gastroenterology. 2001 Oct; 121(4): 799-804.

2

Current therapies and different treatment methods for irritable bowel syndrome

Dharati Rami[1*], Nehal Shah[1], Pinak Patel[1], Vivek Rami[2]

Abstract

Current paper describes potential therapies available to treat Irritable bowel syndrome is a brain gut disorder characterized most commonly by cramping, abdominal pain, bloating, constipation, and diarrhea which is the most common and fatal disease. The pathophysiology provides the rationale for pharmacotherapy: abnormal gastrointestinal motor functions, visceral hypersensitivity, psychosocial factors, autonomic dysfunction, and mucosal immune activation. Understanding the mechanisms, and their mediators or modulators including neurotransmitters and receptors have led to several therapeutic approaches including agents acting on the serotonin receptor or serotonin transporter system, antidepressants, novel selective anticholinergics, α-adrenergic agonists, opioid agents, cholecystokinin-antagonists, neurokinin-antagonists, somatostatin receptor agonists, corticotropin releasing factor antagonists, chloride channel activators, guanylate cyclase-c agonists, melatonin, atypical benzodiazepines, antibiotics, immune modulators and probiotics. The mechanisms and current evidence regarding efficacy of these agents are reviewed.

Introduction

Irritable bowel syndrome is a brain gut disorder characterized most commonly by cramping, abdominal pain, bloating, constipation, and diarrhea. IBS causes a great deal of discomfort and distress, but it does not permanently harm the intestines and does not lead to a serious disease, such as cancer. The pathophysiology of IBS is still not well understood, but is most likely multifactorial. Several factors such as motor and sensory dysfunction, neuroimmune mechanisms, psychological factors, and changes in the intraluminal milieu appear to play a role. The increased release of serotonin in the circulation especially in the IBS-D group and increased serine proteases (derived from mast cells) in stool of patients with IBS provide evidence for the potential role of neurotransmitters or chemical mediators such as proteases in the disorder.[1, 2]

*Corresponding author:

[1]Indubhai Patel College of Pharmacy and Research Centre, Dharmaj, Gujarat-388430, India.

E-mail: dharati_pharma@yahoo.co.in

[2]Internal Medicine Resident, Sheth Vadilal Sarabhai General Hospital, Ahmedabad-380006, Gujarat, India.

There are three types of IBS

1. IBS with Constipation: This comes with stomach pain and discomfort, bloating, abnormally delayed or infrequent bowel movement, or lumpy/hard stool.
2. IBS with Diarrhea: This comes with stomach pain and discomfort, an urgent need to move your bowels, abnormally frequent bowel movements, or loose/watery stool.
3. IBS with alternating constipation and diarrhea[3, 6]

Background of IBS

Irritable bowel syndrome is a functional gastrointestinal disorder affecting up to 3–15% of the general population in western countries. Most people can control their symptoms with diet, stress management, and prescribed medications. For some people, however, IBS can be disabling. They may be unable to work, attend social events, or even travel short distances. It occurs more often in women than in men, and it begins before the age of 35 in about 50 percent of people.[4, 5]

Approaches to treat IBS

This article reviews recent and novel approaches in IBS therapy (Table 1, Figure 2) that have preclinical efficacy, Phase IIa studies of pharmacodynamics or proof of concept, and Phase IIb or phase III studies that show evidence of efficacy.

Serotonergic system

Serotonin (5-hydroxytryptamine) is an important neurotransmitter of the enteric nervous system (ENS), the peristaltic reflex (chiefly 5-HT4-receptor), the brain–gut axis and vagal and visceral afferent cell bodies or pathways, chiefly 5-HT3-receptors [16, 17]. 5-HT plays a pivotal role in the modulation of multiple gut functions such as motility, sensation, blood flow and secretion [18, 19]. In humans, the highest level of specific binding has been found in the amygdalae, which are integral to the emotional responses to visceral stimulation.

Activity at 5-HT-receptors is regulated by the 5-HT reuptake transporter protein (SERT [20]). It is controversial whether there is reduced expression of SERT (mRNA or immunohistochemistry) in IBS [21, 22]

5-HT3 antagonists and 5-HT4 agonists have demonstrated efficacy and effectiveness in the treatment of multiple or global symptoms of IBS. The prototype medications were alosetron and tegaserod.

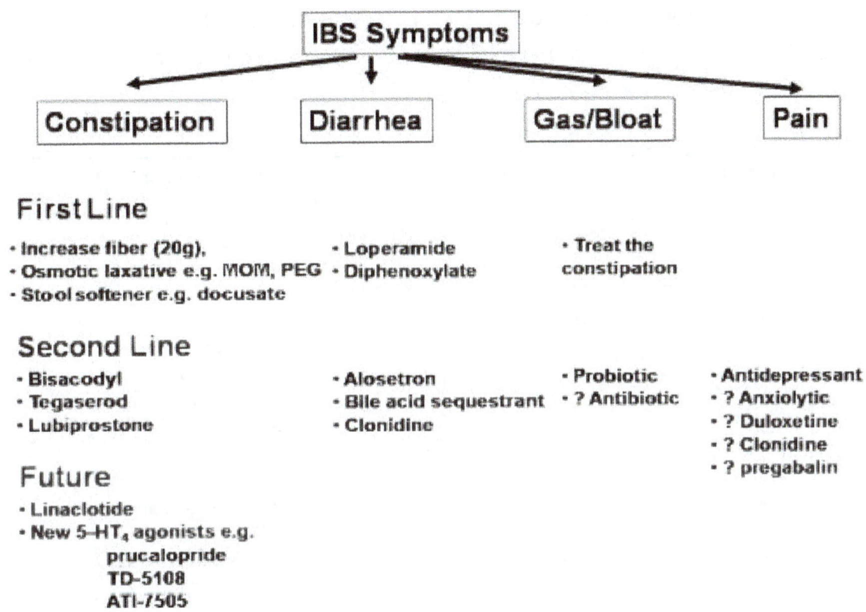

Fig. 1 Current management of IBS and potential role of therapies in pipeline for IBS

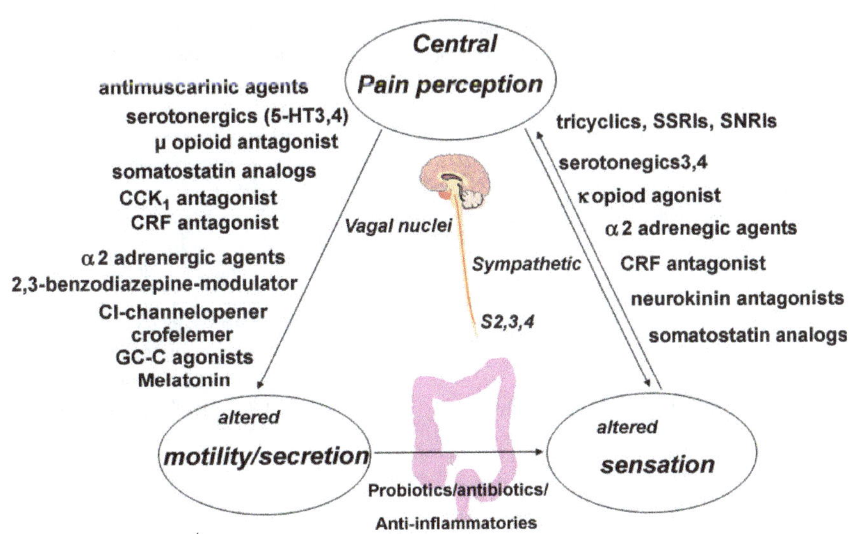

Fig. 2 Current, novel and experimental treatments for IBS.

5-HT3-receptor antagonists

5-HT3-receptor antagonists retard colonic transit, reduce secretion, and increase colonic compliance in response to distension[23] and have central effects that contribute to their beneficial effects on sensation in IBS[24].

Alosetron and subsequently *cilansetron* were efficacious in several large, multicentre, randomised controlled clinical trials, reviewed in an updated meta-analysis[25]. 5-HT3 antagonists more effective than the comparators in achieving global improvement in IBS symptoms (pooled relative risk, 1.60; 95% confidence interval [CI], 1.49–1.72; heterogeneity index, I^2 = 0%) and relief of abdominal pain and discomfort (pooled relative risk, 1.30; 95% CI, 1.22– 1.39; I^2 = 22%). Benefit was apparent for both agents, in both genders. These agents were more likely to cause constipation (pooled relative risk, 4.28; 95% CI, 3.28–5.60, I^2 = 65%); 0.2% using 5-HT3 antagonists had possible ischaemic colitis versus none in control groups. Cilansetron was never approved; alosetron is associated with clear benefits on quality of life[26], but warnings about potential lack of safety has resulted in only a minority of patients being prescribed the medication.

5HT3-receptor Agonists

The 5-HT3 agonist, *MKC-733, also named DDP733 and pumosetrag* in the literature, stimulated fasting antroduodenal migrating motor complex activity and accelerated small intestinal transit [27]. A preliminary report of a phase 2 a study in IBS-C showed a significant overall benefit in overall clinical response rate (54%) in patients receiving 1.4 mg t.i.d. versus to a 15% for placebo[28].

Table 1: Drugs in Use or in Clinical Development for IBS.

Target System	Receptor Activity	Compounds	Human Physiological Effects	Potential or Approved Indication
Serotonergic receptor system	5-HT4-agonists	Prucalopride, ATI-7505 TD-5108	Prokinetic, secretagogue	IBS-C FC
	5-HT3-antagonist	Alosetron, cilansetron	Decrease motility and secretion, increase compliance decrease pain	IBS-D FD
	5-HT3-agonist	DDP-733 e.g. Venlafaxine,	Accelerates small bowel transit	IBS-C FC
Antidepressants	SSRI SNRI		Increase compliance, decrease tone, and sensation	IBS FAP
Cholinergic system	Selective M3-antagonists	Zamifenacin, darifenacin, Clidinium bromide	Reduce colonic motility Decrease Pain?	IBS-D FD
Î±-Adrenergic system	Î±2-agonist	Clonidine	Increases compliance, decreases tone, and sensation	IBS-D FAP
Opioid system	Peripheral Î¼-opioid antagonists	Alvimopan, methylnaltrexone	Prokinetic Increase laxation	IBS-C FC, OIC
	Îº-Opioid-agonist	Asimadoline	Decrease sensation	IBS, FAP
Corticoids	CRH antagonist CRF1 antagonist	Î±hCRH, pexacerfont	Reduce stimulation induced motility and sensitivity	IBS-D FAP
Benzodiazepine	2<comma>3-benzodiazepine receptor	Dexofisopam, Chlordiazepoxide	Reduces stool frequency, Increases stool consistency	IBS-D
Melatonin	Receptor?	Melatonin	Decreases Pain	IBS, FAP
CCK	CCK antagonists	Loxiglumide, dexloxiglumide	Accelerate gastric emptying, Delay prox. colonic transit	IBS
Somatostatin	Somatostatinreceptor agonist	Octreotide	Slows down transit, decreases secretion	IBS-D FD
Neurokinin (NK)	NK antagonists 1 and 2	Ezlopitant, nepadutant	Reduce visceral sensation (NK1) and motility (NK2)	IBS FAP
	NK antagonist 3	Talnetant	Accelerates transit, increases secretion	IBS-C FC
Chloride channel	Activator	Lubiprostone	Decreases stool consistency, increases stool frequency	IBS-C FC
Guanylate cyclase-c	Agonist		Overall symptom relief	IBS-C FC
Antibiotics	Neomycin, rifaximin	Linaclotide	Decrease bloating and pain, slow colon transit	IBS-C FC
Probiotics	Bacterial flora	VSL#3, Lactobacilli bifidobacteriae		IBS bloating flatulence
Proton Pump inhibitor with Antidepressant & anticholinergic	.....	Pantoprazole sodium, Chlordiazepoxide, clidinium bromide	Reduce acid secretion, Reduces stool frequency, Increases stool consistency, Reduce colonic motility Decrease Pain	IBS bloating flatulence

5HT4-receptor agonists

5HT4-receptor agonists generally accelerate small bowel and colonic transit.

Tegaserod: Tegaserod is a selective partial agonist of the 5-HT4-receptor. Several trials in IBS and chronic constipation were summarized in a Cochrane meta-analysis[29]. In IBS-C, tegaserod did not significantly improve the patients' individual symptoms of abdominal pain and discomfort although bowel habit showed a statistically significant improvement with tegaserod 4 mg and there was a non-significant trend in this outcome in favour of tegaserod, 12 mg. In patients with chronic constipation, the RR of being a responder in terms of complete spontaneous bowel movements per week with tegaserod 12 mg was 1.54 (95% CI, 1.35–1.75). The drug was essentially withdrawn because of possible, rare cardiovascular adverse effects.

Newer 5-HT4-receptor agonists

ATI-7505 is a novel, potent agonist of the 5-HT4-receptor and is chemically related to the 5-HT4-receptor agonist, cisapride. However, it has been chemically designed to eliminate cardiac liabilities (e.g., QT prolongation, tachycardia) and CYP450-dependent metabolism at therapeutically relevant concentrations. Pharmacodynamic data in healthy human volunteers [30] indicate prokinetic effects with acceleration of gastric emptying (20 mg t.i.d.) and colonic transit (10 mg t.i.d.; overall and ascending colon emptying), as well as inducing looser stool consistency. Thus, it appears to be promising for IBS-C. Extensive human safety data are not available. To date, there are no reports of adverse cardiac side effects.

Table 2: Comparative Analysis of Pantoprazole with other PPI's

Proton Pump Inhibitor	Bioavailability (%)	Cmax (μmol/L)	Duration of Effect (Hrs)	Protein Binding (%)	Drug Interaction
Pantoprazole	77	5.73 5 (40 mg)	24-72	98	None Diazepam, Warfarin,
Omeprazole	30-40	0.70 5 (20 mg)	24-72	95	Digoxin, Phenytoin, Ketoconazole
Lansoprazole	77-80	2.25 5 (30 mg)	24	97	Ketoconazol Theophylline
Rabeprazole	52	0.48 6 (20 mg) 1.86 2 (20 mg)	24	96	None
Esomeprazole	64	2.38 2 (40 mg)	24-72	97	None

Table 3: Comparison of Pantoprazole Vs Omeprazole

Pantoprazole	Omeprazole
It has least drug interaction	More drug interaction because has greater interaction with cytochrome system. It has drug interaction with Diazepam, Phenytoin, Warfarin.
Bioavailability is 77%	Bioavailability is 30-40%
Pantoprazole is a category-B drug.	Pantoprazole is a category-C drug
Can be used for maintenance therapy in duodenal ulcer.	Can not be used for maintenance therapy in duodenal ulcer

Table 4: Comparison of Pantoprazole Vs Lansoprazole

Pantoprazole	Lansoprazole
It has least drug interaction	It has drug interaction with Ketoconazole, Theophylline.
Duration of action is 24-72 hr.	Duration of action 24 hr.
It does not have drug food interaction	It has drug food interaction

Table 5: Comparison Of Pantoprazole Vs Rabeprazole

Pantoprazole	Rabeprazole
Duration of action is 24-72 hr.	Duration of action 24 hr.
Bioavailability is 77%	Bioavailability is 54%
Protein binding of Pantoprazole is 97%	Protein binding of Rabeprazole is 95%
Mechanism of action is to bind both Cysteine 813 & 833 Cysteine	It binds to Cystein 813 and not to Cysteine 822

Prucalopride is a 5-HT4-receptor agonist that has been extensively studied, including pharmacodynamics and large clinical trials in patients with severe chronic constipation[31, 32, 33, 34]. The medication has greater selectivity (~150-fold) for 5-HT4-receptors than for hERG channel, and it is anticipated that this will be sufficient to prove safely from a cardiac arrhythmia perspective. Certainly, administration for approximately 1 year in more than 80 people with cardiovascular co-morbidity proved safe[35].

TD-5108 (or *velusetrag*) is a potent agonist at human 5-HT4-receptors with high intrinsic activity that displays preferential binding to the 5-HT4-receptor compared with other 5-HT-receptor subtypes or hERG channel[36]. In vivo studies have shown that TD-5108 increases colonic transit in guinea pigs, relaxes oesophageal body musculature in rats, and increases contractility in multiple regions of the GI tract including the gastric antrum, duodenum, jejunum and proximal colon in conscious dogs with implanted strain gauges[37]. In healthy volunteers, single dose, 30- and 50 mg, TD-5108 accelerated colonic and small bowel transit; with multiple doses, TD-5108 30 mg also accelerated colonic transit[38]. A 400-patient, randomised, controlled trial demonstrated efficacy on bowel frequency and consistency in chronic constipation[39].

Antidepressants

Many patients with IBS receive psychoactive agents for their co-morbid psychiatric illnesses, including anxiety, mood, and somatoform disorders, and for the potential effects on visceral sensation. Some SSRIs accelerate small bowel transit; others have effects on colorectal sensation, compliance or tone (e.g., citalopram, venlafaxine,).

There may also be racial or ethnic differences, as efficacy appears greatest in trials conducted in Iran. In intention-to-treat analysis, complete responses were significantly more common in the amitriptyline group. Efficacy of antidepressants in treatment of IBS has been appraised in a recent meta-analysis. At first evaluation, one might conclude that this class of drugs is extremely effective. The calculated relative risk of IBS symptoms persisting or remaining unimproved after treatment with antidepressant therapy versus placebo was 0.66 (95% CI, 0.57–0.78), with the NNT with antidepressant therapy to prevent IBS symptoms persisting of 4 (95% CI, 3–6). However, it is worth noting that very few (typically small single centre) trials individually show significance, and the meta-analysis involves diverse medications and doses, study designs, endpoints, questionable generalizability, and small studies. The analysis included 13 studies comparing antidepressants (total n = 432) to placebo (n = 357) for IBS; 7 studies were in secondary, and 6 in tertiary care with none in primary or community cohorts. Moreover, there was marginal statistically significant heterogeneity detected between studies (I^2 = 26.4%, P = 0.17) and funnel plot asymmetry (P = 0.02), suggestive of publication bias.

In the meta-analysis, only three papers are associated with clear efficacy and they involve small samples of patients: two in Iranian patients and one in German patients. Intriguingly, the most efficacious treatment attributed to a tricyclic agent was reported with a trial of amitryptiline, 10 mg, that did not significantly affect abdominal pain, bloating or diarrhoea, relative to placebo. Similarly, the trial of the SSRI, fluoxetine in 44 patients in Iran shows very large differences in patients with significant abdominal discomfort and bloating, but the proportion of placebo responders over 12 weeks was uncharacteristically low (<15% average), and it is unclear whether these results are generalizable.[40, 41, 42]

Antimuscarinics/Anticholinergics/Smooth muscle relaxants

Gastrointestinal effects of acetylcholine are mediated by nicotinic receptors in the myenteric plexus, and by muscarinic receptor subtypes M1–3, in the myenteric plexus, as well as the neuromuscular junction. Acetylcholine is the main excitatory neurotransmitter in the gastrointestinal (GI) tract. Nonselective anticholinergics or specific antimuscarinic agents reduce bowel motility and associated pain. Relaxant drugs act directly on the smooth muscle e.g. by blocking smooth muscle Ca^{2+} channels. Several compounds (mebeverine, otilinium, pinaverium, and cimetropium), used in Europe, have never been approved in the U.S. Several meta-analyses suggest global improvement with this class of agents, with a mean odds ratio of 2.13 [95% CI, 1.77–2.58]. The low quality (Jadad Scores) of the individual clinical trials compromises the overall interpretation of efficacy of this drug class.

Newer anticholinergics specifically targeting the muscarinic type-3 receptor (M3) on smooth muscle decrease non-specific anticholinergic side effects (dry mouth or increased heart rate) and have promising gastrointestinal effects in animal models. Amongst M3-selective antagonists, darifenacin (used to treat overactive bladder) is associated with constipation, and zamifenacin significantly reduced colonic motility without other anticholinergic effects in 36 IBS patients.[43, 44]

α-Adrenergic agents

The adrenergic nervous system provides extrinsic tonic inhibitory control of non-sphincteric gut motility. The α2-adrenergic agents such as clonidine affect human colonic and rectal motor and sensory functions, increasing colonic compliance, reducing fasting tone without altering the colonic response to a meal or colonic transit, and significantly reducing sensation within a dose range of 0.1–0.3 mg b.i.d. In a study of 44 patients with IBS-D, 67% of the patients treated with clonidine 0.1 mg twice daily compared to 46% in the placebo group achieved satisfactory relief, the primary endpoint. Clonidine also significantly improved bowel functions without altering gastrointestinal transit. Drowsiness, dizziness and dry mouth were observed at doses >0.1 mg b.i.d. This suggests benefits of α2-adrenergic agents in IBS.[45, 46, 47]

Gaba-ergic agents and A2δ ligand

Gabapentin, a 3-alkylated analogue of γ-amino butyric acid (GABA), has been shown to reduce elements of central sensitization in human experimental hyperalgesia. Forty patients with IBS-D were randomised for 5-day treatment with gabapentin, 300 mg/day and then 600 mg/day, which reduced rectal sensory thresholds through attenuating rectal sensitivity to distension and enhancing rectal compliance.

Preclinical studies suggest that the α2δ ligand, pregabalin, reduces both visceral allodynia and hyperalgesia, but is inactive on basal sensitivity. The perception of rectal distension was tested in 26 hypersensitive IBS patients randomised to increasing doses of oral pregabalin for 3 weeks or placebo control. Pregabalin significantly increased the sensory thresholds from baseline for first sensation desire to defecate and pain compared with placebo; it also increased rectal compliance, an effect unrelated to the changes in sensitivity. Studies of GABA-ergic agents and α2δ ligands on clinical outcomes in IBS are not available.[48]

Opioid agents

Three major opioid receptors, μ, δ, and κ, are distributed in the peripheral and central nervous systems. μ-Agonists modulate visceral nociception and to slow down gastrointestinal transit resulting in constipation or central side effects. κ-Opioid receptors are involved in visceral perception.[49]

κ-Opioid agonist

Asimadoline: The κ-opioid agonist, asimadoline, was shown to reduce sensation in response to distensions in the non- noxious range applied to the colon and to relax colonic and gastric tone during fasting. There were no significant effects on gastrointestinal or colonic transit or postprandial tone response to meal ingestion. Delvaux et al. showed that this drug increased sensory thresholds in patients with IBS. On demand treatment of IBS pain with asimadoline was not significantly better than placebo; however, a recent trial using daily administration of asimadoline demonstrated efficacy in patients with IBS-D and IBS with mixed bowel habits (IBS-M).[50]

Peripheral μ-opioid antagonists

Alvimopan: Alvimopan, a novel, peripherally restricted μ- opioid antagonist, is effective in the treatment of opioid- induced constipation and postoperative ileus. It reverses the peripheral effects of narcotics without influencing the pain relief desired by concomitant opioid administration. A pharmacodynamic study in healthy volunteers confirmed that alvimopan normalized the colonic transit delay induced by co-administered codeine. Interestingly, alvimopan alone accelerated colonic transit, suggesting that the μ-opiate mechanisms participate in the physiological control of colonic transit.

Oral *naltrexone* does not accelerate colonic transit, but oral methylnaltrexone accelerated gut transit in opiate-naïve controls and it reversed the prolongation of orocecal transit induced by long-term methadone. Trials to test the effects of peripheral μ-opioid antagonists such as alvimopan and methylnaltrexone in patients with constipation, IBS-C, and opiate-induced constipation are warranted. [51, 52]

CRF receptor antagonists

Corticotropin releasing factor (CRF) is a key mediator of stress response in the brain gut axis. Two CRF receptor subtypes have been cloned: CRF1 and CRF2. In animals, stress activation of the CRF receptors alters gastrointestinal motility, effects that can be blocked with selective CRF1-receptor antagonists (*antalarmin*) and the nonselective CRF receptor antagonist *α-helical CRF9–41* (*αhCRF*). The increased colonic motility response to rectal electrical stimulation in IBS patients was significantly suppressed after αhCRF infusion. However, the CRF1 antagonist, *pexacerafont*, was not effective in normalizing colonic transit or bowel function in patients with diarrhoea-predominant IBS. The role of CRF modulation requires further study.[53, 54]

3-Benzodiazapine receptor modulator

Dextofisopam is the R-enantiomer of the nonsedating homophthalazine anxiolytic, tofisopam. It binds to

2, 3-benzodiazepine receptors located in subcortical and hypothalamic regions. In animal models, dextofisopam reduced stimulation-induced colonic motility and visceral sensitivity. A 12-week, placebo-controlled, phase II study in patients with diarrhoea-predominant or alternating-IBS showed more months with adequate relief in the dextofisopam compared to the placebo group. The effects were most prominent within the first 4 weeks of treatment, and also included an improvement of stool consistency and a reduction of stool frequency. The drug was well tolerated, with only 3% reporting constipation; however, 12% of the patients experienced a worsening of abdominal pain (versus 4% in the placebo group).[55, 56]

Melatonin

Melatonin is a pineal gland neurohormone involved in the regulation of the sleep–wake cycle; it is also synthesized in the gastrointestinal tract, and may participate in the regulation of gastrointestinal motility and sensitivity, possibly by blocking nicotinic channels or Ca^{2+} activated K^{+} channels. Two small studies of the effects of melatonin in IBS patients reported improvement of abdominal pain and IBS symptom score or a reduction of rectal pain sensitivity. This appears to be a peripheral effect, since there was no alteration of sleep or anxiety or depression. The role of melatonin modulation in IBS requires further study.[57, 58]

CCK1 antagonists

Cholecystokinin (CCK), a neuropeptide released by endocrine cells within the duodenal and jejunal mucosa in response to a variety of nutrients, has been proposed as a mediator of IBS symptoms. Colonic responses to CCK *in vivo* and *in vitro* were increased in IBS patients. The effects of CCK are mediated by two distinct receptors, CCK1 and CCK2 and, which are located predominantly in the periphery and the central nervous system respectively. The CCK1 (also called CCKA) receptors are present in gastrointestinal tract smooth muscles and vagal afferents. Blockade of CCK1 receptors in the gastrointestinal tract was proposed as an approach to stimulate gut motility and to change colonic transit time in patients with IBS-C.[59]

Loxiglumide and *Dexloxiglumide*: Loxiglumide is a highly specific, competitive antagonist of the CCK1 receptor. Earlier pharmacodynamic and clinical studies suggested that loxiglumide might improve constipation. A 12-week, phase II trial of 200 mg/day dexloxiglumide in female IBS- C patients showed improvement in abdominal pain and discomfort compared to placebo, but two large phase III trials in IBS-C showed no efficacy for dexloxiglumide. The latter result was consistent with a pharmacodynamics study in IBS-C which showed no significant effect on overall colonic transit or satisfactory relief of IBS. However, in a phase III randomised withdrawal study, dexloxiglumide demonstrated sustained relief of symptoms in female (not male) patients. Further studies with this mediation are awaited.[60]

Somatostatin analogs

The somatostatin analog, *octreotide*, activates predominantly somatostatin type 2 receptors, and reduces gastrointestinal secretion, retards gastrointestinal transit and has antinociceptive properties. Octreotide retards orocecal and small bowel transit time in patients with IBS- D and and normalizes visceral perception and discomfort thresholds in IBS patients without changing rectal compliance and. There are no clinical trials with octreotide in IBS.[61]

Neurokinin-antagonists

NK1-receptors play a role in nociception, whereas NK2 receptors have a greater influence on smooth muscle contractility and of NK2-antagonists on gut motility. In a small pharmacodynamic study of IBS patients, the NK1- receptor antagonist, *ezlozipant*, reduced the emotional response to rectosigmoid distension but did not significantly decrease rectal sensitivity. In healthy controls, the NK2-receptor antagonist, *nepadutant*, reduced contraction frequency and amplitude on migrating motor complexes in the small intestine and effectively antagonized the motility-stimulating effects of infused NKA.

The NK3 antagonist, *talnetant*, was tested in pharmacodynamics and clinical trials, and proved ineffective. [62, 63]

Chloride channel modulators

Cl^{-} Channel (ClC2) Opener

Intestinal Cl^{-} secretion is critical for intestinal fluid and electrolyte transport. In the gastrointestinal tract, chloride channels type 2, ClC2, has been found in gastric parietal cells, small intestinal and colonic epithelia. *Lubiprostone* is a prostone that acts as a selective ClC2 activator and increases intestinal water secretion. In a pharmacodynamic study, lubiprostone was shown to accelerate small bowel and colonic transit time in healthy volunteers. In several clinical trials, lubiprostone, 24 μg b.i.d., had positive effects on stool consistency, frequency and straining, and was safe and effective for treating constipation, . Interestingly, lubiprostone accelerated colonic transit without accelerating ascending colon emptying, suggesting it affects distal colonic function. Lubiprostone also reduced abdominal pain and improved bowel dysfunction in IBS-C. Side effects of lubiprostone include diarrhoea and nausea that is usually mild and transient. In January 2006, the FDA approved lubiprostone.[64]

Guanylate cyclase-c agonist

Linaclotide is a novel agonist of the human guanylate cyclase-c (GC-C), a transmembrane protein located in the gut epithelium. Activation of the GC-C induces secretion of fluid, sodium and bicarbonate in the intestinal lumen. In animal and early human safety studies, linaclotide has been observed to increase stool frequency, decrease stool consistency and decrease visceral pain. A phase IIA pilot, randomised, controlled study shows efficacy of this drug in treatment of chronic constipation. Therefore, the drug seems to be promising for the treatment of IBS-C and chronic constipation.[65]

Crofelemer

Crofelemer reduces excess chloride ion secretion via the CFTR channel. Crofelemer does not affect gut motility and is not absorbed systemically to any significant level. It has been used in the past to treat diarrhoea associated with intestinal secretion. In a dose-ranging study of crofelemer versus placebo b.i.d. for 12 weeks in 242 IBS-D patients, crofelemer did not produce improvement in the primary endpoint related to bowel function, urgency or adequate relief. On the other hand, female IBS-D patients exposed to the highest dose of 500 mg b.i.d. crofelemer had a higher proportion of pain and discomfort free days. These post hoc observations suggest that further studies are indicated to assess the visceral analgesic potential of crofelemer.[66]

Probiotics

Probiotics may have beneficial effects on altered colonic inflammation or barrier function that may be found in some IBS patients. The precise mechanism of action of probiotics is unclear and change of intraluminal milieu and modification of fermentation processes and gas production, inactivation of bile acids with decreased effect of endogenous bile acids on colonic fluid secretion and motility, and alteration of gastrointestinal motility may also contribute to the symptom improvement. A recent meta- analysis identified 19 randomised, controlled trials (18 papers) in 1650 IBS patients. Trial quality was generally good. Amongst 10 randomised, controlled trials involving 918 patients providing outcomes as a dichotomous variable, probiotics were significantly better than placebo with an NNT = 4 (95% CI, 3–12.5); however, there was significant heterogeneity (I^2 = 68%, p = 0.001) and possible funnel plot asymmetry. Amongst 15 trials assessing 1351 patients that reported an improvement in IBS score as a continuous outcome, the standard mean difference was −0.34 (95% CI, −0.60 to −0.07); however, there was statistically significant heterogeneity (I^2 = 79%, p = 0.001). These data suggest overall benefit for probiotics, but the precision of the NNT is uncertain. The safety profile of probiotics suggests they may be considered for the treatment of bloating and flatulence.[67]

Antibiotics

The role of bacterial overgrowth of the small intestine (SIBO) in IBS is controversial. A placebo-controlled study showed that antibiotic treatment with neomycin normalized the lactulose hydrogen breath test (LBT), and this was associated with significant reduction of IBS symptoms over the short term (~1 week). More convincing evidence of the efficacy of antibiotics is provided by the randomised, controlled trials and a preliminary report from Lembo *et al.*. Although there are many unanswered questions, regarding long-term effects, and frequency of retreatment, some patients may benefit from rifaximin treatment.[68]

Immune modulators

Sodium Cromoglycate

Sodium cromoglycate is a mast cell stabilizer; there is experimental evidence of increased mast cell infiltration and greater proximity of mast cells to intramural nerve endings. Proteases that may arise from mast cells have been associated with activation of visceral algesia in experimental studies. Sodium cromoglycate alone or in association with dietary exclusion of suspected allergens has been tested in trials conducted in IBS-D and childhood IBS.[69]

ASA Compounds or Budesonide

Given the efficacy of *budesonide* in microscopic or collagenous colitis and and the increasing evidence of immune activation in IBS, we anticipate more formal trials of these agents, especially in post-infectious IBS. In a recent meta-analysis, Chande *et al.* report that, amongst 3 trials with budesonide for collagenous colitis, the odds ratio for inducing a response was 12.32 (95% CI, 5.53–27.46), maintaining response was OR 8.82, and NNT of 2. Similar efficacy was observed for trials that included both collagenous and lymphocytic colitis (NNT of 3). *Mesalazine* and *bismuth* compounds were less effective for microscopic colitis. However, a small, pilot clinical trial in IBS suggests that mesalazine reduced total number of immune cells and mast cells and pain severity score, and increased global relief relative to placebo treatment. These interesting and provocative data suggest that 5-ASA compounds deserve further study.[70]

New combination therapies available to treat IBS

Pantoprazole Sodium, Clidinium bromide and Chlordiazepoxidem in their combined Capsule dosage form

Literature survey reveled that the newer approaches to treat IBS is the combination of Pantoprazole sodium, clidinium bromide and chlordiazepoxide. The study was done to assesse the IBS efficacy and safety of a combination of 20 mg of Pantoprazole sodium, 2.5mg of clidinium bromide and 5mg of chlordiazepoxide in comparison to Librax(®) (Clidinium bromide and chlordiazepoxide) in patients with acute uncomplicated IBS bloating flatulence. Results of completed the trial in Pantoprazole Sod. Clidinium Bromide, Chlordiazepoxide group while in Librax(®) completed the trial. Less side effects was noted in combination of Pantoprazole Sod. Chlordiazepoxide, clidinium bromide group while its Librax (®) appear side effects as upset stomach, drowsiness, weakness or tiredness, excitement, sleeplessness, dry mouth, heartburn, bloated feeling, eyes more sensitive to sunlight than usual, taste changes, changes in appetite. The available data support the evaluation of drug combination in a larger population as fixed dose combination.

ULRAX [Brand Name]

Composition

Pantoprazole -20mg Chlordiazepoxide- 5 mg Clidinium Bromide-2.5 mg

Pantoprazole

Benzimidazole derivative blocks the proton pump by reacting with (H+/K+)-ATPase enzyme by causing it's inhibition of action resulting long lasting inhibition of gastric acid secretion.

Proton Pump Inhibitor

Proton Pump Inhibitors binds Proton Pump (H+K+(-ATPase enzyme) that results in irreversible inhibition of acid secretion by the proton pump.

Their duration of action is much longer because of their unique mechanism of action:

1. PPI only effective when proton pump is actively making acid.
2. Proton pump is lost after PPI interaction.
3. Proton pumps are reactivated after pumps are renewed.
4. Peak serum level post dose 1.5 hrs.
5. PPI must be closed before a meal for maximal efficacy.

Indications

1. Peptic Ulcers
2. Gastric Ulcers
3. Duodenal Ulcers
4. NSAID Induced gastritis
5. Helicobacter Pylori
6. Reflux Esophagitis
7. Zollinger Elison's Syndrome

Different Proton Pump Inhibitors Available in the Market

1. Omeprazole
2. Lansoprazole
3. Pantoprozole
4. Rabeprazole
5. Esomeprazole

Dose

1. 40 mg once daily for 6-8 week.
2. 20 mg once daily for maintenance therapy for healed esophagitis low grade reflux esophagitis.
3. Do not break, crush or chewtablets.

Advantages

1. Less or no drug interaction.
2. For H Pylori eradication.
3. FDA approved (Feb 2, 2000)
4. No interaction with antacids

Drug Interactions

Not significant, Advise patient to avoid alcohol, products containing NSAIDs and foods that may cause an increase in GI irritation.

Precautions

1. Hepatic impairment
2. Pregnancy

Chlordiazepoxide

Thus chlordiazepoxide is an anxiolytic & act as an agonist at specific benzodiazepine receptor, located on the membrane of GABA neuron which are inhibitory in nervous system, Chlordiazepoxide and GABA forms complex with chloride ion leads to stimulation of benzodiazepine receptors and potentiate the action of GABA which in turn controls the flow of chloride ions across neuron membrane, thereby relieves the patient from anxiety.

Pharmacokinetics

Peak Plasma Level -0.5 – 4 hrs. Protein Binding -96%
Elimination -5 – 30 hrs.

Advantage over other similar drugs

1. Produces a smooth long lasting effect.
2. Preferred in chronic anxiety state.

Dose

15 – 100 (mg/day)

Uses

Treatment of moderate to serve depression associated with moderate to severe anxiety. Symptoms which respond in the first week of treatment are:

1. Insomnia
2. Feeling of guilt
3. Agitation
4. Psychic and somatic anxiety.
5. Anorexia Muscle pain

Alcohol withdrawal syndrome

Side effects

Drowsiness
CNS depression with concomitant alcohol intake

Contraindications

Hypersensitivity to either benzodiazepine or tricyclic antidepressants.

- During acute recovery phase following myocardial infraction.

Precautions

1. Use cautions while driving or performing other tasks requiring alertness.
2. Avoid alcohol and other CNS depressants

Clidinium Bromide

It is an antispasmodic agent, Antispasmodic agents relax smooth muscle in the gut and reduce propulsive contractions, decreasing postprandial abdominal pain, gas, bloating, and fecal urgency. It works through anticholinergic or antimuscarinic properties and may be used in an as-needed or in an anticipatory fashion.

Conclusion

The field of IBS therapeutics is vibrant, with greater understanding of neuroenteric mechanisms, effectors and transmitters in the brain–gut axis. These should provide opportunities for the development of new therapeutic agents for IBS treatment. For almost all of the drug classes described here, rigorous phase III trials and assessment of drug safety are eagerly awaited.Combination therapy more effective and safety rather than single drug therapy.

Abbreviations

- IBS, irritable bowel syndrome;
- IBS-C, irritable bowel syndrome with predominant constipation;
- IBS-D, irritable bowel syndrome with predominant diarrhoea;
- FC, functional constipation;
- FD, functional diarrhoea;
- FAP, functional abdominal pain;
- OR, odds ratio;
- CI, confidence interval;
- SNRI, serotonin and norepinephrine reuptake inhibitor

References

1. D.A. Drossman, Z. Li, E. Andruzzi et al.: U.S. householder survey of functional gastrointestinal disorders. Prevalence, sociodemography, and health impact Dig Dis Sci, 38 (1993), pp. 1569–1580.
2. F. Cremonini, N.J. Talley: Irritable bowel syndrome: epidemiology, natural history, health care seeking and emerging risk factors Gastroenterol Clin North Am, 34:189– 204, 2005.
3. D.A. Drossman, M. Camilleri, E.A. Mayer et al. AGA technical review on irritable bowel syndrome Gastroenterology, 123:2108–2131, 2002.M. Camilleri Mechanisms in IBS: something old, something new, something borrowed Neurogastroenterol Motil, 17:311– 316, 2005.
4. S.P. Dunlop, N.S. Coleman, E. Blackshaw et al. Abnormalities of 5-hydroxytryptamine metabolism in irritable bowel syndrome Clin Gastroenterol Hepatol, 3:349–357, 2005.
5. C.P. Bearcroft, D. Perrett, M.J. Farthing Postprandial plasma 5 hydroxytryptamine in diarrhoea predominant irritable bowel syndrome: a pilot study Gut, 42:42–46, 1998.
6. L.A. Houghton, W. Atkinson, R.P. Whitaker et al.: Increased platelet depleted plasma 5-hydroxytryptamine concentration following meal ingestion in symptomatic female subjects with diarrhoea predominant irritable bowel syndrome Gut, 52:663–670, 2003.
7. R. Roka, A. Rosztoczy, M. Leveque et al.A pilot study of fecal serine-protease activity: a pathophysiological factor in diarrhea-predominant irritable bowel syndrome Clin Gastroenterol Hepatol, 5:550–555, 2007.
8. R. Borman Serotonergic, modulation and irritable bowel syndrome, Expert Opin Emerg Drugs, 6:57–68, 2001.
9. R.C. Spiller, Postinfectious irritable bowel syndrome, Gastroenterology, 124:1662–1671, 2003.
10. R.C. Spiller, D. Jenkins, J.P. Thornley et al., Increased rectal mucosal enteroendocrine cells, T lymphocytes, and increased gut permeability following acute Campylobacter enteritis and in post-dysenteric irritable bowel syndrome, Gut, 47:804–811, 2000.

11. R.C. Spiller, Infection, immune function, and functional gut disorders, Clin Gastroenterol Hepatol, 2:445–455, 2004.
12. G. Barbara, V. Stanghellini, R. De Giorgio et al., Activated mast cells in proximity to colonic nerves correlate with abdominal pain in irritable bowel syndrome, Gastroenterology, 126:693– 702, 2004.
13. L. O'Mahony, J. McCarthy, P. Kelly et al., Lactobacillus and bifidobacterium in irritable bowel syndrome: symptom responses and relationship to cytokine profiles, Gastroenterology, 128:541–551, 2005.
14. J. Aerssens, M. Camilleri, W. Talloen et al., Alterations in mucosal immunity identified in the colon of patients with irritable bowel syndrome, Clin Gastroenterol Hepatol, 6:194– 205, 2008.
15. M.D. Gershon, Review article: roles played by 5- hydroxytryptamine in the physiology of the bowel, Aliment Pharmacol Ther, 13 (Suppl. 2) pp. 15–30, 1999.
16. M.D. Gershon, Review article: serotonin receptors and transporters—roles in normal and abnormal gastrointestinal motility, Aliment Pharmacol Ther, 20 (Suppl. 7) pp. 3–14, 2004.
17. G.A. Hicks, J.R. Coldwell, M. Schindler et al., Excitation of rat colonic afferent fibres by 5-HT(3) receptors, J Physiol, 544 (Pt 3) (2002), pp. 861–869
18. M. Camilleri, Serotonin in the gastrointestinal tract, Curr Opin Endocrinol Diabetes Obes, 16 (2009), pp. 53–59
19. M.D. Gershon, Plasticity in serotonin control mechanisms in the gut, Curr Opin Pharmacol, 3 (2003), pp. 600–607
20. M.D. Coates, C.R. Mahoney, D.R. Linden et al., Molecular defects in mucosal serotonin content and decreased serotonin reuptake transporter in ulcerative colitis and irritable bowel syndrome, Gastroenterology, 126 (2004), pp. 1657–1664
21. C. Andrews, M. Camilleri, A.E. Bharucha et al., Serotonin-transporter (SERT) polymorphism genotype and SERT expression in mucosal biopsies of patients with irritable bowel syndrome, Gastroenterology, 130 (2006), p. A24 [abstract]
22. M.D. Gunput, Review article: clinical pharmacology of alosetron, Aliment Pharmacol Ther, 13 (Suppl. 2) (1999), pp. 70–76
23. E.A. Mayer, S. Berman, S.W. Derbyshire et al., The effect of the 5-HT3 receptor antagonist, alosetron, on brain responses to visceral stimulation in irritable bowel syndrome patients, Aliment Pharmacol Ther, 16 (2002), pp. 1357–1366
24. V. Andresen, V.M. Montori, J. Keller et al.Effects of 5-hydroxytryptamine (serotonin) type 3 antagonists on symptom relief and constipation in nonconstipated irritable bowel syndrome: a systematic review and meta-analysis of randomized controlled trialsClin Gastroenterol Hepatol, 6 (2008), pp. 545–555
25. H.B. El-Serag, K. Olden, D. Bjorkman, Health-related quality of life among persons with irritable bowel syndrome: a systematic review, Aliment Pharmacol Ther, 16 (2002), pp. 1171–1185
26. N.S. Coleman, L. Marciani, E. Blackshaw et al., Effect of a novel 5-HT3 receptor agonist MKC-733 on upper gastrointestinal motility in humans, Aliment Pharmacol Ther, 18 (2003), pp. 1039–1048
27. W.G. Paterson, D. Ford, S.C. Ganguli et al.A novel, oral 5HT3 partial agonist, DDP733, improves overall response in patients with irritable bowel syndrome and constipation (IBS-C): a randomized, double-blind, placebo-controlled, parallel-group, dose-ranging study Gastroenterology, 134 (2008), p. A546- A547 [abstract]
28. B.W. Evans, W.K. Clark, D.J. Moore et al.Tegaserod for the treatment of irritable bowel syndrome and chronic constipation Cochrane Database Syst Rev (2007), p. CD003960
29. M. Camilleri, M.I. Vazquez-Roque, D. Burton et al.Pharmacodynamic effects of a novel prokinetic 5-HT receptor agonist, ATI-7505, in humans Neurogastroenterol Motil, 19 (2007), pp. 30–38
30. E.P. Bouras, M. Camilleri, D.D. Burton et al.Prucalopride accelerates gastrointestinal and colonic transit in patients with constipation without a rectal evacuation disorder Gastroenterology, 120 (2001), pp. 354–360
31. M. Camilleri, R. Kerstens, A. Rykx et al.A placebo-controlled trial of prucalopride for severe chronic constipation N Engl J Med, 358 (2008), pp. 2344–2354
32. J. Tack, M. Van Outryve, G. Beyens et al.Prucalopride (Resolor(R) in the treatment of severe chronic constipation in patients dissatisfied with laxatives Gut (2008) [November 5, Epub ahead of print]
33. E.M. Quigley, L. Vandeplassche, R. Kerstens et al.Clinical trial: the efficacy, impact on quality of life, and safety and tolerability of prucalopride in severe chronic constipation—a 12-week, randomized, double-blind, placebo-controlled study Aliment Pharmacol Ther, 29 (2009), pp. 315–328
34. M. Camilleri, R. Kerstens, G. Beyens et al.A double-blind, placebo-controlled trial to evaluate the safety and tolerability of prucalopride oral solution in constipated elderly patients living in a nursing facility Gastroenterology, 136 (Suppl. 1) (2009), p. 240
35. J.A. Smith, D.T. Beattie, D. Marquess et al.The in vitro pharmacological profile of TD-5108, a selective 5-HT(4) receptor agonist with high intrinsic activity, Naunyn Schmiedebergs Arch Pharmacol, 378 (2008), pp. 125–137
36. D.T. Beattie, S.R. Armstrong, J.P. Shaw et al.The in vivo gastrointestinal activity of TD-5108, a selective 5-HT(4) receptor agonist with high intrinsic activity, Naunyn Schmiedebergs Arch Pharmacol, 378 (2008), pp. 139–147
37. M. Camilleri, M. Manini, S. McKinzie et al.Dose-related effects of TD-5108, a selective 5-HT4 receptor agonist with high intrinsic activity, on gastrointestinal (GI) and colonic transit in healthy volunteers, Neurogastroenterol Motil, 20 (Suppl. 2) (2008), p. 6 [abstract]
38. M.R. Goldberg, Y.-P. Li, K. Pitzer et al.TD-5108, a selective 5- HT4 agonist, is consistently better than placebo regardless of response definition in patients with chronic constipation, Gastroenterology, 134 (2008), p. A 545
39. D.A. Gorard, G.W. Libby, M.J. Farthing, Influence of antidepressants on whole gut and orocaecal transit times in health and irritable bowel syndrome, Aliment Pharmacol Ther, 8 (1994), pp. 159–166
40. J. Tack, A placebo controlled trial of buspirone, a fundus relaxing drug, in functional dyspepsia: effect on symptoms and gastric sensory and motor functions, Gastroenterology, 116 (2000), p. G1423
41. H. Vahedi, S. Merat, A. Rashidioon et al.Effect of fluoxetine in patients with pain and constipation-predominant irritable bowel syndrome: a double-blind randomized-controlled study, Aliment Pharmacol Ther, 22 (2005), pp. 381–385
42. R.K. Goyal, Muscarinic receptor subtypes. Physiology and clinical implications, N Engl J Med, 321 (1989), pp. 1022–1029
43. R.M. Eglen, Muscarinic receptors and gastrointestinal tract smooth muscle function, Life Sci, 68 (2001), pp. 2573–2578
44. A.E. Bharucha, M. Camilleri, A.R. Zinsmeister et al., Adrenergic modulation of human colonic motor and sensory function, Am J Physiol, 273 (5 Pt 1) (1997), pp. G997–1006
45. A. Malcolm, S.F. Phillips, M. Camilleri et al., Pharmacological modulation of rectal tone alters perception of distention in humans, Am J Gastroenterol, 92 (1997), pp. 2073–2079
46. A. Malcolm, M. Camilleri, L. Kost et al., Towards identifying optimal doses for alpha-2 adrenergic modulation of colonic and rectal motor and sensory function, Aliment Pharmacol Ther, 14 (2000), pp. 783–793
47. L.A. Houghton, C. Fell, P.J. Whorwell et al.Effect of a second-generation alpha2delta ligand (pregabalin) on visceral sensation in hypersensitive patients with irritable bowel syndrome, Gut, 56 (2007), pp. 1218–1225
48. T.J. Borody, E.M. Quigley, S.F. Phillips et al.Effects of morphine and atropine on motility and transit in the human ileum, Gastroenterology, 89 (1985), pp. 562–570
49. S. Delgado-Aros, H.J. Chial, F. Cremonini et al., Effects of asimadoline, a kappa-opioid agonist, on satiation and postprandial symptoms in health, Aliment Pharmacol Ther, 18 (2003), pp. 507–514
50. C.P. Delaney, J.L. Weese, N.H. Hyman et al., Phase III trial of

alvimopan, a novel, peripherally acting, mu opioid antagonist, for postoperative ileus after major abdominal surgery, Dis Colon Rectum, 48 (2005), pp. 1114–1125
51. M.J. Owens, C.B. Nemeroff, Physiology and pharmacology of corticotropin-releasing factor, Pharmacol Rev, 43 (1991), pp. 425–473
52. C.S. Yuan, J.F. Foss, M. O'Connor et al., Methylnaltrexone for reversal of constipation due to chronic methadone use: a randomized controlled trial, J Am Med Assoc, 283 (2000), pp. 367–372
53. S.R. Sweetser, S.J. Linker Nord, D.D. Burton et al., Effects of a novel corticotrophin releasing factor receptor-1 antagonist, BMS-562086, on gastrointestinal and colonic transit and bowel habits in patients with diarrhea-predominant irritable bowel syndrome (D-IBS), Gastroenterology, 134 (2008), p. A 548
54. S.M. Leventer, R.F. Kucharik, J.C. Keogh et al., The potential of dextofisopam for treatment of irritable bowel syndrome and inflammatory bowel disease, Am J Gastroenterol, 99 (2004), p. S 279
55. S.M. Leventer, K. Raudibaugh, C.L. Frissora et al., Clinical trial: dextofisopam in the treatment of patients with diarrhoea-predominant or alternating irritable bowel syndrome, Aliment Pharmacol Ther, 27 (2008), pp. 197–206
56. W.Z. Lu, K.A. Gwee, S. Moochhalla et al., Melatonin improves bowel symptoms in female patients with irritable bowel syndrome: a double-blind placebo-controlled study, Aliment Pharmacol Ther, 22 (2005), pp. 927–934
57. G.H. Song, P.H. Leng, K.A. Gwee et al.Melatonin improves abdominal pain in irritable bowel syndrome patients who have sleep disturbances: a randomised, double blind, placebo controlled study, Gut, 54 (2005), pp. 1402–1407
58. S.A. Wank, Cholecystokinin receptors, Am J Physiol, 269 (5 Pt 1) (1995), pp. G628–G646
59. B.M. Meyer, B.A. Werth, C. Beglinger et al., Role of cholecystokinin in regulation of gastrointestinal motor functions, Lancet, 2 (1989), pp. 12–15
60. M.R. von der Ohe, M. Camilleri, G.M. Thomforde et al., Differential regional effects of octreotide on human gastrointestinal motor function, Gut, 36 (1995), pp. 743–748
61. L.A. Houghton, F. Cremonini, M. Camilleri et al., Effect of the NK3 receptor antagonist, talnetant, on rectal sensory function and compliance in healthy humans, Neurogastroenterol Motil, 19 (2007), pp. 732–743
62. G.E. Dukes, O.E. Dewit, G.J. Sanger et al., Lack of effect of the NK3 receptor antagonist, talnetant SB223242 on symptoms of IBS: results of 2 randomized, double-blind, placebo-controlled, dose-ranging trials, Gastroenterology, 132 (2007), p. A60
63. Lubiprostone: RU 0211, SPI 0211, Drugs R D, 6 (2005), pp. 245–258
64. M.G. Currie, K.F. Fok, J. Kato et al., Guanylin: an endogenous activator of intestinal guanylate cyclase, Proc Natl Acad Sci USA, 89 (1992), pp. 947–951
65. A.W. Mangel, P. Chaturvedi, Evaluation of crofelemer in the treatment of diarrhea-predominant irritable bowel syndrome patients, Digestion, 78 (2008), pp. 180–186
66. E.F. Verdu, S.M. Collins, Irritable bowel syndrome and probiotics: from rationale to clinical use, Curr Opin Gastroenterol, 21 (2005), pp. 697–701
67. M. Pimentel, E.J. Chow, H.C. Lin, Normalization of lactulose breath testing correlates with symptom improvement in irritable bowel syndrome. A double-blind, randomized, placebo-controlled study, Am J Gastroenterol, 98 (2003), pp. 412–419
68. O. Leri, S. Tubili, F.G. De Rosa et al., Management of diarrhoeic type of irritable bowel syndrome with exclusion diet and disodium cromoglycate, Inflammo-pharmacology, 5 (1997), pp. 153–158
69. S. Miehlke, A. Madisch, B. Bethke et al., Oral budesonide for maintenance treatment of collagenous colitis: a randomized, double-blind, placebo-controlled trial, Gastroenterology, 135 (2008), pp. 1510–1516.

3

A physician-based study to assess the prevalence, current treatment standards, and therapy need gaps in the management of irritable bowel syndrome in India

Keyur Sheth*

Abstract

Background: Irritable bowel syndrome (IBS) is the most common functional gastrointestinal disorder that can significantly affect quality of life. A physician-based survey was conducted to understand the prevalence, current treatment strategies, and gaps in IBS management in India.

Methods: A total of 197 physicians participated to complete a questionnaire comprising 36 questions related to the prevalence and current treatment of IBS and assess gaps in its management.

Results: Most physicians take a detailed history of the IBS syndrome and association-driven criteria to diagnose IBS. Most physicians reported that >50% of the patients had IBS mixed with anxiety, and most patients with IBS suffered for 2-4 weeks before seeking medical consultation. Most respondents reported that IBS patients took home remedies before consultation. Respondents ranked mebeverine plus chlordiazepoxide, followed by mebeverine monotherapy as preferred treatment for management of IBS symptoms. Mebeverine plus chlordiazepoxide was most preferred for IBS patients with anxiety. More than 70 % of physicians reported that mebeverine and its combination with chlordiazepoxide were efficacious with no adverse events for all subtypes of IBS. Most physicians prescribed probiotics with multiple strains for 2-4 weeks in patients with IBS.

Conclusions: IBS is a common gastrointestinal disorder with no apparent diagnosis and management. The survey findings support the use of mebeverine therapy for the management of IBS symptoms.

Keywords: Irritable bowel syndrome, Mebeverine, Probiotics, Anxiety, Chlordiazepoxide

Introduction

Irritable bowel syndrome (IBS) is the most common functional gastrointestinal disorder that can significantly affect quality of life, including various social and psychological factors.[1,2] The global prevalence of IBS in the general population ranges from 9% to 22%, and its prevalence in India ranges from 4.0% to 7.9%.[3-7] Over the last 20 years, rapid socioeconomic development in Asia has led to a transition in health and environmental status of the general population. The prevalence of IBS among Asian countries appears to be rapidly increasing.[8] Although the etiology of IBS remains elusive, it has a significant impact on quality of life and social functioning of patients.[9] Moreover, a strong association exists between IBS and psychological illnesses, anxiety, and depression.[10,11] According to a meta-analysis, the prevalence of anxiety symptoms in patients with IBS was reported at 39.1%, while the prevalence of depressive symptoms was 28.8%.[12]Other reasons have been proposed, including nutrition, gut bacteria, atypical sensitivity of gut viscera, gut dysmotility, and moderate chronic inflammation. Minimal proportions of patients with IBS seek medical attention, most of whom receive primary care.[13]

According to the Rome III criteria, IBS symptoms are characterized as abdominal pain, discomfort, or bloating accompanied by a change in bowel habit, and these symptoms can resolve by defecation.[14] The symptom of abdominal pain is the most important based on the recently published Rome IV criteria, and it is known to reduce or increase after defecation.[15]

There is no specific test to diagnose IBS definitively. However, physicians need to take a complete medical history and perform physical examination and tests to rule out other gastrointestinal conditions, such as celiac disease.[14,15] IBS can be managed with a range of drugs and nonpharmacological methods in current clinical practice.[16,17] Nonpharmacological methods, including dietary changes, increased physical activity, and psychological counseling, are commonly recommended in the early stages of treatment.[16,17] Pharmacological

*Correspondence:
Dr. Keyur Sheth,
E-mail: itsdr@hotmail.com

psychological counseling, are commonly recommended in the early stages of treatment.[16,17] Pharmacological management is recommended in conjunction with non-pharmacological management, and the drug is chosen based on the presence of constipation or diarrhea and the symptom of bowel habit.[16,17]

Despite the high prevalence, impact on quality of life, and social impact of IBS, physicians' perceptions of the disease and their choice of treatment strategies have not been extensively studied.[18] A key challenge is that physicians and patients with IBS often have differing perspectives on the nature and severity of gastrointestinal symptoms, and many patients with IBS may not be aware of being afflicted with this disorder.[18] Indeed, some physicians may encounter challenges in treating IBS, which has comparable symptoms to ulcerative colitis, Crohn's disease, and celiac disease.

Additionally, counselling and lifestyle modification play a role in management as well. Here, a physician-based survey was conducted to assess the prevalence, current treatment strategies and gaps in the management of patients with IBS in India.

METHODS

Survey

This was a cross-sectional, questionnaire-based survey conducted between March 2021 and December 2021 to assess prevalence of, treatment strategies for, and gaps in the diagnosis and management of patients with IBS across India. A total of 197 physicians involved in the clinical practice of IBS from all 4 zones across India participated in the survey. Participants were invited to complete the internet-based structured survey questionnaire. The survey questionnaire was developed based on a study by Darvish- Damavandi et al and comprised of 36 questions, including questions on understanding IBS prevalence, diagnosis, and current treatment options (Table 1).[19] This survey was performed in accordance with the protocol, International Conference on Harmonization-Good Clinical Practice (ICH-GCP) guidelines. Informed consent was obtained from the participating physicians. Because this survey did not entail any direct patient intervention, ethical clearance by an external ethics review board was not obtained. The confidentiality and identity of the participating physicians were preserved throughout the survey and data processing.

Data analysis

A formal sample size estimate was not done for this survey, but with 197 respondents and 36 questions, a respondent-to-item ratio of >8 was maintained, in line with previous studies recommending a respondent-to-item ratio of >2.[20] The process of data entry and quality checking was performed along with query resolution. Responses to all questions by the 197 survey respondents were expressed as proportions (percentages) across different categories. The rank data were calculated by the weighted linear combination method and determined which answer choice was preferred overall. The response with the largest weighted sum ranking was the most preferred choice, and the weights were applied in reverse. Statistical analyses were performed using statistical package for the social sciences (SPSS) software version 25.0 (IBM Corp., Armonk, NY, USA) and Microsoft excel 2019 (Microsoft Corporation).

RESULTS

Prevalence of patients by IBS subtype

When assessed by clinical presentation of IBS symptoms, IBS-D was present in 10-30% of patients according to 43.7% of physicians, IBS-C was present in 10-30% of patients according to 59.9% of physicians, IBS-mixed was present in 10-30% of patients according to 34.0% of physicians, and IBS with anxiety was present in >50% of patients according to 38.6% of physicians (Figure 1).

Prevalence of IBS by gender

W ith regard to gender-wise prevalence of patients with IBS, 3.6%, 52.3%, 42.1%, and 2.0% of physicians reported that the prevalence of male patients was <25%, 25%-50%, 50%-75%, and >75%, respectively. According to 5.6%, 45.7%, 43.7%, and 5.1% of patients, the prevalence of female patients was 25%, 25-50%, 50-75%, and >75%, respectively.

Consultation, diagnosis, and challenges in the management of IBS

In all, 45.7% of physicians opined that patients typically suffer from IBS for 2-4 weeks before they consult a physician, while 35.5% of physicians reported that this duration was 2-6 months due to lack of awareness (Table 3). Majority of the physicians (61.7%) opined that patients take home remedies before physician consultation.

Regarding the mode adopted by physicians for diagnosis of IBS, 92.9% stated that they first take a detailed history of the IBS syndrome, 87.3% reported that they used association-driven criteria (Rome IV/Manning) to diagnose IBS in their regular practice, and 68.0% implement diagnostic modalities for excluding IBS (Table 2).

Concerning the key challenges in IBS management, 84.8% of physicians faced challenges in history taking and counseling as they believed that patients need extensive support in managing their recurrent symptoms (Table 3).

Regarding support needed to be extended to IBS patients, 95.4% of physicians considered diet and lifestyle counselling, 89.3% considered psychological counselling support, 63.5% considered history taking per Rome IV criteria, and 42.1% considered patient communities as useful strategies. Notably, in the general approach to managing patients with IBS with anxiety, 91.4% of physicians considered the combination of an antispasmodic with chlordiazepoxide to be effective (Table 3).

Preferred pharmacotherapies for reducing IBS symptoms

For management of IBS symptoms, the most preferred pharmacotherapy was mebeverine plus chlordiazepoxide by 40.6% physicians, mebeverine monotherapy by 26.9% physicians, clidinium bromide plus chlordiazepoxide by 11.7% physicians, and clidinium bromide with dicyclomine plus chlordiazepoxide by 15.2% physicians. Moreover, more than half the physicians ranked mebeverine monotherapy (rank 1=26.9% and rank 2=23.9%) or mebeverine plus chlordiazepoxide (rank 1=40.6% and rank 2=33.0%) as the top two preferred therapies. Overall, physicians ranked mebeverine plus chlordiazepoxide as the most preferred therapy, followed by mebeverine (Figure 2).

Prescription pattern and duration of therapies for IBS management

In all, 39.6% of physicians reported that a combination of mebeverine and chlordiazepoxide was prescribed to >50% of IBS patients with anxiety. Concerning the prescription pattern for management of IBS symptoms, mebeverine monotherapy was prescribed to <15% of patients by 45.7% of physicians, mebeverine plus chlordiazepoxide was prescribed to 15-30% of patients by 37.6% of physicians, clidinium bromide plus chlordiazepoxide was prescribed to 15-30% of patients by 39.6% of physicians, and clidinium bromide plus dicyclomine and chlordiazepoxide was prescribed to <15% times of patients by 40.1% of physicians (Table 4).

The preferred average duration of prescription by therapy type was 4 to 8 weeks for duration by 44.7%, 41.6%, and 37.6% of physicians prescribing mebeverine monotherapy, mebeverine plus chlordiazepoxide, and clidinium bromide plus chlordiazepoxide, respectively.

Ov erall, it was observed that >70% of physicians preferred mebeverine or mebeverine plus chlordiazepoxide for at least 4 weeks (Table 4).

Physicians' perspectives on efficacy and tolerability of mebeverine and its combination

When physicians were asked to opine on their perception about efficacy and tolerability of mebeverine monotherapy, 21.3% rated it as extremely efficacious, and 46.2% rated it as efficacious. Mebeverine plus chlordiazepoxide combination was rated as extremely efficacious and efficacious by 27.9% and 49.8% of physicians, respectively (Figure 3). Furthermore, mebeverine was reported to be extremely safe by 40.6% of physicians and safe by 52.8% of the physicians, whereas mebeverine plus chlordiazepoxide was reported as extremely safe and safe by 18.8% and 54.8% of the physicians, respectively (Figure 3).

Majority of the physicians (64.5%) responded that mebeverine or its combination with chlordiazepoxide was useful in all subtypes of IBS, namely, IBS-C, IBS-D, and IBS-mixed. Interestingly, only 29.4% of physicians felt that mebeverine or its combination with chlordiazepoxide was useful in IBS-mixed, and only 21.3% of physicians felt that it was useful in IBS-D (Table 5). Notably, 71.1% of physicians felt that mebeverine or its combination with chlordiazepoxide was not associated with any side effects.

Regarding the advantage of mebeverine, 81.7% of physicians reported that mebeverine had all the listed benefits such as gut-specific antispasmodic action, usefulness in all IBS subtypes, Rome IV recommendation, and absence of anticholinergic side-effects, with 15.7% of physicians reporting that its gut-specific antispasmodic action was an advantage (Figure 4).

Physicians' preference for probiotics

In terms of probiotic preferences for managing various bowel diseases, 72.1%, 65.0%, and 55.3% of physicians prescribed probiotics for IBS with small intestinal bacterial overgrowth (SIBO), IBD, and 55.3% IBS, respectively (Figure 5). On advocating the usage of probiotics, 52.8% of physicians recommended their use for 2-4 weeks, while 25.4% recommended them for 1-2 weeks (Table 6). For patients with IBS, majority of the physicians (53.3%) preferred multiple strains of probiotics, whereas *Lactobacillus*, *Bifidobacterium*, and *Saccharomyces* were preferred by 25.9%, 18.8%, and 2.0% of physicians, respectively (Table 6). For patients with IBS and associated SIBO who are on antibiotics, 48.2% of physicians stated that they prescribed sequential usage of probiotics after antibiotic, 40.6% stated that simultaneous usage along with an antibiotic was preferred, and 11.6% stated that they did not prefer use of probiotics in such patients. Most physicians (79.7%) preferred prescribing a probiotic resistant to rifaximin (Table 6).

Table 1: Survey questionnaire.

Section 1: Prevalence of IBS				
Q1	What is the percentage of patients who present with symptoms of IBS-D?			
	a) <10%	b) 10%-30%	c) 30%-50%	d) >50%
Q2	What is the percentage of patients who present with symptoms of IBS-C?			
	a) <10%	b) 10%-30%	c) 30%-50%	d) >50%
Q3	What is the percentage of patients who present with symptoms of IBS-mixed?			
	a) <10%	b) 10%-30%	c) 30%-50%	d) >50%
Q4	What is the percentage of patients who present with symptoms of IBS with anxiety?			

a) <10% b) 10%-30% c) 30%-50% d) >50%

Q5 What is percentage breakup of male patients with IBS?

a) <25% b) 25%-50% c) 50%-75% d) >75%

Q6 What is percentage breakup of female patients with IBS?

a) <25% b) 25%-50% c) 50%-75% d) >75%

Q7 How long do patients typically suffer from IBS symptoms before they consult you?

a) 2-4 weeks b) 4-8 weeks c) 2-6 months d) >6 months

Q8 Do the patients take home remedy before visiting you?

a) Yes (name____________) b) No

Q9 How do you diagnose IBS (tick all options that apply)?

a) Detailed history taking b) Association driven criteria (Rome IV/Manning, etc.) c) Diagnostic modalities for excluding IBS

Q10 Which of the following are key challenges that you face in managing patients with IBS?

a) History taking as they have a lot to say b) Counseling as they need a lot of support in managing their recurrent symptoms c) Both a & b d) Others ....

Q11 What is the general approach in managing patients with IBS with anxiety?

a) Plain antispasmodic b) Antispasmodic combination with chlordiazepoxide c) Anti-diarrheal or laxatives/fibers as per symptoms

Q12 Rank the following based on your preference to help reduce IBS symptoms? (mention as 1-5; 1 being highest and 5 being lowest)

Drug	Rank (1-5)
Mebeverine	
Mebeverine + chlordiazepoxide	
Clidinium bromide + chlordiazepoxide	
Clidinium bromide + dicyclomine + chlordiazepoxide	
Others	

Q13 To what % of patients with IBS and anxiety do you prescribe a combination of mebeverine and chlordiazepoxide?

a) <15% b) 15%-30% c) 30%-50% d) >50%

Q14 To what % of patients with IBS do you prescribe mebeverine monotherapy?

a) <15% b) 15%-30% c) 30%-50% d) >50%

Q15 To what % of patients with IBS do you prescribe a combination of mebeverine and chlordiazepoxide?

a) <15% b) 15%-30% c) 30%-50% d) >50%

Q16 To what % of patients with IBS do you prescribe a combination of clidinium bromide and chlordiazepoxide?

a) <15% b) 15%-30% c) 30%-50% d) >50%

Q17 To what % of patients with IBS do you prescribe a combination of clidinium bromide + dicyclomine + chlordiazepoxide?

a) <15% b) 15%-30% c) 30%-50% d) >50%

Q18 On an average, for how much duration is mebeverine monotherapy prescribed to a patient with IBS?

a) <2 weeks b) 2-4 weeks c) 4-8 weeks d) >8 weeks

Q19 On an average, for how much duration is a combination of mebeverine and chlordiazepoxide prescribed to a patient with IBS?

a) <2 weeks b) 2-4 weeks c) 4-8 weeks d) >8 weeks

Q20 On an average, for how much duration is a combination of clidinium bromide and chlordiazepoxide prescribed to a patient with IBS?

a) <2 weeks b) 2-4 weeks c) 4-8 weeks d) >8 weeks

Q21 How would you rate the efficacy of mebeverine monotherapy to reduce IBS symptoms?

a) Extremely efficacious b) Efficacious c) Varies from patient to patient d) Poor efficacy e) Very poor efficacy

Continued.

Section 1: Prevalence of IBS					
Q22	How would you rate the efficacy of combination of mebeverine and chlordiazepoxide to reduce IBS symptoms?				
	a) Extremely efficacious	b) Efficacious	c) Varies from patient to patient	d) Poor efficacy	e) Very poor efficacy
Q23	How would you rate the tolerability of mebeverine monotherapy to reduce IBS symptoms?				
	a) Extremely safe	b) Safe	c) Varies from patient to patient	d) Side effects seen in a few	e) Side effects seen in many patients
Q24	How would you rate the tolerability of combination of mebeverine and chlordiazepoxide to reduce IBS symptoms?				
	a) Extremely safe	b) Safe	c) Varies from patient to patient	d) Side effects seen in a few	e) Side effects seen in many patients
Q25	Do your patients who are prescribed mebeverine monotherapy or combination of mebeverine and chlordiazepoxide complain about any side effects?				
	a) Yes – Which ones? ________________			b) No	
Q26	In which subtype of IBS, do you find mebeverine monotherapy or combination of mebeverine and chlordiazepoxide useful (tick all that apply)?				
	a) IBS-C	b) IBS-D		c) IBS-mixed	d) All subtypes
Q27	What according to you are the advantages of mebeverine? (tick all that apply)?				
	a) Gut-specific antispasmodic	b) Useful in all sub types of IBS	c) Rome IV recommended	d) No anti cholinergic side -effects	e) All of the above
Q28	Which of the following would you find useful in extending support to IBS patients (tick all that apply)?				
	a) Diet and lifestyle counseling support	b) Psychological counseling support	c) History taking tracker as per Rome IV criteria	d) Patient c ommunity	e) Others
Q29	Do you prescribe probiotics in patients with IBS?				
	a) Yes		b) No		
Q30	Do you prescribe probiotics in patients with IBD?				
	a) Yes		b) No		
Q31	Do you prescribe probiotics in patients with IBS and SIBO?				
	a) Yes		b) No		
Q32	Do you prescribe probiotics in patients with other GI conditions?				
	a) Yes (please specify________________)		b) No		
Q33	In the above patients, for how long do you advocate usage of probiotics?				
	a) <1 week	b) 1-2 week s	c) 2-4 weeks	d) >4 weeks	
Q34	Which probiotic do you prefer to use in IBS patients?				
	a) Lactobacillus	b) Saccharomyces	c) Bifidobacteriu m	d) Multiple strains	
Q35	Do you prescribe probiotics to patients with IBS and associated SIBO who are on antibiotics?				
	a) Yes, sequential usage of probiotic after antibiotic	b) Yes, simultaneous usage along with antibiotic		c) No	
Q36	Would you prefer to prescribe a probiotic that is resistant to rifaximin (antibiotic)?				
	a) Yes		b) No		

IBS, irritable bowel syndrome; IBS-C, IBS with constipation; IBS-D, IBS with diarrhea; SIBO, small intestinal bacterial overgrowth

Table 2: Features of IBS among Indian patients.

Variables	Frequency, n (%), N=197
Duration of IBS before physician consultation	
2-4 weeks	90 (45.7)
4-8 weeks	12 (6.1)
2-6 months	70 (35.5)

Continued.

Variables	Frequency, n (%), N=197
>6 months	25 (12.7)
Home remedy for IBS before physician consultation	
Yes	122 (61.9)
No	75 (38.1)
Mode of IBS diagnosis	
Detailed history taking	183 (92.9)
Association-driven criteria (Rome IV/Manning, etc.)	172 (87.3)
Diagnostic modalities for excluding IBS	134 (68.0)
Key challenges in IBS management	
History taking as they have a lot to say	7 (3.6)
Counselling as they need a lot of support in managing their recurrent symptoms	23 (11.7)
Both of the above	167 (84.8)
General approach in managing patients with IBS with anxiety	
Plain antispasmodic	5 (2.5)
Antispasmodic combination with chlordiazepoxide	180 (91.4)
Anti-diarrheal or laxatives/fibres as per symptoms	12 (6.1)

IBS: Irritable bowel syndrome

Table 3: Prescription pattern and duration of therapies for patients with IBS.

Parameters	Proportion of physicians, n (%) N=197			
Prescription pattern for IBS with anxiety	**<15%**	**15-30%**	**30-50%**	**>50%**
Mebeverine + chlordiazepoxide for IBS with anxiety	7 (3.5)	50 (25.4)	62 (31.5)	78 (39.6)
Prescription pattern for IBS	**<15%**	**15-30%**	**30-50%**	**>50%**
Mebeverine monotherapy	90 (45.7)	67 (34.0)	30 (15.2)	10 (5.1)
Mebeverine + chlordiazepoxide	35 (17.8)	74 (37.6)	59 (29.9)	29 (14.7)
Clidinium bromide + chlordiazepoxide	40 (20.3)	78 (39.6)	63 (32.0)	16 (8.1)
Clidinium bromide + dicyclomine + chlordiazepoxide	79 (40.1)	45 (22.8)	55 (27.9)	18 (9.1)
Prescription duration for IBS	**<2 weeks**	**2-4 weeks**	**4-8 weeks**	**>8 weeks**
Mebeverine monotherapy	13 (6.6)	39 (19.8)	88 (44.7)	57 (28.9)
Mebeverine + chlordiazepoxide	12 (6.1)	42 (21.3)	82 (41.6)	61 (31.0)
Clidinium bromide + chlordiazepoxide	21 (10.7)	54 (27.4)	74 (37.6)	48 (24.4)

IBS: Irritable bowel syndrome

Table 4: Physicians' perspectives on usefulness, side effects, and advantages of mebeverine or its combination with chlordiazepoxide in patients with IBS.

Proportion of physicians, n (%)	Frequency N=197
Usefulness in	
IBS-C	10 (5.1)
IBS-D	42 (21.3)
IBS-mixed	58 (29.4)
All subtypes	127 (64.5)
Side effects	
Yes	57 (28.9)
No	140 (71.1)

IBS: Irritable bowel syndrome

Table 5: Physicians' experience about the prescribing pattern of probiotics in patients with various gastrointestinal disorders.

Proportion of physicians, n (%)	N=197
Prescribed duration of usage of probiotics (weeks)	
<1	3 (1.5)
1-2	50 (25.4)
2-4	104 (52.8)

Continued.

Proportion of physicians, n (%)	N=197
>4	40 (20.3)
Preferred probiotic for patients with IBS	
Lactobacillus	51 (25.9)
Saccharomyces	4 (2.0)
Bifidobacterium	37 (18.8)
Multiple strains	105 (53.3)
Prescription of probiotics for patients with IBS and associated SIBO who are on antibiotics?	
Sequential usage of probiotic after antibiotic	95 (48.2)
Simultaneous usage of probiotic along with antibiotic	80 (40.6)
No usage of probiotic	22 (11.2)
Prescription of a probiotic that is resistant to rifaximin	
Yes	157 (79.7)
No	40 (20.3)

IBS: Irritable bowel syndrome; SIBO: small intestinal bacterial overgrowth

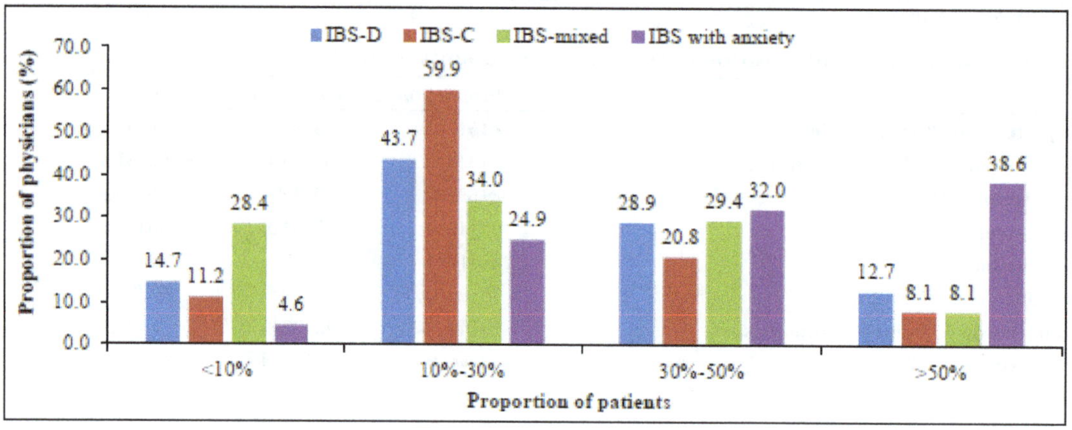

Figure 1: Prevalence of patients with IBS in Indian clinical practice by IBS subtype.

IBS: Irritable bowel syndrome; IBS-C: IBS with constipation; IBS-D: IBS with diarrhoea; SIBO: small intestinal bacterial overgrowth

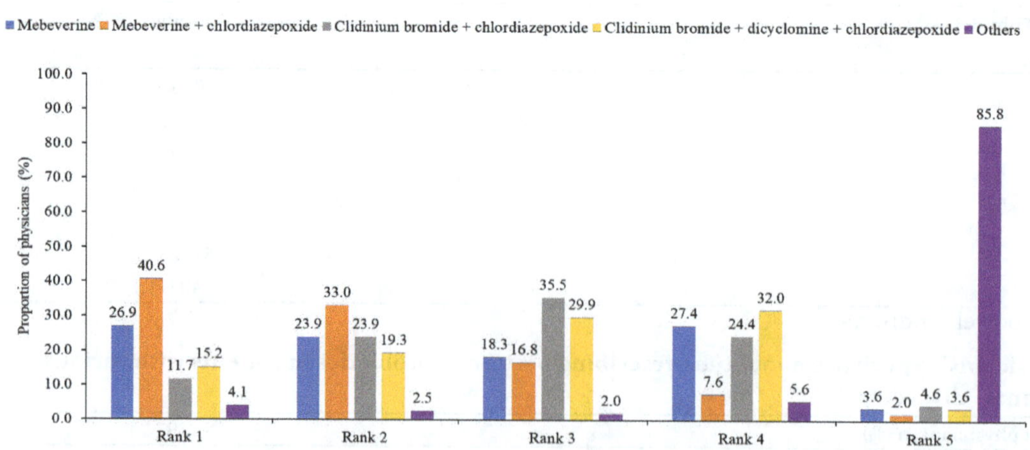

Figure 2: Physicians' ranking preferences for various pharmacotherapies in the management of IBS symptoms.

IBS: Irritable bowel syndrome

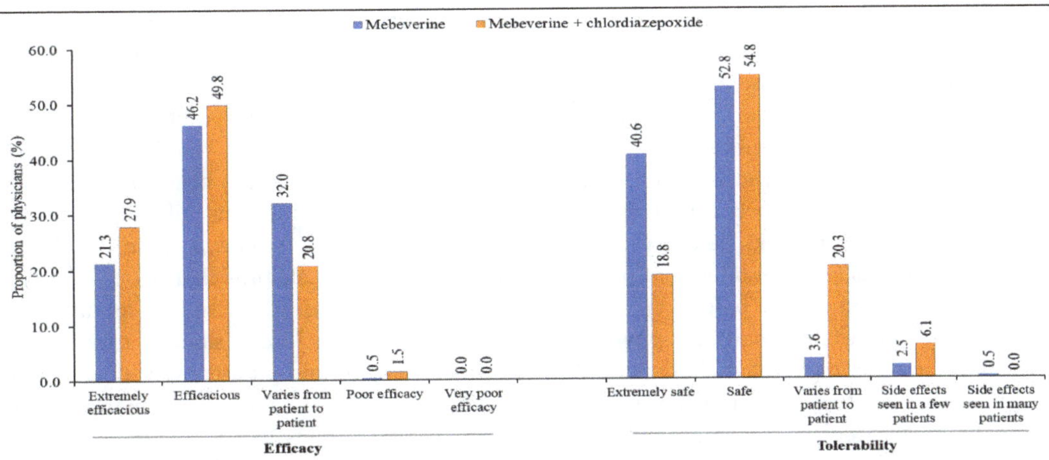

Figure 3: Efficacy and tolerability of mebeverine and mebeverine chlordiazepoxide combination to reduce IBS symptoms.

IBS: Irritable bowel syndrome

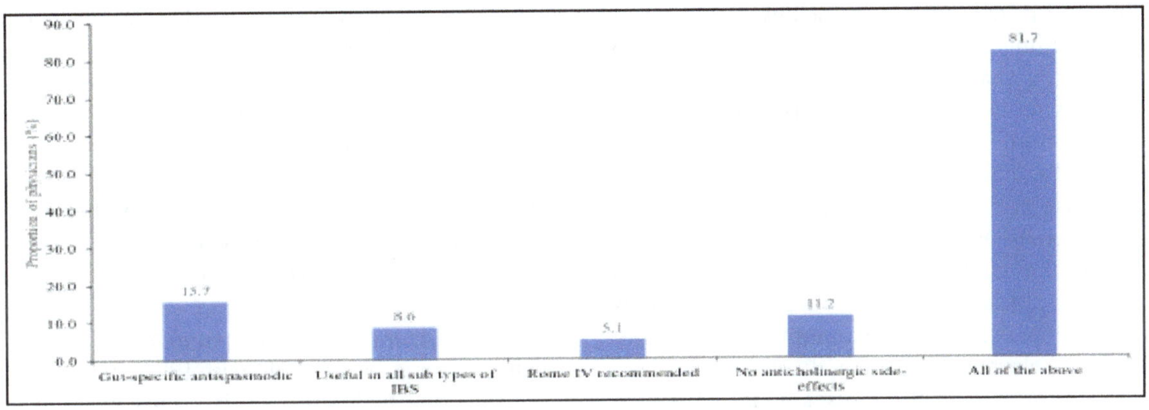

Figure 4: Advantages of mebeverine in reducing IBS symptoms.

IBS: Irritable bowel syndrome

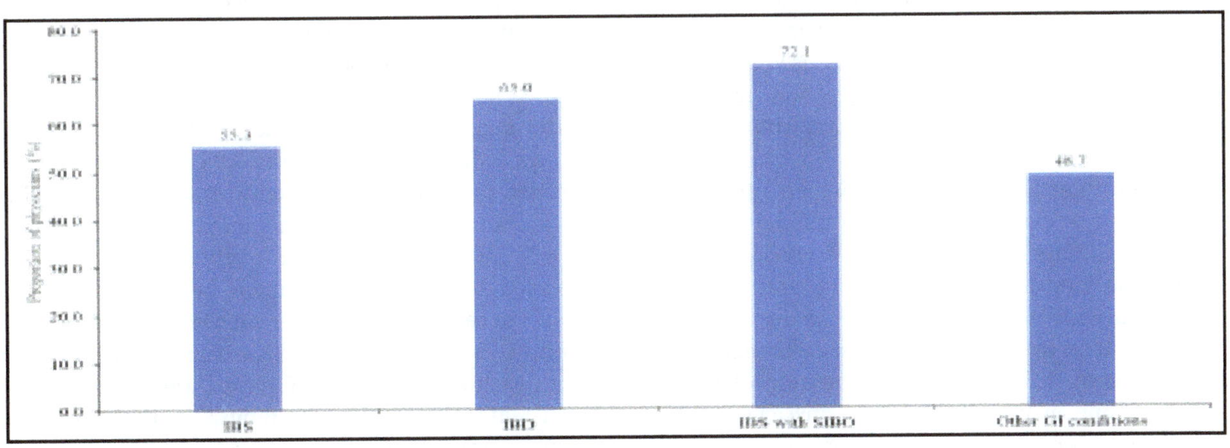

Figure 5: Preference for probiotics by gastrointestinal condition.

GI: Gastrointestinal; IBD: irritable bowel disease IBS: irritable bowel syndrome

Discussion

The present survey demonstrates that most physicians take a detailed history of the IBS syndrome and association-driven criteria to diagnose IBS in their regular clinical practice. More than 50% of the patients had IBS mixed with anxiety as stated by 38.6% physicians, and almost half of the survey responders reported that patients typically suffer with IBS for 2-4 weeks before physician consultation. Most physicians (61.9%) stated that patients with IBS take home remedies before physician consultation. Moreover, more than half the physicians ranked mebeverine monotherapy or mebeverine plus chlordiazepoxide as the top two preferred therapies for IBS management. In particular, the most preferred choice was mebeverine plus chlordiazepoxide for IBS patients with anxiety. Most respondents (81.7%) were convinced of the benefits of mebeverine, majority of the physicians reported that mebeverine or its combination with chlordiazepoxide was efficacious and safe for IBS. Almost all physicians believed that diet and lifestyle counselling and psychological counselling support were useful in extending support to patients with IBS. Most physicians stated that they prescribed probiotics with multiple strains for 2-4 weeks in patients with IBS.

Many studies indicated that IBS is diagnosed based on symptoms, and establishing a definitive diagnosis can be difficult because typical features are not discriminative, and precise biomarkers in clinical practice are lacking.[21] According to the guidelines, IBS is not an excluding diagnosis, and physicians are encouraged to establish a positive diagnosis based on symptom criteria alone.[22] Because of the elevated pre-test risk of celiac disease, serological testing for celiac disease is considered beneficial in individuals with diarrhoea-predominant IBS.[23] The current study did not look into differences in diagnostic approaches based on the IBS subtype. Notably, our survey showed that most physicians reported collecting a detailed history of IBS syndrome and used association-driven criteria to diagnose IBS in their regular practice. Furthermore, most physicians used the Rome criteria in their daily clinical practice and frequently recommended additional tests before confirming an IBS diagnosis.

Physicians in this study opined that most patients with IBS suffered for 2-4 weeks before they consulted a physician and took home remedies before physician consultation. In addition to seeking a diagnosis, testing, and symptom relief, patients with IBS frequently have anxiety concerns about stigma, tend to self-medicate, and rarely express all of their concerns.[24-27] Notably, in the setting of limited consultation time, as mentioned by the physicians in this study, neither doctors nor patients discuss concerns if other, more serious matters relating to diagnosis and treatment remain. However, the lack of discussion does not imply that these factors are unimportant to patients; instead, it may contribute to patients' perceptions of the negative impact of IBS on their quality of life.

Many studies indicate that most patients with IBS in primary care do not require pharmacotherapy.[24,28] However, medications are necessary to address the three most common symptoms of IBS, namely diarrhoea, constipation, and stomach pain.[1,29] Anticholinergics, antispasmodics, calcium channel blockers, prokinetics, and laxatives have been used to modify gastrointestinal motility.[1,29] At the same time, psychotropics, antidepressants, and putative visceral analgesics have also been used.[30] Results of meta-analyses have indicated that antispasmodics like mebeverine are more effective than placebo in treating IBS.[31,32] Smooth muscle relaxants were more helpful than placebo in treating IBS, mainly when stomach discomfort is the primary complaint. Mebeverine hydrochloride is one of the direct-acting intestinal smooth muscle relaxants and may relieve abdominal pain or spasm in IBS. Although the efficacy of bulking drugs is controversial, they may be beneficial for persons with IBS who suffer from constipation or diarrhea as their chief complaint.[33] Consistent with the above findings, our survey results indicate that mebeverine plus chlordiazepoxide combination was the most preferred (40.6%) pharmacotherapy to reduce IBS symptoms, followed by mebeverine monotherapy (26.9%). Combination of mebeverine and chlordiazepoxide was the most preferred choice of physicians (39.6%) for >50% of IBS patients with anxiety. Thus, mebeverine or mebeverine and chlordiazepoxide combination for 4-8 weeks have been recommended to help with IBS symptoms.

Mebeverine hydrochloride is a musculotropic sodium channel antagonist that relieves spasms while maintaining gut motility by acting directly on the smooth muscles of the gastrointestinal system. Mebeverine hydrochloride is an antispasmodic and available in a range of dosages. IBS symptoms have been successfully treated with antispasmodics.[34] A recent observational study suggested that mebeverine hydrochloride treatment was confirmed effective in the treatment of IBS with improvements in all IBS-quality of life subscales and scores. The study findings indicated that the total IBS quality of life score exceeded the minimal important response (>10.2), which was a statistically significant increase from baseline at week 4. At week 8, the IBS quality of life total score increased by 24.3 points, much beyond the clinically significant response. Moreover, mebeverine hydrochloride treatment improved IBS and gastrointestinal symptoms within each subgroup (IBS-C, IBS-D, and IBS-mixed).[35] Consistent with the above findings, our findings indicate that most physicians found mebeverine or its combination with chlordiazepoxide to be efficacious and safe in the management of IBS symptoms. Almost 65% of physicians responded that mebeverine or its combination with chlordiazepoxide is useful in all subtypes of IBS, namely IBS C, IBS D, and IBS-mixed). Most physicians (81.7%) reported that mebeverine has all the listed benefits such as gut-specific antispasmodic action, usefulness in all IBS subtypes, Rome IV recommendation, and absence of anticholinergic side effects.

Studies indicate that a brief psychoeducational intervention in the form of patient counselling for IBS management, which includes diet, lifestyle, and psychological counselling, appears to change IBS cognition and fears effectively, improving disease-related quality of life.[36,37] Consistent with the above findings, our survey indicates that almost all physicians were considered extending patient support such as diet, lifestyle, and psychological counselling to be effective strategies in managing IBS.

Results from an open-label study indicated that supplementation of multistrain probiotics (*Bifidobacterium, Lactobacillus, and Enterococcus*) improved IBS symptoms via associated changes in gastrointestinal flora, and the gradually beneficial effect remained stable for two weeks.[38] Similarly, a double-blind, randomized controlled trial found that multistrain probiotics (one strain of *Lactobacillus* sp. and four strains of *Bifidobacterium* sp.) use improved IBS symptoms and metabolomic characteristics of treated subjects. After eight weeks of treatment, dissatisfaction with bowel habits and stool frequency also greatly improved. In particular, probiotics significantly altered the metabolites, and they could be used as biomarkers to predict probiotic action in patients with IBS-D.[39] In our study, it was observed that most physicians prescribed probiotics for IBS with SIBO, and for a duration of 2-4 weeks.

Our study has certain limitations, which include limited internal validity (generalizability) of the questionnaire. Furthermore, modes of data collection by questionnaire carries a risk of recall bias or contamination by the participants. However, several strengths of this study should be acknowledged, which include exploration from a national perspective and representation of reasonably large sample size of physicians from different zones providing care to patients with IBS.

Conclusion

In conclusion, IBS is a common gastrointestinal disorder that affects people of both genders. Although IBS has been shown to have a detrimental impact on patients' quality of life, many elements of IBS remain unsolved, including the best management option to reduce IBS symptoms. The present survey supports understanding the prevalence, diagnosis, and therapeutic management of IBS in India. In particular, the usefulness of mebeverine therapy in reducing IBS symptoms was also established.

Acknowledgements

The authors would like to thank AlphaMD Private Limited for medical writing support.

Funding: The study was funded by Abbott India Ltd. Conflict of interest: None declared

Ethical approval: The study was approved by the Institutional Ethics Committee

References

1. Bonetto S, Fagoonee S, Battaglia E, Grassini M, Saracco GM, Pellicano R. Recent advances in the treatment of irritable bowel syndrome. Pol Arch Intern Med. 2021;131:709-15.
2. Chey WD. Irritable Bowel Syndrome. Gastroenterol Clin North Am. 2021;50:15-6.
3. Talley NJ. Functional gastrointestinal disorders as a public health problem. Neurogastroenterology & Motility 2008;20:121-9.
4. Minocha A, Johnson WD, Abell TL, Wigington WC. Prevalence, Sociodemography, and QualitLife of Older Versus Younger Patients with Irritable Bowel Syndrome: A Population-Based Study. Digestive Dis Sci. 2006;51:446-53.
5. Hungin APS, Chang L, Locke GR, Dennis EH, Barghout V. Irritable bowel syndrome in the United States: prevalence, symptom patterns and impact. Alimentary Pharmacol Therap. 2005;21:1365-75.
6. Ghoshal UC, Abraham P, Bhatt C, Choudhuri G, Bhatia SJ, Shenoy KT, et al. Epidemiological and clinical profile of irritable bowel syndrome in India: report of the Indian Society of Gastroenterology Task Force. Indian J Gastroenterol. 2008.;27:22-8.
7. Makharia GK, Verma AK, Amarchand R, Goswami A, Singh P, Agnihotri A, et al. Prevalence of Irritable Bowel Syndrome: A Community Based Study From Northern India. J Neurogastroenterol Motility. 2011;17:82-7.
8. Gwee K-A, Bak Y-T, Ghoshal UC, Gonlachanvit S, Lee OY, Fock KM, et al. Asian consensus on irritable bowel syndrome. J Gastroenterol Hepatol. 2010;25:1189-205.
9. Cassar GE, Youssef J G, Knowles SR, Moulding R, Austin D. The Impact of Diagnostic Status on Quality of Life in Irritable Bowel Syndrome. Turkish J Gastroenterol. 2021;32:808-18.
10. Goodoory VC, Mikocka-Walus A, Yiannakou Y, Houghton LA, Black CJ, Ford AC. Impact of Psychological Comorbidity on the Prognosis of Irritable Bowel Syndrome. Am J Gastroenterol. 2021;116:1485-94.
11. Sibelli A, Chalder T, Everitt H, Workman P, Windgassen S, Moss-Morris R. A systematic review with meta-analysis of the role of anxiety and depression in irritable bowel syndrome onset. Psychol Med. 2016;46:3065-80.
12. Zamani M, Alizadeh-Tabari S, Zamani V. Systematic review with meta-analysis: the prevalence of anxiety and depression in patients with irritable bowel syndrome. Alimentary Pharmacol Therap. 2019;50:132-43.
13. Chey WD, Kurlander J, Eswaran S. Irritable Bowel Syndrome. JAMA. 2015;313:949.
14. Drossman DA. Rome III: The new criteria. Chinese J Digestive Dis. 2006;7:181-5.
15. Lacy B, Patel N. Rome Criteria and a Diagnostic Approach to Irritable Bowel Syndrome. J Clin Med. 2017;6:99.
16. Zhou S, Liu X, Wang X, Xi F, Luo X, Yao L, et al. Pharmacological and non-pharmacological treatments for irritable bowel syndrome. Medicine. 2019;98:e16446.
17. Rawla P, Sunkara T, Raj JP. Updated review of current pharmacological

and non-pharmacological management of irritable bowel syndrome. Life Sciences. 2018;212:176-81.

18. Collins J, Farrall E, Turnbull DA, Hetzel DJ, Holtmann G, Andrews JM. Do We Know What Patients Want? The Doctor-Patient Communication Gap in Functional Gastrointestinal Disorders. Clin Gastroenterol Hepatol. 2009;7:1252-4.
19. Darvish-Damavandi M, Nikfar S, Abdollahi M. A systematic review of efficacy and tolerability of mebeverine in irritable bowel syndrome. World J Gastroenterol. 2010;16:547-53.
20. Anthoine E, Moret L, Regnault A, Sébille V, Hardouin JB. Sample size used to validate a scale: a review of publications on newly-developed patient reported outcomes measures. Health Qual Life Outcomes. 2014;12:176.
21. Sood R, Gracie DJ, Law GR, Ford AC. Systematic review with meta-analysis: the accuracy of diagnosing irritable bowel syndrome with symptoms, biomarkers and/or psychological markers. Alimentary Pharmacol Therap. 2015;42:491-503.
22. Palsson OS, Whitehead WE, van Tilburg MAL, Chang L, Chey W, Crowell MD, et al. Development and Validation of the Rome IV Diagnostic Questionnaire for Adults. Gastroenterology. 2016;150:1481-91.
23. Cash BD, Schoenfeld P, Chey WD. The utility of diagnostic tests in irritable bowel syndrome patients: a systematic review. Am J Gastroenterol. 2002;97:2812-9.
24. Bijkerk CJ, Wit NJ de, Stalman WA, Knottnerus JA, Hoes AW, Muris JW. Irritable Bowel Syndrome in Primary Care: The Patients' and Doctors' Views on Symptoms, Etiology and Management. Canad J Gastroenterol. 2003;17:363-8.
25. Casiday RE, Hungin APS, Cornford CS, de Wit NJ, Blell MT. Patients' explanatory models for irritable bowel syndrome: symptoms and treatment more important than explaining aetiology. Fam Pract. 2008;26:40-7. [
26. Niknam R, Mousavi S, Safarpour A, Mahmoudi L, Mahmoudi P. Self-medication of irritable bowel syndrome and dyspepsia: How appropriate is it? J Res Pharm Pract. 2016;5:121.
27. Barry CA. Patients' unvoiced agendas in general practice consultations: qualitative study. BMJ. 2000;320:1246-50.
28. Paterson WG, Thompson WG, Vanner SJ, Faloon TR, Rosser WW, Birtwhistle RW, et al. Recommendations for the management of irritable
29. bowel syndrome in family practice. IBS Consensus Conference Participants. CMAJ. 1999;161:154-60.
30. Defrees DN, Bailey J. Irritable Bowel Syndrome. Primary Care: Clinics in Office Practice. 2017;44:655-71.
31. Törnblom H, Drossman DA. Psychotropics, Antidepressants, and Visceral Analgesics in Functional Gastrointestinal Disorders. Curr Gastroenterol Rep. 2018;20:58.
32. Poynard T, Regimbeau C, Benhamou Y. Meta- analysis of smooth muscle relaxants in the treatment of irritable bowel syndrome. Alimentary Pharmacol Therap. 2001;15:355-61.
33. Poynard T, Naveau S, Mory B, Chaput JC. Meta- analysis of smooth muscle relaxants in the treatment of irritable bowel syndrome. Alimentary Pharmacol Therap. 2007;8:499-510.
34. Jailwala J. Pharmacologic Treatment of the Irritable Bowel Syndrome. Ann Int Med. 2000;133:136.
35. Winsemius A, Meuwsen IM, Boon C, van der Laan A, Brekle A, de Vries M. A pharmacokinetic comparison of the modified release capsule and a plain tablet formulation of mebeverine. Int J Clin Pract. 2002;56:659-62.
36. Hou X, Chen S, Zhang Y, Sha W, Yu X, Elsawah H, et al. Quality of Life in Patients with Irritable Bowel Syndrome (IBS), Assessed Using the IBS–Quality of Life (IBS-QOL) Measure After 4 and 8 Weeks of Treatment with Mebeverine Hydrochloride or Pinaverium Bromide: Results of an International Prospective Observational Cohort Study in Poland, Egypt, Mexico and China. Clinical Drug Investigation. 2014;34:783-93.
37. Hetterich L, Stengel A. Psychotherapeutic Interventions in Irritable Bowel Syndrome. Front Psychiatry 2020;11.
38. Halpert A. Irritable Bowel Syndrome: Patient- Provider Interaction and Patient Education. J Clin Med. 2018;7:3.
39. Fan YJ, Chen SJ, Yu YC, Si JM, Liu B. A probiotic treatment containing Lactobacillus, Bifidobacterium and Enterococcus improves IBS symptoms in an open label trial. J Zhejiang Univ Sci B. 2006;7:987- 91.
40. Kim J, Cho K, Kim JS, Jung HC, Kim B, Park MS, et al. Probiotic treatment induced change of inflammation related metabolites in IBS-D patients/double-blind, randomized, placebo- controlled trial. Food Sci Biotechnol. 2020;29:837- 44.
41. H. Vahedi, S. Merat, A. Rashidioon et al.Effect of fluoxetine in patients with pain and constipation-predominant irritable bowel syndrome: a double-blind randomized-controlled study, Aliment Pharmacol Ther, 22 (2005), pp. 381–385
42. R.K. Goyal, Muscarinic receptor subtypes. Physiology and clinical implications, N Engl J Med, 321 (1989), pp. 1022–1029
43. R.M. Eglen, Muscarinic receptors and gastrointestinal tract smooth muscle function, Life Sci, 68 (2001), pp. 2573–2578
44. A.E. Bharucha, M. Camilleri, A.R. Zinsmeister et al., Adrenergic modulation of human colonic motor and sensory function, Am J Physiol, 273 (5 Pt 1) (1997), pp. G997–1006
45. A. Malcolm, S.F. Phillips, M. Camilleri et al., Pharmacological modulation of rectal tone alters perception of distention in humans, Am J Gastroenterol, 92 (1997), pp. 2073–2079
46. A. Malcolm, M. Camilleri, L. Kost et al., Towards identifying optimal doses for alpha-2 adrenergic modulation of colonic and rectal motor and sensory function, Aliment Pharmacol Ther, 14 (2000), pp. 783–793
47. L.A. Houghton, C. Fell, P.J. Whorwell et al.Effect of a second-generation alpha2delta ligand (pregabalin) on visceral sensation in hypersensitive patients with irritable bowel syndrome, Gut, 56 (2007), pp. 1218–1225
48. T.J. Borody, E.M. Quigley, S.F. Phillips et al.Effects of morphine and atropine on motility and transit in the human ileum, Gastroenterology, 89 (1985), pp. 562–570
49. S. Delgado-Aros, H.J. Chial, F. Cremonini et al., Effects of asimadoline, a kappa-opioid agonist, on satiation and postprandial symptoms in health, Aliment Pharmacol Ther, 18 (2003), pp. 507–514
50. C.P. Delaney, J.L. Weese, N.H. Hyman et al., Phase III trial of alvimopan, a novel, peripherally acting, mu opioid antagonist, for postoperative ileus after major abdominal surgery, Dis Colon Rectum, 48 (2005), pp. 1114–1125
51. M.J. Owens, C.B. Nemeroff, Physiology and pharmacology of corticotropin-releasing factor, Pharmacol Rev, 43 (1991), pp. 425–473
52. C.S. Yuan, J.F. Foss, M. O'Connor et al., Methylnaltrexone for reversal of constipation due to chronic methadone use: a randomized controlled trial, J Am Med Assoc, 283 (2000), pp. 367–372
53. S.R. Sweetser, S.J. Linker Nord, D.D. Burton et al., Effects of a novel corticotrophin releasing factor receptor-1 antagonist, BMS-562086, on gastrointestinal and colonic transit and bowel habits in patients with diarrhea-predominant irritable bowel syndrome (D-IBS), Gastroenterology, 134 (2008), p. A 548
54. S.M. Leventer, R.F. Kucharik, J.C. Keogh et al., The potential of dextofisopam for treatment of irritable bowel syndrome and inflammatory bowel disease, Am J Gastroenterol, 99 (2004), p. S 279

55. S.M. Leventer, K. Raudibaugh, C.L. Frissora et al., Clinical trial: dextofisopam in the treatment of patients with diarrhoea-predominant or alternating irritable bowel syndrome, Aliment Pharmacol Ther, 27 (2008), pp. 197–206
56. W.Z. Lu, K.A. Gwee, S. Moochhalla et al., Melatonin improves bowel symptoms in female patients with irritable bowel syndrome: a double-blind placebo-controlled study, Aliment Pharmacol Ther, 22 (2005), pp. 927–934

4

The role of serotonin and diet in the prevalence of irritable bowel syndrome: A systematic review

Khushi Bruta, Vanshika, Kishnoor Bhasin and Bhawana*

Abstract

Serotonin or 5-hydroxytryptamine (5-HT)- a neurotransmitter of both the Enteric Nervous System and the Central Nervous System is synthesized by the hydroxylation of L- tryptophan to 5-hydroxytryptophan.
Serotonin has been associated with gut functions like assimilation and absorption, alongside the regulation of particle transport and fluid discharge in the gastrointestinal tract and its deficiency is found to be a prominent factor in the prevalence of gut disorders like Irritable Bowel Syndrome.
For this review, we assessed the conventional treatment methods of common drugs, with the recently accredited treatment options like dietary regulation, exercise, meditation, and acupuncture. Having found that the most commonly used drugs exhibited various side effects like nausea, fatigue, rash, and dizziness, an in-depth evaluation of different Indian dietary patterns and their respective effects on tryptophan levels has been highlighted to formulate an ideal diet for patients with Irritable Bowel Syndrome (IBS). This review seeks to explore the numerous studies conducted to link IBS with the lack of serotonin production in the body, alongside exploring the evidence associating certain foods with raised tryptophan levels to hypothesize a suitable Indian diet.
This review, in its essence, stresses the crucial need for further research on the dietary implications of common Indian foods and their FODMAP (Fermented Oligosaccharides, Disaccharides, Monosaccharides, And Polyols) contents, while underscoring the benefits of using unconventional and natural methods for the treatment of tryptophan-related gut disorders.

Keywords: Serotonin, Tryptophan, Irritable bowel syndrome, FODMAP

Background

Serotonin (5-hydroxytryptamine or 5-HT) is a neurotransmitter associated with the Central Nervous System and the Enteric Nervous System. It is produced by a biochemical conversion process (Fig. 1) where tryptophan, a component of proteins, combines with tryptophan hydroxylase, a chemical reactor to produce 5-hydroxytryptamine [1].

It is usually called the happy hormone because it contributes to wellbeing and happiness. A decrease in its level has been seen in various mental illnesses like depression and anxiety.

Apart from this, Serotonin has another crucial role in Gut motility. It was established during the early 1950s that a large amount of Serotonin (5-HT) is released from the mucosa at a comparative time as peristalsis happened within the digestive tract [2]. Since then, numerous studies have been conducted to analyze the relation between 5-HT and motility.

Serotonin and gut

The microorganisms present in the gut are capable of synthesizing 5-HT but this bacterial production is far exceeded by biosynthesis in Enterochromaffin (EC) Cells. Alternatively, these microbes help regulate the gut and plasma 5-HT levels by providing signals to the host

* Correspondence: bhawana.sharma@rajguru.du.ac.in
Department of Biochemistry, Shaheed Rajguru College of Applied Sciences for Women, University of Delhi, Vasundhara Enclave, New Delhi 110096, India

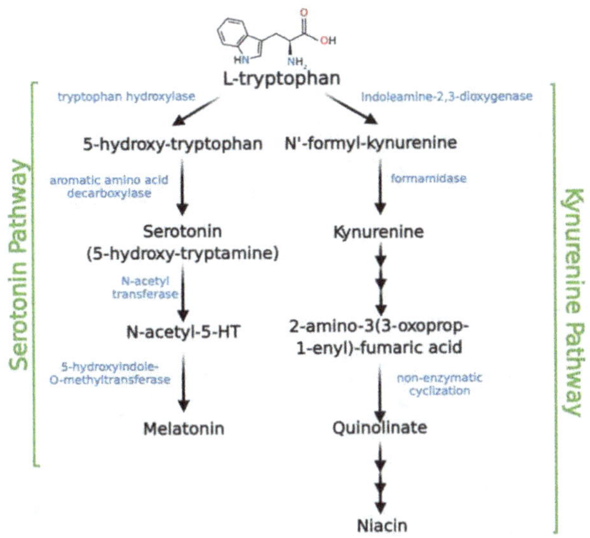

Fig. 1 Tryptophan Metabolism: Tryptophan is a substrate for the large neutral amino-acid transporter system and competes for transport with several other amino acids essential for brain function. Once in the CNS, L-tryptophan is hydroxylated to 5-hydroxytryptophan by the enzyme tryptophan hydroxylase type 2, the rate-limiting step in the brain serotonin synthesis. This is followed by subsequent decarboxylation involving the enzyme L-aromatic acid decarboxylase to serotonin (5-hydroxytryptamine, 5-HT)

mucosal cells in the form of Tryptophan hydroxylase 1 (TPH1) expression [3]. Moreover, it has been directly affirmed that Enterochromaffin (EC) cells are without a doubt mechanically sensitive and express the mechanosensitive molecule channel. (Fig. 2).

Studies like the Tyrode arrangement, utilizing modified Trendelenburg's strategy were conducted in a confined portion of the lumen to study the role of 5-HT in peristaltic reflex [4–6]. Grider, in 1998, illustrated the part of 5-HT-4 receptor ascending contraction and descendingrelaxation in the jejunum of humans, guinea pigs, and rodents. 5-HT3 has to be included in motility and discharge [7]. Luminal 5-HT is required for intestinal supplement and water assimilation, and impacts bicarbonate and electrolyte discharge into the lumen [8–10]. Through stimulation of 5-HT3 receptors on intestinal vagal afferent nerve endings, EC-cell–derived 5-HT increases postprandial pancreatic protein release, synergistically with cholecystokinin [11]. This, in turn, increases absorption and assimilation of additional luminal secretion. Gastrointestinal 5-HT increases bile activity by increasing the expression of the apical sodium-dependent bile salt transporter [12]. As such, 5-HT may act as a referee of several impacts that are credited to both 5-HT and Glucagon-Like Peptide-2, checking restriction of gastric cleansing and nutrient-stimulated gastric release [13–16].

Evidence for direct regulation comes from recent studies on lab-raised and gut microbiome-deficient, germ-free animals. They have high levels of circulating tryptophan and lower levels of serotonin but once gut microbes are introduced, falling levels of circulating tryptophan are observed [17].

Fasting also fortifies the synthesis and discharge of 5-HT from EC cells in mice due to increased translation of TPH1 [18]. Upon detection of low glucose by colonic EC cells, that mirror in-vitro fasting conditions, an increase in TPH1 expression, and 5-HT production and release are observed [19].

Irritable Bowel Syndrome (IBS) is a chronic gastrointestinal disorder affecting about 9–23% of the population in the world. It includes a group of symptoms including abdominal pain and changes in the pattern of bowel movements, without any evidence of underlying damage. IBS has been divided into 4 types depending on whether diarrhea, constipation, both, or neither are common (IBS-D, IBS-C, IBS-M, IBS-U). There is no specific laboratory or imaging test that can be helpful in the diagnosis of IBS. Physicians use 3 sets of diagnostic criteria for IBS which are:

1. **Rome Criteria:** This includes abdominal pain and discomfort lasting on average at least 1 day a week in the last 3 months. Pain and Discomfort are associated with defecation.
2. **Manning Criteria:** This focus on pain relieved by passing stool and on having incomplete bowel movements, mucus in stool, and changes in stool consistency.
3. **Type of IBS:** Symptoms according to the type of IBS are observed.

Relationship between serotonin and irritable bowel syndrome

Numerous studies were done to legitimize the relation of Irritable Bowel Syndrome to the lack of serotonin synthesis and release. Gene knockout and Gene transformation were among the best techniques used to study this relationship. Researchers examined that a decrease in the production of intestinal serotonin leads to the weakening of the intestinal lining, which inevitably results in clogging or constipation and an increment in serotonin levels within the gut [20].

One hypothesis is that the Serotonin Transporter-SERT is deficient in the enterocytes of individuals with IBS. Another hypothesis focuses on diminished numbers of enterochromaffin cells within the GI tract of individuals with IBS.

It was shown that the upregulation of the Indoleamine-pyrrole 2,3-dioxygenase activates a metabolic pathway, which is also likely to be associated with the pathogenesis of IBS. Afterward, considerations have shown that both females [21] and males [22] with IBS have extended kynurenine concentrations compared to controls. Therefore,

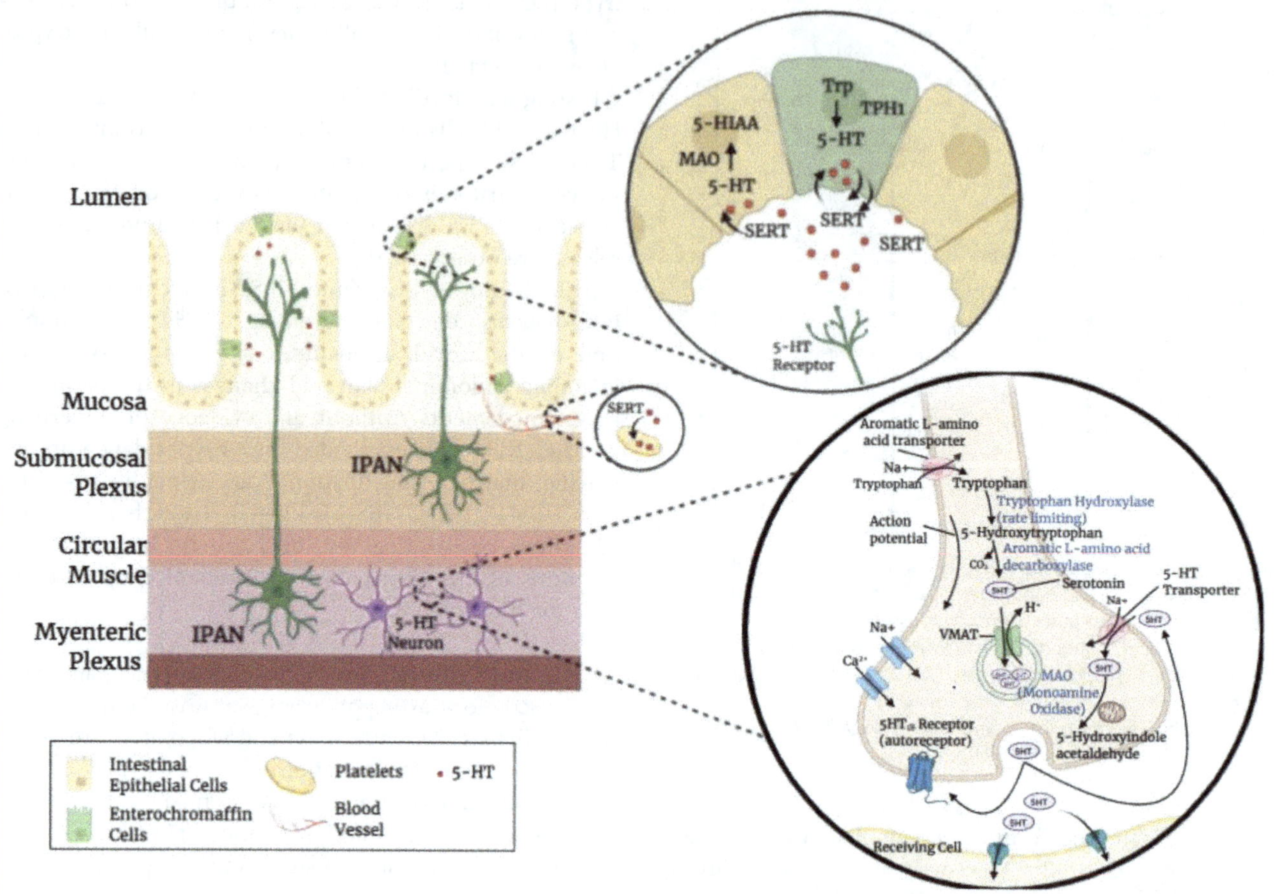

Fig. 2 Serotonin Synthesis, activation, and degradation: 5-HT is synthesized in the intestinal epithelium by enterochromaffin cells from Tryptophan (Trp) by tryptophan hydroxylase (TPH1). Indigenous bacteria (including Streptococcus, Enterococcus, Escherichia, and Clostridium) in human microbiota promote 5-HT biosynthesis from colonic enterochromaffin cells (ECs), which supply 5-HT to the mucosa, lumen, and circulating platelets. Luminal distention results in the basal release of 5-HT into the interstitial space of the mucosa, leading to the activation of 5-HT receptors on intrinsic primary afferent neurons (IPANs) in both submucosal and myenteric plexuses. 5-HT is inactivated through the action of serotonin reuptake transporter (SERT), which is expressed by intestinal epithelial cells. Once intracellular, 5-HT is degraded by monoamine oxidase (MAO) into 5-hydroxyindoleacetic acid (5-HIAA). Platelets also express SERT. Gut Bacterial species involved in Tryptophan metabolism include Streptococcus, Enterococcus, and Escherichia, and Clostridium

a positive relationship was found between IBS and the kynurenine/tryptophan extent. Those with extraordinary IBS side impacts have extended shunting of tryptophan along the kynurenine pathway which contributes to the unusual serotonergic function. SERT expression is seen to be diminished in IBS patients [23]. On the other hand, SSRI administration increases colonic motility and high-amplitude compressions are related to stomach cramping [24]. Chronic treatment of mice with the specific serotonin reuptake inhibitor (SSRI) paroxetine, reduced stool yield, and delayed upper GI tract movement [25]. These discoveries propose that changed mucosal 5-HT signaling seems to contribute to the indications of IBS.

IBS and its subtypes

There are three major subtypes of IBS. IBS-D is associated primarily with diarrhea, IBS-C is concerned with constipation and lastly, the third subtype deals with mixed symptoms of both constipation and diarrhea There have been studies that were conducted to compare the SERT-P polymorphism in IBS patients and sound individuals. This polymorphism comes about in a long (L) and a brief (S) allele. It can occur as homozygous (S/S) genotypes, heterozygous (L/S) SERT genotypes, and homozygous long (L/L) genotypes.

This study demonstrated that the SERT-P polymorphism was related to IBS-C within the Indian populace. The recurrence of the SERT-P S/S genotype was higher in IBS-C patients than in normal individuals [26].

In IBS-D, there has been no identified distinction in the basal or fortified mucosal 5-HT release, despite the finding that both mucosal 5-HT secretion and TpH1 mRNA levels are declined [27]. Postprandial 5-HT levels are elevated in platelet-poor plasma tests from IBS-D [28–30] or post-infectious IBS patients, but they have been reduced or unchanged in IBS-C.

IBS and mental illness

IBS and its symptoms largely impact daily activities and body image and are a cause of worry to patients. IBS is usually related to disgrace, and patients are stigmatized as 'frequent fliers' or 'somatizers'. Cognitive behavior therapy (CBT) could be a psychological or 'talking' therapy, which can be significantly helpful for patients with IBS. Fifty to 90% of IBS patients have a co-existing psychological condition, reminiscent of anxiety or depression (Table 1). Researchers have found high levels of reported sexual and emotional abuse among patients with IBS. Somatization disorder (SD), a psychiatric disorder has a prevalence of around 25% in patients with IBS, compared with around 1% among the overall population [31].

Treatment of IBS

Conventional method

Drugs are the most common treatment options for patients with gut disorders like IBS.

In cases of IBS-D and pain-predominant IBS, antispasmodics are used as the first-line treatments and include calcium channel blockers and neurokinin-type 2 receptor antagonists. Rifaximin is deemed to be the best second-line treatment for IBS-D. Rifaximin (RFX), is a non-absorbable antibiotic that inhibits protein synthesis and translation through binding to the beta subunit of bacterial DNA-dependent RNA polymerase. RFX should be avoided in patients with hepatic impairment and in the case of pregnant women, this medication should be taken with caution due to the potential hazards to the fetus. For patients with IBS-C, besides fiber and laxatives, the most plausible option as a second-line treatment is linaclotide (LIN) [32]. Caution should be taken in pregnant women as it showed severe maternal toxicity in animal studies. Administration of LIN is not affected by renal or hepatic impairment as it is metabolized within GI-tract. Thus, laxatives should be chosen wisely and used with caution.

Ondansetron (OND) helps in relieving stool frequency, stool urgency, colonic transit time, and stool consistency. It is proved to have lower efficacy with disease progression; hence, it is only suitable for IBS with mild diarrhea. However, most of the OND treated patients experience constipation followed by headache, rectal bleeding, abdominal pain and backache.

As with other drugs for IBS-D, constipation and nausea are the first common side effects among patients treated by eluxadoline tablets. Patients without gallbladder tend to have sphincter of Oddi spasm (SOS) and pancreatitis. Eluxadoline should be avoided in patients with any stage of hepatic impairment as the plasma concentration made a 16-fold and 4-fold rise in severe and mild/moderate cases.

Alternative/ complementary treatment

Besides the conventional use of drugs to treat IBS, studies have also focused on many alternative treatments.

For instance, *meditation* was recently linked with an increase in dopamine levels. A study by Perreau-Linck and colleagues was among the first to show that self-induced changes in mood can affect one's serotonin production.

Another approach used in elevating serotonin levels is *exposure to bright light.*

In a study that assessed measurements of the serotonin metabolite 5-hydroxyindoleacetic acid (5-HIAA) in the venous outflow from the brain, a direct relation was observed between the duration of bright sunlight and the rate of serotonin synthesis. Similarly, serotonin levels are higher in the post-mortem brain of humans who died during summers, as compared to those who died during winters. In rats, the highest serotonin levels are observed during the light part of the light-dark cycle. In humans, the effect of tryptophan deficiency on the mood of healthy individuals was seen to be highly diminished under bright light, as opposed to dim light.

Exercise is also believed to increase serotonin function in the brain. Major studies in this matter were initiated under the hypothesis that the fatigue caused by exercise leads to increased plasma tryptophan and diminished levels of branched-chain amino acids (BCAAs) leucine, isoleucine, and valine This causes a significant increase in tryptophan availability as BCCAs can hinder tryptophan transport to the brain.

Post and colleagues assessed the biogenic amine metabolites in cerebrospinal fluid (CSF) of clinically

Table 1 IBS Patients with co-existing Mental illness studies

Study	Number of Patients	Percentage of participants with psychological illness
Blanchard et al (2007)	210	66.6% (DSM-IV Axis type-1 disorder)
Kennedy et al (2005)	149	43% (Any psychological disorder in the past year)
Payne and Blanchard (1995)	34	85% (DSM-IV Axis type-1 disorder)
Tkachuk et al (2003)	28	68% (DSM-IV Axis type-1 disorder)

Deficiency of serotonin is common in IBS and as well as in many mental disorders. Many studies were done to study the existence of mental illness in IBS patients, here are enlisted some of the studies with the percentage of IBS patients with psychological illness [31]

depressed patients before and after an elevation in their physical activity [33].

Patrick and Ames in 2015, studied the effects of aerobic exercise on brain serotonin levels. Exercise has the potential to increase tryptophan's chances of crossing the blood-brain barrier by muscular- uptake of competitive amino acids [34].

Regular exercise (30 min of swimming daily, 4 weeks) was seen to increase serotonin metabolism and production in the brainstem and cerebral cortex but decrease hippocampal serotonin levels.

In another study, the introduction of a low-to-moderate intensity exercise regime significantly improved IBS symptoms and this improvement remained considerable even 60 days post-training. However, signs of inflammation, oxidative stress, antioxidants, and other IBS symptoms were observed 8 weeks post-training. This led to the conclusion that a regular exercise routine is essential to conserve the benefits of exercise training.

Another well-known factor is *diet.* Foods that are rich in tryptophan are often believed to be associated with elevated serotonin levels. Since the early 1970s, nutritional research developments show that brain function is influenced by the availability of various nutrients in the diet. In the mid-1970s, Gessa et al. demonstrated that acute administration of a mixture of essential amino acids lacking Tryptophan (Trp-free mixture) produced a specific and long-lasting reduction of brain tryptophan and serotonin levels in rats [35].

Administration of this Trp-free amino acid mixture in rats produced a sharp drop in the concentration of serum tryptophan associated with a decrease in brain tryptophan, serotonin (5-HT), and 5-hydroxyindoleacetic acid (5-HIAA) levels in rats.

Ingestion of only proteins diminishes rat brain Tryptophan and 5-HT because all of the amino acids compete with tryptophan for transportation across the blood-brain barrier. Conversely, carbohydrate consumption increases Trp and 5-HT levels in the brain as ingestion of carbohydrates increases blood insulin levels which in turn increases the uptake of branched-chain amino acids into muscles, thus decreases their plasmic concentration and competition at the blood-brain barrier.

A minor component of milk, α-Lactalbumin, contains relatively more tryptophan than most proteins. In small quantities, the ingestion of α-lactalbumin is seen to improve mood and cognition under certain circumstances, probably owing to elevated serotonin [36].

Dietary fibre is a safe and cheap way to improve IBS. As an example, bran is proved to be a natural bulking agent [37].

Peppermint oil is a common remedy for IBS and abdominal pain. It counters spasmodic movements by the transport of calcium ions across the cell membrane.

Techniques like *Acupuncture and Colon Hydroscopy* are also considered to help relieve abdominal distress. It has been indicated that several acupoints have distinguished effects on D-IBS, C-IBS, and abdominal irritation. It is known to exhibit certain gut responses that lead to inhibited acid output, reduced rectal hypersensitivity, and normalized motility. However, this effect is not always observed. Nevertheless, the National Institute for Health and Care Excellence (NICE) guidelines do promote the use of acupuncture to treat IBS.

Colon hydrotherapy (CHT) is a minimal access technique widely adopted to treat bowel inconsistencies. However, several side effects such as perforation, rectal bleeding, and pelvic abscess have been reported [38].

Discussion

The relationship between Serotonin and Gut has been stated in various research papers including various Gut-related disorders like Irritable Bowel Syndrome (IBS) and their treatments along with detailed information of Serotonin-rich drugs to improve bodily functions but most of these studies include data based on populations of the countries in the west. Through this review paper, we have tried to discuss such disorders in the context of India's population and dietary routines including food items commonly consumed in different regions of India along with their tryptophan content and hence formulated an ideal diet (as per the data) which in the future, can be introduced to various IBS patients to check its effectiveness in improving their condition.

Serotonin and diet

A considerable amount of studies associate depleting serotonin levels with a dietary tryptophan deficiency. These studies also show that changes in plasma tryptophan influence brain tryptophan and thus, 5-HT concentrations. One such study on rats, at the Institute of Pharmacology and Nutritional Physiology, University of Cagliari, proved that a substantial decline in serum and brain tryptophan levels is followed by a decrease in 5-HT and 5-hydroxyindoleacetic acid (5-HIM), within 2 hours of consuming a tryptophan deficient diet [39]. It was also found that serotonin levels were increased when insulin was ejected into the body. The fatty acid, carbohydrate, protein components of the diet are believed to be responsible for a hike in insulin secretion; which in turn, increases plasma tryptophan levels. The elevation in plasma tryptophan, due to carbohydrates also elicits a simultaneous increase in brain tryptophan, thus raising the brain serotonin concentration [40]. However, a hypercaloric, high-fat-high-sugar diet is seen to significantly decrease SERT-binding by about 30% [41] Thus, diets like the ketogenic diet (KD), which is a low-carbohydrate, high-fat, is shown to affect concentrations of norepinephrine, dopamine, and serotonin, which in turn are proven to modulate seizure susceptibility in many animal models [40]. Such snacking-centric diets can therefore alter the serotonergic system and increase obesity risks.

This relationship between brain-serotonin and diet can also prove to be clinically important. Food items that are known to raise 5-HT levels, can be fed to patients to modulate brain outputs, associated with serotonergic neurons. Drug-efficacy for serotonin-receptor interactions may also be enhanced using this knowledge. Alternatively, the effectiveness of 5-HT blocking drugs can also be increased by the administration of tryptophan-deficient diets [42].

It has been well established that a tryptophan-rich and FODMAP-low diet can aid in alleviating the symptoms of IBS. However, such dietary intervention has mostly been hypothesized for a western diet. In this review, we have discussed a diet based on the daily food intake of an average Indian individual. The daily L-tryptophan requirement for a normal human is 900–1000 mg [43].

The diet of an IBS patient should be developed, keeping in mind the following aspects-

1. Water-soluble fiber- Dietary fiber increases stool bulk by stimulating colonic mucosa. However, consuming water-insoluble fiber, like bran, may further cause abnormal bloating and intestinal discomfort whereas water-soluble fiber like psyllium often aids in relieving symptoms of GI tract disorders [44].
2. Low fat- Patients with IBS are often subjected to gas retention (bloating), nausea, and distension caused by the intraluminal fat in the small intestine. They exhibit abnormal lipid dependent motor dysfunction and increased rectal hypersensitivity. Thus, few patients associate IBS with fat-intake. However, regular differences in dietary fat consumption levels have not been found between sound individuals and IBS patients [45].
3. Gluten-free- Gluten is a mixture of proteins- gliadin and glutenin. It increases intestinal permeability by changing the function of the mucosal barrier. A gluten-free diet would ultimately lead to decreased permeability and reduced bowel frequency in IBS-D patients. This would also cause a reduced intake of FODMAPS which would ultimately aid in relieving IBS symptoms.
4. Low FODMAPs- FODMAPs (Fermented Oligosaccharides, Disaccharides, Monosaccharides, and Polyols), are a group of short-chain carbohydrates that are digested and absorbed poorly in the GI tract. Some examples include fructose, raffinose, nystose, and kestose. A low FODMAP diet has been effectively proven to be effective against IBS symptoms in numerous clinical trials. However, studies are still required for the determination of FODMAP contents in common Indian foods and the tolerance levels in an Asian setting.
5. Tryptophan-rich diet- Elevated serotonin levels are often associated with tryptophan-rich food

Table 2 Tryptophan Content in food items with low FODMAP

Food items with High FODMAP	Tryptophan Content (g) (per 100 g of food item)	Water-Soluble Dietary Fiber (g) (per 100 g of food item)	Food items with Low FODMAP	Tryptophan Content (g) (per 100 g of food item)	Water-Soluble Dietary Fiber (g) (per 100 g of food item)
Apple	0.0030	2.44	**Banana**	0.0118	1.04
Mango	0.0056	1.10	**Orange**	0.0003	0.56
Wheat	0.1168	4.67	**Maize**	0.0632	0.94
Barley	0.2080	3.01	**Rice**	0.0860	0.82
Rye	0.1080	15.1	**Ragi**	0.0664	1.67
Cabbage	0.0230	2.47	**Brinjal**	0.0156	1.20
Cauliflower	0.0291	2.51	**Capsicum**	0.0124	0.73
Cashew	0.2226	3.30	**Almond**	0.1851	2.52
Pistachio	0.2811	10.3	**Walnut**	0.1622	0.65
Cheese	0.2002	0.00	**Yogurt**	0.1550	0.00
Milk	0.0452	0.00	**Oats**	0.1785	3.81
Honey	0.0042	0.23	**Kidney Beans**	0.2790	2.62
Mushroom	0.0356	1.02	**Bitter Gourd**	0.0204	3.10
Beetroot	0.0142	2.84	**Lady Finger**	0.0093	1.33

Along with taking the appropriate amount of Tryptophan, a low FODMAPs (Fermented Oligosaccharides, Disaccharides, Monosaccharides, And Polyols) can also help in improving the condition. A diet with poorly adsorbed FODMAPs is considered as an effective strategy for symptom control in patients with IBS. A reason that contributes to poor absorption of FODMAPs includes the absence of luminal enzymes capable of hydrolyzing glycosidic bonds present in complex carbohydrates and the absence or low activity of brush border enzymes such as GLUT-2 and GLUT-5 [47]

Table 3 An example of Indian ideal diet for IBS patient

Breakfast	Mid-Snack	Lunch	Mid-Snack	Dinner
1 bowl of Greek Yogurt OatMeal 1 cup Oats (0.1785 g Trp and 3.81 g DF) + 1 Banana (0.0139 g Trp and 1.227 g DF) + 1 cup water + ¼ cup Greek yogurt (0.0949 g Trp and 0 g DF)	**1 bowl Nuts** ½ cup Almonds (0.0925 g Trp and 1.26 g DF) + ½ cup Walnuts (0.1054 g Trp and 0.42 g DF)	**Rajma Chawal (Kidney Beans Curry + Rice)** 1 serving Rice (0.1075 g Trp and 1.025 g DF) + 1 cup Rajma (0.1743 g Trp and 1.63 g DF)	**2 Medium Sized Oranges** (0.00084 g Trp and 0.784 g DF)	**3–4 Roti (Indian flat Bread) using Multigrain Flour** ½ cup Maida + ½ cup Ragi (0.1031 g Trp and 2.02 g DF) **With 1 Cup Capsicum Curry** (0.0217 g Trp and 1.27 g DF) Or, **1 Cup Bhindi Fry (Fried Okra)** (0.01729 g Trp and 2.47 g DF) Or, **1 Cup Karela (Bitter Gourd Curry)** (0.0252 g Trp and 3.844 g DF)
Total = 0.2846 g Trp and 5.037 g DF	**Total = 0.1979 g Trp and 1.68 g DF**	**Total = 0.3879 g Trp and 2.655 g DF**	**Total = 0.2846 g Trp and 5.037 g DF**	**Total = 0.125 g Trp (Avg.) and 4 g DF**

**DF*- Dietary Fiber, *Trp*- Tryptophan [45]

consumption. There have been studies that observed a drop in 5- HT serum concentration and reduction in brain-tryptophan, upon administration of a tryptophan-free amino acid mixture.

Diversity in eating habits, patterns, food items, occurs when we move from north to south or east to west India, due to cultural differences, local vegetation, different climatic conditions, social issues, religious beliefs, resources availability, differences in abiotic factors like soil, etc. Many food items, predominant in the Indian diet, possess these qualities and have been listed in (Table 2) [46].

By contrast, about three-fourths of the population in the United States has an eating pattern that is low in vegetables, fruits, dairy, and oils. More than half of the population is exceeding total grain, total protein, saturated fats, sodium, and added sugar recommendations revealing an eating pattern too high in calories.

Along with taking the appropriate amount of Tryptophan, a low FODMAPs (Fermented Oligosaccharides, Disaccharides, Monosaccharides, And Polyols) can also help in improving the condition. A diet with poorly adsorbed FODMAPs is considered as an effective strategy for symptom control in patients with IBS. A reason that contributes to poor absorption of FODMAPs includes the absence of luminal enzymes capable of hydrolyzing glycosidic bonds present in complex carbohydrates and the absence or low activity of brush border enzymes such as GLUT-2 and GLUT-5 [46].

As an example, the above data has been used to formulate an ideal diet for IBS patients in (Table 3) which will fulfill the daily tryptophan requirements (900-1000 mg) and dietary fiber requirements(15-20 g) while keeping the low and high FODMAPs food items in balance.

Conclusion and limitations

The interconnection of all bodily functions is evident when we examine the 'Happy Hormone'- serotonin and trace its functioning from acting as a neurotransmitter to playing an important role in the development of gastrointestinal disorders like Irritable bowel syndrome. Our dietary intake plays a key role in the regulation of IBS, and this information has been utilized to narrow down on food items in the Indian diet which possess all five qualities of being gluten-free, low in fat, low in FODMAP content, rich in tryptophan, and possessing water-soluble fibers.

A limitation of this study would be the absence of a professionally prescribed diet. The regime mentioned in the results of this review is concluded based on readings and analysis of existing literature and is derived from previously-concluded trials.

Abbreviations

5-HT: 5-Hydroxytryptamine; IBS: Irritable Bowel Syndrome; EC: Enterochromaffin; TPH1: Tryptophan hydroxylase-1; CBT: Cognitive Behavior Therapy; FODMAP: Fermented Oligosaccharides, Disaccharides, Monosaccharides, And Polyols; CHT: Colon HydroTherapy; GLUT-1: Glucose Transporter-1; GLUT-2: Glucose Transporter-2; GI: Gastrointestinal; IBS-D: Irritable Bowel Syndrome-Diarrhea; IBS-C: Irritable Bowel Syndrome-Constipation; IBS-M: Irritable Bowel Syndrome-Mixed type; DSM: Diagnostic and Statistical Manual of mental disorders

Acknowledgments

We would like to express our special thanks and gratitude to the Department of Biochemistry, Shaheed Rajguru College of Applied Sciences for Women, University of Delhi, for providing us with valuable opportunities and shaping us into able individuals.

Authors' contributions

The review article was envisaged by Khushi Bruta, Vanshika, Kishnoor Bhasin, Dr. Bhawana and all are equal contributors in drafting the manuscript and performing the literature search. Dr. Bhawana also guided us throughout the process and helped us bridge our idea across to a wider community. The authors read and approved the final manuscript.

References

1. Kendig DM, Grider JR. Serotonin and colonic motility. Neurogastroenterol Motil. 2015;27(7):899–905.
2. Kadowaki M, Wang XO, Shimatani H, Yoneda S, Takaki M. 5-HT4 receptor enhances the propulsive power of the peristaltic reflex in the rat distal colon. Auton Neurosci. 2002;99(1):62–5.
3. Martin AM, Young RL, Leong L, Rogers GB, Spencer NJ, Jessup CF, et al. The diverse metabolic roles of peripheral serotonin. Endocrinology. 2017;158(5): 1049–63.

4. Budhoo MR, Harris RP, Kellum JM. 5-Hydroxytryptamine-induced cl– transport is mediated by 5-HT3 and 5-HT4 receptors in the rat distal colon. Eur J Pharmacol. 1996;298(2):137–44.
5. Burleigh DE, Borman RA. Short-circuit current responses to 5-hydroxytryptamine in human ileal mucosa are mediated by a 5-HT4 receptor. Eur J Pharmacol. 1993;241(1):125–8.
6. Siriwardena A, Kellum JM Jr. A 5-HT2 receptor mediates serotonin-induced electrolyte transport in rat left colon. J Surg Res. 1993;55(3):323–9.
7. Mohammad-Zadeh LF, Moses L, Gwaltney-Brant SM. Serotonin: a review. J Vet Pharmacol Ther. 2008;31(3):187–99.
8. Imada-Shirakata Y, Kotera T, Ueda S, Okuma M. Serotonin activates electrolyte transport via 5-HT2AReceptor in rat colonic crypt cells. Biochem Biophys Res Commun. 1997;230(2):437–41.
9. Tuo BG, Isenberg JI. Effect of 5-hydroxytryptamine on duodenal mucosal bicarbonate secretion in mice. Gastroenterology. 2003;125(3):805–14.
10. Tuo BG, Sellers Z, Paulus P, Barrett KE, Isenberg JI. 5-HT induces duodenal mucosal bicarbonate secretion via cAMP-and Ca2+–dependent signaling pathways and 5-HT4 receptors in mice. Am J Physiol-Gastrointest Liver Physiol. 2004;286(3):G444–51.
11. Cho HJ, Callaghan B, Bron R, Bravo DM, Furness JB. Identification of enteroendocrine cells that express TRPA1 channels in the mouse intestine. Cell Tissue Res. 2014;356(1):77–82.
12. Watanabe H, Akasaka D, Ogasawara H, Sato K, Miyake M, Saito K, et al. Peripheral serotonin enhances lipid metabolism by accelerating bile acid turnover. Endocrinology. 2010;151(10):4776–86.
13. Raybould HE, Glatzle J, Robin C, Meyer JH, Phan T, Wong H, et al. Expression of 5-HT3 receptors by extrinsic duodenal afferents contribute to intestinal inhibition of gastric emptying. Am J Physiol-Gastrointest Liver Physiol. 2003; 284(3):G367–72.
14. LePard KJ, Stephens RL. Serotonin inhibits gastric acid secretion through a 5-hydroxytryptamine1-like receptor in the rat. J Pharmacol Exp Ther. 1994; 270(3):1139–44.
15. Wøjdemann M, Wettergren A, Hartmann B, Holst JJ. Glucagon-like peptide-2 inhibits centrally induced antral motility in pigs. Scand J Gastroenterol. 1998; 33(8):828–32.
16. Wøjdemann M, Wettergren A, Hartmann B, Hilsted L, Holst JJ. Inhibition of sham feeding-stimulated human gastric acid secretion by glucagon-like peptide-2. J Clin Endocrinol Metabol. 1999;84(7):2513–7.
17. Jenkins TA, Nguyen JC, Polglaze KE, Bertrand PP. Influence of tryptophan and serotonin on mood and cognition with a possible role of the gut-brain axis. Nutrients. 2016;8(1):56.
18. Margolis KG, Stevanovic K, Li Z, Yang QM, Oravecz T, Zambrowicz B, et al. Pharmacological reduction of mucosal but not neuronal serotonin opposes inflammation in mouse intestine. Gut. 2014;63(6):928–37.
19. Zelkas L, Raghupathi R, Lumsden AL, Martin AM, Sun E, Spencer NJ, et al. Serotonin-secreting enteroendocrine cells respond via diverse mechanisms to acute and chronic changes in glucose availability. Nutr Metab. 2015;12(1):1–9.
20. Manocha M, Khan WI. Serotonin and GI disorders: an update on clinical and experimental studies. Clin Transl Gastroenterol. 2012;3(4):e13.
21. Fitzgerald P, Cassidy Eugene M, Clarke G, Scully P, Barry S, Quigley Eamonn MM, et al. Tryptophan catabolism in females with irritable bowel syndrome: relationship to interferon-gamma, severity of symptoms and psychiatric co-morbidity. Neurogastroenterol Motil. 2008;20(12):1291–7.
22. Clarke G, Fitzgerald P, Cryan JF, Cassidy EM, Quigley EM, Dinan TG. Tryptophan degradation in irritable bowel syndrome: evidence of indoleamine 2, 3-dioxygenase activation in a male cohort. BMC Gastroenterol. 2009;9(1):1–7.
23. Coates MD, Mahoney CR, Linden DR, Sampson JE, Chen J, Blaszyk H, et al. Molecular defects in mucosal serotonin content and decreased serotonin reuptake transporter in ulcerative colitis and irritable bowel syndrome. Gastroenterology. 2004;126(7):1657–64.
24. Tack J, Broekaert D, Corsetti M, Fischler B, Janssens J. Influence of acute serotonin reuptake inhibition on colonic sensorimotor function in man. Aliment Pharmacol Ther. 2006;23(2):265–74.
25. Coates MD, Johnson AC, Greenwood-van Meerveld B, Mawe GM. Effects of serotonin transporter inhibition on gastrointestinal motility and colonic sensitivity in the mouse. Neurogastroenterol Motil. 2006;18(6):464–71.
26. Sikander A, Rana SV, Sinha SK, Prasad KK, Arora SK, Sharma SK, et al. Serotonin transporter promoter variant: analysis in Indian IBS patients and control population. J Clin Gastroenterol. 2009;43(10):957–61.
27. Houghton LA, Atkinson W, Whitaker RP, Whorwell PJ, Rimmer MJ. Increased platelet depleted plasma 5-hydroxytryptamine concentration following meal ingestion in symptomatic female subjects with diarrhoea predominant irritable bowel syndrome. Gut. 2003;52(5):663–70.
28. Atkinson W, Lockhart S, Whorwell PJ, Keevil B, Houghton LA. Altered 5-hydroxytryptamine signaling in patients with constipation-and diarrhea-predominant irritable bowel syndrome. Gastroenterology. 2006;130(1):34–43.
29. Dunlop SP, Coleman NS, Blackshaw E, Perkins AC, Singh G, Marsden CA, et al. Abnormalities of 5-hydroxytryptamine metabolism in irritable bowel syndrome. Clin Gastroenterol Hepatol. 2005;3(4):349–57.
30. David DA. Irritable bowel syndrome: psychological comorbidities and cognitive behavioural therapy. A review of the literature. Gastrointest Nurs. 2012;10(10):44–50.
31. Mousavi T, Nikfar S, Abdollahi M. An update on efficacy and safety considerations for the latest drugs used to treat irritable bowel syndrome. Expert Opin Drug Metab Toxicol. 2020;16(7):583–604.
32. Young SN. How to increase serotonin in the human brain without drugs. J Psych Neurosci. 2007;32(6):394.
33. Maleki BH, Tartibian B, Mooren FC, FitzGerald LZ, Krüger K, Chehrazi M, et al. Low-to-moderate intensity aerobic exercise training modulates irritable bowel syndrome through antioxidative and inflammatory mechanisms in women: results of a randomized controlled trial. Cytokine. 2018;102:18–25.
34. Fadda F. Tryptophan-free diets: a physiological tool to study brain serotonin function. Physiology. 2000;15(5):260–4.
35. Chang FY, Lu CL. Treatment of irritable bowel syndrome using complementary and alternative medicine. J Chin Med Assoc. 2009;72(6): 294–300.
36. Heijnen S, Hommel B, Kibele A, Colzato LS. Neuromodulation of aerobic exercise—a review. Front Psychol. 2016;6:1890.
37. Thompson WG. Irritable bowel syndrome: a management strategy. Best Pract Res Clin Gastroenterol. 1999;13(3):453–60.
38. Richard DM, Dawes MA, Mathias CW, Acheson A, Hill-Kapturczak N, Dougherty DM. L-tryptophan: basic metabolic functions, behavioral research and therapeutic indications. Int J Tryptophan Res. 2009;2: IJTR-S2129.
39. Biggio G, Fadda F, Fanni P, Tagliamonte A, Gessa GL. Rapid depletion of serum tryptophan, brain tryptophan, serotonin and 5-hydroxyindoleacetic acid by a tryptophan-free diet. Life Sci. 1974;14(7):1321–9.
40. Fernstrom JD, Wurtman RJ. Brain serotonin content: increase following ingestion of carbohydrate diet. Science. 1971;174(4013):1023–5.
41. Koopman KE, Booij J, Fliers E, Serlie MJ, La Fleur SE. Diet-induced changes in the lean brain: hypercaloric high-fat-high-sugar snacking decreases serotonin transporters in the human hypothalamic region. Mol Metab. 2013; 2(4):417–22.
42. Fernstrom JD. Modification of brain serotonin by the diet. Annu Rev Med. 1974;25(1):1–8.
43. El-Salhy M, Ystad SO, Mazzawi T, Gundersen D. Dietary fiber in irritable bowel syndrome. Int J Mol Med. 2017;40(3):607–13.
44. Mullie P, Godderis L, Clarys P. Determinants and nutritional implications associated with low-fat food consumption. Appetite. 2012;58(1):34–8.
45. Longvah T, Anantan I, Bhaskarachary K, Venkaiah K, Longvah T. Indian food composition tables. Hyderabad: National Institute of Nutrition, Indian Council of Medical Research; 2017.
46. Dhingra D, Michael M, Rajput H, Patil RT. Dietary fibre in foods: a review. J Food Sci Technol. 2012;49(3):255–66.
47. Devinder Dhingra, Mona Michael, Hradesh Rajput, R. T. Patil Dietary fibre in foods: a review. J Food Sci Tech. 2012;(3):255–66.

5

Evaluation of the irritable bowel syndrome severity index in Japanese male patients with irritable bowel syndrome with diarrhea

Motoko Ida[1*], Akito Nishida[2], Hiraku Akiho[3], Yoshihiro Nakashima[4], Kei Matsueda[5] and Shin Fukudo[6]

Abstract

Background: Previous studies have indicated that ramosetron, a 5-hydroxytryptamine-3 receptor antagonist, achieves global improvement in irritable bowel syndrome (IBS) symptoms in male patients with IBS with diarrhea (IBS-D). However, in addition to global assessment it was deemed important to assess "clinically meaningful improvements, focusing on the patient's chief complaint and the severity of major IBS symptoms". We performed a randomized, placebo-controlled, phase IV pilot study to explore and examine efficacy variables that allow such evaluation of ramosetron in male patients with IBS-D.

Methods: We performed a prospective study of 115 male outpatients with IBS-D (according to the Rome III criteria), from June 2009 to December 2009 at 25 centers in Japan. After a one-week baseline period, subjects received either 5 μg of ramosetron ($n = 47$) or placebo ($n = 51$) once daily for 12 weeks. To evaluate "clinically meaningful improvements focusing on the severity of major IBS symptoms," the Japanese version of the IBS severity index (IBSSI-J) was used.

Results: Change in IBSSI-J overall score from baseline was −133.5 ± 110.72 in the ramosetron 5 μg group and −108.2 ± 94.44 in the placebo group ($P = 0.228$) at the last evaluation point. Differences in responder rates for at least a 50% reduction from baseline in IBSSI-J between the ramosetron 5 μg group and the placebo group were over 10%, except Month 1. The monthly responder rate for global assessment of relief of overall IBS symptoms in the ramosetron 5 μg group showed a statistically significant improvement compared to placebo at the second month (44.4% vs 18.4%, $P = 0.012$). The proportion of patients who had a ≥ 50% reduction in IBSSI-J overall score was 24/37 (64.9%) in the responder group on global assessment and 18/54 (33.3%) in the non-responder group at Week 12.

Conclusions: Further examination will be needed before IBSSI-J can be used in clinical trials of agents for IBS-D. However, this study revealed that response on global assessment was correlated with improvement in the IBSSI-J, suggesting that global assessment reflects improvement of the symptom severity of patients with IBS-D. (Clinicaltrials.gov ID: NCT00918411 Registered 9 June 2009).

Keywords: 5-hydroxytryptamine (5-HT), Abdominal pain, Abdominal discomfort, Global improvement, Stool consistency, Irritable bowel syndrome severity index

* Correspondence: motoko.ida@astellas.com
[1]Japan-Asia Planning & Administration, Medical & Development, Astellas Pharma Inc., 2-5-1 Nihonbashi-Honcho, Chuo-ku, Tokyo 103-8411, Japan
Full list of author information is available at the end of the article

Background

Irritable bowel syndrome (IBS) is a functional gastrointestinal disorder that is characterized by chronic or recurrent abdominal pain and/or abdominal discomfort associated with abnormal bowel movements [1]. IBS as defined by the Rome III criteria [2] is classified into four subtypes: IBS with diarrhea (IBS-D), IBS with constipation (IBS-C), mixed-type IBS, and unsubtyped IBS. The onset of IBS and its symptoms have for some time been known to be largely associated with various psychosocial stressors. Psychosocial stress causes stimulation of the hypothalamus, releasing corticotropin-releasing hormone (CRH), and causes abnormalities in gastrointestinal motility and lowering of the sensory threshold in the gastrointestinal tract via neurotransmitters, such as 5-hydroxytryptamine (5-HT, serotonin) released from enteric nerves or enterochromaffin cells. Some evidence suggests that 5-HT has a crucial role in IBS-D pathophysiology. Patients with IBS-D show exaggerated colonic motility in response to colonic distention [3] and secretion of 5-HT [4]. Moreover, in animal studies and clinical pharmacological tests, 5-HT_3 receptor antagonists have been reported to suppress abnormalities of gastrointestinal motility (abnormal bowel movements) and a decrease in the sensory threshold in the gastrointestinal tract caused by CRH and stresses [5–7], which suggests involvement of the 5-HT_3 receptor in the occurrence of IBS-D symptoms.

Ramosetron, a potent, selective 5-HT_3 receptor antagonist [5, 8–10], was developed in Japan, initially for the nausea and vomiting of cancer patients receiving chemotherapy and later for IBS-D patients. In clinical studies of IBS-D [11, 12], it was decided that abdominal pain and discomfort, which were the main subjective symptoms of patients with IBS-D, would be assessed by subjects as "global assessment of relief of abdominal pain/discomfort" and that symptoms of diarrhea, such as abnormal stool form, frequent bowel movement and defecation urgency, would be evaluated by patients as "global assessment of improvement in abnormal bowel habits". Furthermore, all subjective symptoms that patients had, including the above symptoms, were comprehensively assessed by the patients as "global assessment of relief of overall IBS symptoms". Of these three global assessments of improvement/relief, the "global assessment of relief of overall IBS symptoms" in particular was considered to be directly linked to therapeutic effects in patients with IBS-D because of the heterogeneity of symptoms, so it was adopted as the primary variable for clinical studies of ramosetron. The efficacy of ramosetron was demonstrated based on the results of this variable in a previous phase III study. However, stratified analysis by sex using the chi-square test (two-sided significance level of 0.05) in the phase III study revealed that ramosetron did not show significant improvement compared to placebo in the global assessment of relief of the overall IBS symptoms of female patients [12]. Based on the above results, marketing approval was granted for the indication of "IBS-D in male patients" in Japan in July 2008. Subsequently, additional clinical studies [13–15] were conducted to evaluate the efficacy and safety of ramosetron for female patients with IBS-D. These studies indicated that 2.5 μg/day of ramosetron was an effective treatment for female patients with IBS-D, in contrast to the optimal dose of ramosetron at 5 μg/day for male patients. Ramosetron was approved for use by women in May, 2015.

The Pharmaceuticals and Medical Devices Agency of Japan has approved the use of global assessment as a primary endpoint for IBS studies since 2002 [11, 12]. However, they also considered it important to assess "clinically meaningful improvements, focusing on the patient's chief complaint and the severity of major IBS symptoms" in addition to the global assessment. The aim of this study was to explore and examine variables that allow such evaluation of ramosetron in patients with IBS-D. The IBS severity index (IBSSI) is a reliable and well-validated instrument for measuring the presence and severity of specific IBS symptoms [16]. Japanese versions of the IBS severity index (IBSSI-J) developed and validated by Shinozaki et al. are available in Japan [17]. Most studies confirming responsiveness of IBSSI were trials aiming at evaluating behavioral interventions. Preliminary evaluation was thought to be needed to assess responsiveness of IBSSI-J in clinical trials using pharmacological agents. This study was conducted as a pilot study for a post marketing study.

Methods

Patient population

This study was conducted from June 2009 to December 2009 at 25 Japanese centers that have departments of gastroenterology. Male outpatients aged 20–64 years were diagnosed with IBS-D based on the Rome III criteria. The study protocol was designed in accordance with the Declaration of Helsinki and was approved by the institutional review board at each site. All patients provided written informed consent prior to participating in study-related procedures.

In the Rome III criteria [2], IBS-D is defined as recurrent abdominal pain/discomfort for at least three days per month in the preceding three months, in association with two or more of the following: improvement with defecation, onset associated with a change in the frequency of stools, and/or onset associated with a change in the form (appearance) of stools. Furthermore, patients have loose (mushy) or watery stools at least 25% of the time and hard or lumpy stools for less than 25% of bowel movements.

Patients were eligible if they fulfilled the criteria for the last three months, with symptom onset at least six months prior to diagnosis. Organic diseases were excluded by colonoscopy or double-contrast barium enema if these examinations had not been performed within five years. Based on a medical interview conducted by the attending physician before provisional registration, patients were excluded if any of the following were evident: a history of resection of the stomach, small intestine, or large intestine (excluding appendicitis or resection of benign polyps); history or current evidence of inflammatory bowel disease; history or current evidence of ischemic colitis, concurrent infectious enteritis, hyperthyroidism, hypothyroidism, or other diseases that may affect gastrointestinal transit or colonic function; history or current evidence of abuse of drugs or alcohol within the previous year; malignant tumors; current evidence of severe depression or a severe anxiety disorder that could potentially affect the evaluation of study drug efficacy; concurrent serious cardiovascular, respiratory, renal, hepatic, gastrointestinal (excluding IBS), hematological, or neurological/psychiatric diseases; or a history of drug allergies. In addition, patients were excluded if they were using drugs or undergoing examinations that could affect the evaluation of study drug efficacy; if they had been enrolled in previous clinical studies of ramosetron or had taken ramosetron; and if they were participating or had participated in other clinical studies within the 12 weeks prior to study initiation.

Patients satisfying the inclusion and exclusion criteria for typical IBS-D symptoms during a one-week baseline period were enrolled. Severity of abdominal pain/discomfort had to exceed mean scores of 0.7 or more assessed daily on a 5-point ordinate (numerical rating) scale (0, none; 1, mild; 2, moderate; 3, severe; and 4, intolerable). The number of bowel movements had to exceed three times or more per week. Stool consistency was assessed with using the Bristol Stool Form Scale (BSFS) [2] as follows; type 1, separate hard lumps, like nuts (hard to pass); type 2, sausage shaped but lumpy; type 3, like a sausage but with cracks on its surface; type 4, like a sausage or snake, smooth and soft; type 5, soft blobs with clear-cut edges (passed easily); type 6, fluffy pieces with ragged edges (mushy stool); or type 7, watery, no solid pieces, and entirely liquid. Following this classification of stool consistency using the BSFS, patients who had either type 1 or type 2 stools were excluded. Patients who had not used drugs or undergone examinations that could affect the evaluation of study drug efficacy within 10 days prior to randomization; who recorded all items in the patient diary for five days or more during the baseline period; and who were not judged ineligible for the study according to the clinical laboratory test results obtained before the baseline period were randomized and then given treatment.

Study design

This randomized, placebo-controlled clinical trial comprised a provisional registration period, a one-week baseline period, and a 12-week treatment period, similar to previous studies [11, 12]. Following the baseline period, eligible patients were randomly assigned to 12-week oral treatment with placebo or ramosetron hydrochloride 5 μg once daily before breakfast. Visits were scheduled at Weeks 2, 4, 8, and 12 (or at discontinuation) to assess treatment efficacy, drug compliance, and occurrence of adverse events. Randomization was performed in a 1:1 ratio using a block size of four based on a randomization list developed by a third-party contract research organization. Placebo tablets were externally distinguishable from ramosetron hydrochloride tablets, however, they were indistinguishable when packaged in press through pack sheets. Patients were prohibited to use drugs or undergo examinations, such as other IBS therapeutic drugs, antidiarrheal drugs, and colonoscopy, that could affect the evaluation of study drug efficacy during the treatment period. All patients, investigators, and sponsors were blinded until all observations and evaluations were completed, the statistical analysis plan was finalized, and all data had been locked. All authors had access to the study data and reviewed and approved the final manuscript.

Data collection

During the baseline and treatment periods, patients recorded their IBS symptoms daily on paper diary cards at bedtime. In the diary, patients recorded the BSFS for every bowel movement throughout the study period. Patients scored severity on a five-point ordinate (numerical rating) scale and the duration of all continuous abdominal pain/discomfort from Week 1 to Week 4, Week8 and Week12 they had experienced. Every seven days during the treatment period, patients also graded summarized IBS symptoms compared with the baseline period on a five-point ordinate scale as follows: relief from overall IBS symptoms and abdominal pain/discomfort (0, completely relieved; 1, considerably relieved; 2, somewhat relieved; 3, unchanged; and 4, worsened) and improvement in abnormal bowel habits (0, nearly normalized; 1, considerably relieved; 2, somewhat relieved; 3, unchanged; and 4, worsened). Patients assessed IBS severity using the Japanese version of the IBS Severity Index (IBSSI-J) every four weeks [16, 17].

Efficacy and safety endpoints

To explore and examine variables that allow evaluation of "clinically meaningful improvements, focusing on the severity of major IBS symptoms" achieved by this drug, the IBSSI-J was assessed as a new measure in this trial in addition to the previous global assessment [11, 12]. IBSSI-J contains five questions that measure, on a 100-point scale, the severity of abdominal pain, the frequency of abdominal pain, the intensity of abdominal distention, dissatisfaction with bowel habits, and interference with QOL. All five components contribute to the score equally, yielding overall scores ranging from 0 to 500. IBS severity is graded as mild (75–174), moderate (175–299), or severe (300–500) on the basis of overall scores [16]. Patients who had at least a 50% reduction from baseline (≥50% reduction) in IBSSI-J overall score were defined as responders at each evaluation point. In the monthly responder rates for global assessment of relief of overall IBS symptoms, relief of abdominal pain/discomfort and improvement in abnormal bowel habits, patients with scores of 0 or 1 at each weekly evaluation point were defined as weekly responders, and patients who were weekly responders for at least two of the four weeks were defined as monthly responders. Change in IBSSI-J score and percent change in the IBSSI-J from baseline were calculated with reference to the category of global assessment of overall IBS symptoms (responder vs. non-responder) at each evaluation point.

Statistical analysis

Sample sizes of 60 patients or more (30 patients/group or more) were set based on the feasibility of a post marketing study to explore and examine the endpoints of the patient's chief complaint or IBS severity. Statistical analysis was performed using SAS Drug Development (ver. 3.4) and PC-SAS (ver. 8.2) (SAS Institute Inc., Cary, NC, USA).

Efficacy analyses included the full analysis set (FAS), which was as complete as possible and as close as possible to the intention-to-treat ideal of including all randomized subjects. The FAS included all patients who received at least one dose of the study drug during the treatment period and for whom at least one endpoint could be evaluated. To determine the robustness of the results, primary analyses were performed according to the per-protocol set. Safety analyses were performed for all patients who received at least one dose of the study drug during the treatment period.

Change from baseline and percent change from baseline in IBSSI-J score were summarized at each evaluation point by treatment group and/or monthly response for global assessment of relief of overall IBS symptoms. Treatment comparison used a *t*-test with a two-sided significance level of 0.05. IBSSI score was categorized and summarized by whether the subject was a monthly responder on global assessment of relief of overall IBS symptoms.

Monthly responder rates for global assessment of relief of overall IBS symptoms are expressed as a percentage of responders, and 95% confidence intervals (95% CIs) are presented. The treatment groups were compared using the chi-square test with a two-sided significance level of 0.05. In addition, responder rates for at least a 50% reduction from baseline (≥50% reduction) in IBSSI-J at each evaluation point are similarly analyzed as an ad hoc analysis.

Results

Overall study population

Written informed consent was provided by 115 patients. Of these, 17 patients dropped out and 98 patients were randomly allocated to the ramosetron 5 μg group ($n = 47$), or the placebo ($n = 51$) group (Fig. 1). Ultimately 44

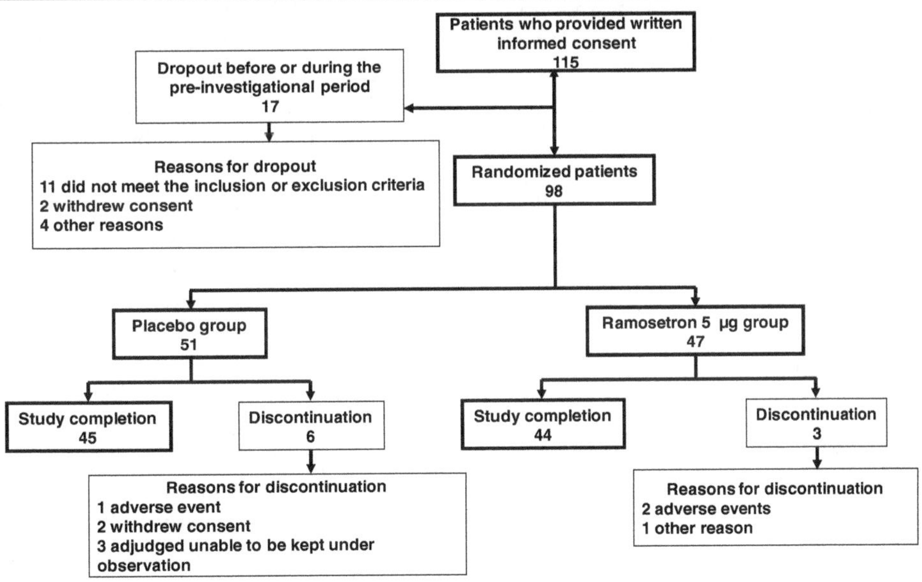

Fig. 1 Flowchart showing patient progress throughout the study. Reasons for dropping out of the study are shown

patients in the ramosetron 5 μg group and 45 patients in the placebo group completed the study. The reasons for discontinuation are shown in Fig. 1. In the placebo group, one patient discontinued by withdrawing consent after randomization, with no data, and was excluded from the FAS used in the efficacy analyses. The decision to exclude this patient from FAS was taken before unblinding, according to the predefined procedure stipulated in the study protocol.

All the demographic and baseline characteristics shown in Table 1 were similar among patients allocated to each group. The medication adherence rates were 97.6% in the ramosetron 5 μg group and 97.9% in the placebo group.

Efficacy

The baseline IBSSI-J overall scores in the ramosetron 5 μg and placebo groups were 267.1 ± 98.75 and 246.6 ± 80.52, respectively (Table 2). The respective first-quartile point and third-quartile points were 180.0 and 355.0 in the ramosetron 5 μg group and 200.0 and 290.0 in the placebo group. Severity of IBS can be graded as mild (75–174), moderate (175–299), or severe (300–500) on the basis of overall IBSSI scores. The proportions of patients with moderate severity at baseline were 29.8% in the ramosetron 5 μg group and 64.0% in the placebo group, with severe grading 46.8 and 22.0%, respectively (Table 1). Most patients enrolled in this study were classified as moderate to severe. Table 2 also shows the baseline score for each of the five components included in the IBSSI-J. The highest score was dissatisfaction with bowel habits, 68.6 ± 25.55 and 66.8 ± 22.78 in the ramosetron 5 μg and placebo groups, respectively. Second was interference with QOL (60.0 ± 27.59 and 54.3 ± 27.39, respectively), followed by frequency of abdominal pain (55.1 ± 33.87 and 57.4 ± 33.61, respectively). Intensity of abdominal distention showed the lowest scores, 35.6 ± 32.25 and 23.8 ± 25.65, respectively. Abdominal pain was assessed from the aspects of severity and frequency in the IBSSI-J. Frequency of abdominal pain was worse than severity of abdominal pain.

Table 1 Demographics and baseline characteristics

Patient background	Placebo (*n* = 50)	Ramosetron 5 μg (*n* = 47)	*P* value
Age (years)	40.9 ± 11.11	41.0 ± 9.31	0.970
Duration of disease (months)	103.9 ± 90.27	111.5 ± 129.10	0.738
Severity of abdominal pain/ discomfort (0–4)	1.43 ± 0.58	1.52 ± 0.61	0.481
Bristol Stool Form Scale (1–7)	5.55 ± 0.66	5.52 ± 0.43	0.764
Stool frequency (times/day)	2.77 ± 1.33	2.44 ± 1.09	0.181
IBSSI-J overall score	246.6 ± 80.52	267.1 ± 98.75	0.264
No symptoms (0–74)	0 (0.0%)	1 (2.1%)	-
Mild (75–174)	7 (14.0%)	10 (21.3%)	-
Moderate (175–299)	32 (64.0%)	14 (29.8%)	-
Severe (300–500)	11 (22.0%)	22 (46.8%)	-

Data are expressed as mean ± standard deviation. *P* values were calculated using analysis of variance

Change in IBSSI-J overall score from baseline (Table 3) was −133.5 ± 110.72 in the ramosetron 5 μg group and −108.2 ± 94.44 in the placebo group (*P* = 0.228) at the last evaluation point. Differences between the ramosetron 5 μg and placebo groups adjusted by baseline scores were −11.51 (95% CI, −43.13–20.11, *P* = 0.471) at Week 4, −14.39 (95% CI, −47.70–18.93, *P* = 0.393) at Week 8, −16.90 (95% CI, −54.80–21.01, *P* = 0. 378) at Week 12 and −13.60 (95% CI, −49.89–22.68, *P* = 0.459) at the last evaluation point (Fig. 2a). Differences in responder rates for at least a 50% reduction from baseline (≥50% reduction) in IBSSI-J between in the ramosetron 5 μg group and the placebo group were over 10%, except Month 1 (Fig. 2b). Changes in each component of the IBSSI-J from baseline in the ramosetron 5 μg and placebo groups at all evaluation points are shown in Table 3.

The monthly responder rate for global assessment of relief of overall IBS symptoms at the last evaluation point was 46.8% (95% CI, 32.1–61.9) in the ramosetron 5 μg group and 34.0% (95% CI, 21.2–48.8, *P* = 0.281) in the placebo group (Fig. 3a). Even though the number of patients enrolled in this study is limited, a statistically significant difference between ramosetron and placebo was shown at the second month (*P* = 0.012). Monthly responder rates for improvement in abnormal bowel habits in the ramosetron 5 μg group were significantly higher than those in the placebo group at the first month (*P* = 0.015) and the third month (*P* = 0.048) (Fig. 3b). On the other hand, monthly responder rates for abdominal pain/discomfort in the ramosetron 5 μg group did not show a statistically significant difference between ramosetron and placebo at any evaluation point (data not shown).

Figure 4 shows the relationship between IBSSI-J and the global assessment of relief of overall IBS symptoms. Mean changes in IBSSI-J overall scores from baseline are categorized into ≤ −200, −200 < and ≤ −80, −80 < and ≤ −50, −50 < and ≤ 0, 0 < and compared by responder/non-responder for global assessment of relief of overall IBS symptoms in Fig. 4a. Patients who had mean changes in IBSSI-J overall scores from baseline exceeding 200 points were more numerous in the responder group on global assessment compared to the non-responder group (45.9% vs 11.1% at Week 12). Patients with a change of over 80 points or over 50 points were also more numerous in the responder group on global assessment than in the non-responder group at all evaluation points.

Table 2 Baseline IBSSI-J score

		N	Mean ± SD	Min	Max	Median	First-quartile points	Third-quartile points	*t*-test
Overall score	Placebo	50	246.6 ± 80.52	80	410	245	200	290	t = −1.123, df = 95, *P* = 0.264
	Ramosetron 5 μg	47	267.1 ± 98.75	60	440	275	180	355	
Severity of abdominal pain	Placebo	50	44.3 ± 26.71	0	100	47.5	20	70	t = −0.647, df = 95, *P* = 0.519
	Ramosetron 5 μg	47	47.8 ± 26.70	0	90	50	30	70	
Frequency of abdominal pain	Placebo	50	57.4 ± 33.61	0	100	60	30	90	t = 0.335, df = 95, *P* = 0.739
	Ramosetron 5 μg	47	55.1 ± 33.87	0	100	60	30	90	
Intensity of abdominal distention	Placebo	50	23.8 ± 25.65	0	80	17.5	0	50	t = −2.007, df = 95, *P* = 0.048
	Ramosetron 5 μg	47	35.6 ± 32.25	0	100	30	0	60	
Dissatisfaction with bowel habits	Placebo	50	66.8 ± 22.78	20	100	60	50	90	t = −0.361, df = 95, *P* = 0.719
	Ramosetron 5 μg	47	68.6 ± 25.55	0	100	70	50	90	
Interference with QOL	Placebo	50	54.3 ± 27.39	0	100	55	30	80	t = −1.013, df = 95, *P* = 0.314
	Ramosetron 5 μg	47	60.0 ± 27.59	0	100	60	40	80	

Data are expressed as mean ± standard deviation. *P* values were calculated using analysis of variance

Similarly, the percent change in IBSSI-J from baseline was categorized into ≤ −75, −75 < and ≤ −50, −50 < and ≤ −30, −30 < and ≤ 0 and 0 < and compared by responder/non-responder for global assessment of relief of overall IBS symptoms (Fig. 4b). The number of patients who had a ≥ 75% reduction in IBSSI-J overall score was higher in the responder group on global assessment than in the non-responder group (35.1% vs 11.1% at Week 12). The rate of patients who had a ≥ 50% reduction or ≥ 30% reduction in IBSSI-J overall score was also higher in the responder group on global assessment than in the non-responder group at all evaluation points.

Safety

Safety was evaluated for all 98 patients. Adverse events were experienced by 27 patients (57.4%) in the ramosetron 5 μg group and by 20 patients (39.2%) in the placebo group (Table 4). The incidence of hard stool was higher in the ramosetron 5 μg group than in the placebo group, which was considered to be caused by the pharmacological action of ramosetron. All the events including constipation and hard stool observed in this study were mild and improved quickly. There was no occurrence of ischemic colitis or serious adverse events.

Discussion

In this clinical study, IBSSI-J was used to explore and examine variables that allow the assessment of "clinically meaningful improvements, focusing on the severity of major IBS symptoms". We showed that most patients enrolled had moderate to severe IBS symptoms in the baseline period. The highest score among each component was for dissatisfaction with bowel habits. Second were interference with QOL and frequency of abdominal pain. It is well known that IBS significantly impairs health related quality of life (QOL) [18]. The patients in this study were considered to have impaired QOL. The lowest score for the five components was for intensity of abdominal distention. Patients with abdominal distention and/or bloating were reported to be more numerous with IBS-C than with IBS-D [19]. The lowest score of intensity of abdominal distention in IBSSI-J in this study might be related to a lower contribution of abdominal distention to IBS symptom severity in IBS-D.

The proportion of patients who had a ≥ 50% reduction in IBSSI-J overall score was more than 10% higher in the ramosetron 5 μg group than in the placebo group, except Month 1. Although significant results were lacking, the graph shape of changes in IBSSI-J score at all evaluation points in the ramosetron 5 μg group seems to be superior to that of the placebo group. Francis et al. suggested that a decrease of 50 points in IBSSI overall score correlated with improvement in clinical symptoms [16]. On the other hand, Whitehead et al. have proposed that ≥ 50% reduction in IBSSI overall score from the baseline score was considered to constitute clinically meaningful improvement of symptoms [20]. We evaluated other categorization to find 'clinically meaningful improvements' by pharmacological agents, and compared responder/non-responder for global assessment of relief of overall IBS symptoms. In Francis's report, mean change of IBSSI from baseline to 3 months later was significantly greater in the patients who became clinically considerably better than little changed (change in score: 83 vs 6) [16]. Based on their reports, we selected −50 and −80 point reductions.

Table 3 Change in each IBSSI-J component score from baseline at each evaluation point

	Week 4		Week 8		Week 12		Last point	
	Placebo	Ramosetron 5 µg	Placebo	Ramosetron 5 µg	Placebo	Ramosetron 5 µg	Placebo	Ramosetron 5 µg
	Mean ± SD *P* value	Mean ± SD *P* value	Mean ± SD *P* value	Mean ± SD *P* value	Mean ± SD *P* value	Mean ± SD *P* value	Mean ± SD *P* value	Mean ± SD *P* value
N	48	46	49	44	47	44	50	47
Overall scores	−75.0 ± 81.52	−95.9 ± 105.12 *P* = 0.283	−103.0 ± 81.81	−130.6 ± 114.27 *P* = 0.181	−110.3 ± 97.04	−137.0 ± 113.18 *P* = 0.231	−108.2 ± 94.44	−133.5 ± 110.72 *P* = 0.228
Severity of abdominal pain	−15.3 ± 25.18	−17.0 ± 25.15 *P* = 0.743	−21.4 ± 28.46	−24.3 ± 27.41 *P* = 0.625	−21.9 ± 30.42	−26.6 ± 27.01 *P* = 0.439	−21.9 ± 29.76	−26.1 ± 26.41 *P* = 0.467
Frequency of abdominal pain	−16.5 ± 25.89	−20.0 ± 32.52 *P* = 0.560	−24.7 ± 29.38	−26.6 ± 35.04 *P* = 0.777	−25.1 ± 32.56	−28.2 ± 35.13 *P* = 0.666	−24.6 ± 31.77	−28.1 ± 33.98 *P* = 0.603
Intensity of abdominal distension	−9.7 ± 23.13	−16.3 ± 27.68 *P* = 0.214	−12.2 ± 24.54	−17.8 ± 26.66 *P* = 0.295	−11.5 ± 25.83	−16.6 ± 29.88 *P* = 0.385	−10.8 ± 25.26	−16.3 ± 29.22 *P* = 0.325
Dissatisfaction with bowel habits	−16.2 ± 31.23	−20.8 ± 28.18 *P* = 0.454	−19.2 ± 33.55	−31.4 ± 29.88 *P* = 0.067	−25.1 ± 33.57	−33.4 ± 31.50 *P* = 0.230	−24.8 ± 33.84	−32.5 ± 30.63 *P* = 0.243
Interference with QOL	−17.3 ± 27.76	−21.8 ± 29.94 *P* = 0.454	−25.5 ± 27.75	−30.5 ± 34.84 *P* = 0.445	−26.7 ± 28.67	−32.2 ± 32.53 *P* = 0.396	−26.1 ± 28.04	−30.6 ± 32.44 *P* = 0.470

Data are expressed as mean ± standard deviation. *P* values were calculated using analysis of variance

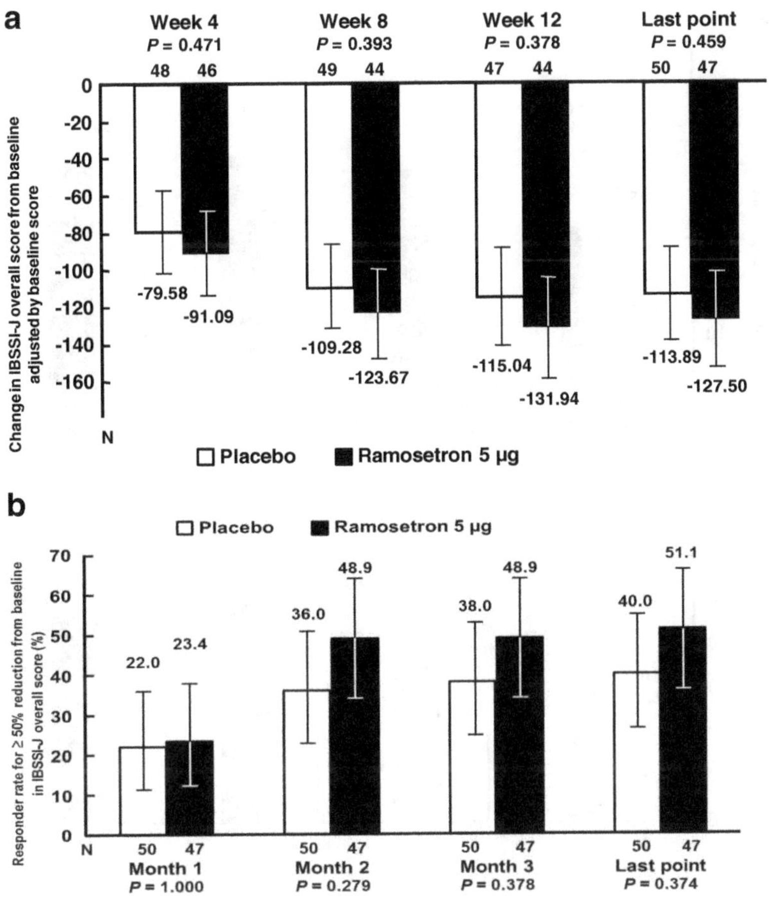

Fig. 2 Change in IBSSI-J overall scores. **a** Change in IBSSI-J overall scores from baseline, adjusted by baseline score. Column height: the values adjusted using the baseline score as a covariate. Error bar: 95% CI. *P* values were calculated using analysis of covariance with the treatment group as a factor and baseline score as a covariate. **b** Responder rates for at least a 50% reduction from baseline in IBSSI-J overall score. Column height: responder rate (%). Error bar: 95% CI

The baseline IBSSI-J overall scores in our ramosetron 5 μg and placebo groups were 267.1 ± 98.75 and 246.6 ± 80.52, respectively (Table 1). Because IBS severity is rated as No symptoms (0–74), we set a −200 point reduction as the score at which the symptoms were eliminated. Similarly, in addition to 50% reduction, we examined 3/4 and 1/3 reduction categories to explore the clinical meaningful change. Our study showed patients who had changes in their overall IBSSI-J scores from baseline of over 50 points were more numerous in the monthly responder group based on global assessment of relief of overall IBS symptoms than in the non-responder group. This finding is in accordance with the results of Francis. The proportion of patients who had a ≥ 50% reduction in IBSSI-J overall score was also higher in the responder group on global assessment (24/37, 64.9%) than in the non-responder group (18/54, 33.3%) at Week 12. The studies by Francis et al. and Whitehead et al. were trials aiming to evaluate behavioral interventions, and these effects were not compared to placebo. In patients with IBS-C, it was recently reported that linaclotide showed a statistically significantly higher change in IBSSI overall score from baseline as well as in the percentage of patients with ≥ 50% reduction in IBSSI overall score compared to placebo [21]. Nevertheless, those data suggest that the IBSSI could be used for measuring response to pharmacological agents for patients with IBS-C; there is little data used for measuring the response of patients with IBS-D. This study was the first trial to use the IBSSI-J to measure the response to pharmacological agents in patients with IBS-D.

Despite the limited patient number in this study, statistically significant differences between ramosetron and placebo were shown in the monthly responder rate for global assessment of relief of overall IBS symptoms at the second month and in the monthly responder rates for improvement in abnormal bowel habits at the first

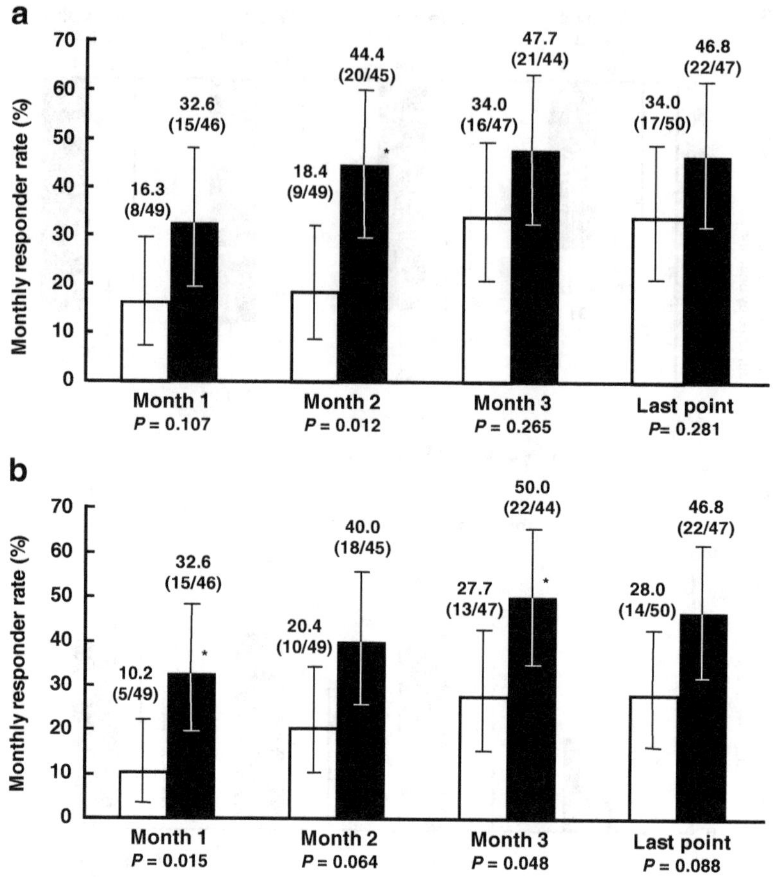

Fig. 3 Global assessments. **a** Monthly responder rates for global assessments of relief of overall IBS symptoms. **b** Monthly responder rates for improvement in abnormal bowel habits. Column height: responder rate (%). Error bar: 95% CI. *P* values were calculated using the chi-square test, as follows: $^{*}P < 0.05$

and the third months. Improvement in bowel habits was shown to contribute to improvement of global assessment of relief of overall IBS symptoms, as in previous studies [12]. The differences between ramosetron and placebo were more evident than those in the IBSSI-J overall scores.

Whitehead et al. reported that patients with milder symptoms at baseline were more likely to report satisfactory relief than patients with moderate or severe symptoms in a usual care study [20]. On the other hand, Drossman et al. reported that baseline symptom severity was no longer confounded with a report of adequate relief (AR) at the study end point, if patients who reported AR at baseline were excluded from study participation [22]. A meta-analysis involving 10,066 IBS patients to investigate whether improvement of symptoms depends on their severity showed no correlation between the severity of IBS and the improvement of symptoms in a binary assessment [23]. In this study, the sample size of each severity group was too small to permit assessment of the relationship between baseline severity and global assessment. AR was not used.

In this study, the monthly responder group with respect of global assessment of relief of overall IBS symptoms showed a greater change in the IBSSI-J overall score and percent change from baseline than did the non-responder group. This study thus revealed that responses on global assessment were correlated with improvement in IBSSI-J, suggesting that global assessment reflects improvement of the symptom severity of patients with IBS-D. IBS is a syndrome that includes multiple symptoms (abdominal pain/discomfort, stool form, stool frequency, etc.) [1]. Global assessments of relief of overall IBS symptoms allow patients to assess improvement in multiple IBS symptoms [11–15]. The Japanese Society of Gastroenterology (JSGE) developed evidence-based clinical practice guidelines for IBS [24]. They recommend treating IBS patients as they can feel improvement in IBS symptoms based on the assessment of patient-reported outcomes. Global assessment of relief

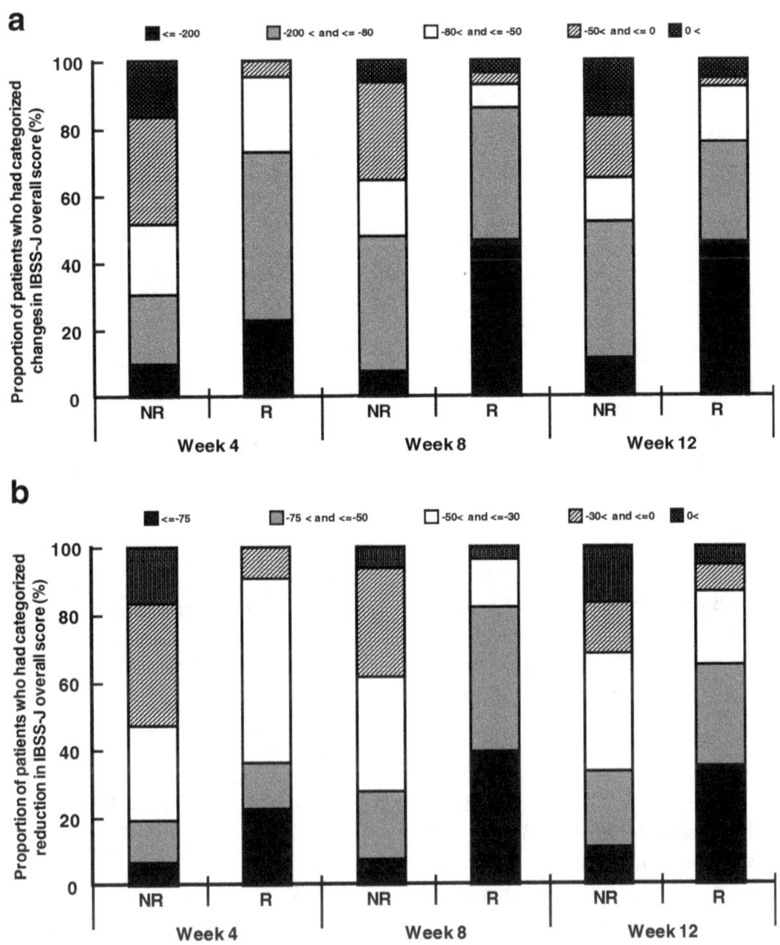

Fig. 4 Relationship between IBSSI-J and global assessment. **a** Changes in IBSSI-J overall scores from baseline were compared by responder/non-responder for global assessment of relief of overall IBS symptoms. Mean changes in IBSSI-J overall scores from baseline were categorized into the following groups: ≤ −200, −200 < and ≤ −80, −80 < and ≤ −50, −50 < and ≤ 0, 0 <. **b** Percent change in IBSSI-J overall score from baseline was compared by responder/non-responder for global assessment of relief of overall IBS symptoms. Percent change in IBSSI-J from baseline was categorized into the following groups: ≤ −75, −75 < and ≤ −50, −50 < and ≤ −30, −30 < and ≤ 0 and 0 <

of overall IBS symptoms can be a useful efficacy variable in IBS-D.

IBSSI-J showed that the patients in this study have impaired QOL. For the improvement of QOL, it is important for IBS patients to evaluate 'clinically meaningful improvements', because it was reported IBS patients impaired their QOL [18]. Although generic QOL instruments like SF-36 can be good measurement tools for comparing the impact of different conditions on health status, disease-specific QOL is considered to be sensitive for measuring the impact of treatment. IBS-QOL is a reliable and well-validated outcome for assessing the QOL of IBS patients. We used IBS-QOL and obtained the result that ramosetron significantly improved IBS-QOL compared to placebo in the following post marketing study for male patients with IBS-D [25].

This study was a pilot study and has some limitations. First, the sample size was not sufficient to detect a statistically significant difference between ramosetron and placebo. Second, this study was conducted with only male patients with IBS-D. Third, psychosocial factors may have affected to the response to the drug. Especially, expectations of the drug efficacy, which differs among patients, is likely to affect the drug effects [26]. The effect of expectations can be tested by use of placebo [26]. Therefore, the drug effect seen in clinical trials are supposed to be a summation of placebo effects and real pharmacological effects. Because we included a placebo group in this study, it is easier to assume a real pharmacological effect of ramosetron. Further experience will be needed to use this questionnaire as a primary endpoint in clinical studies

Table 4 Incidence of adverse events

Event	Placebo (*n* = 51)	Ramosetron 5 μg (*n* = 47)
All adverse events	20 (39.2%)	27 (57.4%)
Gastrointestinal disorders	8 (15.7%)	13 (27.7%)
Abdominal discomfort	0 (0.0%)	2 (4.3%)
Constipation	2 (3.9%)	0 (0.0%)
Hard stool	3 (5.9%)	9 (19.1%)
Nausea	2 (3.9%)	0 (0.0%)
Infections and infestations	4 (7.8%)	5 (10.6%)
Nasopharyngitis	4 (7.8%)	3 (6.4%)
Gastroenteritis	0 (0.0%)	2 (4.3%)
Hepatobiliary disorders	2 (3.9%)	2 (4.3%)
Hepatic function abnormal	2 (3.9%)	1 (2.1%)
Skin and subcutaneous tissue disorder	2 (3.9%)	3 (6.4%)
Dermatitis contact	1 (2.0%)	2 (4.3%)

Data are expressed as number (%). Events with an incidence of ≥ 3% in any of the groups are listed

related to the development of the pharmacological agents for IBS-D patients.

Conclusions

Further examination will be needed before IBSSI-J can be used in clinical trials of agents for IBS-D. However, this study revealed that the responses on global assessment were correlated with improvement in the IBSSI-J, suggesting that global assessment reflects improvement of the symptom severity of patients with IBS-D.

Abbreviations

BSFS: Bristol Stool Form Scale; 95% CI: 95% confidence interval; CRH: Corticotropin-releasing hormone; FAS: Full analysis set, 5-HT, 5-hydroxytryptamine; 5-HT_3: 5-hydroxytryptamine receptor 3; IBS: Irritable bowel syndrome; IBS-C: Irritable bowel syndrome with constipation; IBS-D: Irritable bowel syndrome with diarrhea and IBSSI-J, Japanese version of IBS Severity Index

Acknowledgments

The authors thank the investigators for participating in the study. English translation assistance was provided by SunFlare Co., Ltd. and funded by Astellas Pharma Inc.

Authors' contributions

MI, HA and AN designed the study, assessed the data, and wrote the manuscript. YN performed statistical analyses. SF and KM provided important scientific comments on study design, data analysis and manuscript content. All authors have approved the final version of the article, including the authorship list.

Authorship statement

Guarantor of the article: Motoko Ida.

Author details

[1]Japan-Asia Planning & Administration, Medical & Development, Astellas Pharma Inc., 2-5-1 Nihonbashi-Honcho, Chuo-ku, Tokyo 103-8411, Japan. [2]Development Project Management, Astellas Pharma Inc., Tokyo, Japan. [3]Japan-Asia Clinical Development 2, Development, Astellas Pharma Inc., Tokyo, Japan. [4]Japan-Asia Data Science, Development, Astellas Pharma Inc., Tokyo, Japan. [5]Sakura Life Clinic, Tokyo, Japan. [6]Department of Behavioral Medicine, Tohoku University Graduate School of Medicine, Sendai, Japan.

References

1. Drossman DA. The functional gastrointestinal disorders and the Rome III process. Gastroenterology. 2006;130:1377–90.
2. Longstreth GF, Thompson WG, Chey WD, Houghton LA, Mearin F, Spiller RC. Functional bowel disorders. Gastroenterology. 2006;130:1480–91.
3. Kanazawa M, Palsson OS, Thiwan SO, Turner MJ, van Tilburg MA, Gangarosa LM, et al. Contributions of pain sensitivity and colonic motility to IBS symptom severity and predominant bowel habits. Am J Gastroenterol. 2008;103:2550–61.
4. Dunlop SP, Coleman NS, Blackshaw E, Perkins AC, Singh G, Marsden CA, et al. Abnormalities of 5-hydroxytryptamine metabolism in irritable bowel syndrome. Clin Gastroenterol Hepatol. 2005;3:349–57.
5. Miyata K, Ito H, Fukudo S. Involvement of the 5-HT_3 receptor in CRH-induced defecation in rats. Am J Physiol. 1998;274:G827–31.
6. Goldberg PA, Kamm MA, Setti-Carraro P, van der Sijp JR, Roth C. Modification of visceral sensitivity and pain in irritable bowel syndrome by 5-HT_3 antagonism (Ondansetron). Digestion. 1996;57:478–83.
7. Delvaux M, Louvel D, Mamet JP, Campos-Oriola R, Frexinos J. Effect of alosetron on responses to colonic distension in patients with irritable bowel syndrome. Aliment Pharmacol Ther. 1998;12:849–55.
8. Miyata K, Kamato T, Nishida A, Ito H, Katsuyama Y, Iwai A, et al. Pharmacologic profile of (R)-5-[(1-methyl-3-indolyl)carbonyl]-4,5,6,7-tetrahydro-1H-benzimidazole hydrochloride (YM060), a potent and selective 5-hydroxytryptamine3 receptor antagonist, and its enantiomer in the isolated tissue. J Pharmacol Exp Ther. 1991; 259:15–21.
9. Miyata K, Kamato T, Nishida A, Ito H, Yuki H, Yamano M, et al. Role of the serotonin 3 receptor in stress-induced defecation. J Pharmacol Exp Ther. 1992;261:297–303.
10. Miyata K, Yamana M, Kamato T, Akuzawa S. Effect of serotonin (5-HT)3-receptor antagonists YM060, YM114 (KAE-393), ondansetron and granisetron on 5-HT4 receptors and gastric emptying in rodents. Jpn J Pharmacol. 1995;69:205–14.
11. Matsueda K, Harasawa S, Hongo M, Hiwatashi N, Sasaki D. A phase II trial of the novel serotonin type 3 receptor antagonist ramosetron in Japanese male and female patients with diarrhea-predominant irritable bowel syndrome. Digestion. 2008;77:225–35.
12. Matsueda K, Harasawa S, Hongo M, Hiwatashi N, Sasaki D. A randomized, double-blind, placebo-controlled clinical trial of the effectiveness of the novel serotonin type 3 receptor antagonist ramosetron in both male and female Japanese patients with diarrhea-predominant irritable bowel syndrome. Scand J Gastroenterol. 2008;43:1202–11.
13. Fukudo S, Matsueda K, Haruma K, Ida M, Hayase H, Akiho H, et al. Optimal dose of ramosetron in female patients with irritable bowel syndrome with diarrhea: a randomized, placebo-controlled phase II trial. Neurogastroenterol Motil. 2017. doi:10.1111/nmo.13023.
14. Fukudo S, Kinoshita Y, Okumura T, Ida M, Akiho H, Nakashima Y, et al. Ramosetron reduces symptoms of irritable bowel syndrome with diarrhea and improves quality of life in women. Gastroenterology. 2016;150:358–66.
15. Fukudo S, Kinoshita Y, Okumura T, Ida M, Hayashi K, Akiho H, et al. Effect of ramosetron in female patients with irritable bowel syndrome with diarrhea: a phase III long-term study. J Gastroenterol. 2016;9:874–82.
16. Francis CY, Morris J, Whorwell PJ. The irritable bowel severity scoring system: a simple method of monitoring irritable bowel syndrome and its progress. Aliment Pharmacol Ther. 1997;11:396–402.
17. Shinozaki M, Kanazawa M, Sagami Y, Endo Y, Hongo M, Drossman DA, et al. Validation of the Japanese version of the Rome II modulator questionnaire and irritable bowel syndrome severity index. J Gastroenterol. 2006;40:491–4.
18. Gralnek IM, Hays RD, Kilbourne A, Naliboff B, Mayer EA. The impact of irritable bowel syndrome on health-related quality of life. Gastroenterology. 2000;119:654–60.
19. Chang L, Lee OY, Nalicoff B, Schmulson M, Mayer EA. Sensation of bloating and visible abdominal distension in patients with irritable bowel syndrome. Am J Gastroenterol. 2001;96:3341–7.
20. Whitehead WE, Palsson OS, Levy RL, Feld AD, Vonkorff M, Turner M. Reports of "satisfactory relief" by IBS patients receiving usual medical care are confounded by baseline symptom severity and do not accurately reflect symptom improvement. Am J Gastroenterol. 2006;101:1057–65.

21. Johnston JM, Kurtz CB, Macdougall JE, Lavins BJ, Currie MG, Fitch DA, et al. Linaclotide improves abdominal pain and bowel habits in a phase IIb study of patients with irritable bowel syndrome with constipation. Gastroenterology. 2010;139:1877–86.
22. Passos MC, Lembo AJ, Conboy LA, Kaptchuk TJ, Kelly JM, Quilty MT, et al. Adequate relief in a treatment trial with IBS patients: a prospective assessment. Am J Gastroenterol. 2009;104:912–9.
23. Spiegel B, Camilleri M, Bolus R, Andresen V, Chey WD, Fehnel S, et al. Psychometric evaluation of patient-reported outcomes in irritable bowel syndrome randomized controlled trials: A Rome Foundation report. Gastroenterology. 2009;137:1944–53.
24. Fukudo S, Kaneko H, Akiho H, Inamori M, Endo Y, Okumura T, et al. Evidence-based clinical practice guidelines for irritable bowel syndrome. J Gastroenterol. 2015;50:11–30.
25. Fukudo S, Ida M, Akiho H, Nakashima Y, Matsueda K. Effect of ramosetron on stool consistency in male patients with irritable bowel syndrome with diarrhea. Clin Gastroenterol Hepatol. 2014;12:953–9.
26. Marchant J. Placebos: Honest fakery. Nature. 2016;535:S14–5.

6

Cognitive behavioral treatment for irritable bowel syndrome: A recent literature review

Nagisa Sugaya[1*], Kentaro Shirotsuki[2] and Mutsuhiro Nakao[3]

Abstract

Irritable bowel syndrome (IBS) is a gastrointestinal psychosomatic disorder that often develops and worsens with stress. Hence, it is important to treat it from both, its physical and mental aspects. We reviewed recent research on cognitive-behavioral therapy (CBT)—one of the most widely studied psychological treatments for IBS—since it focuses on addressing the cognitions and behaviors associated with IBS symptoms, and combines diverse content, such as cognitive techniques, exposure, stress management, and mindfulness, whose effects have been widely studied. Research on CBT for IBS varies not only in terms of content of the interventions, but also in terms of implementation (individual or group, face-to-face or online). Internet-delivered CBT has recently shown the possibility of providing more accessible and cost-effective psychological intervention to IBS patients in formats, other than face-to-face. In recent years, many standardized scales that allow for IBS-specific psychological assessments have been used in clinical studies of CBT for IBS. Tools that competently deliver effective interventions and properly measure their effectiveness are expected to spread to many people suffering from IBS.

Keywords: Irritable bowel syndrome, Cognitive behavior therapy, Psychological assessment, Brain-gut axis

Introduction

Irritable bowel syndrome (IBS) is one of the most common functional gastrointestinal disorders. Since its prevalence in the general population is as high as 5–10% [1], its associated medical and economic problems have also been pointed out [2]. The Rome IV criteria [3], the diagnostic criteria currently used internationally, defines IBS as recurrent abdominal pain occurring on an average, at least 1 day per week in the last 3 months, and associated with at least two of the following three abnormalities: (1) defecation-related, (2) change in defecation frequency, or (3) change in stool characteristics (appearance). The pathogenesis of IBS includes: (1) abnormalities in gastrointestinal motility, (2) lowered gastrointestinal sensory threshold, and (3) psychological abnormalities (anxiety, depression, etc.). The pathophysiology of IBS includes: (1) abnormalities in gastrointestinal motility, (2) decreased gastrointestinal sensory threshold, and (3) psychological abnormalities (anxiety, depression, etc.), all of which, are related to abnormalities in the functional relationship between the brain and intestine (brain-gut connection). Since IBS is a gastrointestinal psychosomatic disorder that often develops and worsens with stress, it is important to treat it from both the physical and mental aspects [4]. We shall review recent research on cognitive-behavioral therapy—one of the most widely studied psychological treatments for IBS.

Application of cognitive behavioral therapy for IBS

Guidelines for the treatment of IBS [4] recommend psychological interventions for patients, who do not respond to standard pharmacotherapy. Psychological interventions, such as cognitive behavioral therapy (CBT), relaxation, hypnotherapy, and dynamic psychotherapy have been reported to be effective for treating IBS [5]. Since it has been reported that cognitions and behaviors

* Correspondence: nagisa618@gmail.com
[1]Unit of Public Health and Preventive Medicine, School of Medicine, Yokohama City University, 3-9 Fukuura, Kanazawa-ku, Yokohama City 236-0004, Japan
Full list of author information is available at the end of the article

associated with IBS symptoms are involved in unpleasant emotions, such as anxiety and abdominal symptoms [6, 7], CBT targeting cognitions and behaviors associated with such symptoms have been widely tested for efficacy. Toner et al. [8] stated that the purpose of CBT in IBS is to reconfigure how IBS is viewed, given that, its purpose is to help patients to: (1) reframe their view of IBS from helplessness and hopelessness to resourcefulness and hopefulness, (2) identify the relationship between their thoughts, feelings, and behaviors with the environment and IBS symptoms, and (3) identify and implement more effective coping strategies to improve the quality of life (QOL). A recent meta-analysis reported that IBS patients' pretreatment cognitive-emotional characteristics (comorbidity of mood or anxiety disorder, symptom catastrophizing and worries, tendencies of somatosensory amplification, low symptom acceptance, or self-efficacy) predict bad patient outcomes in CBT [9].

Various forms of CBT for IBS

CBT for IBS focuses on addressing the cognitions and behaviors associated with IBS symptoms and combines diverse content, such as cognitive techniques, exposure, stress management, and mindfulness, the effects of which, have been widely studied. For example, CBT for IBS conducted in a previous study by Lackner et al. [10] consisted of the provision of information regarding brain-gut interactions; self-monitoring of gastrointestinal symptoms, their antecedents (i.e., triggers) and consequences; muscle relaxation to dampen physiological arousal and increase control over gastrointestinal symptoms; worry control to challenge and dispute negatively skewed thinking patterns; flexible problem solving to aid in the deployment of more effective ways of managing realistic stressors; and relapse prevention training to maintain treatment gains. In addition, CBT combined with exposure has been reported to be effective, especially in patients with significant avoidance behaviors related to IBS symptoms [11]. Several studies have also demonstrated the effectiveness of CBT combined with mindfulness [12], and the addition of exposure has been reported to increase IBS symptoms and related anxiety as well as QOL improvements [13]. Recently, several studies have demonstrated the efficacy of CBT with interoceptive exposure in IBS patients [14, 15]. Interoceptive exposure involves exposing one's self to self-induced abdominal sensations (e.g., tightening abdominal muscles, consuming foods that are to be avoided, etc.) to reduce anxiety in response to abdominal disturbance common in IBS [15].

Research on CBT for IBS varies not only in terms of the interventions' contents, but also in terms of its implementation (individual or group, face-to-face or online). Research on internet-delivered CBT has been increasing in recent years (Table 1), and its effects on IBS and functional abdominal pain have been seen not only in adults, but also in children [16–19]. CBT delivered through the telephone and internet has been shown to be effective, suggesting the usefulness of conducting it remotely [20]. Furthermore, internet-delivered CBT has been reported to be effective not only in improving abdominal pain, QOL, and psychological symptoms, but also in reducing health care costs [18], and is expected to become more widespread in the future. Home and clinic-based CBT have been reported to result in substantial and enduring relief of multiple IBS symptoms for patients with treatment-refractory IBS, and its effects generally extended post treatment, for a 12-month period [10]. CBT with minimal medical visits has also been shown to be cost-effective [21]. Therefore, if CBT—conducted at home via the internet or other means, as well at medical institutions—becomes widespread, it may make it easier for IBS patients, who have difficulty visiting medical institutions frequently to access appropriate and cost-effective treatments. With the use of internet or telephone-delivered CBT, however, we should be prepared with countermeasures if symptoms worsen. For example, for a child patient, a guardian should accompany and then monitor the child closely. A hotline should be set up in case of emergency.

Psychological assessment tools of CBT for IBS

Psychological interventions to alter cognition and behaviors specific to IBS, require appropriate psychological assessment. Some of the scales commonly used in recent research on CBT for IBS are presented below.

Visceral sensitivity index

The Visceral Sensitivity Index is a unidimensional 15-item scale that measures gastrointestinal symptom–specific anxiety (e.g., "I often fear that I will not be able to have normal bowel movements") [22]. Items are rated on a Likert scale ranging from 0 (strongly disagree) to 5 (strongly agree). It has a high internal consistency (Cronbach's $\alpha = 0.93$) [23]. Its qualitative score was classified as: 0–10 (minimal or mild), 11–30 (moderate), and 31–75 (severe).

Cognitive scale for functional bowel disorder

The Cognitive Scale for Functional Bowel Disorder [8] includes 25 items that measure maladaptive cognition related to abdominal symptoms (e.g., "I am always sick with bowel problems"). The items are rated from 1 (strongly disagree) to 7 (strongly agree). Its total score ranges from 25 to 175, and it has a high internal consistency (Cronbach's $\alpha = 0.93$).

Table 1 Recent research on the effect of internet-delivered CBT for IBS patients

Author	Year	Participants	Interventions	Results
Bonnert et al	2017	Internet-CBT group: $N = 47$ Waitlist control group: $N = 54$ Age range: 13–17 years.	The internet-CBT spanned over 10 weeks and included 10 weekly modules directed at adolescents, and five modules directed at parents. The main principle of the treatment was to use exposure exercises to reduce symptom-fear and avoidance. The modules consisted of short texts, examples, audio-files, and videos. Clinical psychologists with CBT-training provided online support to adolescents and parents.	1) Pretreatment to post-treatment changes on gastrointestinal symptoms as the primary outcome and on almost all secondary outcomes was significantly larger for the internet-CBT group as compared with the control group. 2) After 6 months, the results were stable or significantly improved.
Lalouni et al	2019	Internet-CBT group: $N = 46$ Treatment as usual group: $N = 44$ Age range: 8–12 years.	The children's exercises included exposure to symptom-provoking stimuli (e.g., eating certain foods) and situations in which they feared having symptoms (e.g., physical exercise), and those that decreased their symptom-controlling strategies (e.g., precautionary toilet visits). A short mindfulness exercise was taught as a means to increase awareness of the abdominal symptoms. The parents encouraged their children to work on exposure exercises that decreased their attention from symptom complaints, and increased their attention toward more adaptive behaviors. Licensed psychologists who specialized in CBT provided online support to children and their parents.	1) Gastrointestinal symptom severity, quality of life, gastrointestinal-specific anxiety, avoidance behaviors, and parental responses to children's symptoms improved significantly in the internet-CBT group, as compared with the group that received treatment as usual . 2) The effects of internet-CBT persisted through 36 weeks of follow-up evaluation. 3) The internet-CBT group had significantly less health care usage than group that received treatment as usual, with an average cost difference of US $137.
Hughes et al	2020	Internet-CBT group: $N = 17$ Telephone-CBT group: $N = 17$ Mean age (SD): 39.94 (11.71) years.	Internet-CBT program consisted of eight web-based sessions to be completed on a weekly basis, three 30-min telephone support sessions over 9 weeks. The telephone-CBT group received six one-hour telephone-based CBT sessions over 9 weeks. The same CBT content was delivered via telephone and website, with only the mode of delivery being different. The CBT content was based on an empirical cognitive behavioral model of IBS, and comprised educational, behavioral, and cognitive techniques aimed at improving bowel habits, developing stable healthy eating patterns, addressing unhelpful thoughts, managing stress, reducing symptom that focused on preventing relapse. Trained CBT therapists provided telephone support.	(Inductive thematic analysis was used to analyze the data). 1) Participants liked the flexibility of CBT via internet and telephone-, and this facilitated engagement. 2) Potential barriers to engagement in both the groups included: initial skepticism and concerns about the biopsychosocial nature of CBT; initial concerns about telephone-delivered talking therapy; challenges of maintaining motivation and self-discipline given their already busy lives, and finding nothing new in the internet-CBT. 3) Participants described helpful changes in their understanding of IBS, attitudes toward IBS, ability to recognize IBS patterns, and IBS-related behaviors. 4) Consistent with the trial results, participants described lasting positive effects on their symptoms, work, and social lives.
Hunt et al	2021	Internet-CBT group: $N = 62$ Waitlist control group: $N = 59$ Age range: 18–63 years.	The application program of internet-CBT consists of eight weekly modules focusing on psychoeducation, relaxation training, exercise, the cognitive model of stress management, applying CBT to IBS symptoms, reducing avoidance through exposure therapy, behavioral experiments, and information about diet.	Gastrointestinal symptoms, IBS-related quality of life and cognition, visceral sensitivity, and fear of foods improved significantly in the internet-CBT group.
Owusu et al	2021	Internet-CBT group: $N = 25$ Control group: $N = 11$ Age range: 19–61 years.	The internet-CBT program is self-paced. It consists of eight sessions, designed to be completed within 12 weeks. Therapeutic targets include: knowledge of the biopsychosocial model of IBS and the brain-gut connection; improving bowel habits; developing a stable eating routine; reducing hypervigilance to IBS symptoms; identifying unhelpful gastrointestinal-related thoughts; recognizing how these automatic thoughts affect behaviors, emotions, and gastrointestinal symptoms; and accepting and processing emotions. The internet-CBT program delivers cognitive and behavioral skills and techniques in an interactive manner through repetition of brief learnings and exercises.	1) IBS symptom severity significantly improved at 2-month and 3-month follow-up. The within-group effect size between baseline and 3-month follow-up gastrointestinal symptom scores was large and 63.6% experienced a clinically meaningful improvement. 2) Gastrointestinal-specific anxiety symptoms and cognitions significantly improved at 2-month follow-up, as did unhelpful IBS safety behaviors. 3) Clinically meaningful improvement was observed in depressive and anxiety symptoms at 3-month follow-up among participants with symptoms above the clinical threshold at baseline.

CBT cognitive behavior therapy, *IBS* irritable bowel syndrome

Gastrointestinal cognitions questionnaire

The Gastrointestinal Cognitions Questionnaire consists of 16 self-report items rated on a 5-point Likert scale, ranging from 0 (hardly) to 4 (very much). Individual items are summed, and the total scores range from 0 to 64. The questionnaire consists of three subscales: the pain/life interference subscale (e.g., "When I feel my GI symptoms acting up, I am afraid the pain will be excruciating and intolerable"), the social anxiety subscale (e.g., "If I have to get up and leave an event, meeting, or social gathering, to go to the bathroom, people will think there is something wrong with me"), and the disgust sensitivity subscale (e.g., "The thought of fecal incontinence is terrifying. If it happened, it would be awful"). The scale has been shown to have good internal consistency (Cronbach's $\alpha = 0.92$) [24]. Its qualitative score was classified as: 0–19 (minimal or mild), 20–39 (moderate), and 40–64 (severe).

Irritable bowel syndrome-behavioral responses questionnaire

The Irritable Bowel Syndrome-Behavioral Responses Questionnaire [25] includes 26 items with responses ranging from 1 (never) to 7 (always), and its total score ranges from 26 to 182. It consists of two factors: avoidance behavior scale (e.g., "I avoid going out in case I have problems with my IBS") and control behavior scale (e.g., "After opening my bowels, I check my stool for abnormalities"), and has sufficient internal consistency (Cronbach's $\alpha = 0.86$).

The irritable bowel syndrome quality of life questionnaire

The Irritable Bowel Syndrome Quality of Life questionnaire is a 34-item self-report measure, specifically designed to assess the impact of IBS on QOL (e.g., "I am bothered by how much time I spend on the toilet") [26, 27]. It has a high internal consistency (Cronbach's $\alpha = 0.95$) [27]. Its qualitative score was classified as: 0–31 (minimal or mild), 32–66 (moderate), and 67–100 (severe impairment).

The effect of CBT for IBS and its psychobiological mechanism

A number of previous studies have demonstrated that CBT improves anxiety, depression, QOL, and abdominal symptoms in patients with IBS [28–30]. It has also been reported that CBT reduces neural activity in the parahippocampal gyrus and lower right cingulate cortex, and that changes in limbic activity are associated with improvements in abdominal symptoms and anxiety [31]. These brain regions are associated with excessive vigilance and emotional memory [32]. Some previous studies reported that CBT has a direct effect on IBS symptoms, that were independent of its effect on psychological distress, suggesting that the reduction of IBS symptoms improve psychological distress, rather than vice versa [33]. Furthermore, a meta-analysis of CBT for IBS reported more efficacy for abdominal symptoms rather than psychological symptoms [30]. In other words, it is interesting to note, that cognitive and behavioral transformation in IBS may contribute to the improvement of abdominal symptoms through direct involvement in the brain-gut correlation process of IBS, and thus alleviate psychological distress, such as anxiety and depression.

Conclusion

We reviewed recent research on the characteristics and effects of CBT for IBS, its mechanism, and tools for measuring its effectiveness. The biopsychological mechanisms underlying the effects of CBT have been gradually elucidated in parallel with the elucidation of the biological characteristics of IBS. In addition, internet-delivered CBT has recently shown the possibility of providing more accessible and cost-effective psychological interventions to IBS patients, in formats other than face-to-face. These tools are expected to spread to many IBS patients, including those, suffering from IBS, but who do not visit medical institutions.

Abbreviations

IBS: Irritable bowel syndrome; CBT: Cognitive behavior therapy; QOL: Quality of life

Acknowledgments

None.

Authors' contributions

NS organized the project and wrote the manuscript. KS and MN conducted the literature search and were involved in the conceptualization of the review. All the authors (NS, KS, and MN) read and approved the final manuscript, and share the final responsibility for the decision to submit it for publication.

Author details

[1]Unit of Public Health and Preventive Medicine, School of Medicine, Yokohama City University, 3-9 Fukuura, Kanazawa-ku, Yokohama City 236-0004, Japan. [2]Graduate School of Human and Social Sciences, Musashino University, Tokyo, Japan. [3]Department of Psychosomatic Medicine, School of Medicine, International University of Health and Welfare, Chiba, Japan.

References

1. Palsson OS, Whitehead WE, Van Tilburg MAL, Chang L, Chey W, Crowell MD, et al. Development and validation of the Rome IV diagnostic questionnaire for adults. Gastroenterology. 2016;150(6):1481–91.
2. Black CJ, Ford AC. Global burden of irritable bowel syndrome: trends, predictions and risk factors. Nat Rev Gastroenterol Hepatol. 2020;17(8):473–86. https://doi.org/10.1038/s41575-020-0286-8.
3. Drossman DA. Functional gastrointestinal disorders: history, pathophysiology, clinical features, and Rome IV. Gastroenterology. 2016;150: 1262e79 Retrieved from: https://theromefoundation.org/rome-iv/.
4. Fukudo S, Okumura T, Inamori M, Okuyama Y, Kanazawa M, Kamiya T, et al. Evidence-based clinical practice guidelines for irritable bowel syndrome 2020. J Gastroenterol. 2021;56(3):193–217.
5. Ford AC, Lacy BE, Harris LA, Quigley EMM, Moayyedi P. Effect of antidepressants and psychological therapies in irritable bowel syndrome: an updated systematic review and meta-analysis. Am J Gastroenterol. 2019; 114(1):21–39.
6. Sugaya N, Nomura S, Shimada H. Relationship between cognitive factors and anxiety in individuals with irritable bowel syndrome. Int J Behav Med. 2012;19(3):308–15.
7. Windgassen S, Moss-Morris R, Goldsmith K, Chalder T. Key mechanisms of cognitive behavioural therapy in irritable bowel syndrome: the importance of gastrointestinal related cognitions, behaviours and general anxiety. J Psychosom Res. 2019;118:73–82.
8. Toner BB, Stuckless N, Ali A, Downie F, Emmott S, Akman D. The development of a cognitive scale for functional bowel disorders. Psychosom Med. 1998;60:492–7.

9. Sarter L, Heider J, Kirchner L, Schenkel S, Witthöft M, Rief W, et al. Cognitive and emotional variables predicting treatment outcome of cognitive behavior therapies for patients with medically unexplained symptoms: a meta-analysis. J Psychosom Res. 2021;146:110486. https://doi.org/10.1016/j.jpsychores.2021.110486.
10. Lackner JM, Jaccard J, Radziwon CD, Firth RS, Gudleski GD, Hamilton F, et al. Durability and decay of treatment benefit of cognitive behavioral therapy for irritable bowel syndrome: 12-month follow-up. Am J Gastroenterol. 2019 Feb;114(2):330–8. https://doi.org/10.1038/s41395-018-0396-x.
11. Hesser H, Hedman-Lagerlöf E, Lindfors P, Andersson E, Ljótsson B. Behavioral avoidance moderates the effect of exposure therapy for irritable bowel syndrome: a secondary analysis of results from a randomized component trial. Behav Res Ther. 2021;141:103862.
12. Billones R, Saligan L. What works in mindfulness interventions for medically unexplained symptoms? A systematic review. Asian Pac Isl Nurs J. 2020;5:1–11.
13. Ljótsson B, Hesser H, Andersson E, Lackner JM, El Alaoui S, Falk L, et al. Provoking symptoms to relieve symptoms: a randomized controlled dismantling study of exposure therapy in irritable bowel syndrome. Behav Res Ther. 2014;55:27–39.
14. Craske MG, Wolitzky-Taylor KB, Labus J, Wu S, Frese M, Mayer EA, et al. A cognitive-behavioral treatment for irritable bowel syndrome using interoceptive exposure to visceral sensations. Behav Res Ther. 2011;49: 413–21.
15. Kawanishi H, Sekiguchi A, Funaba M, Fujii Y, Yoshiuchi K, Kikuchi H, et al. Cognitive behavioral therapy with interoceptive exposure and complementary video materials for irritable bowel syndrome (IBS): protocol for a multicenter randomized controlled trial in Japan. Biopsychosoc Med. 2019;13:14.
16. Bonnert M, Olén O, Lalouni M, Benninga MA, Bottai M, Engelbrektsson J, et al. Internet-delivered cognitive behavior therapy for adolescents with irritable bowel syndrome: a randomized controlled trial. Am J Gastroenterol. 2017;112(1):152–62.
17. Hunt M, Miguez S, Dukas B, Onwude O, White S. Efficacy of Zemedy, a mobile digital therapeutic for the self-management of irritable bowel syndrome: crossover randomized controlled trial. JMIR MHealth UHealth. 2021;9(5):e26152.
18. Lalouni M, Ljótsson B, Bonnert M, Ssegonja R, Benninga M, Bjureberg J, et al. Clinical and cost effectiveness of online cognitive behavioral therapy in children with functional abdominal pain disorders. Clin Gastroenterol Hepatol. 2019;17(11):2236–2244.e11.
19. Owusu JT, Sibelli A, Moss-Morris R, van Tilburg MAL, Levy RL, Oser M. A pilot feasibility study of an unguided, internet-delivered cognitive behavioral therapy program for irritable bowel syndrome. Neurogastroenterol Motil. 2021:e14108.
20. Hughes S, Sibelli A, Everitt HA, Moss-Morris R, Chalder T, Harvey JM, et al. Patients' experiences of telephone-based and web-based cognitive behavioral therapy for irritable bowel syndrome: longitudinal qualitative study. J Med Internet Res. 2020;22(11):e18691.
21. Dunlap LJ, Jaccard J, Lackner JM. Minimal-contact versus standard cognitive behavioral therapy for with irritable bowel syndrome: cost-effectiveness results of a multisite trial. Ann Behav Med. 2021:kaaa119.
22. Labus JS, Mayer EA, Chang L, Bolus R, Naliboff BD. The central role of gastrointestinal-specific anxiety in irritable bowel syndrome: further validation of the visceral sensitivity index. Psychosom Med. 2007;69(1): 89–98.
23. Labus JS, Bolus R, Chang L, Wiklund I, Naesdal J, Mayer EA, et al. The visceral sensitivity index: development and validation of a gastrointestinal symptom-specific anxiety scale. Aliment Pharmacol Ther. 2004;20(1):89–97.
24. Hunt MG, Ertel E, Coello JA, Rodriguez L. Development and validation of the GI-cognitions questionnaire. Cognit Ther Res. 2014;38(4):472–82.
25. Reme SE, Darnley S, Kennedy T, Chalder T. The development of the irritable bowel syndrome-behavioral responses questionnaire. J Psychosom Res. 2010;69:319–25.
26. Drossman DA, Patrick DL, Whitehead WE, Toner BB, Diamant NE, Hu Y, et al. Further validation of the IBS-QOL: a disease-specific quality-of-life questionnaire. Am J Gastroenterol. 2000;95(4):999–1007.
27. Patrick DL, Drossman DA, Frederick IO, DiCesare J, Puder KL. Quality of life in persons with irritable bowel syndrome: development and validation of a new measure. Dig Dis Sci. 1998;43(2):400–11.
28. Lackner JM, Jaccard J, Krasner SS, Katz LA, Gudleski GD, Holroyd K. Self-administered cognitive behavior therapy for moderate to severe irritable bowel syndrome: clinical efficacy, tolerability, feasibility. Clin Gastroenterol Hepatol. 2008;6:899–906.
29. Leibbrand R, Hiller W. Cognitive behavior therapy for functional gastrointestinal disorders: is group treatment effective? Acta Neuropsychiatr. 2003;15:242–8.
30. Radu M, Moldovan R, Pintea S, Băban A, Dumitrascu D. Predictors of outcome in cognitive and behavioural interventions for irritable bowel syndrome. A meta-analysis. J Gastrointestin Liver Dis. 2018;27(3):257–63.
31. Lackner JM, Lou Coad M, Mertz HR, Wack DS, Katz LA, Krasner SS, et al. Cognitive therapy for irritable bowel syndrome is associated with reduced limbic activity, GI symptoms, and anxiety. Behav Res Ther. 2006;44:621–38.
32. Kennedy PJ, Clarke G, Quigley EM, Groeger JA, Dinan TG, Cryan JF. Gut memories: towards a cognitive neurobiology of irritable bowel syndrome. Neurosci Biobehav Rev. 2012;36:310–40.
33. Lackner JM, Jaccard J, Krasner SS, Katz LA, Gudleski GD, Blanchard EB. How does cognitive behavior therapy for irritable bowel syndrome work? A mediational analysis of a randomized clinical trial. Gastroenterology. 2007; 133:433–44.

7

Validity and reliability of the Japanese versions of cognitive and behavioral scales for irritable bowel syndrome

Nagisa Sugaya[1*], Yoshitoshi Tomita[2], Misako Funaba[3], Hiroshi Iida[4], Kentaro Shirotsuki[5], Fumiyuki Chin Gardner[6], Toshinari Odawara[7], Tetsuya Ando[3,8] and Masahiko Inamori[4]

Abstract

Background: The Cognitive Scale for Functional Bowel Disorders (CS-FBD) and Irritable Bowel Syndrome-Behavioral Responses Questionnaire (IBS-BRQ) are a useful measures to assess cognitive-behavioral aspects in individuals with IBS. This study aimed to confirm the reliability and validity of the Japanese versions of the CS-FBD (CS-FBD-J) and IBS-BRQ (IBS-BRQ-J).

Methods: Participants comprised 192 students and 22 outpatients diagnosed with irritable bowel syndrome (IBS). There were 76 students who met the diagnostic criteria for IBS and two students who received treatment for IBS. Participants completed questionnaires containing the CS-FBD-J, IBS Severity Index (IBS-SI), Visceral Sensitivity Index (VSI), 24-item Dysfunctional Attitudes Scale (DAS-24), Hospital Anxiety and Depression Scale (HADS), and Social Adaptation Self-evaluation Scale (SASS).

Results: Our exploratory factor analysis revealed that the CS-FBD-J had a unidimensional factor structure and that the factor loadings for two of the 25 items were less than 0.4. The IBS-BRQ-J had a two-factor structure, and the factor loadings for eight of the 26 items were less than 0.4. The confirmatory factor analysis for the 18-item version of IBS-BRQ-J showed that the model fit indices were not sufficient. The CS-FBD-J and IBS-BRQ-J had significant, moderate correlations with the IBS-SI and VSI in the IBS and control groups. Correlation between the DAS-24 and the CS-FBD-J was not significant. The CS-FBD-J and IBS-BRQ-J were significantly correlated to the HADS and SASS (IBS-BRQ-J) only in the IBS group. The scores of CS-FBD-J and IBS-BRQ-J showed significant group differences between the IBS patient group, non-patient IBS group, and control group. The internal consistencies of the CS-FBD-J and IBS-BRQ-J were high. The item-total correlation analysis for the CS-FBD-J and IBS-BRQ-J showed that the correlations between each item and the total score were significant.

Conclusion: This study confirmed the reliability and validity of the 23-item version of the CS-FBS-J and the 18-item version of the IBS-BRQ-J with the deletion of items with low factor loadings. Regarding the IBS-BRQ-J, two factor structures were confirmed (factor 1: behavior obsessed with abdominal symptoms, factor 2: avoidance of abdominal symptoms and associated difficulties) although the model fit of the structure needs further study.

*Correspondence: nagisa618@gmail.com

[1] Unit of Public Health and Preventive Medicine, School of Medicine, Yokohama City University, 3-9 Fukuura, Kanazawa-ku, Yokohama 236-0004, Japan

Full list of author information is available at the end of the article

Keywords: Irritable bowel syndrome, Cognitive scale for functional bowel disorders, Irritable bowel syndrome-behavioral responses questionnaire, Japanese version

Background

Irritable bowel syndrome (IBS) is a functional gastrointestinal disorder characterized by persistent chronic abdominal pain and disturbance of bowel movements [1]. It is a typical psychosomatic disorder of the digestive system that is exacerbated by psychological stress. Our previous study [2] reported that the cognitive-emotion process is related to the aggravation of anxiety in individuals with IBS; severe anxiety sensitivity in individuals with IBS related to their symptom-related cognition and the altered cognition associated with increased anxiety can lead to the development of a disabling condition, including avoidant behavior. Behavioral problems also related to gastrointestinal symptoms play an important role in the pathophysiology of IBS. The majority of participants with IBS are reported to have a high level of impairment or avoidance of daily activities [3].

Based on the above characteristics of individuals with IBS, many previous studies have reported the effect of cognitive-behavioral (CBT) or cognitive therapy on the abdominal symptoms and emotional distress of patients with IBS [4, 5]. Furthermore, various measures explicitly developed for IBS, such as the Visceral Sensitivity Index (VSI [6]) and the IBS-QOL [7], have been used as outcomes of such IBS intervention studies, including gastrointestinal symptoms and general anxiety and depression. Additionally, it is essential in CBT to assess the cognitive-behavioral aspects of IBS appropriately because these are variables directly targeted for such intervention.

The Cognitive Scale for Functional Bowel Disorders (CS-FBD [8]) is a useful measure to assess maladaptive cognitions, focusing on functional bowel disorders related to negative thoughts, perfectionism, and social desirability. The CS-FBD is a valid and reliable scale that can be used as an outcome measure in evaluating the efficacy of different forms of psychotherapeutic intervention for functional bowel disorders (e.g., IBS, functional diarrhea/constipation), and can also serve as a helpful assessment tool for health professionals working with patients diagnosed with IBS [8]. CS-FBD has been used in many previous studies, including clinical trials of CBT [9–14]. The VSI [6] has been developed to assess gastrointestinal-specific anxiety, cognitive, affective, and behavioral responses to fear of GI sensations, symptoms, and the context in which they occur, and it has been translated into Japanese [15]. The CS-FBD focuses on maladaptive cognition that is not specific to anxiety, and its content is differentiated from the VSI. CS-FBD items were generated from the diaries of automatic thought records in patients with functional gastrointestinal disorders, and included a variety of themes: bowel performance anxiety, out of control, perfectionism, anger/frustration, self-efficacy, social approval, embarrassment/shame, heightened sensitivity to social rules and norms, and self-nurturance. Unlike the VSI, the CS-FBD is a "cognition"-specific scale. It has the advantage of precisely assessing the role of cognition in the cognitive-behavioral model of IBS and the degree of cognitive transformation achieved in CBT. The CS-FBD was utilized along with the VSI in previous studies (e.g., [13]).

Additionally, the irritable bowel syndrome-behavioral responses questionnaire (IBS-BRQ) [16] was developed to assess the IBS-specific pattern of avoidance and control behavior, and has been validated for individuals with IBS and has convergent validity and good test-retest reliability. IBS-BRQ has been used in many previous studies [14, 17–22]. Bonnert et al. [17] reported that changes in IBS-related unhelpful behavior assessed by the IBS-BRQ [16] mediated the effect of exposure-based Internet-CBT on gastro-intestinal (GI) symptoms. The decrease in avoidance behavior explained a large portion (67%) of the total treatment effect. They also observed a unidirectional relation over time between avoidance behavior and GI symptoms, corroborating a causal effect. Additionally, Windgassen et al. [22] found that an increased avoidance behavior score, one of the subscales of the IBS-BRQ, was associated with an increased frequency of diarrhea symptoms, and that a higher control behavior score, another subscale of the IBS-BRQ, was associated with a higher frequency of hard/lumpy stools.

Hence, the CS-FBD and IBS-BRQ may contribute to develop cognitive-behavioral model of IBS and to refining the assessment of effect of psychological treatment for IBS. However, the Japanese versions of CS-FBD and IBS-BRQ have not been fully assessed.

The purpose of this study is to confirm the reliability and validity of the Japanese version of the CS-FBD (CS-FBD-J) [Study 1] and IBS-BRQ (IBS-BRQ-J) [Study 2].

Methods

Participants

Participants were recruited between September 2013 and March 2021. They were outpatients who were diagnosed with IBS in the gastroenterology and psychosomatic medicine departments of hospitals in Tokyo and Kanagawa and college students, including patients with

IBS who met the diagnostic criteria (Rome III criteria) and others who did not meet the diagnostic criteria. The present study was approved by the ethics committee of Yokohama City University (B130905050) and the National Center of Neurology and Psychiatry (A2018-046). Written informed consent was obtained from all participants.

Measures

Cognitive Scale for Functional Bowel Disorders translated into Japanese

The Cognitive Scale for Functional Bowel Disorders (CS-FBD) [8] includes 25 items that measure maladaptive cognition related to abdominal symptoms, with responses ranging from 1 (*strongly disagree*) to 7 (*strongly agree*). The total score for this scale ranges from 25 to 175. One of the authors (N.S.), who is a psychologist knowledgeable about functional gastrointestinal disorders and psychosomatic medicine, translated the original version into Japanese. Another author (F.G.) who is bilingual in English and Japanese, back-translated the Japanese items into English. We compared the results of the back translation to the original version and confirmed agreement among the researchers about the nuances.

Irritable bowel syndrome-behavioral responses questionnaire translated into Japanese

The IBS-BRQ [16] includes 26 items with responses ranging from 1 (never) to 7 (always). It has two factors: avoidance behavior scale and control behavior scale. The IBS-BRQ was translated into Japanese using a standard method. One of the authors (N.S.), who is a psychologist well versed in functional gastrointestinal disorders and psychosomatic medicine, translated the original version into Japanese. Another author (F.G.) who is bilingual in English and Japanese, back-translated the Japanese items into English. We compared the results of the back translation to the original version and confirmed the agreement among the researchers about the nuances.

Japanese version of the Rome III modular questionnaire (only items related to IBS)

The Rome III Diagnostic Criteria for Functional Gastrointestinal Disorders [23] have been widely used to define IBS. Rome IV had not been published at the start of this investigation. Using the Rome III modular questionnaire [24, 25], the presence of IBS was determined if the participants had abdominal pain or discomfort for at least three weeks (at least once per week) in the previous three months and two of the three following symptoms: (1) pain or discomfort that improves or stops after a bowel movement, (2) a change in the number of bowel movements when the pain or discomfort starts, and (3) either softer or harder stools than usual when the pain or discomfort starts. There are four defined subtypes of IBS. The diarrhea-predominant IBS (IBS-D) group includes individuals with loose, mushy, or watery stools more than 25% of the time and no or rare hard or lumpy stools. In constipation-predominant IBS (IBS-C), individuals pass hard or lumpy stools more than about 25% of the time and no or rare loose, mushy, or watery stools. The mixed type IBS (IBS-M) group includes individuals with loose, mushy or watery stools and hard or lumpy stools more than 25% of the time. Finally, individuals with unclassifiable IBS (IBS-U) pass rare loose, mushy or watery stools or rare hard or lumpy stools or none at all.

IBS severity index

The IBS Severity Index (IBS-SI) [26, 27] was used to assess the severity of gastrointestinal symptoms. This scale consists of 5 items: abdominal pain (2 items), abdominal distension, bowel movements, and quality of life, and the total score ranges from 0 to 500. The IBS-SI classifies the severity of IBS as mild (75–174), moderate (175–299), or severe (300–500) based on clinical observations of patients with IBS.

Japanese version of the Visceral Sensitivity Index

The Visceral Sensitivity Index (VSI) [6, 15] is a self-reported measure of gastrointestinal symptom-specific anxiety in patients with IBS. The VSI includes 15 items with responses ranging from 1 (*strongly agree*) to 6 (*strongly disagree*) and scores ranging from 0 to 5.

Japanese version of the 24-item Dysfunctional Attitudes Scale

The 24-item Dysfunctional Attitudes Scale (DAS-24) [28, 29] is a self-report scale for depression schemata with responses ranging from 1 (*strongly disagree*) to 7 (*strongly agree*). The DAS-24 contains three factors: "achievement," "self-control," and "dependency." The achievement subscale consists of eight items, for example, "If I fail partly, it is as bad as being a complete failure." The dependency subscale consists of eight items, for example, "I am nothing if a person I love doesn't love me." The self-control subscale consists of eight items, for example, "A person should do well at everything he undertakes."

Hospital Anxiety and Depression Scale

The Hospital Anxiety and Depression Scale (HADS) [30, 31] is a self-report questionnaire for anxiety and depression. The HADS includes 14 questions on a 4-point scale, consisting of an anxiety subscale with seven items and a depression subscale with seven items. This psychometric instrument was chosen because all its items refer solely to an emotional state and do not consider somatic symptoms.

Japanese version of the Social Adaptation Self-evaluation Scale

The Social Adaptation Self-Evaluation Scale (SASS) [32, 33] was developed to assess social impairment caused by depression. This scale has 21 items, with scores ranging from 0 to 3. Lower SASS score indicates impaired social adaptation.

Procedure

Patients

Patients with IBS were given written and oral explanations about the purpose of this study, the protection of their personal information, and that participation was voluntary. Patients with IBS who agreed to participate provided informed consent. Participants then completed questionnaires containing the physical and psychological scales mentioned above.

College students

The researchers recruited college students after class hours or via the university's online bulletin board. Participants recruited by the latter method were limited to those who met the diagnostic criteria for IBS. Informed consent was obtained using the same procedures as for patients.

Statistical analysis

The factor structure of the CS-FBD-J and the IBS-BRQ-J was confirmed by exploratory factor analysis. For the IBS-BRQ-J, confirmatory factor analysis using the Structure Equation Model (SEM) was conducted. In the SEM, assessment of model fit was based on multiple indicators; Goodness-of-Fit Index (GFI), Adjusted goodness-of-Fit Index (AGFI), Comparative fit index (CFI), and Root-mean-square error of approximation (RMSEA). Construct validity was confirmed using Pearson's correlation coefficient analysis between the CS-FBD-J and scores on the IBS-SI, VSI, DAS, and HADS and between the IBS-BRQ-J and scores on the IBS-SI, the item of disruption to daily life (IBS-SI), VSI, HADS, and SASS in the IBS and control groups. Criterion-related validity was confirmed using analysis of covariance to compare the CS-FBD-J score and the IBS-BRQ-J between the IBS patient group, the non-patient IBS group, and the control group after adjusting age, and a post-hoc test with Bonferroni's method was employed to test the differences between groups. We compared these three groups to investigate criterion-related validity more precisely because the IBS patient and non-patient IBS groups were expected to have different severity of psychosomatic symptoms. The internal consistency reliability of the CS-FBD-J and the IBS-BRQ-J was determined using Cronbach's α. The correlations between each item and the total score of the CS-FBD-J were used to conduct item-total correlation analysis. The comparisons of sex ratio between the IBS patient, non-patient IBS, and control groups were conducted using the χ^2 test. One-way analysis of variance was applied to compare age between these groups. Analysis of covariance was used to compare IBS-SI, the item of disruption to daily life (IBS-SI), VSI, HADS, and SASS between these groups after adjusting age. The significance level was set at less than 5%. Data analyses were performed using SPSS software (version 25.0; IBM Corp., NY, USA).

Results

Descriptive results

Table 1 presents the descriptive results for the participants. In our study, 203 college students were enrolled, and 192 students (53 male and 139 female, 20.2±3.0 yrs.) provided valid data. There were 76 students who met the diagnostic criteria for IBS, and two students received treatment for IBS. Twenty-two outpatients who were diagnosed with IBS in the gastroenterology or psychosomatic medicine departments of hospitals in Tokyo and Kanagawa (17 male and 5 female, 38.0±13.0 yrs.) provided valid data. Eleven participants who received treatment for IBS received psychiatric medication. Two IBS patients did not meet the presence of abdominal discomfort or pain for at least six months criterion of IBS. This may have been due to a period of symptom resolution with treatment. However, because they met all other criteria during the survey period, they were included in the IBS patient group. The IBS group (IBS patients and

Table 1 Descriptive results of the study participants

		N(%)			
	Total	**Male**		**Female**	
IBS patient	**24**	**17**	**(70.8)**	**7**	**(29.2)**
Non-patient IBS	74	21	(28.4)	53	(71.6)
Control	116	32	(27.6)	84	(72.4)
IBS-D	28	13	(46.4)	15	(53.6)
IBS-C	9	1	(11.1)	8	(88.9)
IBS-M	55	22	(40.0)	33	(60.0)
IBS-U	6	2	(33.3)	4	(66.7)

IBS Irritable bowel syndrome
IBS-D Diarrhea-predominant IBS
IBS-C Constipation-predominant IBS
IBS-M Mixed-type IBS
IBS-U Unclassifiable IBS

non-IBS patients) included 28 participants with diarrhea-predominant IBS (IBS-D), 9 with constipation-predominant IBS (IBS-C), 55 with mixed-type IBS (IBS-M), and 6 with unclassifiable IBS (IBS-U). There was a significant difference of sex ratio between the IBS patient, non-patient IBS, and control groups (χ^2 = 17.86, $p <$ 0.001, Cramer's V = 0.289). The prevalence of male sex was higher among IBS patients than in the other groups. Table 2 shows the differences in each variable between the IBS patient (n =24), non-patient IBS (n =74), and control groups (n =116) after adjusting for age. Figure 1 shows the plot of the CS-FBD-J score and the IBS-BRQ-J score in each group. There was a significant difference of age between groups (F [2, 211] = 102.88, $p < 0.001$). The IBS patient group had a higher mean age than other groups. After adjusting for age, there were significant group effects in the IBS-SI, disruption to daily life, VSI, and SASS. Multiple comparison analysis showed higher scores of the IBS-SI and disruption to daily life in the IBS patient and non-patient groups than in the control group. There was a significant difference in the VSI between all groups. The SASS score of the IBS patients was lower than that of the non-patient IBS and control groups. Although there was a significant group effect of the DAS, multiple comparison analysis did not show any significant differences among the groups.

Study 1 (validity and reliability of the CS-FBD-J)

Factor analysis

Exploratory factor analysis (using maximum likelihood estimation and promax rotation) without assigning the number of factors revealed the presence of five components with eigenvalues exceeding 1. However, inspection of the scree plot revealed a break after the first component. Therefore, we decided to retain a unidimensional factor structure for further investigation (Table 3). Factor analysis showed that the factor loadings for two items (items 6 and 18) were less than 0.4. After excluding these items from the analysis, the factor loadings for all items were above 0.4, and a single factor of the 23-item version accounted for 45.85% of the total variance.

Construct validity

The results of the correlation analysis between the CS-FBD-J and other variables in the IBS and control groups confirmed the construct validity (Table 4). The scores of the 25-item and 23-item versions of CS-FBD-J had significant moderate correlations with the IBS-SI and VSI scores in all participants, the IBS group, and the control group. The DAS-24 score was significantly correlated with the 25-item version of CS-FBD-J in both the IBS and control groups, but the correlations were low. Moreover, correlations between the 23-item version of

Table 2 Comparison of each variable between IBS patient, non-patient IBS, and control groups after adjusting for age

	Mean (*SD*)								
	IBS patient (n = 24)		Non-patient IBS (n – 74)		Control (n = 116)		F	p	η_p^2
CS-FBD (25 items)	103.5	(30.2)	78.6	(25.1)	57.1	(21.9)	29.01	< 0.001	0.216
CS-FBD (23 items)	93.7	(29.2)	69.8	(24.6)	49.4	(20.7)	28.40	< 0.001	0.213
IBS-BRQ (26 items)	84.7	(32.4)	62.4	(22.8)	46.7	(19.8)	21.91	<0.001	0.173
IBS-BRQ (18 items)	60.2	(24.0)	42.2	(17.0)	30.0	(14.2)	24.50	<0.001	0.189
IBS-SI	193.3	(109.7)	193.9	(80.7)	116.1	(86.6)	18.96	< 0.001	0.153
Disruption to daily life (IBS-SI)	56.9	(30.4)	43.4	(25.3)	25.4	(27.0)	11.58	< 0.001	0.101
VSI	52.4	(14.7)	23.2	(19.8)	13.6	(17.0)	22.69	< 0.001	0.197
DAS	92.1	(24.4)	93.1	(24.5)	87.3	(20.7)	3.50	0.032	0.033
HADS (Anxiety)	7.4	(4.8)	7.3	(3.6)	6.4	(3.8)	2.73	0.067	0.026
HADS (Depression)	5.3	(4.8)	4.8	(3.0)	4.9	(3.8)	0.21	0.811	0.002
HADS (Total)	12.7	(9.1)	12.1	(6.0)	11.3	(7.0)	1.08	0.342	0.010
SASS	29.9	(7.8)	35.9	(6.4)	37.4	(6.5)	6.24	0.002	0.058

IBS irritable bowel syndrome

CS-FBD-J Japanese version of Cognitive Scale for Functional Bowel Disorders

IBS-BRQ Irritable Bowel Syndrome-Behavioral Responses Questionnaire

IBS-SI IBS Severity Index

VSI Visceral Sensitivity Index

DAS-24 24-item Dysfunctional Attitudes Scale

HADS Hospital Anxiety and Depression Scale

SASS Social Adaptation Self-evaluation Scale

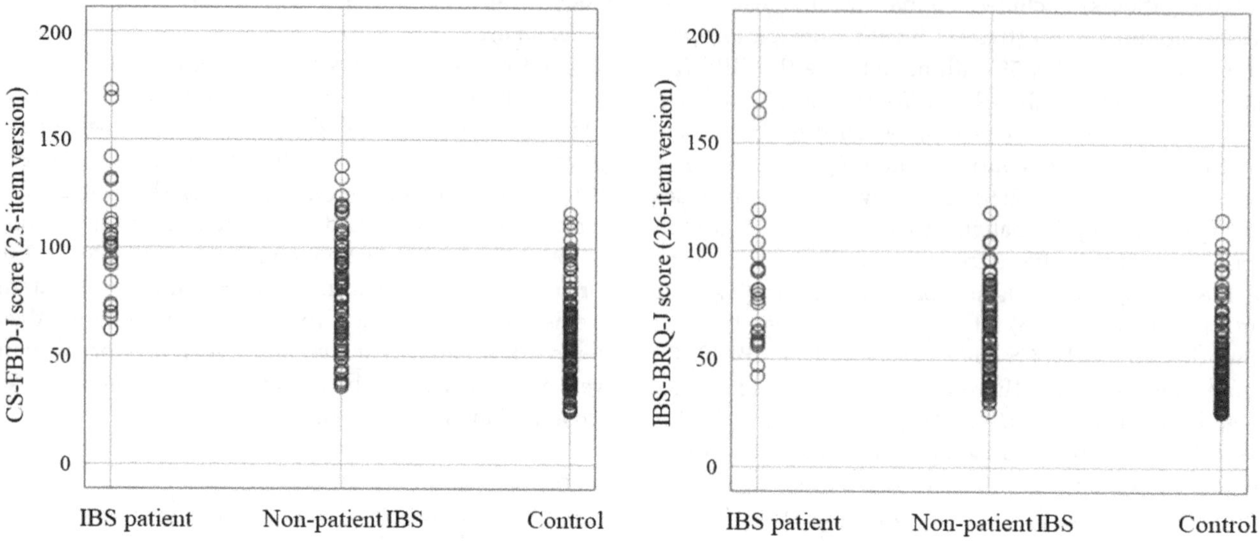

Fig. 1 Plots of the CS-FBD-J and IBS-BRQ-J scores of IBS patient, non-patient IBS, and control groups. IBS: irritable bowel syndrome. CS-FBD-J: Japanese version of Cognitive Scale for Functional Bowel Disorders. IBS-BRQ: Irritable Bowel Syndrome-Behavioral Responses Questionnaire

CS-FBD-J and DAS-24 did not reach a significant level. Regarding the HADS, although the 25-item and 23-item versions of the CS-FBD-J in the IBS group were significantly correlated with the HADS-anxiety and depression scores, their intercorrelations in the control group were not significant.

Criterion-related validity

We compared the scores of the 25-item and 23-item versions of the CS-FBD-J between the IBS patient, non-patient IBS, and control groups after adjusting for age to confirm the criterion-related validity (Table 2). There were significant group effects in both versions of the CS-FBD-J, and multiple comparison analysis showed significant differences between all groups (i.e., IBS patient > non-patient IBS > control).

Reliability

Cronbach's α was calculated to estimate the reliability of the CS-FBD-J. The internal consistencies of the 25-item and 23-item versions (excluding items 6 and 18) in all participants, the IBS group, and the control group were high (25-item version: all participants: $\alpha = 0.94$, IBS group: $\alpha = 0.94$, control group: $\alpha = 0.92$; 23-item version: all participants: $\alpha = 0.95$, IBS group: $\alpha = 0.94$, control group: $\alpha = 0.92$).

The item-total correlation analysis for the 25-item and 23-item versions of the CS-FBD-J (Table 3) showed that the correlations between each item and the total score were significant (25-item version: $ps < 0.001$, $rs = 0.323$–0.810; 23-item version: $ps < 0.001$, $rs = 0.433$–0.812).

Study 2 (validity and reliability of the IBS-BRQ-J)

Factor analysis

Exploratory factor analysis (using maximum likelihood estimation and promax rotation) without assigning the number of factors revealed the presence of six components with eigenvalues exceeding 1. However, inspection of the scree plot revealed a break after the second component. Therefore, we decided to retain a two-factor structure for further investigation (Table 5). Factor analysis showed that the factor loadings for eight items (items 1, 2, 8, 9, 10, 11, 23, and 24) were less than 0.4. After excluding these items from the analysis, the factor loadings for all items were above 0.4, and two factors of the 18-item version accounted for 43.84% and 51.51 % of the total variance, respectively.

In the results of the SEM for the 18-tem version (Fig. 2), the model fit indices were not sufficient (GFI = 0.749, AGFI = 0.680, CFI = 0.797, RMSEA = 0.133).

Construct validity

The results of the correlation analysis between IBS-BRQ-J and other variables in the IBS and control groups were examined for construct validity. Regarding both the 26-item and 18-item versions of IBS-BRQ-J, the scores of IBS-SI, disruption to daily life, and VSI showed significant, positive correlations with the IBS-BRQ-J scores in both the IBS and control groups, while the scores of anxiety (HADS), depression (HADS), and SASS were significantly correlated to the IBS-BRQ-J score only in the IBS group.

Table 3 Results of the item-total analysis and factor analysis

Items	25-item version		23-item version	
	Item-total correlation	Factor loadings	Item-total correlation	Factor loadings
19. Not take advantage of opportunities due to bowel problems	0.720	0.785	0.727	0.786
16. Concern about lasting through events	0.802	0.781	0.817	0.782
23. Worry about losing control of bowels in public	0.810	0.770	0.812	0.768
12. Bowel problems interfere with feeling good about myself	0.761	0.769	0.763	0.769
14. Can't concentrate due to pain	0.767	0.766	0.780	0.767
13. Worry about my bowel symptoms on a trip	0.789	0.763	0.800	0.763
9. I feel very down about my bowel symptoms	0.712	0.756	0.730	0.759
7. Frustrated by bowel symptoms	0.722	0.754	0.734	0.755
5. Bowel symptoms are agony	0.763	0.733	0.763	0.732
8. Pain will never go away	0.700	0.724	0.717	0.727
20. Symptoms make me feel out of control	0.686	0.724	0.693	0.726
11. Worry about not finding a bathroom when I need one	0.774	0.714	0.776	0.712
2. I'm always sick with bowel problems	0.686	0.705	0.688	0.705
4. Can't function normally when sick with bowel problems	0.731	0.696	0.735	0.695
3. Symptoms are too much to handle	0.692	0.693	0.698	0.696
21. Bowel symptoms in restaurant	0.639	0.635	0.653	0.636
22. With frequent bathroom visits, others think something is wrong	0.668	0.627	0.663	0.622
15. Embarrassing to keep going to bathroom	0.611	0.581	0.607	0.576
25. Must get home when 1 have symptoms	0.553	0.541	0.563	0.542
1. Not getting to bathroom in time	0.483	0.490	0.489	0.491
17. Being late upsets me	0.567	0.480	0.541	0.472
24. Feeling guilt if I nurture myself	0.431	0.452	0.433	0.450
10. Passing gas in public	0.471	0.416	0.473	0.414
18. Hate making a fool of myself	0.389	0.313	-	-
6. Do my absolute best at everything	0.323	0.262	-	-
	Eigenvalue	10.72	Eigenvalue	10.54
	Variance (%)	42.87%	Variance (%)	45.85%

Criterion-related validity

We compared the scores of the 26-item and 18-item versions of the IBS-BRQ-J between the IBS patient, non-patient IBS, and control groups after adjusting for age to confirm the criterion-related validity (Table 2). The scores of both versions of the IBS-BRQ-J showed significant group differences, and the multiple comparison test showed that the IBS patient and non-patient IBS groups had higher scores than the control group and that the IBS patient group had a higher score than the non-patient IBS group.

Reliability

We calculated Cronbach's α to estimate the reliability of the IBS-BRQ-J. The internal consistencies of the 26-item version and the 18-item version in all participants, the IBS group, and the control group were high (26-item version: all participants: $\alpha = 0.93$, IBS group: $\alpha = 0.92$, control group: $\alpha = 0.92$; 18-item version: all participants: $\alpha = 0.92$, IBS group: $\alpha = 0.91$, control group: $\alpha = 0.91$). Regarding the 18-item version, the internal consistencies of factor 1 (all participants: $\alpha = 0.92$, IBS group: $\alpha = 0.91$, control group: $\alpha = 0.93$) and factor 2 (all participants: $\alpha = 0.83$, IBS group: $\alpha = 0.77$, control group: $\alpha = 0.79$) were sufficient.

The item-total correlation analysis for the 26-item and 18-item versions of the IBS-BRQ-J (Table 6) showed that the correlations between each item and the total score were significant (26-item version: $ps < 0.001$, $rs = 0.453–0.752$; 18-item version: $ps < 0.001$, $rs = 0.487–0.759$).

Table 4 Correlations between the CS-FBD-J (25-item and 23-item version) and other variables

25-item version		IBS-SI	VSI	DAS-24	HADS (Anxiety)	HADS (Depression)	HADS (Total)
Total	*r*	0.617	0.625	0.249	0.335	0.219	0.305
	p	< 0.001	< 0.001	< 0.001	< 0.001	0.001	< 0.001
IBS group	*r*	0.569	0.553	0.213	0.455	0.361	0.444
	p	< 0.001	< 0.001	0.035	< 0.001	< 0.001	< 0.001
Control group	*r*	0.488	0.515	0.224	0.162	0.144	0.169
	p	< 0.001	< 0.001	0.017	0.084	0.127	0.073
23-item version		IBS-SI	VSI	DAS-24	HADS (Anxiety)	HADS (Depression)	HADS (Total)
Total	*r*	0.620	0.632	0.221	0.336	0.222	0.307
	p	< 0.001	< 0.001	0.001	< 0.001	0.001	< 0.001
IBS group	*r*	0.574	0.557	0.191	0.450	0.357	0.440
	p	< 0.001	< 0.001	0.059	< 0.001	< 0.001	< 0.001
Control group	*r*	0.492	0.531	0.179	0.167	0.150	0.175
	p	< 0.001	< 0.001	0.058	0.075	0.111	0.062

IBS irritable bowel syndrome

CS-FBD-J Japanese version of Cognitive Scale for Functional Bowel Disorders

IBS-SI IBS Severity Index

VSI Visceral Sensitivity Index

DAS-24 24-item Dysfunctional Attitudes Scale

HADS Hospital Anxiety and Depression Scale

Discussion

Study 1 (validity and reliability of the CS-FBD-J)

While the CS-FBD-J had a one-factor structure in common with the original version, items 6 and 18 of the Japanese version had low factor loadings and were deleted from this version. For the original version of the CS-FBD, although factor loadings for these two items were below 0.4, the authors determined to retain them based on their relevance to a priori themes (Toner et al., 1998). However, in the present study, we could find no reason to retain these items. Because the automatic thoughts referenced in these two items could not be interpreted by some people as being related to abdominal symptoms, the factor loadings of the two items were lower in this study (Table 3).

We confirm that the construct validity of the CS-FBD-J is sufficient. Regardless of the presence or absence of IBS in the participants, the CS-FBD-J and IBS symptom-related scales (IBS-SI and VSI) were positively correlated. Thus, the CS-FBD-J was shown to reflect gastrointestinal symptom-specific cognition. In contrast, general dysfunctional cognition not specific to gastrointestinal symptoms (DAS-24) was not prominently correlated with CS-FBD-J. Although this result differs from the original version, it may indicate a difference between general dysfunctional cognition and IBS-specific cognition. The difference in correlation coefficients between the CS-FBD-J and DAS-24 in the IBS group was slight in the 25-item and 23-item versions. This difference may relate to the finding that the DAS-24 scores were not significantly different in the presence of IBS. In addition, anxiety and depression (HADS) were correlated with CS-FBD-J only in the IBS group. Cognition of abdominal symptoms has been reported to be associated with anxiety and depression in IBS patients [3, 12], and the CS-FBD-J may reflect cognition specific to gastrointestinal symptoms that affect the emotions of individuals with IBS. Thus, the CS-FBD-J could be beneficial exclusively for individuals experiencing abdominal symptoms. In both the previous study [12] and the present data, the VSI was correlated with anxiety but not with depression, whereas the CS-FBD-J was correlated not only with anxiety but also with depression. Therefore, the CS-FBD can be distinguished from the concept measured by the VSI in that it reflects cognitions that affect both anxiety and depression. The CS-FBD and the VSI can be used for different purposes or can be combined to elaborate on cognitions related to gastrointestinal symptoms.

Sufficient criterion-related validity of the CS-FBD-J was also confirmed. The CS-FBD-J scores were higher in IBS patients, non-IBS patients, and the control group, in that order. In this study, the intensity of IBS symptoms (IBS-SI) by group was also in this order. This suggests that there is a large difference in CS-FBD-J scores, not only in the presence or absence of IBS but also in the high- and low-severity groups.

Table 5 Results of the item-total analysis and factor analysis

Items	26-item version			18-item version		
		Factor loadings			Factor loadings	
	Item-total correlation	Factor 1	Factor 2	Item-total correlation	Factor 1	Factor 2
13. I avoid making plans in case I have problems with my IBS	0.706	**0.936**	-0.075	0.699	**0.950**	-0.083
12. I avoid going out in case I have problems with my IBS	0.726	**0.894**	-0.020	0.721	**0.909**	-0.033
26. I avoid staying away from home overnight in case my IBS flares up	0.579	**0.859**	-0.159	0.595	**0.847**	-0.130
21. I avoid certain social situations (e.g., restaurants) because of my IBS	0.655	**0.794**	-0.016	0.668	**0.758**	0.035
20. I avoid certain work situations (e.g., meetings) because of my IBS	0.736	**0.794**	0.086	0.752	**0.758**	0.146
14. I carry other items (e.g., wet wipes, sanitary towels, spare underwear) in case my IBS flares up	0.617	**0.683**	-0.110	0.608	**0.682**	-0.121
17. I avoid sex in case my IBS flares up (and causes embarrassment)	0.559	**0.682**	-0.161	0.551	**0.716**	-0.207
15. I take medication (e.g., before going out) just in case my IBS flares up	0.683	**0.665**	0.017	0.704	**0.599**	0.100
22. I avoid certain foods (e.g., dairy products, spicy foods) because of my IBS	0.665	**0.626**	0.114	0.667	**0.586**	0.155
19. I ask for reassurance about my IBS	0.690	**0.610**	0.267	0.706	**0.559**	0.341
16. I carry medication with me in case my IBS flares up	0.693	**0.516**	0.125	0.725	**0.439**	0.221
24. When I have diarrhea I do things to ease it (e.g. take prescribed medication, take alternative medication)	0.623	**0.436**	0.122		-	-
10. I avoid certain foods when I have bowel problems	0.600	**0.301**	0.211		-	-
9. I avoid exercise when I have stomach pains	0.511	**0.290**	0.151		-	-
11. I wear baggy clothing when my stomach feels bloated or distended	0.463	**0.252**	0.112		-	-
6. I spend more time on the toilet than I ideally would like	0.632	-0.087	**0.733**	0.655	-0.068	**0.694**
4. After opening my bowels I check for blood	0.453	-0.170	**0.703**	0.487	-0.167	**0.686**
5. After opening my bowels I check my stool for abnormalities	0.526	-0.170	**0.701**	0.574	-0.188	**0.712**
3. I strain when opening my bowels	0.635	0.107	**0.650**	0.640	0.127	**0.603**
25. I am constantly aware of my stomach	0.752	0.117	**0.639**	0.759	0.032	**0.733**
7. I often go to the toilet to open my bowels and then do not pass anything	0.564	0.019	**0.545**	0.581	0.053	**0.482**
18. When I go out, I make sure I know where the nearest toilet is	0.741	0.366	**0.441**	0.746	0.295	**0.525**
8. I often go to the toilet to pass water and find I open my bowels	0.476	0.125	**0.426**		-	-
1. I eat specific foods to help me open my bowels more	0.481	0.022	**0.399**		-	-
2. I eat specific foods to help me open my bowels less	0.491	0.240	**0.393**		-	-
23. After I open my bowels, I wipe more than I would like	0.609	0.264	**0.390**		-	-
	Eigenvalue	9.63	1.57	Eigenvalue	7.89	1.38
	Variance (%)	37.03%	43.06%	Variance (%)	43.84%	51.51%
	Cronbach's α =0.93			Cronbach's α = 0.92		

The high reliability of the CS-FBD-J was confirmed. The alpha coefficient was greater than 0.9, indicating a high internal consistency. The item-total correlation was significant for all items and exceeded 0.4 for the 23-item version.

Study 2 (validity and reliability of the IBS-BRQ-J)

As in the original version, two factors were extracted: factor 1 consisted mainly of items related to avoidance of abdominal symptoms and associated difficulties, and factor 2 consisted mainly of items related to behavior

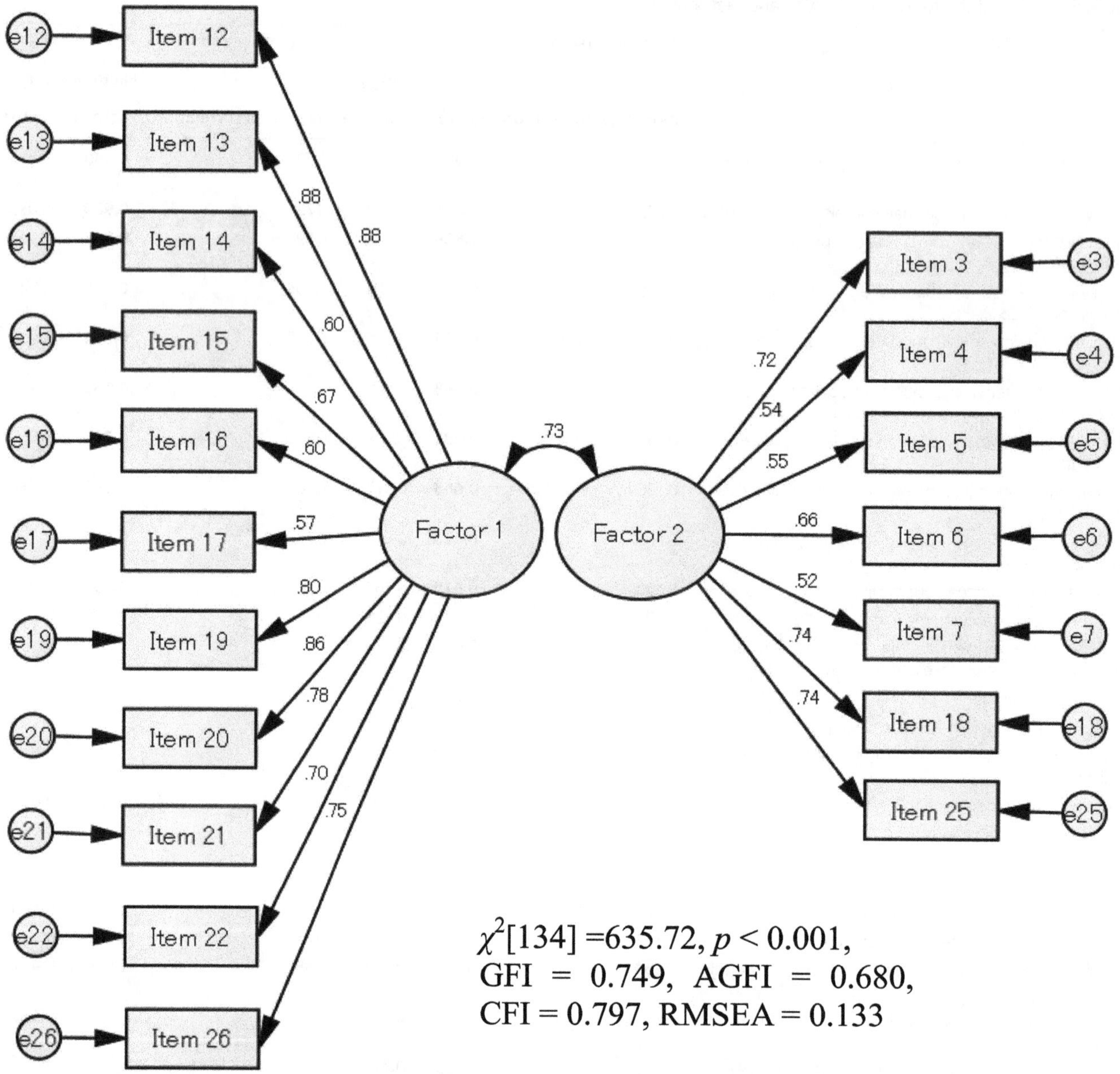

Fig. 2 The results of the SEM. GFI: Goodness-of-Fit Index, AGFI: Adjusted goodness-of-Fit Index, CFI: Comparative fit index, RMSEA: Root-mean-square error of approximation

obsessed with abdominal symptoms. The items comprising each factor were similar to those in the original version. However, the names of these factors in the original version of the IBS-BRQ were "avoidance behavior" and "control behavior," but because items related to eating behavior for the purpose of controlling defecation were deleted, the content was closer to "obsession" than "control." In the Japanese version, eight items with low factor loadings were deleted from the 26 items of the original version of the IBS-BRQ. This suggests that there may be cultural differences in the behavioral responses associated with abdominal symptoms. However, confirmatory factor analysis of the IBS-BRQ-J, which consists of 18 items and two factors, showed that the model fit was not satisfactory. Therefore, the factorial validity of the IBS-BRQ-J is unstable and needs to be further investigated.

In contrast, the construct validity and criterion-related validity of the IBS-BRQ-J were adequate, and correlations between the IBS-BRQ-J and general

Table 6 Correlations between the IBS-BRQ-J (26-item and 18-item version) and other variables

26 items		IBS-SI	Disruption to daily life (IBS-SI)	VSI	HADS (Anxiety)	HADS (Depression)	HADS (Total)	SASS
Total	*r*	0.556	0.538	0.598	0.316	0.233	0.302	-0.269
	p	<0.001	<0.001	<0.001	<0.001	<0.001	<0.001	<0.001
IBS group	*r*	0.488	0.464	0.518	0.449	0.386	0.454	-0.290
	p	<0.001	<0.001	<0.001	<0.001	<0.001	<0.001	0.004
Control group	*r*	0.452	0.461	0.518	0.113	0.127	0.133	-0.082
	p	<0.001	<0.001	<0.001	0.229	0.177	0.159	0.396
18 items		IBS-SI	Disruption to daily life (IBS-SI)	VSI	HADS (Anxiety)	HADS (Depression)	HADS (Total)	SASS
Total	*r*	0.560	0.533	0.610	0.305	0.240	0.300	-0.262
	p	<0.001	<0.001	<0.001	<0.001	<0.001	<0.001	<0.001
IBS group	*r*	0.491	0.464	0.533	0.434	0.399	0.452	-0.282
	p	<0.001	<0.001	<0.001	<0.001	<0.001	<0.001	0.005
Control group	*r*	0.450	0.442	0.521	0.098	0.131	0.126	-0.061
	p	<0.001	<0.001	<0.001	0.300	0.166	0.181	0.524

IBS irritable bowel syndrome
IBS-BRQ-J Japanese version of Irritable Bowel Syndrome-Behavioral Responses Questionnaire
IBS-SI IBS Severity Index
VSI Visceral Sensitivity Index
HADS Hospital Anxiety and Depression Scale
SASS Social Adaptation Self-evaluation Scale

measures not related to IBS were significant only in the IBS group. The correlations between the IBS-BRQ-J and general scales not related to IBS were significant only in the IBS group, suggesting that negative emotions and maladjustment in people with IBS are likely to be symptom-driven, which explains the difference between the correlations in the IBS and control groups. Therefore, the results suggest that the IBS-BRQ-J may be an appropriate tool for assessing behavioral responses specific to IBS. Additionally, the IBS-BRQ-J would benefit only those suffering from abdominal symptoms, not healthy individuals, as the CS-FBD-J is.

The reliability of the IBS-BRQ-J was shown to be sufficiently high by the alpha coefficient and the item-total test; the alpha coefficient of factor 2 (behavior obsessed with abdominal symptoms) was lower because of a smaller number of items (seven items), but the reliability of both the IBS and control groups exceeded 0.7, and thus the reliability was considered to be sufficient.

Although the IBS-BRQ-J needs further study for the model fit of the two-factor structure, the results of other reliability and validity indices were sufficient. Currently, there is no other tool for assessing behavioral responses related to IBS other than the IBS-BRQ. The IBS-BRQ-J is expected to be an extremely useful and indispensable tool for research examining the psychological aspects of IBS and for assessment in the clinical practice of IBS using cognitive-behavioral therapy.

The study limitations

The present study has several limitations. First, there were few patients with IBS among the participants in this study. In the previous studies of the original versions, all participants were patients with IBS (For the CS-FBD, 3 of 75 participants had other functional bowel disorders). As shown by the data of this study, the severity of IBS and non-IBS patients may differ. If we collect data from a sufficient number of patients with IBS or FBD and conduct factor analysis, the results may be different from those of this study. Second, in the assessment of the presence of IBS, the diagnostic criteria for IBS used in this study were not the latest Rome-IV criteria, which had not been published at the time the study started. In the latest diagnostic criteria, the presence of abdominal pain is essential for the diagnosis of IBS. Based on the above issues, further validation of CS-FBD-J and IBS-BRQ is required by extracting individuals with IBS using the latest diagnostic criteria and collecting sufficient data from IBS patients. Third, for the CS-FBD-J and IBS-BRQ-J, the number of items in the original and Japanese versions do not match, making a strict comparison with previous studies difficult. Fourth, the VSI used for construct validity is not a cognition-specific scale. Because we were unable to verify the significant correlation between the CS-FBD-J and the DAS-24 in the present study, we could not rigorously confirm whether the CS-FBD-J adequately measures the concept of cognition. Fifth, we did not determine the coexistence of organic gastrointestinal diseases among the study participants.

Conclusion

The CS-FBD-J and IBS-BRQ-J are useful scales for assessing non-functional cognition and behavioral problems specific to gastrointestinal symptoms. The present study confirmed the reliability and validity of the 23-item version of the CS-FBS after the deletion of two items with low factor loadings. Regarding the IBS-BRQ-J, eight items with low factor loadings were deleted from the 26 items of the original version, and two factor structures were confirmed: Factor 1 consisted mainly of items related to behavior obsessed with abdominal symptoms, and factor 2 consisted mainly of items related to avoidance of abdominal symptoms and associated difficulties. Although the IBS-BRQ-J needs further study for the model fit of the two-factor structure, the results of other reliability and validity indices were sufficient. These scales are expected to contribute to a more precise assessment of patients in research on and clinical practice of functional gastrointestinal disorders.

Abbreviations

IBS: Irritable bowel syndrome; CS-FBD-J: Japanese version of Cognitive Scale for Functional Bowel Disorders; IBS-BRQ-J: Japanese version of Irritable Bowel Syndrome-Behavioral Responses Questionnaire; IBS-SI: IBS Severity Index; VSI: Visceral Sensitivity Index; DAS-24: 24-item Dysfunctional Attitudes Scale; HADS: Hospital Anxiety and Depression Scale; SASS: Social Adaptation Self-evaluation Scale.

Acknowledgments

None.

Authors' contributions

NS organized the project, analyzed the data, and wrote the manuscript. NS, HI, and MI designed the study. NS and FG translated the CS-FBD and IBS-BRQ into Japanese. NS, YT, MF, HI, KS, TO, TA, and MI collected the data. All the authors read, revised, and approved the final manuscript, and share the final responsibility for the decision to submit it for publication. The author(s) read and approved the final manuscript.

Author details

[1]Unit of Public Health and Preventive Medicine, School of Medicine, Yokohama City University, 3-9 Fukuura, Kanazawa-ku, Yokohama 236-0004, Japan. [2]Department of Psychosomatic Medicine, National Center Hospital, National Center of Neurology and Psychiatry, 4-1-1 Ogawahigashi, Kodaira, Tokyo 187-8553, Japan. [3]Department of Behavioral Medicine, National Institute of Mental Health, National Center of Neurology and Psychiatry, 4-1-1 Ogawahigashi, Kodaira, Tokyo 187-8553, Japan. [4]Department of Medical Education, School of Medicine, Yokohama City University, 3-9 Fukuura, Kanazawa-ku, Yokohama 236-0004, Japan. [5]Faculty of Human Sciences, Musashino University, 3-3-3 Ariake, Koto-ku, Tokyo 135-8181, Japan. [6]Department of Pediatrics, The Pennsylvania State University, 500 University Drive, Hershey, PA 17033, USA. [7]Health Management Center, Yokohama City University, 22-2 Seto, Kanazawa-ku, Yokohama 236-0027, Japan. [8]Department of Psychosomatic Medicine, Narita Hospital, International University of Health and Welfare, 852 Hatakeda, Narita, Chiba 286-8686, Japan.

References

1. Longstreth GF, Thompson WG, Chey WD, Houghton LA, Mearin F, Spiller RC. Functional bowel disorders. Gastroenterology. 2006;130:1480–91.
2. Sugaya N, Nomura S, Shimada H. Relationship between cognitive factors and anxiety in individuals with irritable bowel syndrome. Int J Behav Med. 2012;19:308–15.
3. Ballou S, Keefer L. The impact of irritable bowel syndrome on daily functioning: characterizing and understanding daily consequences of IBS. Neurogastroenterol Motil. 2017;29(4):e12982.
4. Leibbrand R, Hiller W. Cognitive behavior therapy for functional gastrointestinal disorders: is group treatment effective? Acta Neuropsychiatr. 2003;15:242–8.
5. Lackner JM, Jaccard J, Krasner SS, Katz LA, Gudleski GD, Holroyd K. Self-administered cognitive behavior therapy for moderate to severe irritable bowel syndrome: clinical efficacy, tolerability, feasibility. Clin Gastroenterol Hepatol. 2008;6:899–906.
6. Labus JS, Bolus R, Chang L, Wiklund I, Naesdal J, Mayer EA, et al. The Visceral Sensitivity Index: development and validation of a gastrointestinal symptom-specific anxiety scale. Aliment Pharmacol Ther. 2004;20(1):89–97.
7. Patrick DL, Drossman D, Frederick IO, Dicesare J, Puder KL. Quality of life in persons with irritable bowel syndrome. Development and validation of a new measure. Dig Dis Sci. 1998;43:400–11.
8. Toner BB, Stuckless N, Ali A, Downie F, Emmott S, Akman D. The development of a cognitive scale for functional bowel disorders. Psychosom Med. 1998;60:492–7.
9. Everitt H, Landau S, Little P, Bishop FL, McCrone P, O'Reilly G, et al. ACTIB trial team. Assessing Cognitive behavioural Therapy in Irritable Bowel (ACTIB): protocol for a randomised controlled trial of clinical-effectiveness and cost-effectiveness of therapist delivered cognitive behavioural therapy and web-based self-management in irritable bowel syndrome in adults. BMJ Open. 2015;5:e008622.
10. Halpert A, Rybin D, Doros G. Expressive writing is a promising therapeutic modality for the management of IBS: A pilot study. Am J Gastroenterol. 2010;105:2440–8.
11. Han CJ, Dong C, Jarrett ME, Heitkemper MM. Symptom comparisons between Asian American and white American women with irritable bowel syndrome. Gastroenterol Nurs. 2018;41:223–32.
12. Jarrett ME, Cain KC, Barney PG, Burr RL, Naliboff BD, Shulman R, et al. Balance of autonomic nervous system predicts who benefits from a self-management intervention Program for Irritable Bowel Syndrome. J Neurogastroenterol Motil. 2016;22:102–11.
13. Ljótsson B, Hesser H, Andersson E, Lackner JM, El Alaoui SE, Falk L, et al. Provoking symptoms to relieve symptoms: A randomized controlled dismantling study of exposure therapy in irritable bowel syndrome. Behav Res Ther. 2014;55:27–39.
14. Reme SE, Stahl D, Kennedy T, Jones R, Darnley S, Chalder T. Mediators of change in cognitive behaviour therapy and mebeverine for irritable bowel syndrome. Psychol Med. 2011;41:2669–79.
15. Saigo T, Tayama J, Hamaguchi T, Nakaya N, Tomiie T, Bernick PJ, et al. Gastrointestinal specific anxiety in irritable bowel syndrome: validation of the Japanese version of the visceral sensitivity index for university students. Biopsychosoc Med. 2014;8(1):10.
16. Reme SE, Darnley S, Kennedy T, Chalder T. The development of the irritable bowel syndrome-behavioral responses questionnaire. J Psychosom Res. 2010;69:319–25. https://doi.org/10.1016/j.jpsychores.2010.01.025.
17. Bonnert M, Olén O, Bjureberg J, Lalouni M, Hedman-Lagerlöf E, Serlachius E, et al. The role of avoidance behavior in the treatment of adolescents with irritable bowel syndrome: A mediation analysis. Behav Res Ther. 2018;105:27–35. https://doi.org/10.1016/j.brat.2018.03.006.
18. Everitt H, Landau S, Little P, Bishop FL, McCrone P, O'Reilly G, et al. Assessing cognitive behavioural therapy in irritable bowel (ACTIB): protocol for a randomised controlled trial of clinical-effectiveness and cost-effectiveness of therapist delivered cognitive behavioural therapy and web-based self-management in irritable bowel syndrome in adults. BMJ Open. 2015;5:e008622. https://doi.org/10.1136/bmjopen-2015-008622.
19. Ferreira NB, Gillanders D, Morris PG, Eugenicos M. Pilot study of acceptance and commitment therapy for irritable bowel syndrome: A preliminary analysis of treatment outcomes and processes of change. Clin Psychol. 2018;22:241–50. https://doi.org/10.1111/cp.12123

20. Gillanders D, Ferreira NB, Angioni E, Carvalho SA, Eugenicos MP. An implementation trial of ACT-based bibliotherapy for irritable bowel syndrome. J Contextual Behav Sci. 2017;6:172–7. https://doi.org/10.1016/j.jcbs.2017.04.006.
21. Lalouni M, Ljótsson B, Bonnert M, Hedman-Lagerlöf E, Högström J, Serlachius E, et al. Internet-delivered cognitive behavioral therapy for children with pain-related functional gastrointestinal disorders: feasibility study. JMIR Ment Health. 2017;4:e32. https://doi.org/10.2196/mental.7985.
22. Windgassen S, Moss-Morris R, Everitt H, Sibelli A, Goldsmith K, Chalder T. Cognitive and behavioral differences between subtypes in refractory irritable bowel syndrome. Behav Ther. 2019;50:594–607. https://doi.org/10.1016/j.beth.2018.09.006.
23. Drossman DA, Corazziari E, Delvaux M, Spiller RC, Talley NJ, Thompson WG, et al. Rome III: the functional gastrointestinal disorders. 3rd ed. McLean: Degnon Associates; 2006.
24. Kanazawa M, Nakajima S, Oshima T, Whitehead WE, Sperber AD, Palsson OS, et al. Validity and reliability of the Japanese version of the Rome III diagnostic questionnaire for irritable bowel syndrome and functional dyspepsia. J Neurogastroenterol Motil. 2015;21(4):537–44.
25. Whitehead WE, Validation Working Team. Development and validation of the Rome III diagnostic questionnaire. In: association with the Rome Questionnaire Committee, Drossman DA, Corazziari E, Rome DM III, editors. The functional gastrointestinal disorders. McLean: VA: Degnon Associates, Inc; 2006. p. 835–65.
26. Shinozaki M, Kanazawa M, Sagami Y, Endo Y, Hongo M, Drossman DA, et al. Validation of the Japanese version of the Rome II modular questionnaire and irritable bowel syndrome severity index. J Gastroenterol. 2006;41(5):491–4.
27. Francis CY, Morris J, Whorwell PJ. The irritable bowel severity scoring system: a simple method of monitoring irritable bowel syndrome and its progress. Aliment Pharmacol Ther. 1997;11:395–402.
28. Tajima M, Akiyama T, Numa H, Kawamura Y, Okada Y, Sakai Y, Miyake Y, Ono Y, Power MJ. Reliability and validity of the Japanese version of the 24-item Dysfunctional Attitude Scale. Acta Neuropsychiatr. 2007;19:362–7.
29. Power MJ, Katz R, McGuffin P, Duggan CF, Lam D, Beck AT. The Dysfunctional Attitude Scale (DAS). J Res Pers. 1994;28:263–76.
30. Zigmond AS, Snaith RP. The hospital anxiety and depression scale. Acta Psychiatr Scand. 1983;67:361–70.
31. Zigmond AS, Snaith RP, Kitamura T. Hospital anxiety and depression scale (HAD). Arch Psychiatr Diagn Clin Eval. 1993;4:371–2.
32. Goto M, Ueda N, Yoshimura R, Kakihara S, Kaji K, Yamada Y, et al. Reliability and validity of the Japanese version of the Social Adaptation Self-Evaluation Scale (SASS). Clin Psychiatr. 2005;47:483–9.
33. Bosc M, Dubini A, Polin V. Development and validation of a social functioning scale, the Social Adaptation Self-evaluation Scale. Eur Neropsychopharmacol. 1997;7(Supple.1):S57–70.

8

Restrictive diet in a patient with irritable bowel syndrome leading to Wernicke encephalopathy

Qiang Wang[1], Zeinab Charmchi[1] and Ilena C. George[2*]

Abstract

Background: We present a case of a woman with a past medical history of irritable bowel syndrome (IBS) and anxiety, who presents with ophthalmoplegia, ataxia and memory loss, characteristic of Wernicke encephalopathy.

Case presentation: A 64-year-old woman presented with double vision, unsteady gait and memory loss. These symptoms began after 3 months on an unfortified restricted diet, which she initiated to alleviate IBS symptoms. Magnetic resonance imaging of the brain demonstrated hyperintense T2-weighted signal in the dorsomedial aspect of bilateral thalami, periaqueductal grey matter and around the third ventricle. The patient's visual symptoms improved significantly after thiamine supplementation, although her memory deficits persisted.

Conclusion: Although WE is often associated with chronic alcohol abuse, this case demonstrates the importance of recognizing WE in any patient with a restricted diet and subsequent timely initiation of thiamine.

Keywords: Case report, Wernicke encephalopathy, Thiamine deficiency, Irritable bowel syndrome

Background

Wernicke encephalopathy (WE) is a neurological emergency resulting from thiamine deficiency, which impairs thiamine-dependent glucose and nucleic acid metabolism and in turn causes apoptosis due to *N*-methyl-D-aspartate (NMDA) toxicity, especially in the thalamus and the mammillary bodies [1]. Although WE is most commonly seen in patients with chronic alcohol abuse, other causes include bariatric surgery, hyperemesis gravidarum and malnutrition [2]. WE is easily misdiagnosed due to clinical variance; the classic clinical triad of ocular abnormalities, ataxia, and confusion is only seen in approximately 24–38% of patients [3, 4]. Brain MRI typically reveals hyperintense signal in T2 and fluid-attenuated inversion recovery (FLAIR) and diffusion abnormality in the periaqueductal area, within the dorsomedial thalami, dorsal medulla, and mammillary bodies [5].

WE can be lethal or cause irreversible neurologic sequelae if left untreated, however, outcomes data on WE are limited. A multicenter observational study of 468 WE patients from 2000 to 2012, out of which only 34 cases were non-alcohol related, demonstrated a mortality rate during hospitalization of 5.3% [4] with a majority of these deaths due to infection or liver disease. Another study reported a 45% mortality rate after a median follow-up period of 5 years, largely due to bacterial infections and cancer [3]. Data on appropriate dosing of thiamine is similarly limited. A small case series of WE demonstrated 73% of patients had symptom improvement or resolution after rapid initiation of high dose thiamine (> 500 mg) for a median of 3 days [6].

*Correspondence: igeorge@mgh.harvard.edu
[2] Department of Neurology, Massachusetts General Hospital, 55 Fruit St, Boston, MA 02114, USA
Full list of author information is available at the end of the article

Case presentation

A 64-year-old female with past medical history of hypothyroidism, irritable bowel syndrome (IBS) and panic attacks presented with double vision, unsteady gait and memory loss. She had been experiencing abdominal bloating for the past 3 months, associated with nausea and vomiting, and modified her diet to consist solely of small amounts of unfortified farina. She had similar gastrointestinal symptoms 10 years ago, for which an evaluation including endoscopy and colonoscopy was unrevealing. At that time, she was started on paroxetine for a presumptive diagnosis of IBS and her symptoms resolved after 6 months. She reported no other risk factors for thiamine deficiency, such as alcohol use, or excessive tea and/or coffee consumption. Three months prior to admission, when her symptoms recurred, her psychiatrist empirically reinitiated her on paroxetine, but discontinued this medication when her symptoms did not improve. Three weeks prior to presenting to our institution, she was noted to have double vision and inability to move her eyes laterally. A week later, she experienced a decline in her memory, and was unable to remember recent events and recognize family members. Concurrently, she developed an unsteady gait with frequent falls, which prompted an admission to a community hospital. Computed tomography of the head and abdomen were performed which were unremarkable. She was subsequently transferred to our institution for further workup including a brain MRI. The neurological exam demonstrated impaired short-term and long-term memory, near absence of horizontal eye movements with maintenance of vertical gaze, bilateral dysmetria, diminished sensation to all modalities, as well as an inability to ambulate. MRI of the brain with and without gadolinium (Fig. 1) demonstrated symmetrical hyperintense signal in fluid-attenuated inversion recovery (FLAIR) sequences around the periaqueductal grey matter, third ventricle and bilateral dorsomedial thalami. Serum thiamine level at admission was 26.8 nmol/L (normal range 66.5–200 nmol/L). Folate, vitamins B2 and B12, copper and zinc levels as well as thyroid and liver function tests were within normal range. With a clinical diagnosis of WE, she was started on high dose thiamine supplementation of 500 mg three times daily. After the first dose of thiamine, the patient's horizontal eye movements greatly improved and returned to near-normal within 3 days of supplementation. Her memory impairment did not significantly change with thiamine administration.

Discussion and conclusions

Wernicke encephalopathy (WE) is a relatively uncommon and potentially lethal neurological disorder with estimated prevalence between 0.8 and 2.8% [7, 8] among the general population based on autopsy studies. The actual prevalence is thought to be higher considering significant clinical variance which easily leads to misdiagnosis, however, more recent epidemiology data is limited. Proposed diagnostic criteria require two out of four signs: (a) dietary deficiencies, (b) oculomotor abnormalities, (c) cerebellar dysfunction, and (d) either an altered mental state or mild memory impairment [9]. Brain MRI can also aid in diagnosis [5]. In practice, empirical treatment of high dose thiamine has been standard management for patients with risk of nutrition deficiency who

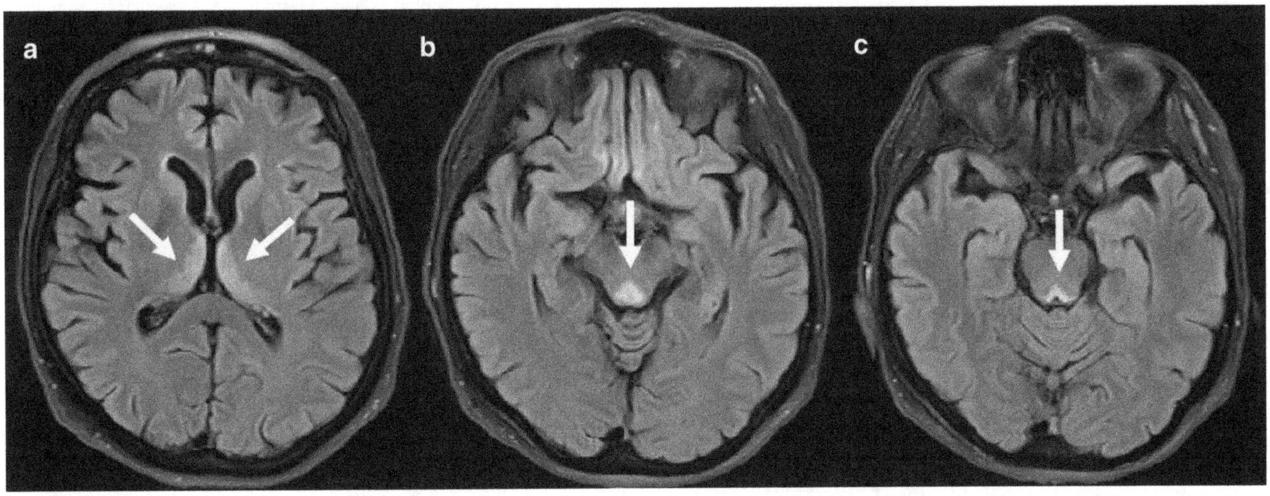

Fig. 1 Fluid-attenuated inversion recovery imaging demonstrating characteristic changes of Wernicke encephalopathy including hyperintense signal changes in the bilateral dorsomedial thalami (**a**), inferior tectal plate (**b**) and around the periaqueductal gray matter within the dorsal midbrain (**c**)

present with altered mental status, considering the low risk associated with supplementation and the extremely high risk of disease burden if misdiagnosed. The differential diagnosis is broad in such cases, including cerebrovascular event, seizures, other causes of toxic-metabolic encephalopathy, and meningoencephalitis. In cases where the diagnosis is uncertain, the workup should continue while patients receive high dose thiamine.

WE is caused by limited thiamine intake or absorption, due to conditions such as alcoholism, bariatric surgery and hyperemesis gravidarum [2]. Thiamine deficiency may alter gut microbial composition, potentially contributing to small intestine bacterial overgrowth (SIBO), a condition whose symptoms include nausea, decreased appetite, bloating, flatulence and malnutrition [10, 11]. Furthermore, IBS and SIBO are frequently co-morbid. The prevalence of SIBO increases in patients with IBS, particularly in the elderly female population [12–15]. Given her symptoms, we speculate that our patient may have had IBS/SIBO with subsequent thiamine deficiency [16], however, confirmatory testing of SIBO with a breath test or jejunal aspirate was not completed. From the available testing, the patient appeared to have an isolated thiamine deficiency as a result of her restrictive diet of unfortified farina. Unfortified farina contains common minerals including iron and vitamin D, whereas fortified farina contains additional vitamins including thiamine and niacin.

In this case, we highlight the importance of early detection and treatment of thiamine deficiency and the need for a high index of suspicion in patients with restricted diets to prevent permanent neurological sequelae. Moreover, it is paramount for patients on a restricted diet to incorporate a supplemental multivitamin including thiamine on a daily basis to prevent nutritional deficiency.

Abbreviations

IBS: Irritable bowel syndrome; FLAIR: Fluid-attenuated inversion recovery; GI: Gastrointestinal; MRI: Magnetic resonance imaging; SIBO: Small intestine bacterial overgrowth; WE: Wernicke's encephalopathy.

Acknowledgements

Not applicable.

Authors' contributions

QW contributed to history taking and examination of the patient and wrote the introduction and case presentation section. ZC contributed to history taking and examination of the patient and wrote the discussion and conclusions section. ICG supervised the team, verified the accuracy of the case presentation and the citing references as well and completed the final revision of the manuscript. All authors have read and approved this manuscript.

Author details

[1] Department of Neurology, Kings County Hospital Center, SUNY Downstate Medical Center and Maimonides Medical Center, SUNY Downstate Health Sciences University, Brooklyn, NY, USA. [2] Department of Neurology, Massachusetts General Hospital, 55 Fruit St, Boston, MA 02114, USA.

References

1. Calderón-Ospina CA, Nava-Mesa MO. B Vitamins in the nervous system: current knowledge of the biochemical modes of action and synergies of thiamine, pyridoxine, and cobalamin. CNS Neurosci Ther. 2020;26(1):5–13.
2. Oudman E, Wijnia JW, Oey M, van Dam M, Painter RC, Postma A. Wernicke's encephalopathy in hyperemesis gravidarum: a systematic review. Eur J Obstet Gynecol Reprod Biol. 2019;236:84–93.
3. Sanvisens A, Zuluaga P, Fuster D, Rivas I, Tor J, Marcos M, et al. Long-term mortality of patients with an alcohol-related Wernicke–Korsakoff syndrome. Alcohol Alcohol. 2017;52(4):466–71.
4. Chamorro AJ, Rosón-Hernández B, Medina-García JA, Muga-Bustamante R, Fernández-Solá J, Martín-González MC, et al. Differences between alcoholic and nonalcoholic patients with Wernicke encephalopathy: a multicenter observational study. Mayo Clin Proc. 2017;92(6):899–907.
5. Manzo G, De Gennaro A, Cozzolino A, Serino A, Fenza G, Manto A. MR imaging findings in alcoholic and nonalcoholic acute Wernicke's encephalopathy: a review. Biomed Res Int. 2014;2014:503596.
6. Nishimoto A, Usery J, Winton JC, Twilla J. High-dose parenteral thiamine in treatment of Wernicke's encephalopathy: case series and review of the literature. In Vivo. 2017;31(1):121–4.
7. Harper C. The incidence of Wernicke's encephalopathy in Australia—a neuropathological study of 131 cases. J Neurol Neurosurg Psychiatry. 1983;46(7):593–8. https://doi.org/10.1136/jnnp.46.7.593.
8. Torvik A. Wernicke's encephalopathy–prevalence and clinical spectrum. Alcohol Alcohol Suppl. 1991;1:381–4.
9. Caine D, Halliday GM, Kril JJ, Harper CG. Operational criteria for the classification of chronic alcoholics: identification of Wernicke's encephalopathy. J Neurol Neurosurg Psychiatry. 1997;62(1):51–60. https://doi.org/10.1136/jnnp.62.1.51.
10. Costliow ZA, Degnan PH. Thiamine acquisition strategies impact metabolism and competition in the gut microbe *Bacteroides thetaiotaomicron*. mSystems. 2017;2(5):e00116–7.
11. Bures J, Cyrany J, Kohoutova D, Förstl M, Rejchrt S, Kvetina J, et al. Small intestinal bacterial overgrowth syndrome. World J Gastroenterol. 2010;16(24):2978–90.
12. Chen B, Kim JJ, Zhang Y, Du L, Dai N. Prevalence and predictors of small intestinal bacterial overgrowth in irritable bowel syndrome: a systematic review and meta-analysis. J Gastroenterol. 2018;53(7):807–18.
13. Shah ED, Basseri RJ, Chong K, Pimentel M. Abnormal breath testing in IBS: a meta-analysis. Dig Dis Sci. 2010;55(9):2441–9. https://doi.org/10.1007/s10620-010-1276-4.
14. Pyleris E, Giamarellos-Bourboulis EJ, Tzivras D, Koussoulas V, Barbatzas C, Pimentel M. The prevalence of overgrowth by aerobic bacteria in the small intestine by small bowel culture: relationship with irritable bowel syndrome. Dig Dis Sci. 2012;57(5):1321–9. https://doi.org/10.1007/s10620-012-2033-7.
15. Giamarellos-Bourboulis E, Tang J, Pyleris E, et al. Molecular assessment of differences in the duodenal microbiome in subjects with irritable bowel syndrome. Scand J Gastroenterol. 2015;50(9):1076–87. https://doi.org/10.3109/00365521.2015.1027261.
16. Lakhani SV, Shah HN, Alexander K, Finelli FC, Kirkpatrick JR, Koch TR. Small intestinal bacterial overgrowth and thiamine deficiency after Roux-en-Y gastric bypass surgery in obese patients. Nutr Res. 2008;28(5):293–8. https://doi.org/10.1016/j.nutres.2008.03.002.

9

Alterations in short-chain fatty acids and serotonin in irritable bowel syndrome: A systematic review and meta-analysis

Mei Luo†, Xiaojun Zhuang†, Zhenyi Tian and Lishou Xiong*

Abstract

Background: Short-chain fatty acids (SCFAs) and serotonin (5-hydroxytryptamine, 5-HT) may be associated with the pathogenesis of irritable bowel syndrome (IBS). There are some reports of alterations in SCFAs and 5-HT in IBS, but their results are inconsistent. We aimed to perform a meta-analysis to assess alterations in SCFAs and 5-HT in IBS patients and their potential role in the abnormal brain-gut-microbiota (BGM) axis.

Methods: Case–control studies detecting SCFAs and 5-HT in IBS patients were identified from PubMed, Web of Science, Cochrane Library, and Scopus databases to identify relevant articles up to September 2018. The standardized mean differences (SMDs) with 95% confidence intervals (CIs) of SCFAs and 5-HT were calculated by REVIEW MANAGER 5.3 to evaluate the alterations of 5-HT and SCFAs in IBS.

Results: Five studies on SCFAs and 5 on 5-HT in IBS patients were included. As compared to healthy controls (HCs), the SMDs of 5-HT in IBS patients was 2.35 (95% CI 0.46–4.24) and the SMDs of total SCFAs, acetic acid, propionic acid, and butyric acid in IBS patients were − 0.01 (95% CI − 0.57–0.55), − 0.04 (95% CI − 0.55–0.47), 0.07 (95% CI − 0.45–0.60), and − 0.00 (95% CI − 0.49–0.49), respectively.

Conclusions: There was an increase in 5-HT in blood of IBS patients, indicating the increased 5-HT in blood may be involved in IBS pathogenesis. However, there were no significant differences in SCFAs in feces between IBS patients and HCs. But the study did not differentiate between subgroups of IBS. These findings might provide insight for future studies of the BGM axis in the pathogenesis of IBS.

Mei Luo and Xiaojun Zhuang contributed equally to the writing of this article

Keywords: Irritable bowel syndrome, Short-chain fatty acids, Serotonin, Brain-gut-microbiota axis, Meta-analysis

Background

Irritable bowel syndrome (IBS) is one of the most common functional gastrointestinal disorders with uncertain pathogenesis, and serious clinical symptoms (such as abdominal pain, diarrhoea or constipation) will have a significant impact on the quality of life in IBS patients [1, 2]. Visceral hypersensitivity, altered gastrointestinal permeability, immune dysfunction or psychological disorder have been generally accepted as potential contributors to the pathogenesis of IBS [3]. Accumulating evidence has demonstrated that alterations in gut microbiota and dysregulation of the brain-gut axis may be associated with IBS pathogenesis [4–7]. Moreover, the gut microbiota may be involved in IBS pathogenesis through the production of metabolites such as short-chain fatty acids (SCFAs) [8]. In the brain-gut axis, the neurotransmitter serotonin (5-hydroxytryptamine, 5-HT), associated with visceral hypersensitivity and

*Correspondence: xionglishou@163.com
†Mei Luo and Xiaojun Zhuang contributed equally to the writing of this article
Department of Gastroenterology and Hepatology, the First Affiliated Hospital of Sun Yat-Sen University, Guangzhou, China

gastrointestinal permeability, has attracted much attention [9, 10]. Mounting evidence detailing the bidirectional interactions between the gut microbiota and the brain supports the concept of the brain-gut-microbiota (BGM) axis, integrating the central nervous system (CNS), gastrointestinal tract (GIT), and microbiota [11, 12].

The brain-gut axis is the interactional two-way regulating axis of the CNS and gastrointestinal function which comprises the CNS, enteric nervous system (ENS), neuroendocrine and immune system [13]. 5-HT, as an important neurotransmitter in the brain-gut axis, may regulate gastrointestinal motility, visceral sensing, and mucosal secretion by activating both intrinsic excitatory and inhibitory enteric motor neurons. While cholinergic neurons can be stimulated by 5-HT to release acetylcholine and further contract smooth muscle, 5-HT can also irritate inhibitory nitrergic neurons to produce nitric oxide to relax smooth muscle [7]. An excess of 5-HT may trigger primary neuronal afferents, leading to visceral hyperalgesia [14]. Thus, in recent years, 5-HT has attracted considerable attention due to its potential effects on gastrointestinal motility, visceral sensory function, and psychophysiology in IBS [15].

Studies worldwide have provided convincing evidence that gut microbiota alterations may be associated with IBS [3, 4, 16]. However, the causal relationship remains unclear. Interactions between the gut microbiota and host cells on the gut mucosal surface could affect the intestinal microenvironment. Conversely, an altered intestinal microenvironment could modify the gut microbiota [17]. SCFAs are the main metabolites of the gut microbiota and may stabilize the intestinal microenvironment and modulate the gut microbiota [18]. Chassard et al. [19] reported dysbiosis of multiple microbes in IBS patients, and a reduction in *Rhodobacillus coli* may directly lead to SCFA deficiency, ultimately resulting in the visceral pain of IBS. In addition, with elevated concentrations of SCFAs, the pH of the intestinal tract could be reduced. At low pH, the proliferation of probiotic bacteria may be promoted while some pathogenic bacteria may be inhibited [20].

It has been reported that SCFAs and 5-HT might be involved in the bidirectional interactions of the BGM axis [21, 22]. Alterations in SCFAs and 5-HT in IBS patients have been demonstrated in some studies, and these alterations may influence gut motor activity and induce various physical symptoms [10, 23, 24]. However, there remains no consensus regarding the role of alterations in SCFAs and 5-HT in the pathogenesis of IBS. Therefore, we aimed to compare alterations in SCFAs and 5-HT in IBS patients and healthy controls (HCs) to explore their potential involvement in the BGM axis in IBS. We performed a meta-analysis to provide more definitive information on whether alterations in SCFAs and 5-HT between IBS patients and HCs contribute to IBS. Our findings provide insight for further explorations of the roles of SCFAs and 5-HT in the BGM axis and their participation in the pathogenesis of IBS.

Methods

Information sources and search strategy

In this meta-analysis, we searched the PubMed, Web of Science, Cochrane Library, and Scopus databases to identify relevant articles up to September 2018. We used "irritable bowel syndrome", "IBS", "short-chain fatty acids", "SCFAs", "serotonin", "5-hydroxytryptamine", and "5-HT" as the search terms. We further retrieved the references from included studies to search potential articles. Finally we selected articles according to the following inclusion and exclusion criteria.

Inclusion and exclusion criteria

Studies were included if they were case–control studies detecting SCFAs and 5-HT in IBS patients and HCs. Below are the inclusion criteria to our meta analysis: (a) studies about IBS patients and HCs; (b) the participants are adults (both IBS patients and HCs); (c) studies measuring SCFAs or 5-HT; (d) available data in the articles and can eventually be expressed as mean ± SD; and (e) sufficient data to calculate the standardized mean difference (SMD) with 95% confidence interval (CI) between the IBS patients and HCs. Two researchers selected the studies that met the predetermined inclusion criteria independently. All potentially relevant papers were obtained and evaluated in detail. Any disagreement between researchers was resolved through discussion until consensus.

Below are the exclusion criteria to our meta analysis: (a) not a case–control study; (b) not adult participants; (c) no full text; and (d) no available or enough data. According to the inclusion and exclusion criteria, 10 articles (5 articles on SCFAs and 5 on 5-HT) were selected for our meta-analysis.

Data extraction

We extracted the following data after reviewed every article: title of the article, name of the first author, year of publication, country, diagnostic criteria of IBS, age and sex of participants, number of IBS patients, number of HCs, methods by which levels of SCFAs and 5-HT were analyzed, available data expressed as mean ± SD (Tables 1, 2, 3, 4, 5), and study samples of the article. Disagreements regarding data extraction were resolved through discussion until consensus.

Table 1 The total SCFAs in IBS patient and HC

References	IBS patient			HC		
	Mean (mmol/l)	SD	Number	Mean (mmol/l)	SD	Number
Kopecny and Simunek [27]	88.15	207.44	16	108.95	60.01	5
Mortensen et al. [8]	96.89	3.64	18	114.00	19.00	9
Ringel-Kulka et al. [26]	92.10	44.10	114	92.00	33.30	33
Tana et al. [25]	107.10	31.10	26	85.80	28.60	26
Vernia et al. [28]	131.40	62.60	38	108.50	58.30	50

SCFAs, short-chain fatty acids; IBS, irritable bowel syndrome; HC, healthy control

Table 2 The acetic acid in IBS patient and HC

References	IBS patient			HC		
	Mean (mmol/l)	SD	Number	Mean (mmol/l)	SD	Number
Kopecny and Simunek [27]	60.16	126.08	16	73.26	44.70	5
Mortensen et al. [8]	62.67	3.14	18	73.00	11.00	9
Ringel-Kulka et al. [26]	58.00	25.80	114	56.60	18.50	33
Tana et al. [25]	67.00	18.80	26	56.70	18.00	26
Vernia et al. [28]	83.20	43.70	38	70.00	49.80	50

IBS, irritable bowel syndrome; HC, healthy control

Table 3 The propionic acid in IBS patient and HC

References	IBS patient			HC		
	Mean (mmol/l)	SD	Number	Mean (mmol/l)	SD	Number
Kopecny and Simunek [27]	18.06	45.00	16	26.08	13.53	5
Mortensen et al. [8]	18.11	2.05	18	21.00	5.00	9
Ringel-Kulka et al. [26]	18.20	9.80	114	20.00	8.00	33
Tana et al. [25]	20.50	9.20	26	15.30	6.60	26
Vernia et al. [28]	23.70	13.10	38	17.10	8.00	50

IBS, irritable bowel syndrome; HC, healthy control

Table 4 The butyric acid in IBS patient and HC

References	IBS patient			HC		
	Mean (mmol/l)	SD	Number	Mean (mmol/l)	SD	Number
Kopecny and Simunek [27]	9.93	23.92	16	9.16	4.94	5
Mortensen et al. [8]	10.00	1.67	18	12.00	3.00	9
Ringel-Kulka et al. [26]	15.80	12.10	114	15.40	8.90	33
Vernia et al. [25]	18.60	15.10	38	13.00	8.50	50

IBS, irritable bowel syndrome; HC, healthy control

Table 5 The 5-HT in IBS patient and HC

References	IBS patient			HC		
	Mean (nmol/l)	SD	Number	Mean (nmol/l)	SD	Number
Thijssen et al. [32]	10.99	22.75	154	10.84	13.44	137
Keszthelyi et al. [33]	26.20	18.20	15	1.90	1.36	15
Yu et al. [30]	35.31	2.15	30	10.55	1.35	30
Park et al. [29]	85.75	76.67	21	31.49	23.49	13
Dunlop et al. [31]	29.53	7.35	15	41.00	6.90	15

5-HT, 5-hydroxytryptamine; IBS, irritable bowel syndrome; HC, healthy control

Quality assessment of included studies

The quality of each study was assessed by our study team according to the Newcastle–Ottawa Scale for case–control studies, which includes three aspects: selection, comparability, and exposure or outcome evaluation in the study population. The selection criteria comprise four items: (a) is the case definition adequate? (b) representativeness of the cases, (c) selection of the controls, and (d) determination of controls. The comparability criteria include comparability of cases and controls on the basis of the design or analysis. The exposure criteria comprise three items: (a) ascertainment of exposure, (b) same method of ascertainment for cases and controls, and (c) non-response rate. Disagreements were resolved through discussion until consensus.

Statistical analysis

We performed a meta-analysis of alterations in SCFAs and 5-HT in IBS patients. REVIEW MANAGER 5.3, developed by staff at the Australasian Cochrane Centre in 2008 and revised in June 2014 to incorporate new features, was used for statistical analysis of continuous data. When the necessary continuous data were available, we calculated the SMD with 95% CI for the data. The I^2 statistic was used to examine heterogeneity across studies. An I^2 value close to 0% implies low heterogeneity, while an I^2 value close to 100% implies high heterogeneity. In cases of obvious heterogeneity (I^2 value > 50%), a random effects meta-analysis model was used.

Funnel plot analysis for publication bias

A funnel plot was used to assess publication bias. Publication bias leads to asymmetry of the funnel plot, as the dispersion of smaller samples is larger and scatters more widely at the bottom of the graph, while the dispersion of larger sample is smaller, resulting in a narrower spread at the top of the plot.

Results

Study selection

As shown in Fig. 1, a total of 2813 citations were obtained for review of titles and abstracts. After excluding duplicate and irrelevant articles, the remaining 13 articles on SCFAs and 20 articles on 5-HT was retrieved for review. Twenty-three studies were excluded for various reasons, as described in the flowchart (Fig. 1). Finally, five articles [8, 25–28] on SCFAs and five articles [29–33] on 5-HT were included in our meta-analysis. The two reviewers from our team were in full agreement in selecting these 10 studies.

Study characteristics

The characteristics of the studies are summarized in Tables 6 and 7. A total of 212 IBS patients and 123 HCs were included in the 5 studies on SCFAs. In all studies, SCFAs were analyzed from fecal samples. Four studies measured SCFA levels by gas chromatography, while one used high-pressure liquid chromatography (HPLC). Data from four studies were expressed in the form of mean ± SD and from one study as mean ± SEM. We then converted the mean ± SEM into the mean ± SD. SCFA levels are expressed as concentrations in mmol L^{-1}. We analyzed alterations in total SCFAs, acetic acid, propionic acid, and butyric acid in IBS patients.

For the five studies on 5-HT, 235 IBS patients and 210 HCs were included in our study. In all studies, 5-HT was analyzed in blood samples (four in plasma samples and one in serum sample) and measured by HPLC. The data from three studies were expressed as the mean ± SD, one study as the mean ± SEM, and one study as the median and range. We converted the available data to the form of mean ± SD where necessary. Concentrations of 5-HT are expressed as nmol L^{-1}. Among the 10 articles included in our study, IBS patients and HCs were age- and sex-matched in 7 studies.

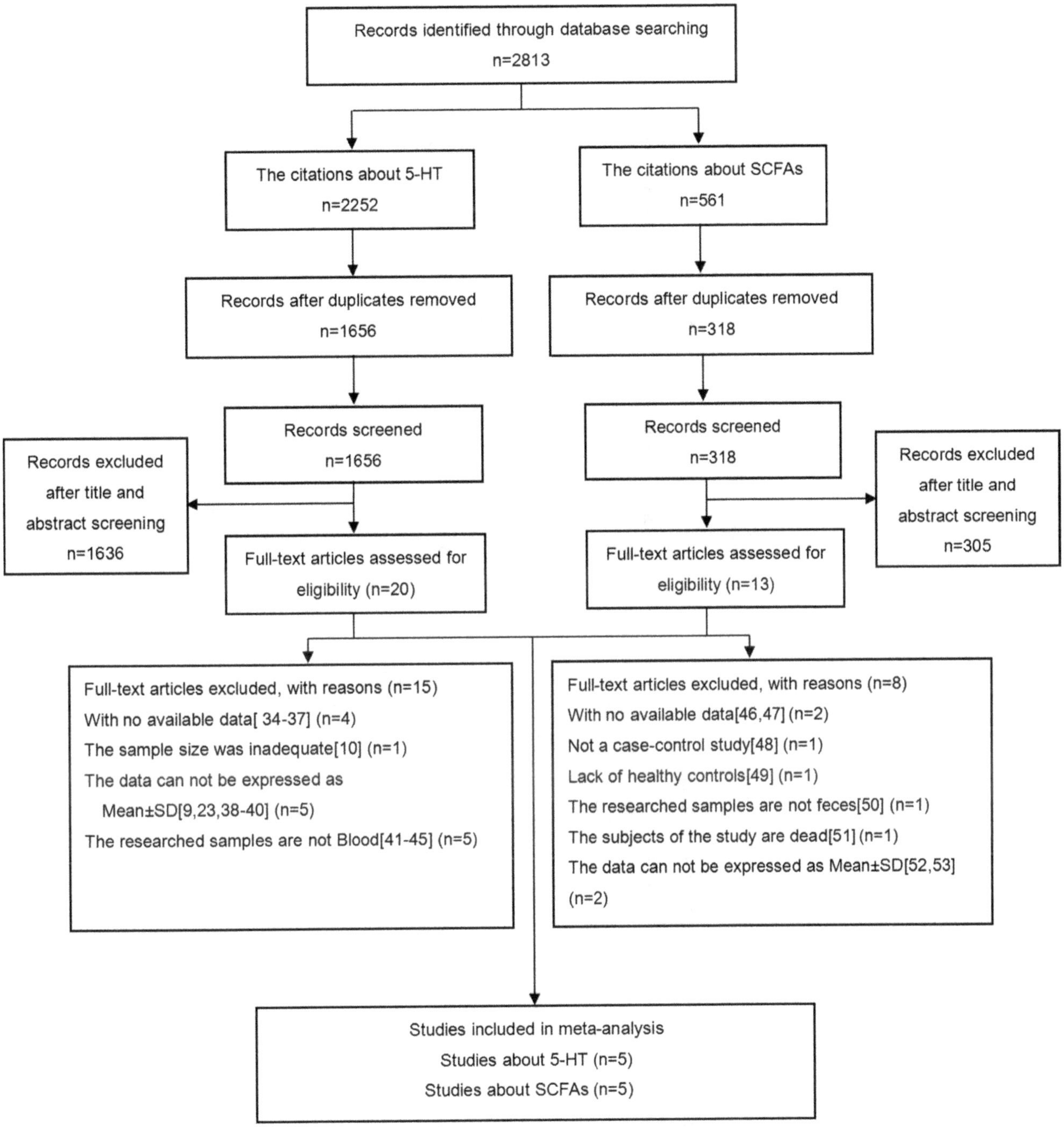

Fig. 1 Flow diagram of assessment of studies identified in the meta-analysis

Assessment of study quality

As shown in Table 8, we used Newcastle–Ottawa Scale to evaluate the quality of each case–control study. All studies included were of moderate quality but did not influence the eligibility of the studies.

Meta-analysis of SMD

Our meta-analysis analyzed alterations in SCFAs (total SCFAs, acetic acid, propionic acid, and butyric acid) and 5-HT in IBS patients from feces and blood respectively. As compared to HCs, the SMD of total SCFAs

Table 6 Characteristics of the five studies of SCFAs in the meta-analysis

References	Year	Location	n, IBS	n, Control	IBS diagnosis	Control composition	Age, IBS (range, $\bar{x} + s$)	Female IBS, n	Age, HC (range, $\bar{x} + s$)	Female HC, n	Sample	Technique
Ringel-Kulka et al. [26]	2015	America	114	33	Rome III	Healthy controls	35.4 ± 11.3	98	33.9 ± 13.0	29	Feces	Gas chromatography
Tana et al. [25]	2010	Japan	26	26	Rome II	Healthy controls	21.7 ± 2.0	13	21.9 ± 3.9	13	Feces	HPLC
Kopecny and Simunek [27]	2002	Czech	16	5	Not reported	Healthy controls	Not reported	Not reported	Not reported	Not reported	Feces	Gas chromatography
Vernia et al. [28]	1987	Italy	38	50	Not reported	Healthy controls	Not reported	Not reported	Not reported	Not reported	Feces	Gas liquid chromatograph
Mortensen et al. [8]	1987	Denmark	18	9	Not reported	Healthy controls	26–68	14	Not reported	Not reported	Feces	Gas liquid chromatography

SCFAs, short-chain fatty acids; IBS, irritable bowel syndrome; HC, healthy control; HPLC, high-pressure liquid chromatography

Table 7 Chracteristics of the included studies of 5-HT in this meta-analysis

References	Year	Location	n, IBS	n, Control	IBS diagnosis	Control Composition	Age, IBS (range, $\bar{x} + s$)	Female IBS, n	Age, HC (range, $\bar{x} + s$)	Female HC, n	Sample	Technique
Yu et al. [30]	2016	China	30	30	Not reported	Healthy controls	39 ± 21	14	42.5 ± 19.5	15	Serum	HPLC
Dunlop et al. [31]	2005	Britain	15	15	Rome II	Healthy controls	35.1 ± 2.9	15	35.9 ± 2.6	10	Plasma	HPLC
Thijssen et al. [32]	2015	Netherlands	154	137	Rome III	Healthy controls	44.5 ± 16.3	108	44.2 ± 19.3	84	Plasma	HPLC
Park et al. [29]	2009	Korea	21	13	Rome II	Healthy controls	24–78	13	29–68	6	Plasma	HPLC
Keszthelyi et al. [33]	2013	Netherlands	15	15	Rome III	Healthy controls	44 ± 13	8	33 ± 17	10	Plasma	HPLC

5-HT, 5-hydroxytryptamine; IBS, irritable bowel syndrome; HC, healthy control; HPLC, high-pressure liquid chromatography

Table 8 Quality assessment of the included studies

References	Year	Selection	Comparability	Exposure	Total
Ringel-Kulka et al. [26]	2015	4	1	2	7
Tana et al. [25]	2010	4	1	2	7
Kopecny and Simunek [27]	2002	2	1	2	5
Vernia et al. [28]	1987	2	1	2	5
Mortensen et al. [8]	1987	2	1	2	5
Yu et al. [30]	2016	2	1	2	5
Dunlop et al. [31]	2005	4	1	2	7
Thijssen et al. [32]	2015	4	1	2	7
Park et al. [29]	2009	4	1	2	7
Keszthelyi et al. [33]	2013	4	1	2	7

Selection includes four criteria: (1) is the determination of case adequate? (2) the representation of the cases, (3) the selection of the controls, (4) The determination of the controls; Comparability criteria include the Comparability of cases and controls is taken into account in design and statistical analysis; Exposure contains three criteria: (1) determination of exposure factors, (2) use the same method to determine the exposure factors in case and control group, (3) non-response rate

was − 0.01 (95% CI − 0.57–0.55), that of acetic acid was − 0.04 (95% CI − 0.55–0.47), that of propionic acid was 0.07 (95% CI − 0.45–0.60), and that of butyric acid was − 0.00 (95% CI − 0.49–0.49), as shown in Fig. 2a–d. There was significant heterogeneity in the studies included, with I^2 values over 50%.

As shown in Fig. 2e, the SMD of 5-HT in IBS patients was 2.35 (95% CI 0.46–4.24). There was also significant heterogeneity in the studies included, with an I^2 value of 97%.

Analysis of funnel plots for publication bias

As shown in Fig. 3a–e, funnel plots were used to assess publication bias among the studies included. However, as the number of included studies was below 10, the ability of these funnel plots to detect publication bias is limited.

Discussion

In recent years, alterations in bidirectional brain-gut interactions have been considered to play a vital role in IBS and some related functional gastrointestinal diseases [18, 54]. Alterations in the gut microbiota have also been confirmed as mechanisms of IBS pathogenesis worldwide [3]. It has been generally accepted that a stable gut microbiota is essential for normal gut physiology and contributes to appropriate signaling along the brain-gut axis [55]. SCFAs, as the main metabolites of the gut microbiota, and 5-HT, as an important regulatory factor of the brain-gut axis, may be involved in the abnormal BGM axis of IBS. Alterations in SCFAs in feces and 5-HT in blood have been found in IBS patients in some studies [27, 28, 30–32]. This is the first meta-analysis to explore the alterations in SCFAs and 5-HT in IBS, and some interesting findings were observed in our meta-analysis. We found that 5-HT levels in the blood in IBS patients were increased compared to those in HCs. However, we found no significant differences in SCFAs in feces between IBS patients and HCs.

Ninety-five percent of human 5-HT comes from the intestines, mainly the intestinal EC cells of the mucous layer, which contains tryptophan hydroxylase (TPH), necessary for the synthesis of 5-HT. The release of 5-HT in EC cells is sensitive to the pressure and chemical stimulation in the lumen [56]. In our study, we found that 5-HT levels were increased in the blood in IBS patients compared to those in HCs. Only one study by Dunlop et al. [31] reported lower 5-HT levels in IBS patients. In the 5 studies on 5-HT in our meta-analysis, all researchers used high-pressure liquid chromatography (HPLC) to measure 5-HT levels in subjects. However, their findings were inconsistent, which may imply that the HPLC method is unstable and has poor repeatability. We did not analyze 5-HT levels among different subtypes of IBS patients in our study. However, some studies have found that differential alterations in 5-HT in various IBS subtypes. Atkinson et al. [9] reported that 5-HT levels were reduced in patients with constipation-predominant IBS (IBS-C). Bearcroft et al. [10] and Houghton et al. [24] found increased 5-HT levels in patients with diarrhea-predominant IBS (IBS-D). These inconsistent findings indicate that alterations in 5-HT may be related to the symptoms of constipation or diarrhea in IBS patients. Houghton et al. [24] also reported that food intake could stimulate colonic motor activity, alter visceral sensitivity, increase blood 5-HT levels, and lead to abdominal pain or diarrhea in IBS patients. Hence, we speculate that alterations in 5-HT may be related to IBS pathogenesis. Our findings support the idea that 5-HT may be a therapeutic target for IBS. In fact, some drugs that act on 5-HT signaling

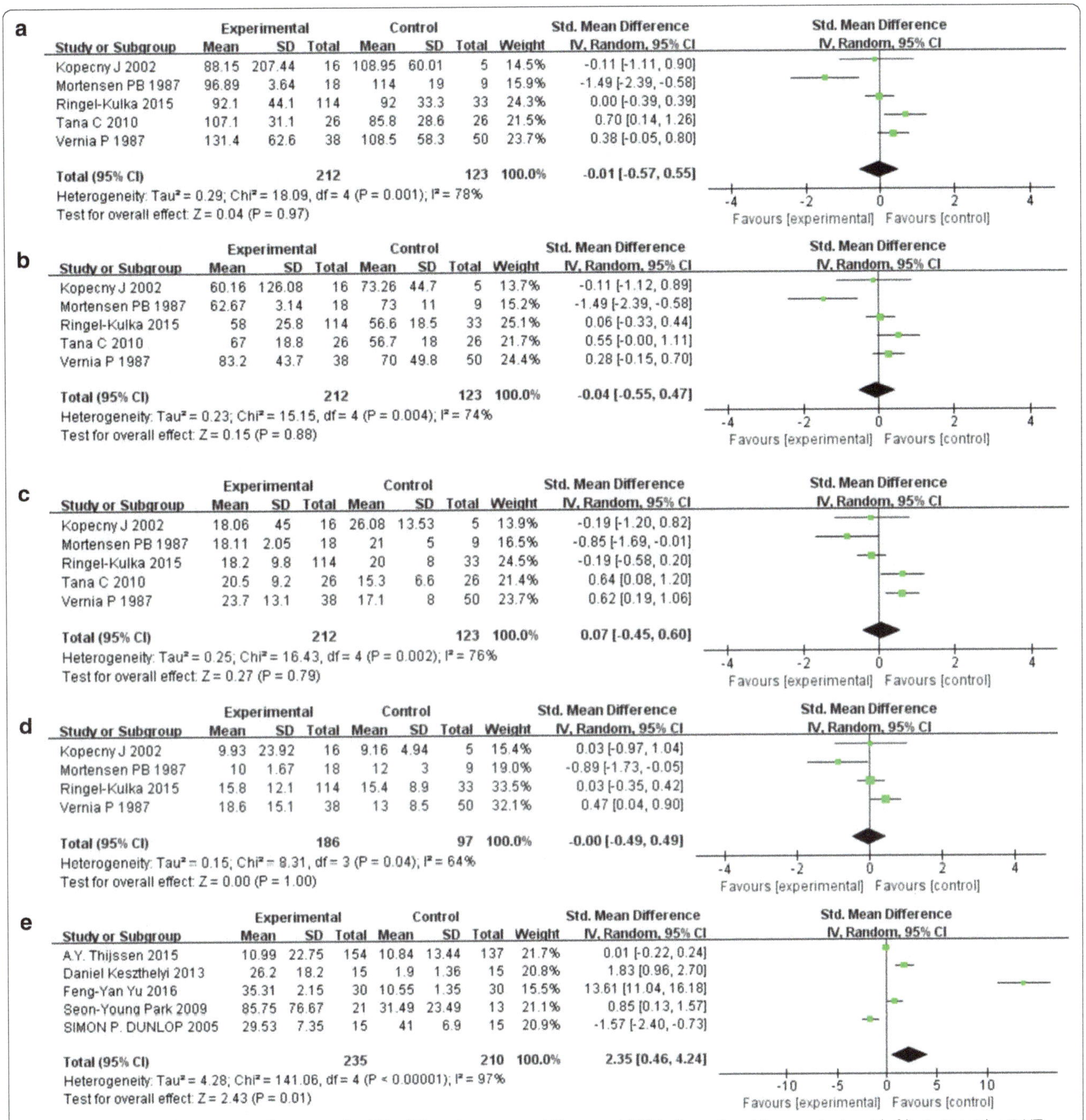

Fig. 2 Forest plots of alterations of SCFAs and 5-HT in IBS patients versus HCs: **a** total SCFAs, **b** acetic acid, **c** propionic acid, **d** butyric acid, **e** 5-HT

are currently used to treat IBS. Tegaserod, a 5-HT4 partial agonist and alosetron, a 5-HT3 antagonist is used in IBS-C and IBS-D to relieve symptoms, respectively. Other agents regulating the levels of 5-HT, such as tricyclic antidepressants and serotonin selective reuptake inhibitors, have also been used in some patients with IBS [56]. Although we found differences in 5-HT levels in blood between IBS patients and HCs, further studies to explore the correlation between altered 5-HT levels and IBS symptoms are warranted.

SCFAs are a type of saturated fatty acids which including acetic acid, propionic acid, butyric acid, isobutyric acid, isopentoic acid, caproic acid, and isocaproic acid. The main SCFAs distributed in the intestines are acetic acid, propionic acid, and butyric acid. Most SCFAs are absorbed by the intestines, while only low levels of

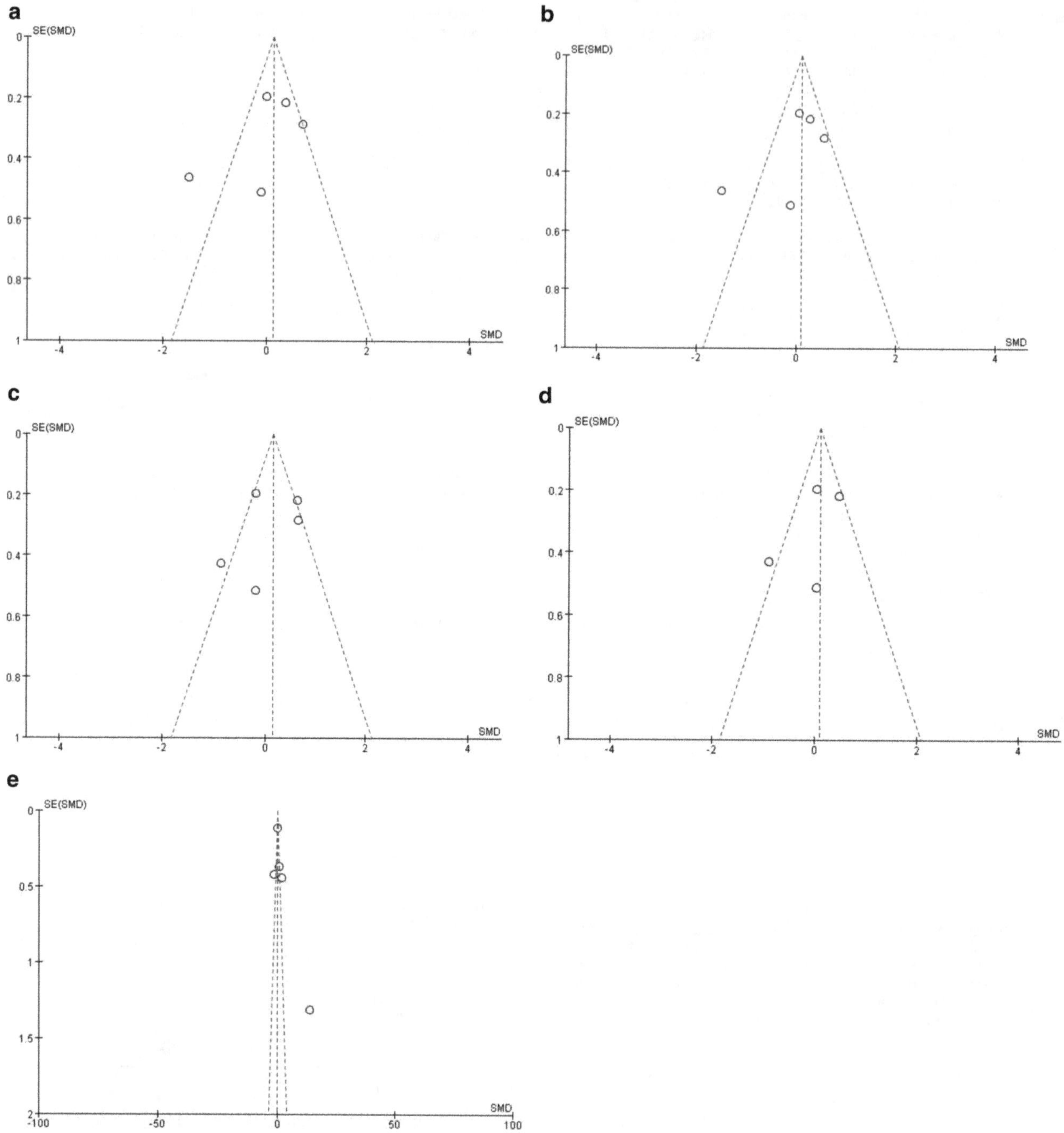

Fig. 3 Funnel plots of alterations of SCFAs and 5-HT in IBS patients versus HCs: **a** total SCFAs, **b** acetic acid, **c** propionic acid, **d** butyric acid, **e** 5-HT

SCFAs escape absorption and can be detected in fecal samples [57]. In our study, we found there were no significant differences in total SCFAs in the feces between the IBS patients and HCs from the available data. We then explored differences in acetic acid, propionic acid, and butyric acid between IBS patients and HCs. Similarly, there were no significant differences in acetic acid, propionic acid, or butyric acid between IBS patients and HCs. Although there were no significant alterations in SCFAs in IBS patients, some studies have reported that SCFAs are altered in the feces of IBS patients [25, 27, 28]. Tana et al. [25] found that levels of acetic acid, propionic acid, and total SCFAs were significantly higher in IBS patients than in controls. These findings were similar to the results reported by Vernia et al. [28]. However, Kopecny et al. [27] found that the fecal SCFAs of IBS patients were characterized by lower levels of total SCFAs, acetic acid, and propionic acid and by higher levels of butyric acid. Although there is no consensus regarding alterations in SCFAs in IBS patients, the altered SCFAs reported in the abovementioned studies may imply their involvement in the pathogenesis of IBS. Interestingly, some studies have reported that SCFAs are associated with symptoms in IBS patients. Soret et al. [58] found that SCFAs could induce plasticity of intestinal myometrial neurons and promote colonic motility, which may cause diarrhea in IBS patients. In addition, Cherbut et al. [59] and Grider et al. [60] reported that the activity of SCFAs in regulating colonic motility may be affected by their concentrations. Thus, a low concentration (10–100 mmol L^{-1}) of SCFAs could increase colonic motility or have no effect, while a high concentration (>100 mmol L^{-1}) of SCFAs could inhibit colonic motility. Maintenance of gut microbiota homeostasis could release SCFAs to maintain intestinal mucosal permeability [61]. Dysbiosis of the gut microbiota may lead to insufficient SCFA intake in IBS patients, which directly constrains the distribution of compact connexin and then increases intestinal mucosal permeability [62]. Regulating SCFAs through the intestinal microenvironment may be a potential therapeutic target for IBS. Clinical trials have found that relevant SCFA products can improve IBS symptoms; for example, sodium butyrate reduced visceral pain in IBS patients [53, 63]. Although some studies have reported alterations in SCFAs in feces of IBS patients and the association of these alterations with symptoms in IBS patients, we found no significant differences in SCFA levels in feces in IBS patients and HCs in our meta-analysis. This implies that the gut microbiota may be involved in the pathogenesis of IBS through pathways other than SCFAs, such as alterations in immune profiles, effects on the CNS, or modulation of the gut neuromuscular function [62], or most SCFAs are absorbed in the colon and the analyzed results from feces are not representative for SCFAs in other parts of the gastrointestinal tract. However, the lack of significant differences in SCFAs between IBS patients and HCs in our meta-analysis may also be due to inadequate sample sizes in the original studies. The analytical methods or samples used to measure SCFA levels also need improvement and optimization in future studies.

As our study indicated that the 5-HT was increased in blood with IBS patients. 5-HT is the significant signaling molecule in the BGM axis and Clarke et al. [64] found the gut microbiota regulated the synthesis of 5-HT in CNS, which might further suggest that the disorder of the BGM axis may be the pathogenesis of IBS.

There are some limitations to our study. First, the statistical heterogeneity was significant among the included studies. This could be explained by differences in analytical methods, sample size, and diagnostic criteria for IBS in the included studies. Second, some studies used intestinal mucosal tissues as samples to analyze 5-HT levels in IBS patients and HCs [33, 40–45]. Data from these studies could not be processed effectively and were not included in our meta-analysis. This may lead to a bias in our meta-analysis results. Lastly, there are four subtypes of IBS, including IBS-C and IBS-D. However, our meta-analysis did not analyze the various subtypes of IBS owing to the limited number of samples but just analyze the IBS-D, the validity of the results could be questioned. More complete profiles of alterations in fecal, blood, or mucosal metabolites in various IBS subtypes are need for a better understanding of their roles in the BGM axis of IBS.

Conclusions

In conclusion, we found increased levels of 5-HT in IBS patients in our meta-analysis. However, there was no significant alteration of SCFAs between IBS patients and HCs. Our findings imply that alterations in 5-HT may be associated with the pathogenesis of IBS and affect the symptoms of IBS patients. Although we found no significant differences in SCFAs between IBS patients and HCs in our meta-analysis, some studies have reported that SCFAs are altered in IBS; such alterations in SCFAs may be a potential mechanism for the development or maintenance of symptoms in IBS patients. The findings of our study warrant further exploration of the relationship between the BGM axis and IBS. Therefore, further studies involving advanced molecular techniques and more strict experimental design are needed to explore alterations in SCFAs in IBS patients, which study samples would not just confined to feces.

Abbreviations

SCFAs: Short-chain fatty acids; 5-HT: 5-Hydroxytryptamine; IBS: Irritable bowel syndrome; BGM: Brain-gut-microbiota; SMDs: Standardized mean differences; CIs: Confidence intervals; HCs: Healthy controls; CNS: Central nervous system; GIT: Gastrointestinal tract; ENS: Enteric nervous system; SMD: Standardized mean difference; CI: Confidence interval; TPH: Tryptophan hydroxylase; IBS-C: Patients with constipation-predominant IBS; IBS-D: Patients with diarrhea-predominant IBS.

Acknowledgements

None.

Authors' contributions

ML, XZ and LX conceived and designed the study; ML and XZ collected the data, refined the acquired data for inclusion and analysed the data; ZT assisted in data interpretation; ML, XZ and LX drafted the manuscript. All the authors have approved the final version of the manuscript.

References

1. Longstreth GF, Thompson WG, Chey WD, Houghton LA, Mearin F, Spiller RC. Functional bowel disorders. Gastroenterology. 2006;130:1480–91.
2. Xiong LS, Chen MH, Chen HX, Xu AG, Wang WA, Hu PJ. A population-based epidemiologic study of irritable bowel syndrome in South China: stratified randomized study by cluster sampling. Aliment Pharmacol Ther. 2004;19:1217–24.
3. Zhuang XJ, Xiong LS, Li L, Li M, Chen M. Alterations of gut microbiota in patients with irritable bowel syndrome: a systematic review and meta-analysis. J Gastroenterol Hepatol. 2017;32:28–38.
4. Zhuang XJ, Tian ZY, Li L, Zeng ZR, Chen MH, Xiong LS. Fecal microbiota alterations associated with diarrhea-predominant irritable bowel syndrome. Front Microbiol. 2018;9:1600.
5. Moraes-Filho JP, Quigley MM. The intestinal microbiota and the role of probiotics in irritable bowel syndrome: a review. Arq Gastroenterol. 2015;52:331–8.
6. Jeffery IB, Otoole PW, Ohman L, Claesson MJ, Deane J, Quigley EMM, et al. An irritable bowel syndrome subtype defined by species-specific alterations in faecal microbiota. Gut. 2012;61:997–1006.
7. Kim DY, Camilleri M. Serotonin: a mediator of the brain-gut connection. Am J Gastroenterol. 2000;95:2698–709.
8. Mortensen PB, Andersen JR, Arffmann S, Krag E. Short-chain fatty acids and the irritable bowel syndrome: the effect of wheat bran. Scand J Gastroenterol. 1987;22:185–92.
9. Atkinson W, Lockhart S, Whorwell PJ, Keevil B, Houghton LA. Altered 5-hydroxytryptamine signaling in patients with constipation- and diarrhea-predominant irritable bowel syndrome. Gastroenterology. 2006;130:34–43.
10. Bearcroft CP, Perrett D, Farthing MJ. Postprandial plasma 5-hydroxytryptamine in diarrhoea predominant irritable bowel syndrome: a pilot study. Gut. 1998;42:42–6.
11. Kennedy PJ, Cryan JF, Dinan TG, Clarke G. Irritable bowel syndrome: a microbiome-gut-brain axis disorder? World J Gastroenterol. 2014;20(39):14105–25.
12. Martin CR, Osadchiy V, Kalani A, Mayer EA. The brain-gut-microbiome axis. Cell Mol Gastroenterol Hepatol. 2018;6:133–48.
13. Grenham S, Clarke G, Cryan J, Dinan TG. Brain-gut-microbe communication in health and disease. Front Physiol. 2011;2:94.
14. Barbara G, Cremon C, Giorgio RD, Dothel G, Zecchi L, Bellacosa L, et al. Mechanisms underlying visceral hypersensitivity in irritable bowel syndrome. Curr Gastroenterol Rep. 2011;13:308–15.
15. Bixquert JM. Treatment of irritable bowel syndrome with probiotics: an etiopathogenic approach at last? Rev Esp Enferm Dig. 2009;101:553–64.
16. Lyra A, Rinttila T, Nikkila J, Kurikka LK, Kajander K, Malinen E, et al. Diarrhoea-predominant irritable bowel syndrome distinguishable by 16S rRNA gene phylotype quantification. World J Gastroenterol. 2009;15:5936–45.
17. Ohman L, Tornblom H, Simren M. Crosstalk at the mucosal border: importance of the gut microenvironment in IBS. Nat Rev Gastroenterol Hepatol. 2015;12:36–49.
18. Rhee SH, Pothoulakis C, Mayer EA. Principles and clinical implications of the brain-gut-enteric microbiota axis. Nat Rev Gastroenterol Hepatol. 2009;6:306–14.
19. Chassard C, Dapoigny M, Scott KP, Crouzet L, Delhomme C, Marquet P, et al. Functional dysbiosis within the gut microbiota of patients with constipated-irritable bowel syndrome. Aliment Pharmacol Ther. 2012;35:828–38.
20. Eswaran S, Muir J, Chey WD. Fiber and functional gastrointestinal disorders. Am J Gastroenterol. 2013;108:718–27.
21. Dass NB, John AK, Bassil AK, Crumbley CW, Whehee WR, Maurio FP, et al. The relationship between the effects of short chain fatty acids on intestinal motility in vitro and GPR43 receptor activation. Neurogastroenterol Motil. 2007;19:66–74.
22. Dinan TG, Cryan JF. The microbiome-gut-brain axis in health and disease. Gastroenterol Clin N Am. 2017;46:77–89.
23. King TS, Elia M, Hunter JO. Abnormal colonic fermentation in irritable bowel syndrome. Lancet. 1998;352:1187–9.
24. Houghton LA, Atkinson W, Whitaker RP, Whorwell PJ, Rimmer MJ. Increased platelet depleted plasma 5-hydroxytryptamine concentration following meal ingestion in symptomatic female subjects with diarrhoea predominant irritable bowel syndrome. Gut. 2003;52:663–70.
25. Tana C, Umesaki Y, Imaoka A, Handa T, Kanazawa M, Fukudo S. Altered profiles of intestinal microbiota and organic acids may be the origin of symptoms in irritable bowel syndrome. Neurogastroenterol Motil. 2010;22:512-e115.
26. Ringel-Kulk T, Choi CH, Temas D, Kim A, Maier DM, Scott K, et al. Altered colonic bacterial fermentation as a potential pathophysiological factor in irritable bowel syndrome. Am J Gastroenterol. 2015;110:1339–46.
27. Kopecny J, Simunek J. Cellulolytic bacteria in human gut and irritable bowel syndrom. Acta Vet Brno. 2002;71:421–7.
28. Vernia P, Latella G, Magliocca FM, Mancuso G, Caprilli R. Seeking clues for a positive diagnosis of the irritable bowel syndrome. Eur J Clin Investig. 1987;17:189–93.
29. Park SY, Park MH, Yoon KW, Cho SB, Lee WS, Park CH, et al. Plasma 5-hydroxytryptamine concentration and its correlation with psychopathology in patients with irritable bowel syndrome. Gut Liver. 2009;3:26–30.
30. Yu FY, Huang SG, Zhang HY, Ye H, Chi HG, Zou Y, et al. Comparison of 5-hydroxytryptophan signaling pathway characteristics in diarrhea-predominant irritable bowel syndrome and ulcerative colitis. World J Gastroenterol. 2016;22:3451–9.
31. Dunlop SP, Coleman NS, Blackshaw E, Perkins AC, Singh G, Marsden CA, et al. Abnormalities of 5-hydroxytryptamine metabolism in irritable bowel syndrome. Clin Gastroenterol Hepatol. 2005;3:349–57.
32. Thijssen AY, Mujagic Z, Jonkers DM, Ludidi S, Keszthelyi D, Hesselink MA. Alterations in serotonin metabolism in the irritable bowel syndrome. Aliment Pharmacol Ther. 2016;43:272–82.
33. Keszthelyi D, Troost FJ, Jonkers DM, Kruimel JW, Leue C, Masclee AM. Decreased levels of kynurenic acid in the intestinal mucosa of IBS patients: Relation to serotonin and psychological state. J Psychosom Res. 2013;74:501–4.
34. Coates MD, Mahoney CR, Linden DR, Sampson JE, Chen J, Blaszyk H, et al. Molecular defects in mucosal serotonin content and decreased serotonin reuptake transporter in ulcerative colitis and irritable bowel syndrome. Gastroenterology. 2004;126:1657–64.
35. Cheung CKY, Lee YY, Chan Y, Cheong PK, Law WT, Lee SF, et al. Decreased basal and postprandial plasma serotonin levels in patients with functional dyspepsia. Clin Gastroenterol Hepatol. 2013;11:1125–9.
36. Faure C, Patey N, Gauthier C, Brooks EM, Mawe GM. Serotonin signaling is altered in irritable bowel syndrome with diarrhea but not in functional dyspepsia in pediatric age patients. Gastroenterology. 2010;139:249–58.
37. Kumar S, Ranjan P, Mittal B, Ghoshal UC. Serotonin transporter gene (SLC6A4) polymorphism in patients with irritable bowel syndrome and healthy controls. J Gastrointest Liver Dis. 2012;21:31–8.
38. Houghton LA, Atkinson W, Lockhart S, Fell C, Whorwell PJ, Keevil B. Sigmoid-colonic motility in health and irritable bowel syndrome: a role for 5-hydroxytryptamine. Neurogastroenterol Motil. 2007;19:724–31.
39. Stasi C, Bellini M, Gambaccini D, Duranti E, Bortoli ND, Fani B, et al. Neuroendocrine dysregulation in irritable bowel syndrome patients: a pilot study. J Neurogastroenterol. 2017;23:428–34.
40. Zuo XL, Li YQ, Yang XZ, Guo M, Guo YT, Lu XF, et al. Plasma and gastric mucosal 5-hydroxytryptamine concentrations following cold water intake in patients with diarrhea-predominant irritable bowel syndrome. J Gastroenterol Hepatol. 2007;22:2330–7.
41. Cremon C, Carini G, Wang BX, Vasina V, Cogliandro RF, Giorgio RD, et al. Intestinal serotonin release, sensory neuron activation, and abdominal pain in irritable bowel syndrome. Am J Gastroenterol. 2011;106:1290–8.
42. Kerckhoffs AP, Terlinde JJ, Akkermans LM, Samsom M. Trypsinogen IV, serotonin transporter transcript levels and serotonin content are increased in small intestine of irritable bowel syndrome patients. Neurogastroenterol Motil. 2008;20:900–7.
43. Wang SH, Dong L, Luo JH, Gong J, Li L, Lu XL, et al. Decreased expression of serotonin in the jejunum and increased numbers of mast cells in the terminal ileum in patients with irritable bowel syndrome. World J Gastroenterol. 2007;13:6041–7.
44. Miwa J, Echizen H, Matsueda K, Umeda N. Patients with constipation-predominant irritable bowel syndrome (IBS) may have elevated serotonin concentrations in colonic mucosa as compared with diarrhea-pre-

dominant patients and subjects with normal bowel habits. Digestion. 2001;63:188–94.
45. El-salhy M, Wendelbo I, GundersenU D. Serotonin and serotonin transporter in the rectum of patients with irritable bowel disease. Mol Med Rep. 2013;8:451–5.
46. Morken MH, Valeur J, Norin E, Midtvedt T, Nysaeter G, Berstad A. Antibiotic or bacterial therapy in post giardiasis irritable bowel syndrome. Scand J Gastroenterol. 2009;44:1296–303.
47. Treem WR, Ahsan N, Kastoff G, Hyams JS. Fecal short-chain fatty acids in patients with diarrhea-predominant irritable bowel syndrome: in vitro studies of carbohydrate fermentation. J Pediatr Gastroenterol Nutr. 1996;23:280–6.
48. Valeur J, Roseth AG, Knudsen T, Malmstrom GH, Fiennes JT, Midtvedt T, et al. Fecal fermentation in irritable bowel syndrome: influence of dietary restriction of fermentable oligosaccharides, disaccharides, monosaccharides and polyols. Digestion. 2016;94:50–6.
49. Kajander K, Krogius-kurikka L, Rinttila T, Karjalainen H, Palva A, Korpela R. Effects of multispecies probiotic supplementation on intestinal microbiota in irritable bowel syndrome. Aliment Pharmacol Ther. 2007;26:463–73.
50. Undseth R, Jakobsdottir G, Nyman M, Berstad A, Valeur J. Low serum levels of short-chain fatty acids after lactulose ingestion may indicate impaired colonic fermentation in patients with irritable bowel syndrome. Clin Exp Gastroenterol. 2015;8:303–8.
51. Cummings JH, Pomare EW, Branch HW, Naylor CP, Macfarlane GT. Short chain fatty acids in human large intestine, portal, hepatic and venous blood. Gut. 1987;28:1221–7.
52. Eastwood MA, Walton BA, Brydon WG, Anderson JR. Faecal weight, constituents, colonic motility, and lactose tolerance in the irritable bowel syndrome. Digestion. 1984;30:7–12.
53. Kang DW, DiBaise JK, Ilhan ZE, Crowell MD, Rideout JR, Caporaso JG, et al. Gut microbial and short-chain fatty acid profiles in adults with chronic constipation before and after treatment with lubiprostone. Anaerobe. 2015;33:33–41.
54. Mayer EA. Gut feelings: the emerging biology of gut-brain communication. Nat Rev Neurosci. 2011;12:453–66.
55. Cryan JF, Dinan TG. Mind-altering microorganisms: the impact of the gut microbiota on brain and behaviour. Nat Rev Neurosci. 2012;13:701–12.
56. Sikander A, Rana SV, Prasad KK. Role of serotonin in gastrointestinal motility and irritable bowel syndrome. Clin Chim Acta. 2009;403:47–55.
57. Besten GD, Eunen KV, Groen AK, Venema K, Reijngoud DJ, Bakkeret BM. The role of short-chain fatty acids in the interplay between diet, gut microbiota, and host energy metabolism. J Lipid Res. 2013;54:2325–40.
58. Soret R, Chevalier J, De Coppet P, Poupeau G, Derkinderen P, Segain JP, et al. Short-chain fatty acids regulate the en-teric neurons and control gastrointestinal motility in rats. Gastroenterology. 2010;138:1772–82.
59. Cherbut C, Ferrier L, Roze C, Anini Y, Blottiere H, Lecannu G, et al. Short-chain fatty acids modify colonic motility through nerves and polypeptide YY release in the rat. Am J Physiol. 1998;275:1415–22.
60. Grider JR, Piland BE. The peristaltic reflex induced by short-chain fatty acids is mediated by sequential release of 5-HT and neuronal CGRP but not BDNF. Am J Physiol Gastrointest Liver Physiol. 2007;292:429–37.
61. Suzuki T, Yoshida S, Hara H. Physiological concentrations of short-chain fatty acids immediately suppress colonic epithelial permeability. Br J Nutr. 2008;100:297–305.
62. Hyland NP, Quigley EM, Brint E. Microbiotahost interactions in irritable bowel syndrome: epithelial barrier, immune regulation and braingut interactions. World J Gastroenterol. 2014;20:8859–66.
63. Banasiewicz T, Krokowicz L, Stojcev Z, Kaczmarek BF, Kaczmarek E, Maik J, et al. Microencapsulated sodium butyrate reduces the frequency of abdominal pain in patients with irritable bowel syndrome. Colorectal Dis. 2013;15:204–9.
64. Clarke G, Grenham S, Scully P, Fitzgerald P, Moloney RD, Shanahan F, et al. The microbiome-gut-brain axis during early life regulates the hippocampal serotonergic system in a sex-dependent manner. Mol Psychiatr. 2013;18:666–73.

Chaihu-Guizhi-Ganjiang Decoction is more efficacious in treating irritable bowel syndrome than Dicetel according to metabolomics analysis

Mingming Li[1,2†], Jiawei Zhu[1†], Xuan Liu[3†], Zhiying Dong[1], Jigui Tang[3], Cian Zhang[3], Jianpeng Jiao[3], Jiani Chen[2], Fenghao Yin[4], Shi Qiu[5], Feng Zhang[2,6], Shouhong Gao[2,6], Zhipeng Wang[2], Xia Tao[2], Xiaoqiang Yue[3*], Lianna Sun[1*] and Wansheng Chen[1,2,5,6*]

Abstract

Background: Chaihu-Guizhi-Ganjiang Decoction (CGGD) is a traditional Chinese medicine (TCM) prescription used to treat viral influenza. There is evidence that CGGD can be used to treat irritable bowel syndrome (IBS) but the potential mechanism of action and metabolites produced upon CGGD treatment remains elusive.

Methods: Patients with IBS were treated with pinaverium bromide (Dicetel™) and then CGGD after a washout period of 1 week. Both treatments lasted for 30 days. The efficacy and changes of metabolites in plasma after the two treatments were compared. Plasma samples were acquired before and after each treatment, and untargeted metabolics analysis was performed.

Results: Efficacy was measured according to the Rome IV criteria and TCM theory. Our results indicated that CGGD showed significantly better efficacy than Dicetel in the treatment of IBS utilizing each criterion. CGGD exerted greater effects on plasma metabolism than Dicetel. Dicetel treatment led to increased tryptophan metabolism (increased levels of 5-Hydroxyindoleacetaldehyde) and increased protein metabolism (increased levels of L-arginine). CGGD treatment significantly ($p < 0.05$) increased carnitine metabolism, with elevated levels of L-carnitine and acylcarnitine in plasma. Such changes in these metabolites could exert effects against IBS by improving gastrointestinal motility and suppressing pain, depression, and inflammation.

Conclusions: CGGD appeared to be more efficacious than Dicetel for treating patients with IBS. The findings provide a sound support for the underlying biomolecular mechanism of CGGD in the prevention and treatment of IBS.

Keywords: Irritable bowel syndrome, Metabolomics analysis, Chaihu-Guizhi-Ganjiang Decoction, Dicetel, Carnitine

[†]Mingming Li, Jiawei Zhu and Xuan Liu have contributed equally to this work

*Correspondence: yuexiaoqiang@163.com; sssnmr@163.com; chenwansheng@smmu.edu.cn

[1] School of Pharmacy, Shanghai University of Traditional Chinese Medicine, Shanghai 201203, People's Republic of China
[2] Department of Pharmacy, Second Affiliated Hospital of Naval Medical University, Shanghai 200003, China
[3] Department of Traditional Chinese Medicine, Second Affiliated Hospital of Naval Medical University, Shanghai 200003, China
Full list of author information is available at the end of the article

Background

Irritable bowel syndrome (IBS) is a debilitating, chronic, and highly prevalent disorder of gut–brain interaction [1, 2]. In routine clinical practice, IBS symptoms include recurrent disordered defecation and abdominal pain [3].

According to the Rome IV criteria, IBS is defined as that patients with IBS recurrent abdominal pain symptoms at least once a week on average [4]. The Rome IV criteria were derived by consensus from a multinational group of experts in disorders of gut–brain interaction [4].

IBS is a common disease with a prevalence of approximately 4.4–4.8% in the USA, UK, and Canada. IBS is more common in females and individuals younger than 50 years [5]. IBS is a highly burdensome condition for healthcare systems, families, and society worldwide. Direct medical costs attributed to IBS in the USA (excluding prescription and over-the-counter medications) have been estimated to be $1.5–$10 billion per year [6]. The direct and indirect costs related to IBS has been estimated to be up to ¥123 billion in China [7]. According to a meta-analysis of 80 clinical studies involving 260,960 individuals in 2012 [8], the IBS prevalence in China was 6.5%. The overall prevalence of IBS in the Chinese population was $\leq 10\%$ in 2016, and the peak age of onset was 30–59 years. Female gender, alcohol drinking, history of intestinal infection, anxiety, depression, or food allergy, and certain living conditions are risk factors for Chinese IBS patients [8–11]. Therefore, the prevention and treatment of IBS is quite important.

The factors leading to susceptibility to IBS are diverse. Despite clearly established symptoms, the pathology of IBS is complicated and loosely understood. In general, it is believed that IBS is a result of a combination of multiple factors, including mental/psychological disorders, visceral hypersensitivity, intestinal infection, and disorders in gastrointestinal (GI) motility [12–14]. In routine practice, drugs such as pinaverium bromide (Dicetel™) and Alosetron™ play roles in intestinal movement. These medication diminish visceral hypersensitivity, improve emotions, and regulate intestinal flora. Dicetel and Alosetron are used commonly to relieve IBS symptoms [15–18]. Dicetel reduces the plateau phase of slow waves in the electrical activity of the smooth muscle cells, thereby inhibiting influx of calcium ions (Ca2+) and preventing consequent contractions of intestinal smooth muscle [19, 20]. Therefore, Dicetel is recommended as a first-line therapy for short-term relief from IBS symptoms [21]. However, due to side effects over a long-term use of Dicetel and Alosetron, efficacious therapy of IBS warrants further investigation.

Traditional Chinese medicine (TCM) formulations have shown favorable effects in IBS treatment [22–24]. According to TCM theory, the etiology of IBS is attributed mainly to the weakness of Pi (spleen) and Wei (stomach) or damage to the Gan (liver) [7, 25], which is summarized as "Dan Re Pi Han" in TCM theory.

Recently, Chaihu Guizhi Ganjiang Decoction (CGGD) has been developed and used to treat liver/spleen deficiency, abdominal pain, and diarrhea [26]. CGGD is composed of Chinese thorowax, Ramulus cinnamomi, Rhizoma Zingiberis, root of Trichosanthes species, Scutellaria baicalensis, oyster shell, and Radix Glycyrrhizae Preparata. CGGD has been shown to have a promising effect against IBS, but its underlying pharmacological mechanism of action remains elusive.

Metabolomics is a comprehensive study of low-molecular-weight metabolites in biological systems, which offers extensive phenotypic information not available by genetic testing [27]. TCM theory focus on the diagnosis and treatment of diseases based on understanding of the overall dynamic state of patients. Hence, metabolomics analysis could provide more direct and important information for deciphering the pharmacological mechanism of action of TCM formulations [28]. Up to now, several studies of CGGD have been reported; however, the effect of CGGD on the plasma metabolome in IBS patients remains unclear.

In this study, we determined the effect of CGGD against IBS compared with that of Dicetel. Moreover, we analyzed the effect of CGGD on the plasma metabolome in IBS patients and explored the potential pharmacological mechanism of action of CGGD against IBS.

Materials and methods

Ethical approval of the study protocol

The study protocol was granted by the Biomedical Research Ethics Committee of Shanghai Changzheng Hospital (Shanghai, China) (No. 2019SL033). Written informed consent was obtained from all participants in the study [10].

Study design

This was a prospective study (Fig. 1A). Patients were treated with two drugs successively and divided into two groups: the positive drug group (Dicetel) and the CGGD control group. The duration of these two treatments was 1 month. A washout period of 1 week was setup to determine the Symptom Index score. The plasma samples of patients were collected across four time periods.

Diagnosis of IBS

The diagnosis of IBS was based on the Rome IV criteria. The typical clinical manifestations of IBS are recurrent abdominal pain (≥ 1 day a week in the last

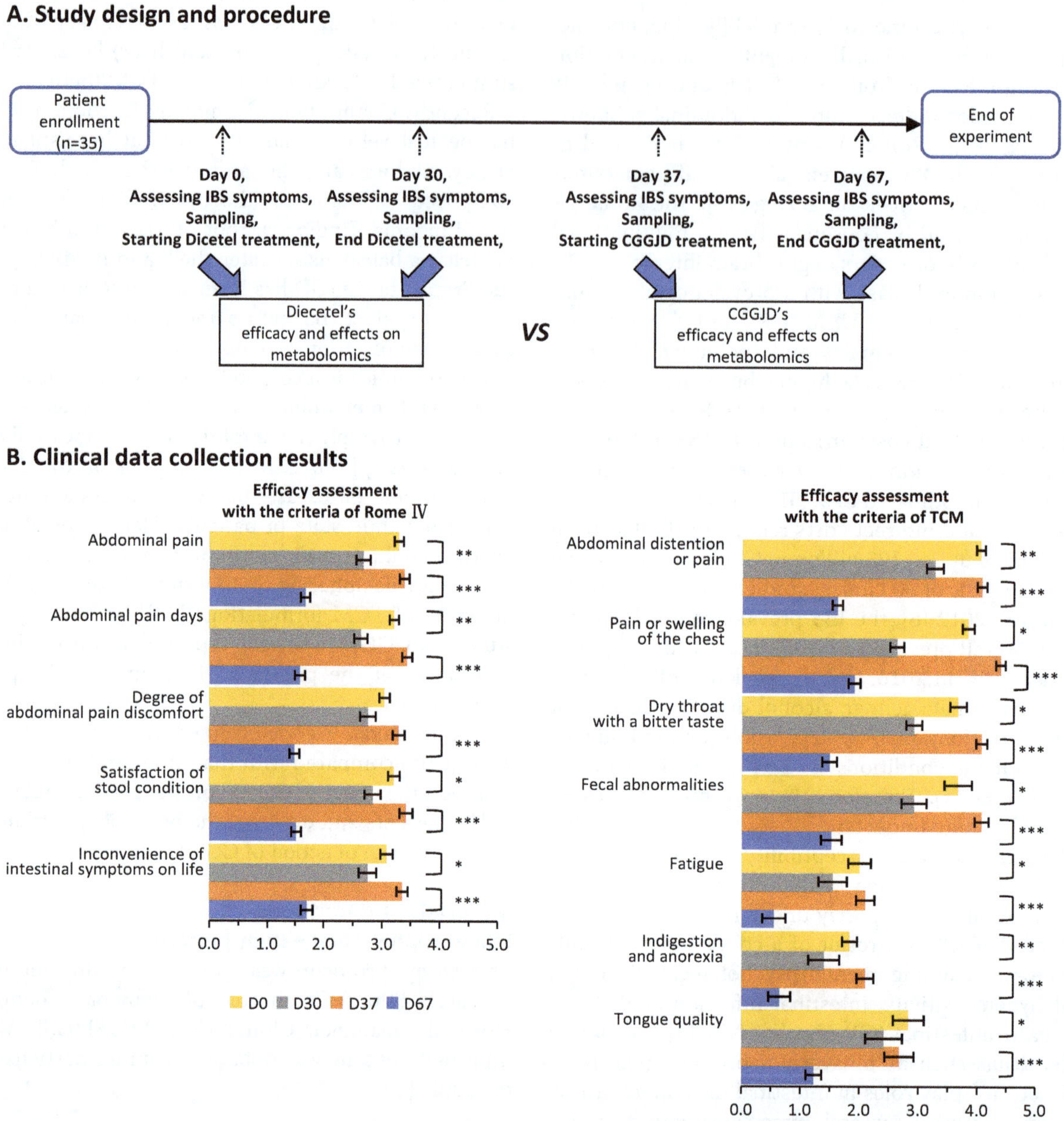

Fig. 1 Experimental design and collection of clinical data. **A** Study design. Patients were enrolled for eligibility assessment based on inclusion criteria. Thirty-five patients were enrolled. "D0–D30" denotes from Day 0 (D0) to Day 30 (D30), and represents differences in patients before and after Dicetel treatment in terms of the Symptom Index score as well as collected blood samples before and after treatment. Eventually, 24 patients provided Discomfort Index scores before and after treatment. D37–D67 represents differences in patients before and after CGGD treatment in terms of the Symptom Index score and collected blood samples before and after treatment. In the middle of these two periods is a 1-week washout period. Thirty-one patients provided scores for the Discomfort Index before and after treatment. "D30 vs. D0" denotes the procedure of exploring the therapeutic effect of Dicetel and the effect of the human metabolome. "D67 vs. D37" refers to the procedure of exploring the therapeutic effect of CGGD and the effect of the human metabolome. **B** Clinical data. The numerical mean of the Symptom Index score and error bar, and P-value are shown. *Represents differences between different groups of the same target. *$p < 0.05$, **$p < 0.01$, ***$p < 0.001$. P-value was calculated by the Student's t-test. Y-axis represents the symptom under different criteria. The X-axis represents the average Symptom Index score when taking different drugs at different stages. Criteria are divided into Rome IV and TCM. The Symptom Index score of patients under different criteria (Rome IV or TCM) is selected, followed by selected by different reference indicators under these two criteria (Additional file 1: Table S1). First, the enrollment time was recorded as "D0" and the Symptom Index was recorded. Second, after 4 weeks of treatment with Dicetel, the Symptom Index score of patients condition at this time was recorded as "D30". Third, after the washout period (1 week), the Symptom Index score was recorded as "D37". Finally, after 4 weeks of treatment with CGGD, the Symptom Index score was recorded as "D67"

3 months) accompanied by changes in defecation frequency and fecal traits (appearance). Symptoms appear for ≥ 6 months and persist for the previous 3 months [29].

The diagnosis of IBS based on TCM theory was also used for efficacy evaluation. It was formulated according to the *Clinical research of new Chinese medicine and the consensus of TCM Diagnosis* [30] and *Treatment of irritable bowel syndrome* (2017) [31]. The main criteria were: (1) pain or swelling of the chest; (2) distension/pain in the abdomen, emotional relapse/aggravation; (3) fecal abnormalities; (4) dry throat with a bitter taste, or dizziness. Secondary criteria were: (i) indigestion and anorexia; (ii) fatigue; (iii) tongue quality. Patients with (3) and at least one of (1), (2), or (4) of the main criteria were diagnosed as having IBS. Patients with two features of secondary criteria and more than one of (1), (2) and (4) of the main criteria were assessed to have IBS.

Inclusion criteria

The inclusion criteria were: (1) meeting the diagnostic criteria for IBS; (2) aged between 18 and 75 years old; (3) providing written informed consent to participate in the study.

Exclusion criteria

The exclusion criteria were: (1) constipation in IBS; (2) patients with other chronic or serious diseases (e.g., heart disease, renal failure); (3) patients with other diseases that affect normal physician–patient communication; (4) combination of two or more diseases meeting the inclusion criteria; (5) long-term use of similar drugs used in our study.

Elimination criteria

The criteria for elimination from this study were: (1) patients failing to receive medication as planned; (2) patients taking drugs other than the study drugs (including TCM formulations or drugs with anti-tumor effects); (3) treatment ceased due to suspected safety issues.

Collection of plasma samples and treatment

Thirty-three patients aged 23–72 years diagnosed with IBS were enrolled from 2020 to 2021. The study lasted for 17 weeks as follows: Dicetel treatment (4 weeks), washout period (1 week), CGGD treatment (4 weeks), and follow-up (8 weeks). During the entire observation period, living conditions and dietary habits remain unchanged according to self-reporting by patients (Table 1).

Patients were treated with Dicetel (50 mg, t.d.s., p.o. [with food]; Abbott Healthcare SAS, Paris, France). The treatment spanned 4 weeks, followed by 1 week of rest without treatment. Then, they were treated with CGGD (1 bag, t.d.s., p.o. [post-prandial]; Guangdong Yifang Pharmaceuticals, Foshan, Guangdong) for 4 weeks. Before and after each treatment, the Discomfort Index of patients according to TCM theory and the Rome IV criteria was obtained. The Discomfort Index was completed by patients and follow-up was conducted in the outpatient setting, inpatient setting, and by telephone consultation. Data input and verification were completed and checked by two individual researchers. Finally, clinical data were obtained for statistical analyses and clinical observations were recorded.

Table 1 Basic information of patients

Age (years)	
< 50	30
50–59	4
60–69	2
> =70	2
Sex	
Male	23
Female	15
Total	38

Simultaneously, plasma samples (5 mL) from each patient at D0 (before Dicetel treatment), D30 (after Dicetel treatment), D37 (before CGGD treatment), and D67 (after CGGD treatment) were collected. Samples were stored at − 80 °C for subsequent analyses.

Metabolomics analysis

Untargeted metabolomic analysis was modified according to our previous work [32]. Sample pretreatment was carried out by protein precipitation. Ultra-high-performance liquid chromatography-quadruple-time of flight-mass spectrometry (UHPLC-Q-TOF–MS) was undertaken on a 1290 Series UHPLC system (Agilent Technologies, Santa Clara, CA, USA) coupled with a 6530 Accurate-Mass Q-TOF LC/MS system (Agilent Technologies) in positive electrospray-ionization mode (Dual Jet Stream; Agilent Technologies).

For chromatography analysis, metabolites separation was performed using a HSS T3 (3.5 μm, 2.1 × 100 mm) column (Waters, Milford, MA, USA), and the flow rate was maintained at 0.4 mL/min. The mobile phase A was water with formic acid (0.1% v/v), and mobile phase B was acetonitrile with formic acid (0.1% v/v). The temperature was maintained at 30 °C. The gradient started with 5% B, increased to 10% at 3.5 min, 40% at 6 min, 60% at 16 min, 80% at 20 min, 100% at 20.3 min, and a post-run of 5 min. The injection volume was 3 μL. The results of chromatography analysis are shown in the Additional files 2.

For mass spectrometry analysis, the capillary voltage was 3500 V, and the nozzle voltage was 500 V. The gas temperature was set at 300 °C with a gas flow of 11 L/min and nebulizer pressure of 35 psi; and a sheath gas temperature was set at 300 °C with a sheath gas flow of 11 L/min. For MS acquisition, centroid data were acquired from 100 to 1100 m/z at 0.5-s intervals. For MS/MS acquisition, data were obtained from 0.33-s intervals with collision energy 0, 10, 20 and 40 eV. A reference solution (m/z 121.0509 and m/z 922.0098) was used to correct small mass drifts during the acquisition [33]. Quality control (QC) samples were injected at the beginning of the run and after every eight samples during sequence analysis to assess the analytical performance [34]. The basic information of results of mass spectrometry analysis are shown in the Additional files 3.

Statistical analyses

Semi-quantitative levels of the plasma metabolome were extracted by MS-DIAL 4.48 (http://prime.psc.riken.jp). All ions were normalized to the internal standard. Ion peaks with a coefficient of variation < 30% in QC samples and co-expressed with additional ions were filtered. The filtered ions were identified by MSFINDER 3.50 (http://prime.psc.riken.jp). Metabolites with the highest identification score encoded by the Human Metabolome Database (https://hmdb.ca) and METLIN (http://metlin.scripps.edu/) were selected for subsequent analyses. Then, data were processed through multiple steps: (1) quantile normalization, (2) $\log_2$ transformation, (3) Pareto Norm sequentially, (4) IQR filtering of metabolites with large within-group variances, and (5) data imputation using K-nearest neighbor [35]. Differential analyses were performed using limma [36]. All clinical covariates were adjusted. Gephi v0.9.2 (https://gephi.org) was used to generate a network based on the results of correlation analyses [37]. The Student's t-test was used to screen CGGD- and Dicetel-related endogenous metabolites. Statistical analyses were carried out using R software (v3.6.3), and $P < 0.05$ was considered to indicate statistical significance. The code of R are shown in the Additional files 4, 5, and 6.

Results

Beneficial effect of CGGD against IBS compared with Dicetel

CGGD showed significantly better efficacy than Dicetel against IBS, according to whether the Rome IV criteria or TCM theory. Efficacy assessment according to the Rome IV criteria is based on five criteria (Fig. 1B): Dicetel improved four of the symptoms and CGGD improved all five ones. In addition, for each criterion, a greater statistical significance in the above changes from CGGD was observed compared with Dicetel. The maximal, median, and minimal degree in improvement of all Rome IV criteria for Dicetel was 0.63, 0.38, and 0.29, and for CGGD was 1.90, 1.81, and 1.64, respectively.

For Dicetel, the least-improved criterion was "Inconvenience of intestinal symptoms on life" (average Symptom Index score decreased from 3.08 to 2.75). The most-improved criterion was "Abdominal pain" (average Symptom Index score decreased from 3.29 to 2.65).

For CGGD, the least-improved criterion was "Satisfaction of stool condition" (average Symptom Index score decreased from 3.42 to 1.52). The most-improved criterion was "Abdominal pain" (average symptom index decreased from 3.29 to 2.65).

Similar results were obtained using TCM theory. Efficacy assessment using TCM theory contains seven criteria (Fig. 1B): Dicetel and CGGD improved all of them. For each criterion, CGGD caused larger changes with greater statistical significance than Dicetel. The maximal, median, and minimal degree of improvement of all TCM-theory criteria for Dicetel was 1.21, 0.75, and 0.42, and for CGGD was 2.58, 2.45, and 1.45, respectively.

For Dicetel, the least-improved criterion was "Tongue quality" (average Symptom Index score decreased from 2.83 to 2.42). The most-improved criterion was "Pain or swelling of the chest" (average Symptom Index decreased from 3.83 to 2.63).

For CGGD, the least-improved criterion was "Indigestion and anorexia" (average Symptom Index score decreased from 2.10 to 0.65). The most-improved criterion was "Dry throat with a bitter taste" (average symptom index decreased from 4.06 to 1.48).

Influence of Dicetel and CGGD on the plasma metabolome

A total of 643 plasma metabolites were identified using untargeted metabolome analysis. Among them, four categories of endogenous metabolites were related to the effect of Dicetel (significant difference between D30 vs. D0). The largest category was "organic acids and derivatives", which contained metabolites such as N-acetyltryptophan, and L-arginine. The second largest category was "lipids and lipid-like molecules", including metabolites such as malonylcarnitine (AC_4-OH) and pimelylcarnitine (AC_6-COOH). The third largest category was "organoheterocyclic compounds", containing metabolites such as 5-Hydroxyindoleacetaldehyde (5-HIAA). In line with this, the plasma levels of most of these metabolites were also increased upon Dicetel treatment.

Seven categories of endogenous metabolites were related to the effect of CGGD (significant difference between D67 vs. D37). The largest category was "lipids and lipid-like molecules", involving metabolites such as hydroxyisovaleroyl carnitine (AC_4–CH_3), 3-hydroxyoctanoyl carnitine (AC_8–OH), phosphatidylethanolamine (35:0), 3-hydroxydecanoyl carnitine (AC_{10}–OH), and phosphatidylcholine (40:7). The second largest category was "organic acids and derivatives", including metabolites such as L-arginine. The third largest category was "organoheterocyclic metabolites", which contained metabolites such as 5-HIAA. Consistently, the plasma levels of most of these metabolites were increased upon CGGD treatment.

According to principal components analysis (PCA) and partial least squares-discriminant analysis (PLS-DA) for these treatment effect-related metabolites, it was revealed that the CGGD-group samples showed better separation compared with the Dicetel-group samples (Fig. 1B). The first principal component (PC1) for the CGGD group and Dicetel group was 33.5%, 37.8% The PC1 of PLS-DA for the CGGD group and the Dicetel group was 32.6%, 36.5%, respectively.

Analysis of enrichment of biological pathways on CGGD and Dicetel-related differential metabolites

Differential metabolites were subjected to further analysis to reveal their biological function in a phenotypic context. In this way, we clarified the reason of the difference in efficacy between CGGD and Dicetel for treating IBS (Fig. 2).

Biological pathway enrichment was carried out using the Reactome Pathway Database (https://reactome.org/) for metabolites associated with efficacy in the Dicetel group and CGGD group (Fig. 3). Overall, the above metabolites enriched in pathways mainly regulate "Metabolism of amino acids and derivatives". All enriched biological pathways were upregulated in the CGGD group and Dicetel group (Fig. 3A). It is noteworthy that "Phase I—Functionalization of metabolites" and "Biological oxidations" were the shared biological pathways between the CGGD group and Dicetel group.

Furthermore, the metabolites from the shared biological pathways between the Dicetel group and CGGD group were subjected to subsequent analysis. 5-HIAA and arginine were enriched in the CGGD group and Dicetel group. Phenylethylamine (PEA) was enriched only in the CGGD group.

Correlation analyses between CGGD- and Dicetel-related differential metabolites

Correlation analysis and a metabolite-metabolite network were performed to assess the associations between CGGD- and Dicetel-related differential metabolites. Correlation analysis demonstrated that the most correlated metabolites in the Dicetel group were N-acetyltryptophan, AC_6-COOH, and arginine (Fig. 4A). The most correlated metabolites in the CGGD group were biotin sulfone, leucylproline, and AC_4-CH_3 (Fig. 4B). These highly correlated metabolites may have important roles in the pharmacological effect of Dicetel and CGGD against IBS.

Discussion

Conventional mechanism of action of IBS

Traditionally, the diagnosis of IBS has been based on identification of symptoms that correlate with several different syndromes associated with disorders such as IBS diarrhea, IBS constipation, functional diarrhea, functional constipation, chronic functional abdominal pain, or bloating [38]. Several peripheral and central mechanisms initiate disorders of GI motor and sensory functions leading to IBS symptoms [39]. The predominant pathophysiological mechanisms in IBS are abnormalities of gut smooth muscle, visceral hypersensitivity, and central nervous system (CNS) hypervigilance. IBS symptoms are not specific to a single etiologic mechanism but are manifestations of several peripheral mechanisms that perturb motor and sensory functions [39]. Our study lacked a healthy control group to elucidate directly the metabolomic basis of IBS, which should be conduct in the future. Nevertheless, anti-IBS drugs induced metabolomics changes in regulation of biological pathways based on abnormalities of gut smooth muscle and CNS

(See figure on next page.)
Fig. 2 Differences in metabolites after treatment with Dicetel and CGGD. **A** Number of metabolites associated with a significantly altered treatment effect. Patients was divided into a Dicetel group (D30 vs. D0) and CGGD group (D67 vs. D37). The part of the axis that is > 0 indicates the number of metabolites whose concentration exhibits an increasing trend. The part of the axis that is < 0 indicates the number of metabolites whose concentration exhibits a decreasing trend. The ordinate expresses a simplified "super-class" of metabolites. The abscissa expresses the number of these simplified super-classes exhibiting high/low expression at different stages. These metabolites were divided into seven species according to their superclass from an Internet website (https://hmdb.ca/): "benzenoids"; "lipids and lipid-like molecules"; "organic acids and their derivatives"; "organoheterocyclic metabolites"; "organic nitrogen metabolites"; "organic oxygen metabolites"; "alkaloids and their derivatives". **B** Sample distributions based on differences in efficacy-related metabolites. The positions of the different-colored spheres represent the distribution of different metabolites at different stages. PCA and PLS-DA plots using differential metabolites associated with treatment efficacy show different sample distributions in the Dicetel group and CGGD group

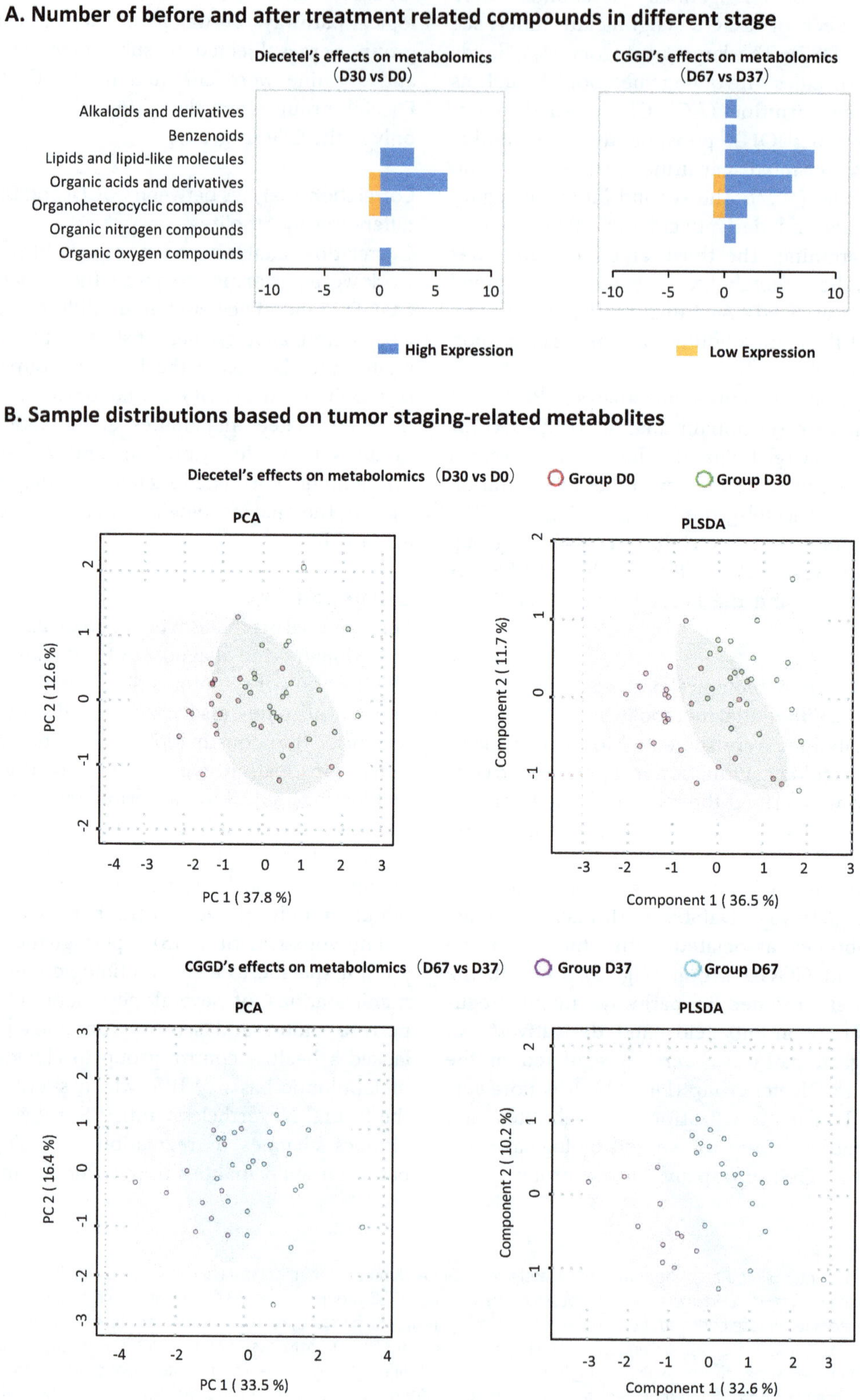

Fig. 2 (See legend on previous page.)

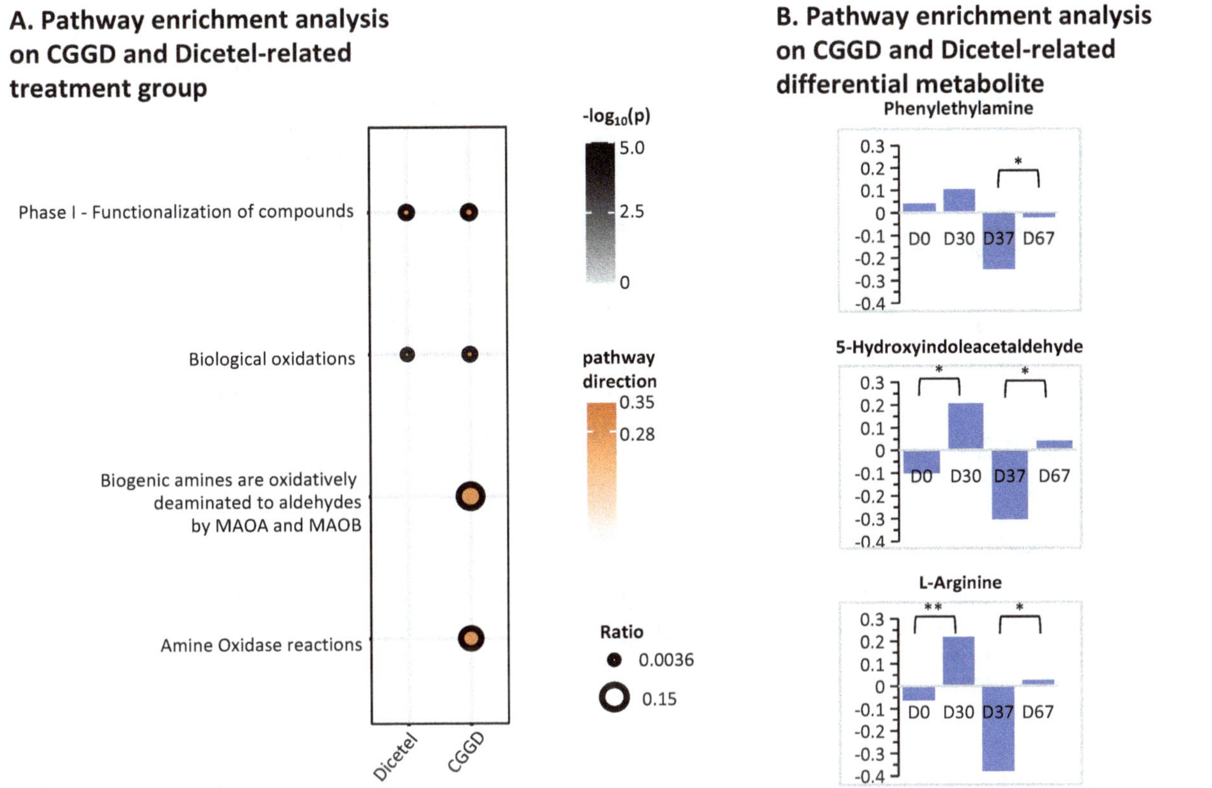

Fig. 3 Analysis of biological pathway enrichment. **A** Biological pathway enrichment analyses in the CGGD group and Dicetel group. The p-value was set at 0.05. The dot border color represents the significance value of pathway enrichment. "Pathway weight" is defined as the number of entities found/total number of entities. The size of the dot represents the pathway weight. "Pathway direction" is the median $\log_2$ fold change (FC) of metabolites in the pathway (red = upregulated). $*p < 0.05$ for D67 vs. D37 and D30 vs. D0. **B** Biological pathway enrichment analyses in the CGGD group and Dicetel group according to differential metabolites. The evaluation criteria were identical to those shown in Fig. 1B. The number on the Y-axis and length of the column represent the concentration of the metabolite at this stage. The X-axis represents the different stages (D0, D30, D37, and D67)

hypervigilance. These biological pathways included the metabolism of tryptophan, arginine, and L-carnitine-regulated lipid metabolism (Additional files 2, 3, 4, 5, 6).

Pharmacological mechanism of action of Dicetel in the body

Dicetel is a GI-selective antagonist of Ca^{2+} channels. It has highly selective spasmolytic activity in the GI tract. Dicetel helps to lessen the discomfort and abdominal pain associated with functional intestinal disturbances (e.g., IBS) by inhibiting Ca^{2+} influx into intestinal smooth muscle cells [40]. Dicetel also inhibits the contractile effect of digestive hormones and proinflammatory mediators such as cholecystokinin, gastrin, and substance P. These metabolites play a key part in the contraction of intestinal smooth muscles, and are linked to defecation-associated abdominal pain and discomfort in patients with IBS.

The beneficial effect of Dicetel arose from two biological pathways. First, Dicetel improved tryptophan metabolism, especially the production of 5-HIAA and N-acetyltryptophan (Fig. 5). Tryptophan can be converted to N-acetyltryptophan by N-Acetyltransferase or into 5-hydroxytryptophan (5-HTP) by tryptophan hydroxylase (TPH) 1 and TPH2. Dicetel is a blocker of L-type Ca^{2+} channels, and Ca^{2+} influx through L-type high-voltage-activated calcium channels is essential for full activation of TPH [19, 41]. Hence, inhibiting Ca^{2+} influx using Dicetel would lead to more N-acetyltryptophan. Conversely, 5-HTP can be converted to 5-hydroxytryptamine (5-HT). Once bound to target receptors or taken-up by 5-HT transporters, internalized 5-HT can be metabolized by monoamine oxidase, thereby leading to 5-HIAA generation. Often, the 5-HIAA concentration is used to detect changes in the whole-body 5-HT level [42]. An increased 5-HIAA level cannot be explained directly by the negative influence on TPH by Dicetel. Another compensatory mechanism (e.g., suppressed 5-HT internalization by cells) may also lead to an increased plasma level of 5-HIAA. The Ca^{2+}-channel blockers isradipine

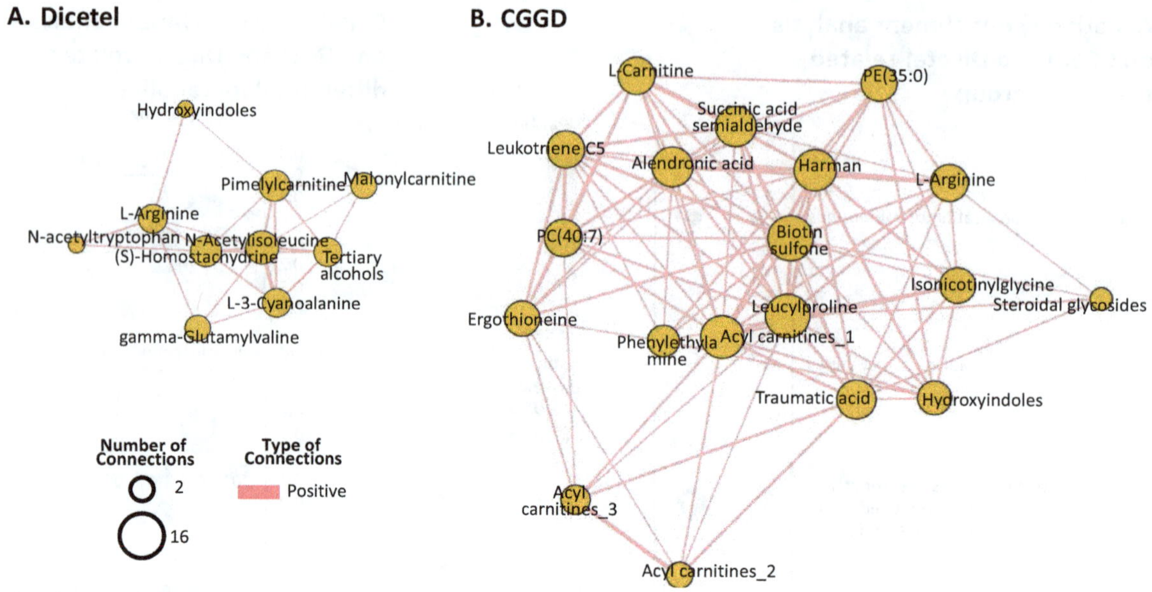

Fig. 4 Correlation analyses. The correlation network reflects the correlation of compounds in the certain pathway. The metabolite–metabolite correlation network comprised only paired metabolites with a significant correlations ($p \leq 0.05$). The degree of thickness, degree of edge, and diameter of the node show the importance of metabolites

and darodipine can increase the 5-HIAA: 5-HT ratio in mouse brains [43].

A low 5-HT level can cause depression [44], which is one of the causes leading to IBS. IBS has been postulated to be the most clinically important peripheral disease associated with 5-HT levels [45]. In addition, 5-HIAA and N-acetyltryptophan cause cell toxicity at high concentrations. 5-HIAA can inhibit the growth of the ovary cells of Chinese hamsters [46] and suppresses normal neuronal function by inducing production of oligomerized alpha-synuclein [47]. N-acetyltryptophan is classified as a "uremic toxin" if present in high abundance in sera or plasma [48, 49]. N-acetyltryptophan has been identified as a catabolite of tryptophan generated by the gut microbiota. After absorption through the intestinal epithelium, tryptophan catabolites enter the bloodstream and are excreted subsequently in urine [50]. Uremic toxins are a diverse group of endogenously produced molecules that, if not cleared appropriately or eliminated by the kidneys, can cause kidney damage, cardiovascular disease, and neurological deficits [51]. The overall negative influence of Dicetel on neurons may suppress IBS-related CNS hypervigilance, and improve GI motility and secretion of the enterochromaffin cells [52, 53].

Apart from tryptophan metabolism, Dicetel can alter the arginine level in blood, which can increase protein synthesis and suppress inflammation. These actions also help to relieve IBS symptoms [54].

Potential pharmacological mechanism of action of CGGD

CGGD has been used in the treatment of liver/spleen deficiency, abdominal pain, and diarrhea [26]. The potential pharmacological mechanism of action of CGGD is more extensive and complex than that of Dicetel. The beneficial effect of CGGD by regulating three biological pathways. Notably, in addition to increased metabolism of tryptophan and arginine (also documented for Dicetel), CGGD improved carnitine-mediated lipid metabolism.

With respect to tryptophan metabolism, CGGD could increase the blood level of PEA, which functions as a neuromodulator or neurotransmitter [55]. PEA is a direct stimulator of 5-HT biosynthesis, thereby regulating GI transit and colonic secretion in vivo and ex vivo. PEA can improve depression [56, 57]. It can activate the G-protein coupled receptor trace amine-associated receptor 1 (TAAR1) which, in turn, mediates 5-HT biosynthesis by stimulating TPH1/ amino acid decarboxylase activities. Zhai and colleagues [58] showed that PEA production stimulates 5-HT biosynthesis to accelerate GI transit via a TAAR1-dependent mechanism. They demonstrated that PEA could relieve constipation [58]. CGGD also increases the blood level of 5-HIAA, which can suppress CNS hypervigilance. baicalin and Chinese thorowax exert positive influence on the concentration of mono amines, including PEA and 5-HT, as reported in the previous study [59], but the exact biological mechanism is

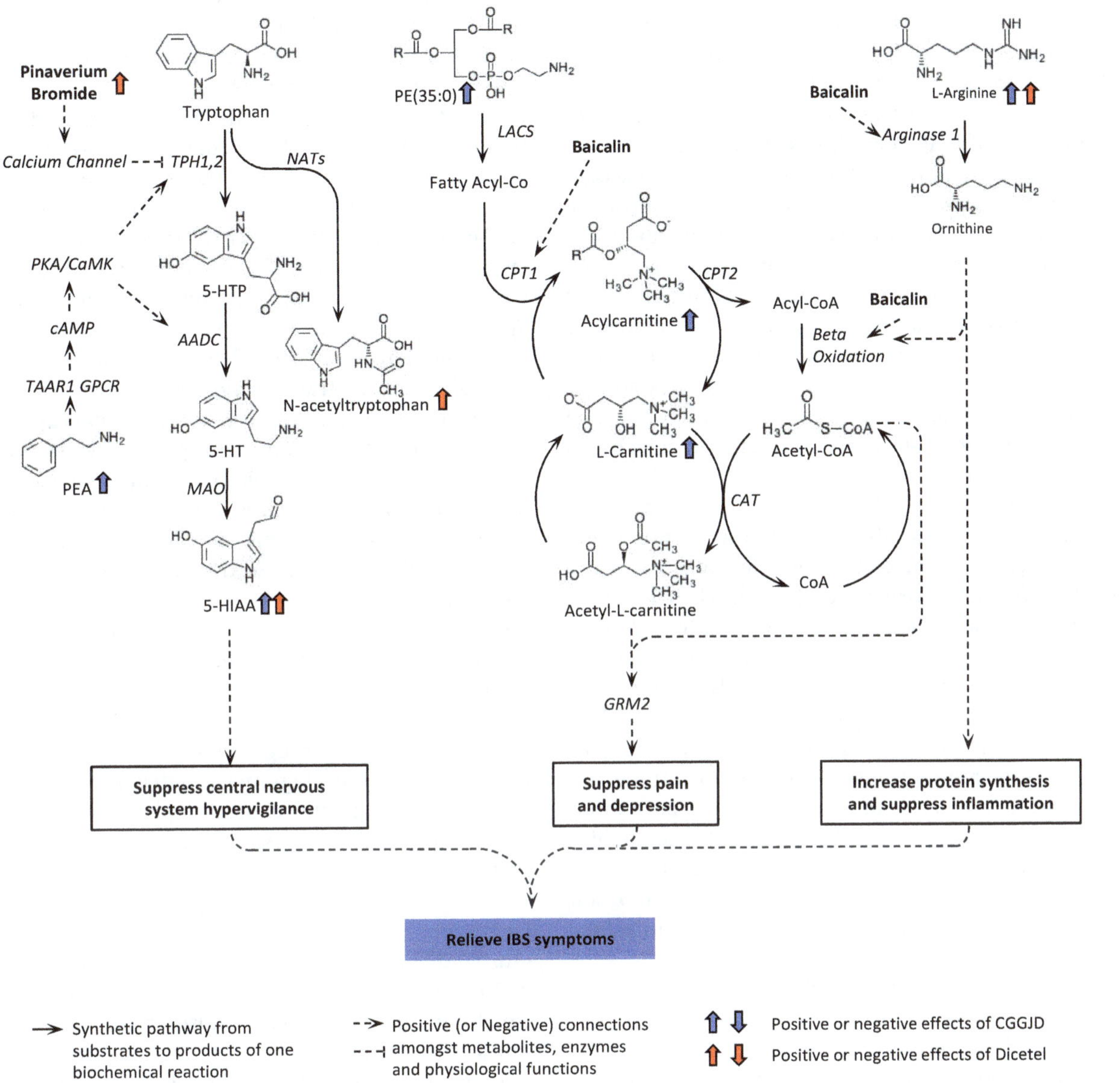

Fig. 5 Metabolism and related metabolic processes. Solid arrows denote the positive connections of substrate and products of a single biochemical reaction. Dotted arrows denote positive connections among metabolites, enzymes, and physiological functions. Blue arrows denote the concentration change of metabolites in the CGGD group. Blue arrows denote the concentration change of metabolites in the Dicetel group. The direction of arrows denotes the change in trend

under investigation. It is speculated that the Ca^{2+} present in oyster shells can also promote tryptophan to be converted to 5-HTP by TPH1/2 [60, 61], thereby resulting in increased metabolic output [62].

The overall effect of CGGD seemed to increase the availability of acetyl groups, which can suppress pain and depression. L-carnitine is transported across cell membranes primarily by two organic cation transporters (OCTNs): OCTN1 and OCTN2. Once inside a cell, the main physiological function of L-carnitine is to shuttle long-chain fatty acids across mitochondrial membranes with the aid of carnitine palmitoyl transferase 1 (CPT1). The latter is located on the internal side of the external mitochondrial membrane and converts activated fatty acyl-coenzyme A (acyl-CoA) from acyl-CoA to acyl-carnitine. Carnitine translocase exchanges acylcarnitine for carnitine from the matrix via the internal mitochondrial membrane. On the internal side of the inner mitochondrial membrane, CPT2 catalyzes acyl-CoA synthesis from acylcarnitine and a matrix pool of

CoA [71]. Acyl-CoA is processed by beta-oxidation to produce energy in the form of adenosine triphosphate [63]. As demonstrated in vitro and in vivo, S. baicalensis and baicalin can activate CPT directly and accelerate the β-oxidation of lipids [24, 64, 65]. CGGD increases the blood level of long-chain lipids such as PE(35:0) and PC(40:7), as well as acylcarnitine. Acetyl-CoA and acetyl-L-carnitine are important providers of acetyl groups. The latter can activate the glutamate receptor metabotropic 2 gene through epigenetic regulation to suppress pain and depression [66, 67]. Studies [67, 68] have shown that carnitine supplementation can improve the depressive state of male patients suffering from uremia and cancer patients. In addition, the root of Trichosanthes species and oyster shells can supplement levels of lysine and aspartate as synthetic substrates of carnitine, which can increase the carnitine content directly [69, 70]. Therefore, combining our results with previous studies, we speculated that CGGD might also exert its therapeutic effect through the carnitine-mediated lipid metabolism.

CGGD can also increase the blood level of arginine, which can activate adenosine monophosphate kinase, then stimulating fatty-acid oxidation in skeletal muscle and glucose uptake in muscles [56, 57]. This phenomenon can be explained (at least in part) by the existence of baicalin. Baicalin can increase expression of arginase-1 [71], which converts arginine into ornithine. Ornithine has been shown to have a role in regulation of cellular immunity in the micro-environment [72], and its metabolites can stimulate protein synthesis and suppress inflammation. Arginine and its metabolites also have important roles in regulation of esophageal, gastric, and intestinal motility [58].

In fact, phytogenic baicalin, a dominant flavonoid isolated from the roots of Scutellaria baicalensis Georgi, is currently used as a promising complementary agent for prevention and treatment of IBS, as well as other intestinal and neurological diseases based on its neuroprotective, anti-inflammatory, and regulating intestinal flora effects [73–75]. Lei and his colleagues found that baicalin could significantly increase the serum levels of 5-HT in the IBS model mice group compared with the control group [76]. In terms of IBS-related phenotype, after IBS induction modeling, the Bristol fecal character score and abdominal withdrawal reflex (AWR) score were significantly elevated in IBS model group (Bristol fecal character score: 6.40 ± 0.28, AWR score: 2.55 ± 0.21) compared with the health control group (Bristol fecal character score: 3.55 ± 0.45, AWR score: 1.75 ± 0.24) ($P < 0.05$). Depression, easy stimulation, loss of appetite, varying degrees of loose stools and body hair contaminated by loose stool were observed to occur in the IBS group. After baicalin treatment, symptoms in the IBS group were alleviated. Besides, there was a significant decrease in the Bristol fecal character score and AWR score in the baicalin treatment group (Bristol fecal character score: 5.28 ± 0.39, AWR score: 2.09 ± 0.35, $P < 0.05$, respectively) compared with the IBS model group compared with IBS model group (Bristol fecal character score: 6.35 ± 0.36, AWR score: 2.67 ± 0.31, $P < 0.05$, respectively) [76].

In addition to baicalin, other ingredients also had beneficial effects against IBS. First, Rhizoma Zingiberis can supplement ergothioneine directly [77]. According to Cheah and colleagues, ergothioneine can relieve the symptoms of several cognitive diseases [78]. Fond and coworkers have suggested that ergothioneine expression through OCTN1 transporters can protect the nervous system from oxidative stress, maintain energy reserves, provide nutritional and neuroprotective factors, and inhibit abnormal brain excitation, combined with the risk factors of IBS [79], which is also an important reason to relieve patients' symptoms. Second, Radix Glycyrrhizae Preparata also has roles in treating depression [59] and IBS [80].

Collectively, combined with the risk factors of IBS, CGGD can improve the mental state of patients by regulating lipid metabolism. We elucidated the pharmacological mechanism of action of CGGD in regulating lipid metabolism through network pharmacology and lipidomics. This strategy may contribute to the discovery of new drugs and clinical application of CGGD in IBS as well as diseases associated with disorders of lipid metabolism.

Limitations

Our study has several limitations, which can be explored in future research. First, the sample size was relatively small for such complicated disease and syndrome. A multi-center study on a larger scale is required to provide stronger and more precise metabolomics results.

Secondly, other potential intrinsic and environmental factors that can influence IBS were not assessed in this study. What's more, only positive results were compared with other positive results from the literature. The metabolites between healthy human and patients with IBD should be further explored, which is necessary for better evaluation of the therapeutic effects of two drugs based on metabolomics. Moreover, the therapeutic effects and biomolecular mechanism of CGGD in treating IBS should been further clarified in the future experiments.

Conclusions

CGGD was more efficacious than Dicetel for treating IBS according to metabolomics analysis. Dicetel could induce tryptophan metabolism leading to increased blood levels of N-acetyltryptophan and 5-HIAA. Dicetel could also improve arginine metabolism. These Dicetel-related biological pathways could suppress CNS hypervigilance and inflammation and increase protein synthesis. CGGD elicited similar changes to pathways involving acetyltryptophan and 5-HIAA, but also induced carnitine-mediated lipid metabolism to suppress pain and depression. The most efficacious active ingredient of CGGD may be baicalin.

Supplementary Information

Additional file 1: Table S1. Symptom index score. The table contained patient's symptom index score under CGGD and Dicetel. The figure for TCM criteria comprises: pain or swelling of the chest; abdominal distension or pain; fecal abnormalities; dry throat with a bitter taste; indigestion and anorexia; fatigue; tongue quality. The figure for Rome IV criteria comprises: abdominal pain, abdominal pain days, degree of abdominal pain discomfort, satisfaction of stool condition, inconvenience of intestinal symptoms on life.

Additional file 2. MS/MS spectral information of significant metabolites. The table included details for the identification results including MS/MS spectral information (MS1 isotopic spectrum and MS/MS spectrum in column K and L separately).

Additional file 3. Total ion chromatogram of different stages. The figure included total ion chromatogram of D0, D30, D37, D67, and QC in this file.

Additional file 4. Codes for statistical analyses. The codes in this file uploaded was used for carrying out statistical analyses.

Additional file 5. Codes for drawing Figure 3. The codes in this file uploaded was used for drawing our Figure 3.

Additional file 6. Codes for drawing Figure 4. The codes in this file we uploaded is used for drawing our Figure 4.

Acknowledgements

We sincerely thank the grants supported by the National Key R&D Program of China (2019YFC1711100), the Jin-Zi-Ta Talent projects, China (0806, YQ672), National Natural Science Foundation of China (81830109 and 81804008), Project of Bethune Exploration: the capacity establishment of pharmaceutical research, China (B-19-H-20200622), and Clinical Medical Technology Incubation Project of Shanghai Changzheng Hospital (YLJS2021A-03).

Author contributions

WSC, LNS, and XQY conceived and designed this study. XL recruited participants. MML and XL designed and carried out the research. JWZ, ZYD, and JPJ collected and prepared samples. MML, JWZ, ZYD, and JGT performed the experiments. MML, JNC, JWZ, and FHY contributed to statistical and bioinformatics analyses. MML, XL and JWZ drafted the manuscript. FZ, SQ, SHG, and ZPW provided constructive suggestions for the study. All authors contributed to the writing of this manuscript. All authors read and approved the final version of the manuscript.

Author details

[1]School of Pharmacy, Shanghai University of Traditional Chinese Medicine, Shanghai 201203, People's Republic of China. [2]Department of Pharmacy, Second Affiliated Hospital of Naval Medical University, Shanghai 200003, China. [3]Department of Traditional Chinese Medicine, Second Affiliated Hospital of Naval Medical University, Shanghai 200003, China. [4]Department of Pharmacy, 905 Hospital of People's Liberation Army Navy, Shanghai 200050, China. [5]Traditional Chinese Medicine Resource and Technology Center, Shanghai University of Traditional Chinese Medicine, Shanghai 201203, China. [6]Shanghai Key Laboratory for Pharmaceutical Metabolite Research, Shanghai 200433, China.

References

1. Ford AC, Lacy BE, Talley NJ. Irritable bowel syndrome. N Engl J Med. 2017;376:2566–78. https://doi.org/10.1056/NEJMra1607547.
2. Drossman DA, Hasler WL. Rome IV—functional GI disorders: disorders of gut-brain interaction. Gastroenterology. 2016;150:1257–61. https://doi.org/10.1053/j.gastro.2016.03.035.
3. Ford AC, Moayyedi P, Lacy BE, et al. American College of Gastroenterology Monograph on the management of irritable bowel syndrome and chronic idiopathic constipation. Am J Gastroenterol. 2014;109:S2–26. https://doi.org/10.1038/ajg.2014.187.
4. Lacy BE, Mearin F, Chang L, et al. Bowel disorders. Gastroenterology. 2016;150:1393-1407.e5. https://doi.org/10.1053/j.gastro.2016.02.031.
5. Palsson OS, Whitehead W, Törnblom H, et al. Prevalence of rome IV functional bowel disorders among adults in the United States, Canada, and the United Kingdom. Gastroenterology. 2020;158:1262-1273.e3. https://doi.org/10.1053/j.gastro.2019.12.021.
6. Canavan C, West J, Card T. Review article: the economic impact of the irritable bowel syndrome. Aliment Pharmacol Ther. 2014;40:1023–34. https://doi.org/10.1111/apt.12938.
7. Chen G, Xie X, Peng C. Treatment of irritable bowel syndrome by CHINESE medicine: a review. Chin J Integr Med. 2021. https://doi.org/10.1007/s11655-021-3521-4.
8. Lovell RM, Ford AC. Global prevalence of and risk factors for irritable bowel syndrome: a meta-analysis. Clin Gastroenterol Hepatol. 2012;10:712-721.e4. https://doi.org/10.1016/j.cgh.2012.02.029.
9. Zhang L, Duan L, Liu Y, et al. A meta-analysis of the prevalence and risk factors of irritable bowel syndrome in Chinese community. Zhonghua Nei Ke Za Zhi. 2014;53:969–75.
10. Zhu J-J, Liu S, Su X-L, et al. Efficacy of Chinese herbal medicine for diarrhea-predominant irritable bowel syndrome: a meta-analysis of randomized, double-blind, placebo-controlled trials. Evid-Based Complement Altern Med. 2016;2016:1–15. https://doi.org/10.1155/2016/4071260.
11. Long Y, Huang Z, Deng Y, et al. Prevalence and risk factors for functional bowel disorders in South China: a population based study using the Rome III criteria. Neurogastroenterol Motil. 2017;29: e12897. https://doi.org/10.1111/nmo.12897.
12. Holtmann GJ, Ford AC, Talley NJ. Pathophysiology of irritable bowel syndrome. Lancet Gastroenterol Hepatol. 2016;1:133–46. https://doi.org/10.1016/S2468-1253(16)30023-1.
13. Wall GC, Bryant GA, Bottenberg MM, et al. Irritable bowel syndrome: a concise review of current treatment concepts. World J Gastroenterol. 2014;20:8796–806. https://doi.org/10.3748/wjg.v20.i27.8796.
14. Radovanovic-Dinic B, Tesic-Rajkovic S, Grgov S, et al. Irritable bowel syndrome—from etiopathogenesis to therapy. Biomed Pap Med Fac Univ Palacky Olomouc Czech Repub. 2018;162:1–9. https://doi.org/10.5507/bp.2017.057.
15. Adriani A, Ribaldone DG, Astegiano M, et al. Irritable bowel syndrome: the clinical approach. Panminerva Med. 2018;60:213–22. https://doi.org/10.23736/S0031-0808.18.03541-3.
16. Corsetti M, Whorwell P. Novel pharmacological therapies for irritable bowel syndrome. Expert Rev Gastroenterol Hepatol. 2016;10:807–15. https://doi.org/10.1586/17474124.2016.1158099.
17. Alammar N, Stein E. Irritable bowel syndrome: what treatments really work. Med Clin North Am. 2019;103:137–52. https://doi.org/10.1016/j.mcna.2018.08.006.
18. Surdea-Blaga T, Baban A, Nedelcu L, Dumitrascu DL. Psychological Interventions for Irritable Bowel Syndrome. J Gastrointestin Liver Dis. 2016;25:359–66. https://doi.org/10.15403/jgld.2014.1121.253.ibs.
19. Malysz J, Farraway LA, Christen M-O, Huizinga JD. Pinaverium acts as L-type calcium channel blocker on smooth muscle of colon. Can J Physiol Pharmacol. 1997;75:969–75. https://doi.org/10.1139/y97-117.
20. Baumgartner A, Drack E, Halter F, Scheurer U. Effects of pinaverium bromide and verapamil on the motility of the rat isolated colon. Br J Pharmacol. 1985;86:89–94. https://doi.org/10.1111/j.1476-5381.1985.tb09438.x.
21. Quigley EMM, Fried M, Gwee K-A, et al. World Gastroenterology Organisation Global Guidelines Irritable Bowel Syndrome: a global perspective update September 2015. J Clin Gastroenterol. 2016;50:704–13. https://doi.org/10.1097/MCG.0000000000000653.

22. Leung WK, Wu JCY, Liang SM, et al. Treatment of diarrhea-predominant irritable bowel syndrome with traditional Chinese herbal medicine: a randomized placebo-controlled trial. Am J Gastroenterol. 2006;101:1574–80. https://doi.org/10.1111/j.1572-0241.2006.00576.x.
23. Teschke R, Wolff A, Frenzel C, et al. Herbal traditional Chinese medicine and its evidence base in gastrointestinal disorders. World J Gastroenterol. 2015;21:4466–90. https://doi.org/10.3748/wjg.v21.i15.4466.
24. Bi Z, Zheng Y, Yuan J, Bian Z. The efficacy and potential mechanisms of Chinese herbal medicine on irritable bowel syndrome. CPD. 2018. https://doi.org/10.2174/1381612823666170822101606.
25. Xu G-Z, Xue Y, Wei S-Q, et al. Valproate reverses stress-induced somatic hyperalgesia and visceral hypersensitivity by up-regulating spinal 5-HT2C receptor expression in female rats. Neuropharmacology. 2020;165: 107926. https://doi.org/10.1016/j.neuropharm.2019.107926.
26. Yang X. Syndrome differentiation and treatment of Taiyang disease in Shanghan Lun. J Chin Integr Med. 2009;7:171–4. https://doi.org/10.3736/jcim20090215.
27. Hollywood K, Brison DR, Goodacre R. Metabolomics: current technologies and future trends. Proteomics. 2006;6:4716–23. https://doi.org/10.1002/pmic.200600106.
28. Xuan Q, Ouyang Y, Wang Y, et al. Multiplatform metabolomics reveals novel serum metabolite biomarkers in diabetic retinopathy subjects. Adv Sci. 2020;7:2001714. https://doi.org/10.1002/advs.202001714.
29. Camilleri M. Irritable bowel syndrome: straightening the road from the Rome criteria. Neurogastroenterol Motil. 2020. https://doi.org/10.1111/nmo.13957.
30. Xiaoyu Zheng, et al (2002) Clinical research of new Chinese medicine and the consensus of TCM Diagnosis. China medical scinece press
31. Spleen and Stomach diseases branch of Chinese Society of Traditional Chinese Medicine. Consensus of experts on diagnosis and treatment of irritable bowel syndrome in Traditional Chinese Medicine. J Tradit Chin Med. 2017;58(18):1614–1620.
32. Deng Y, Yao H, Chen W, et al. Profiling of polar urine metabolite extracts from Chinese colorectal cancer patients to screen for potential diagnostic and adverse-effect biomarkers. J Cancer. 2020;11:6925–38. https://doi.org/10.7150/jca.47631.
33. Gika HG, Theodoridis GA, Wingate JE, Wilson ID. Within-day reproducibility of an HPLC-MS-based method for metabonomic analysis: application to human urine. J Proteome Res. 2007;6:3291–303. https://doi.org/10.1021/pr070183p.
34. Tan Y, Yin P, Tang L, et al. Metabolomics study of stepwise hepatocarcinogenesis from the model rats to patients: potential biomarkers effective for small hepatocellular carcinoma diagnosis. Mol Cell Proteomics. 2012;11(M111): 010694. https://doi.org/10.1074/mcp.M111.010694.
35. Li M, Chen J, Deng Y, et al (2021) Risk prediction models based on hematological/body parameters for chemotherapy-induced adverse effects in Chinese colorectal cancer patients. Support Care Cancer 29:7931–7947. https://doi.org/10.1007/s00520-021-06337-z.
36. Ritchie ME, Phipson B, Wu D, et al. limma powers differential expression analyses for RNA-sequencing and microarray studies. Nucleic Acids Res. 2015;43:e47–e47. https://doi.org/10.1093/nar/gkv007.
37. Li M, Chen J, Liu S, et al. Spermine-related DNA hypermethylation and elevated expression of genes for collagen formation are susceptible factors for chemotherapy-induced hand-foot syndrome in Chinese colorectal cancer patients. Front Pharmacol. 2021;12: 746910. https://doi.org/10.3389/fphar.2021.746910.
38. Longstreth GF, Thompson WG, Chey WD et al (2006) Functional Bowel Disorders. Gastroenterology 130:1480–1491. https://doi.org/10.1053/j.gastro.2005.11.061.
39. Camilleri M. Peripheral mechanisms in irritable bowel syndrome. N Engl J Med. 2012;367:1626–35. https://doi.org/10.1056/NEJMra1207068.
40. Christen MO. Action of pinaverium bromide, a calcium-antagonist, on gastrointestinal motility disorders. General Pharmacol Vasc Syst. 1990;21:821–5. https://doi.org/10.1016/0306-3623(90)90439-S.
41. Maffei ME. 5-Hydroxytryptophan (5-HTP): natural occurrence, analysis, biosynthesis, biotechnology. Physiol Toxicol IJMS. 2020;22:181. https://doi.org/10.3390/ijms22010181.
42. de Herder WW. Biochemistry of neuroendocrine tumours. Best Pract Res Clin Endocrinol Metab. 2007;21:33–41. https://doi.org/10.1016/j.beem.2006.12.002.
43. Gaggi R, Dall'Olio R, Roncada P, Gianni AM. Effects of isradipine and darodipine on serotonergic system of the rat brain. Pharmacol Biochem Behav. 1995;51:183–7. https://doi.org/10.1016/0091-3057(94)00389-z.
44. Firk C, Markus CR. Review: serotonin by stress interaction: a susceptibility factor for the development of depression? J Psychopharmacol. 2007;21:538–44. https://doi.org/10.1177/0269881106075588.
45. Crowell MD, Wessinger SB. 5-HT and the brain-gut axis: opportunities for pharmacologic intervention. Expert Opin Investig Drugs. 2007;16:761–5. https://doi.org/10.1517/13543784.16.6.761.
46. Alden N, Raju R, McElearney K, et al. Using metabolomics to identify cell line-independent indicators of growth inhibition for Chinese hamster ovary cell-based bioprocesses. Metabolites. 2020;10:E199. https://doi.org/10.3390/metabo10050199.
47. Jinsmaa Y, Cooney A, Sullivan P, et al. The serotonin aldehyde, 5-HIAL, oligomerizes alpha-synuclein. Neurosci Lett. 2015;590:134–7. https://doi.org/10.1016/j.neulet.2015.01.064.
48. Tanaka H, Sirich TL, Plummer NS, et al. An enlarged profile of uremic solutes. PLoS ONE. 2015;10: e0135657. https://doi.org/10.1371/journal.pone.0135657.
49. Toyohara T, Akiyama Y, Suzuki T, et al. Metabolomic profiling of uremic solutes in CKD patients. Hypertens Res. 2010;33:944–52. https://doi.org/10.1038/hr.2010.113.
50. Pavlova T, Vidova V, Bienertova-Vasku J, et al. Urinary intermediates of tryptophan as indicators of the gut microbial metabolism. Anal Chim Acta. 2017;987:72–80. https://doi.org/10.1016/j.aca.2017.08.022.
51. Vanholder R, Baurmeister U, Brunet P, et al. A bench to bedside view of uremic toxins. J Am Soc Nephrol. 2008;19:863–70. https://doi.org/10.1681/ASN.2007121377.
52. Ruddell RG, Mann DA, Ramm GA. The function of serotonin within the liver. J Hepatol. 2008;48:666–75. https://doi.org/10.1016/j.jhep.2008.01.006.
53. Thijssen AY, Mujagic Z, Jonkers DMAE, et al. Alterations in serotonin metabolism in the irritable bowel syndrome. Aliment Pharmacol Ther. 2016;43:272–82. https://doi.org/10.1111/apt.13459.
54. Witte MB, Barbul A. Arginine physiology and its implication for wound healing. Wound Repair Regen. 2003;11:419–23. https://doi.org/10.1046/j.1524-475X.2003.11605.x.
55. Oanca G, Stare J, Vianello R, Mavri J. Multiscale simulation of monoamine oxidase catalyzed decomposition of phenylethylamine analogs. Eur J Pharmacol. 2017;817:46–50. https://doi.org/10.1016/j.ejphar.2017.05.061.
56. Mulinari S. Monoamine theories of depression: historical impact on biomedical research. J Hist Neurosci. 2012;21:366–92. https://doi.org/10.1080/0964704X.2011.623917.
57. Violante S, Achetib N, van Roermund CWT, et al. Peroxisomes can oxidize medium- and long-chain fatty acids through a pathway involving ABCD3 and HSD17B4. FASEB J. 2019;33:4355–64. https://doi.org/10.1096/fj.201801498R.
58. Zhai L, Huang C, Ning Z, et al. Phenethylamine-producing gut bacteria induces diarrhea-predominant irritable bowel syndrome by increasing serotonin biosynthesis. Microbiology. 2022. http://biorxiv.org/lookup/doi/10.1101/2022.03.05.483096.
59. Su GY, Yang JY, Wang F, et al. Antidepressant-like effects of Xiaochaihu-tang in a rat model of chronic unpredictable mild stress. J Ethnopharmacol. 2014;152:217–26. https://doi.org/10.1016/j.jep.2014.01.006.
60. Kumer SC, Mockus SM, Rucker PJ, Vrana KE. Amino-terminal analysis of tryptophan hydroxylase: protein kinase phosphorylation occurs at serine-58. J Neurochem. 1997;69:1738–45. https://doi.org/10.1046/j.1471-4159.1997.69041738.x.
61. Duchemin AM, Berry MD, Neff NH, Hadjiconstantinou M. Phosphorylation and activation of brain aromatic L-amino acid decarboxylase by cyclic AMP-dependent protein kinase. J Neurochem. 2000;75:725–31. https://doi.org/10.1046/j.1471-4159.2000.0750725.x.
62. O'Mahony SM, Clarke G, Borre YE, et al. Serotonin, tryptophan metabolism and the brain-gut-microbiome axis. Behav Brain Res. 2015;277:32–48. https://doi.org/10.1016/j.bbr.2014.07.027.
63. Fortin G. l-Carnitine and intestinal inflammation. In: Vitamins and hormones. Elsevier, Amsterdam; 2011, pp 353–366
64. Li C, Zhang H, Li X. The mechanism of traditional Chinese medicine for the treatment of obesity. Diabetes Metab Syndr Obes. 2020;13:3371–81. https://doi.org/10.2147/DMSO.S274534.

65. Wang Z-Y, Jiang Z-M, Xiao P-T, et al. The mechanisms of baicalin ameliorate obesity and hyperlipidemia through a network pharmacology approach. Eur J Pharmacol. 2020;878: 173103. https://doi.org/10.1016/j.ejphar.2020.173103.
66. Adachi T, Fukami K, Yamagishi S-I, et al. Decreased serum carnitine is independently correlated with increased tissue accumulation levels of advanced glycation end products in haemodialysis patients: correlation between carnitine and tissue AGE. Nephrology. 2012;17:689–94. https://doi.org/10.1111/j.1440-1797.2012.01642.x.
67. Tashiro K, Kaida Y, Yamagishi S, et al. L-Carnitine supplementation improves self-rating depression scale scores in uremic male patients undergoing hemodialysis. LDDD. 2017. https://doi.org/10.2174/1570180814666170216102632.
68. Cruciani RA, Dvorkin E, Homel P, et al. l-Carnitine supplementation for the treatment of fatigue and depressed mood in cancer patients with carnitine deficiency: a preliminary analysis. Ann N Y Acad Sci. 2004;1033:168–76. https://doi.org/10.1196/annals.1320.016.
69. Chen Y, Jiang Y, Liao L, et al. Inhibition of 4NQO-induced oral carcinogenesis by dietary oyster shell calcium. Integr Cancer Ther. 2016;15:96–101. https://doi.org/10.1177/1534735415596572.
70. Fang FE, Ng BT, Shaw CP, Wong NSR. Recent progress in medicinal investigations on trichosanthin and other ribosome inactivating proteins from the plant genus Trichosanthes. CMC. 2011;18:4410–7. https://doi.org/10.2174/092986711797200499.
71. Zhu W, Jin Z, Yu J, et al. Baicalin ameliorates experimental inflammatory bowel disease through polarization of macrophages to an M2 phenotype. Int Immunopharmacol. 2016;35:119–26. https://doi.org/10.1016/j.intimp.2016.03.030.
72. Grobben Y, Willemsen-Seegers N, Uitdehaag JCM, et al. High-throughput fluorescence-based activity assay for arginase-1. SLAS Discov. 2020;25:1018–25. https://doi.org/10.1177/2472555220919340.
73. Liang S, Deng X, Lei L, et al. The comparative study of the therapeutic effects and mechanism of baicalin, baicalein, and their combination on ulcerative colitis rat. Front Pharmacol. 2019;10:1466. https://doi.org/10.3389/fphar.2019.01466.
74. Zhang C-Y-Y, Zeng M-J, Zhou L-P, et al. Baicalin exerts neuroprotective effects via inhibiting activation of GSK3β/NF-κB/NLRP3 signal pathway in a rat model of depression. Int Immunopharmacol. 2018;64:175–82. https://doi.org/10.1016/j.intimp.2018.09.001.
75. Ye Y, Huang C, Jiang L, et al. Huanglian-Jie-Du-Tang extract protects against chronic brain injury after focal cerebral ischemia via hypoxia-inducible-factor-1α-regulated vascular endothelial growth factor signaling in mice. Biol Pharm Bull. 2012;35:355–61. https://doi.org/10.1248/bpb.35.355.
76. Li L, Cui H, Li T, et al. Synergistic effect of berberine-based Chinese medicine assembled nanostructures on diarrhea-predominant irritable bowel syndrome in vivo. Front Pharmacol. 2020;11:1210. https://doi.org/10.3389/fphar.2020.01210.
77. Halliwell B, Cheah IK, Tang RMY. Ergothioneine—a diet-derived antioxidant with therapeutic potential. FEBS Lett. 2018;592:3357–66. https://doi.org/10.1002/1873-3468.13123.
78. Cheah IK, Feng L, Tang RMY, et al. Ergothioneine levels in an elderly population decrease with age and incidence of cognitive decline; a risk factor for neurodegeneration? Biochem Biophys Res Commun. 2016;478:162–7. https://doi.org/10.1016/j.bbrc.2016.07.074.
79. Fond G, Loundou A, Hamdani N, et al. Anxiety and depression comorbidities in irritable bowel syndrome (IBS): a systematic review and meta-analysis. Eur Arch Psychiatry Clin Neurosci. 2014;264:651–60. https://doi.org/10.1007/s00406-014-0502-z.
80. Shao Y-Y, Guo Y-T, Gao J, et al. Shaoyao-Gancao Decoction relieves visceral hyperalgesia in TNBS-Induced postinflammatory irritable bowel syndrome via inactivating transient receptor potential vanilloid type 1 and reducing serotonin synthesis. Evid-Based Complement Altern Med. 2020;2020:1–12. https://doi.org/10.1155/2020/7830280.

11

Golden bifid might improve diarrhea-predominant irritable bowel syndrome via microbiota modulation

Mei Luo, Qin Liu, Lin Xiao and Li-Shou Xiong*

Abstract

Objective: Gut microbiota might play a crucial role in the pathogenesis of irritable bowel syndrome (IBS), and probiotics supplement may be an effective treatment option. This study aims to explore the therapeutic effects of Golden bifid on the diarrhea-predominant IBS (IBS-D).

Methods: Twenty-one consecutive IBS-D patients were recruited based on Rome IV criteria. All patients took 2000 mg Golden bifid triple daily for 4 weeks. Gastrointestinal (GI) symptoms, psychological symptoms, small intestine bacterial overgrowth (SIBO) and fecal microbiota characteristics were evaluated in IBS-D patients before and after treatment.

Results: After 4-week treatment of Golden bifid, the GI symptoms such as abdominal pain (2.90 ± 1.04 vs. 1.90 ± 1.26, $P = 0.002$), abdominal distension (2.00 ± 1.34 vs. 1.29 ± 1.31, $P = 0.007$), diarrhea (3.24 ± 1.37 vs. 1.81 ± 1.21, $P = 0.001$), defecatory urgency (3.48 ± 1.03 vs. 2.33 ± 1.35, $P = 0.000$) and incomplete evacuation (2.71 ± 1.15 vs. 1.76 ± 1.26, $P = 0.003$) were significantly alleviated in IBS-D patients. The Self-Rating Depression Scale (SDS) decreased significantly (46.19 ± 11.36 vs. 43.33 ± 9.65, $P = 0.041$), and SIBO could be eradicated in 25% (4/16) of IBS-D patients with SIBO. Meanwhile, the abundance of *Unclassified Lachnospiraceae* and *Dorea* in genus level and *Unclassified Lachnospiraceae, Bacterium Dorea, Bacterium Butyricicoccus* and *Dorea formicigenerans ATCC 27755* in species level were increased in fecal microbiota ($P < 0.05$).

Conclusions: Golden bifid could improve most of GI symptoms and depressive symptoms in IBS-D patients and eradicate a small proportion of SIBO in those IBS-D patients with SIBO. What's more, Golden bifid could also modulate the fecal microbiota in IBS-D patients, which implied that the Golden bifid might improve IBS-D via microbiota modulation.

Keywords: Fecal microbiota, Golden bifid, Self-Rating Anxiety Scale, Self-Rating Depression Scale, 16S rRNA gene-targeted pyrosequencing

Introduction

Irritable bowel syndrome (IBS) is one of the most common globally functional bowel disorders (FBDs). The characteristics of IBS include abdominal pain, abdominal distension, changes in defecation habits, insignificant morphology and biochemics, and its pathogenesis is unclear now [1]. The global prevalence of IBS is as high as 3.3–31.6% with an average prevalence of 8.8% [2], and about 6.5% in China [3]. Although the pathogenesis of IBS is unclear, gut microbiota dysbiosis was found to be associated with the pathogenesis of IBS [4].

The alterations of gut microbiota could damage the intestinal mucosal barrier function, intestinal

*Correspondence: xionglsh@mail.sysu.edu.cn

Department of Gastroenterology and Hepatology, The First Affiliated Hospital of Sun Yat-Sen University, Guangzhou 510080, China permeability, immunity, releasing histamine, 5-hydroxytryptamine, prostaglandins and tryptase and other active substances. The microbiota-derived metabolites eventually cause abdominal pain, diarrhea and other intestinal symptoms [5–8]. Therefore, probiotics intervention has become a significant therapeutic method of IBS for gut microbiota disorder in recent years. Probiotics treatment might be a novel approach to improve the intestinal epithelial barrier function, inhibit the adhesion of pathogenic bacteria and mediate the regulation of immune system. Moreover, research have shown that probiotics therapy could modulate the gut microbiota of IBS patients [9]. *Bifidobacterium bifidum* could effectively alleviate IBS and improve IBS symptoms, including abdominal pain, discomfort, bloating, urgency and digestive disorder simultaneously with an improvement of quality of life [10]. After probiotics treatment, the number of *Lactobacillus* and *Bifidobacterium* in the feces of IBS patients increased significantly [9]. Meanwhile, Ma et al. [11] put forwarded that probiotics supplement might improve the psychological symptoms of IBS patients by regulating the balance of gut microbiota and gut–brain axis. Small intestinal bacterial overgrowth (SIBO) is a clinical syndrome that changes the characteristic or quantity of bacteria in the small intestine. Lactulose hydrogen breath test (LHBT) is a safe, convenient, efficient and noninvasive diagnostic method for SIBO. Study has found that SIBO was one of the pathogenesises of IBS, as eradicating SIBO could alleviate the symptoms of IBS patients [12].

Although some studies have shown that probiotic treatment could improve the IBS and regulate the gut microbiota disorders, there is no consensus on its therapeutic effect and mechanisms. The purpose of this study was to evaluate whether Golden bifid treatment could modulate the fecal microbiota of IBS-D patients by 16S rRNA gene-targeted pyrosequencing technology and explore its therapeutic effect on GI symptoms, SIBO eradication rate and psychological problems of IBS-D patients.

Methods

Study subjects

IBS-D patients were recruited from the Department of Gastroenterology and Hepatology, The First Affiliated Hospital of Sun Yat-sen University, from June 2019 to December 2020. All patients met Rome IV criteria and aged between 18 and 65. They were required to perform a colonoscopy to exclude organic diseases. The protocol was approved by the Medical Ethics Committee of the First Affiliated Hospital of Sun Yat-sen University, and all patients had signed informed consent.

Study design and procedure

All patients took 2000 mg Golden bifid (INNER MONGOLIA Shuangqi Pharmaceutical Co., Ltd., Inner Mongolia, China. 1×10^7 CFU/g *Bifidobacterium Longum*, 1×10^6 CFU/g *Lactobacillus bulgaricus* and 1×10^6 CFU/g *Streptococcus thermophilus*) triple daily for 4 weeks. One fasting fecal sample was collected from all patients for 16S rRNA gene-targeted pyrosequencing at baseline (T0) and the end of treatment (T28) to evaluate the characteristics of gut microbiota. Meantime, all patients completed GI symptom severity scale, Self-Rating Anxiety Scale (SAS), Self-Rating Depression Scale (SDS) questionnaires and lactulose hydrogen breath test (LHBT).

Small intestinal bacterial overgrowth

The LHBT was completed for all IBS-D patients according to a standard procedure. And according to our previous research [13], when the baseline value of $H2 \geq 20$ p.p.m and/or a rise of > 20 p.p.m. from baseline in H2 within 90 min of lactulose administration, the LHBT should be considered a presence of SIBO.

GI symptoms and psychological symptoms

Three questionnaires including GI symptom severity scale [13], SAS [14] and SDS [14] were performed in all IBS-D patients at T0 and T28. The questionnaire of GI symptom severity scale includes abdominal discomfort, abdominal distension, abdominal pain, diarrhea, defecatory urgency and incomplete evacuation, six GI symptoms with seven-point Likert responses, and the final score is negatively correlated with GI symptoms. The SAS and SDS contain 20 items with four-point Likert responses about anxiety and depression, respectively, and the final score is negatively correlated with anxiety or depression symptoms too.

16S rRNA gene-targeted pyrosequencing

Fecal sample collection and DNA extraction

Fecal samples were collected by germ-free disposable sampling spoon and frozen immediately at − 80 °C. Fecal microbial DNA was extracted from 180–220 mg feces using E.Z.N.A.® soil Kit (Omega Bio-tek, Norcross, GA, USA) according to manufacturer's protocols. The DNA concentration and purification were determined by NanoDrop 2000 UV–Vis spectrophotometer (Thermo Scientific, Wilmington, USA), and DNA quality was checked by 1% agarose gel electrophoresis. The qualified fecal bacterial genomic DNA samples were stored in Tris–HCl buffer, pH 8.0, at − 20 °C.

PCR amplification

The V3-V4 hypervariable regions of the bacteria 16S rRNA gene were amplified with primers 338F (5′-ACT CCTACGGGAGGCAGCAG-3′) and 806R (5′-GGA CTACHVGGGTWTCTAAT-3′) by thermocycler PCR system (GeneAmp 9700, ABI, USA). The PCR reactions were conducted using the following program: 3 min of denaturation at 95 °C, 27 cycles of 30 s at 95 °C, 30 s for annealing at 55 °C, and 45 s for elongation at 72 °C, and a final extension at 72 °C for 10 min. PCR reactions were performed in triplicate 20 μL mixture containing 4 μL of 5 × FastPfu Buffer, 2 μL of 2.5 mM dNTPs, 0.8 μL of each primer (5 μM), 0.4 μL of FastPfu Polymerase and 10 ng of template DNA. The resulted PCR products were extracted from a 2% agarose gel and further purified using the AxyPrep DNA Gel Extraction Kit (Axygen Biosciences, Union City, CA, USA) and quantified using QuantiFluor™-ST (Promega, USA) according to the manufacturer's protocol.

Illumina MiSeq sequencing

Purified amplicons were pooled in equimolar and paired-end sequenced (2 × 300) on an Illumina MiSeq platform (Major Bio-Pharm Technology, Shanghai, China) according to the standard protocols by Majorbio Bio-Pharm Technology Co. , Ltd. (Shanghai, China).

Processing of sequencing data

Raw fastq files were demultiplexed, quality-filtered by Trimmomatic and merged by FLASH with the following criteria: (i) The reads were truncated at any site receiving an average quality score < 20 over a 50 bp sliding window. (ii) Primers were exactly matched allowing 2 nucleotide mismatching, and reads containing ambiguous bases were removed. (iii) Sequences whose overlap is longer than 10 bp were merged according to their overlap sequence. Operational taxonomic units (OTUs) were clustered with 97% similarity cutoff using UPARSE, and chimeric sequences were identified and removed using UCHIME. The taxonomy of each 16S rRNA gene sequence was analyzed by RDP Classifier algorithm against the Silva (SSU123) 16S rRNA database using confidence threshold of 70%.

Microbiological analysis

Operational taxonomic units (OTUs) were clustered with 97% similarity cutoff using UPARSE version 7.1, and chimeric sequences were identified and removed using UCHIME. The taxonomy of each 16S rRNA gene sequence was analyzed by RDP Classifier algorithm against the Silva (138/16s_bacteria) 16S rRNA database using confidence threshold of 70%. Then, the rank abundance curves, rarefaction curves, Alpha-diversity analysis, Beta-diversity analysis and community bar chart were used to analyze and compare the characteristics of fecal microbiota in patients with IBS-D before and after Golden bifid treatment. The rank abundance curves were plotted to determine the species abundance and community evenness of each sample, and the range of the curve on the horizontal axis and the gentle degree of the curve on the vertical axis reflect the species abundance and community evenness of the sample, respectively. Rarefaction curves were drawn to determine whether the sample size is sufficient and sequencing data of each sample. Alpha-diversity analyses including community richness parameters (Sobs, Ace, Chao1), community diversity parameters (Shannon, Simpson) and community coverage parameters (Good's coverage) were calculated using the Mothur software. Principal coordinates analysis (PCoA), which is a Beta-diversity analyses, was used to compare the community composition of different samples. Community composition analysis (community bar chart) was used to analyze the species composition drawn with R package software (version 3.3.1). In addition, bacterial taxonomic distributions of sample communities were visualized using the R package software. Microbiome features differences between two groups (before and after Golden bifid treatment) were analyzed with Wilcoxon signed-rank test. PICRUSt2 analysis (KEGG level) was used to predict the functional profiling of microbial communities [12, 15].

Statistical analysis

SPSS 23.0 (SPSS, Inc., Chicago, IL, USA) and Graph Prism version 7.0 (GraphPad Software, Inc., La Jolla, CA, USA) were used for statistical analysis and chart making. The measurement data were expressed in mean differences ± standard deviation ($\overline{x} \pm s$). Paired T test or Wilcoxon test was used for comparison. For all results of statistical analysis, $P < 0.05$ was considered statistically significant and if $P < 0.01$, the difference was statistically significant.

Results

Study subjects

Twenty-one consecutive IBS-D patients (5F, 16 M; age 31.38 ± 8.31 year, BMI 21.06 ± 2.11 kg/m^2) who met Rome IV diagnostic criteria, excluded organic diseases, fulfilled inclusion criteria and agreed to participate in this study were recruited in our study. Table 1 summarizes the demographic and clinical characteristics of all IBS-D patients at baseline.

Table 1 Demographic and clinical characteristics of IBS-D patients at baseline

	IBS-D ($n=21$)
Variable	
Gender (n, %)	
Female	5 (23.81)
Male	16 (76.19)
Age, year (mean ± SD)	31.38 ± 8.31
BMI, kg/m^2 (mean ± SD)	21.06 ± 2.11
Duration, year (n, %)	
< 1	0 (0)
1–3	7 (33.33)
4–10	9 (42.86)
11–20	3 (14.29)
> 20	2 (9.52)
LHBT† (n, %)	
LHBT (+)	16 (76.19)
LHBT (−)	5 (23.81)
Symptoms score (mean ± SD)	
Abdominal pain	2.90 ± 1.04
Abdominal distension	2.00 ± 1.34
Abdominal discomfort	2.29 ± 1.19
Diarrhea	3.24 ± 1.37
Defecatory urgency	3.48 ± 1.03
Incomplete evacuation	2.71 ± 1.15
SAS‡	44.43 ± 6.38
SDS§	46.19 ± 11.36

† *LHBT* Lactulose hydrogen breath test

‡ *SAS* Self-Rating Anxiety Scale

§ *SDS* Self-Rating Depression Scale

Table 2 GI symptoms scores and psychological symptoms scores of IBS-D patients: pre-treatment and post-treatment

Symptoms	Pre-treatment	Post-treatment	*P* value
Abdominal pain	2.90 ± 1.04	1.90 ± 1.26	0.002*
Abdominal distension	2.00 ± 1.34	1.29 ± 1.31	0.007*
Abdominal discomfort	2.29 ± 1.19	1.86 ± 1.06	0.140
Diarrhea	3.24 ± 1.37	1.81 ± 1.21	0.001*
Defecatory urgency	3.48 ± 1.03	2.33 ± 1.35	0.000*
Incomplete evacuation	2.71 ± 1.15	1.76 ± 1.26	0.003*
SAS†	44.43 ± 6.38	43.71 ± 6.54	0.485
SDS‡	46.19 ± 11.36	43.33 ± 9.65	0.041*

† *SAS* Self-Rating Anxiety Scale

‡ *SDS* Self-Rating Depression Scale

*$P < 0.05$ was considered statistically significant

Lactulose hydrogen breath test

After a LHBT at T0, sixteen IBS-D patients had a positive LHBT (six patients have a baseline value of H2 ≥ 20 p.p.m, while the rest have a rise of > 20 p.p.m from baseline in H2 within 90 min of lactulose administration) and were considered a presence of SIBO. After 4-week treatment with Golden bifid, 4 of the 16 (25%) patients with SIBO had a negative LHBT, which implied that the SIBO could be partially eradicated by Golden bifid.

GI symptoms and psychological symptoms

After a 4-week treatment of Golden bifid, the GI symptoms in IBS-D patients including abdominal pain (2.90 ± 1.04 vs. 1.90 ± 1.26), abdominal distension (2.00 ± 1.34 vs. 1.29 ± 1.31), diarrhea (3.24 ± 1.37 vs. 1.81 ± 1.21), defecatory urgency (3.48 ± 1.03 vs. 2.33 ± 1.35) and incomplete evacuation (2.71 ± 1.15 vs. 1.76 ± 1.26) were improved significantly ($P < 0.05$) (Table 2). In psychological symptoms, the SDS was decreased significantly (46.19 ± 11.36 vs. 43.33 ± 9.65, $P < 0.05$), while there was no significant difference in SAS (Table 2).

Characterization of gut microbiota in IBS-D

A total of 42 fecal samples of 21 IBS-D patients before and after Golden bifid treatment were analyzed by 16S rRNA gene-targeted pyrosequencing to observe and compare the characterization of fecal microbiota in IBS-D patients at T0 and T28. After demultiplexing and quality-filtering the original sequencing data, 2,046,464 high-quality sequences were obtained with an average of 48,725 sequences per sample. The sequences with 97% similarity cutoff were clustered, and 715 OTUs were obtained.

The rarefaction curve (Fig. 1A) and rank abundance curves (Fig. 1B) for the 42 samples generated using R software were clustered at the 97% phylotype similarity level. Thus, the sequencing depth was sufficient for exploring the microbial community and the species abundance, and community evenness was suitable for further analysis.

The fecal microbiota richness, evenness and community coverage before and after Golden bifid treatment of IBS-D patients are shown in Table 3. No significant differences in the richness parameters (Sobs, Ace, Chao1) and community diversity parameters (Shannon, Simpson) ($P > 0.05$) were found in IBS-D patients before and after treatment. Meanwhile, the sequencing depth was sufficient for analyzing fecal microbiota according to the coverage parameters values (> 99.9%).

Hierarchical clustering dendrogram and PCoA were used to analyze the similarity between microbial communities in the 42 fecal samples (Fig. 2). The overall trend of the hierarchical clustering dendrogram was that gut microbiota of one IBS-D patients before and after Golden bifid treatment clustered together firstly and then clustered with other patients, which indicated that the fecal

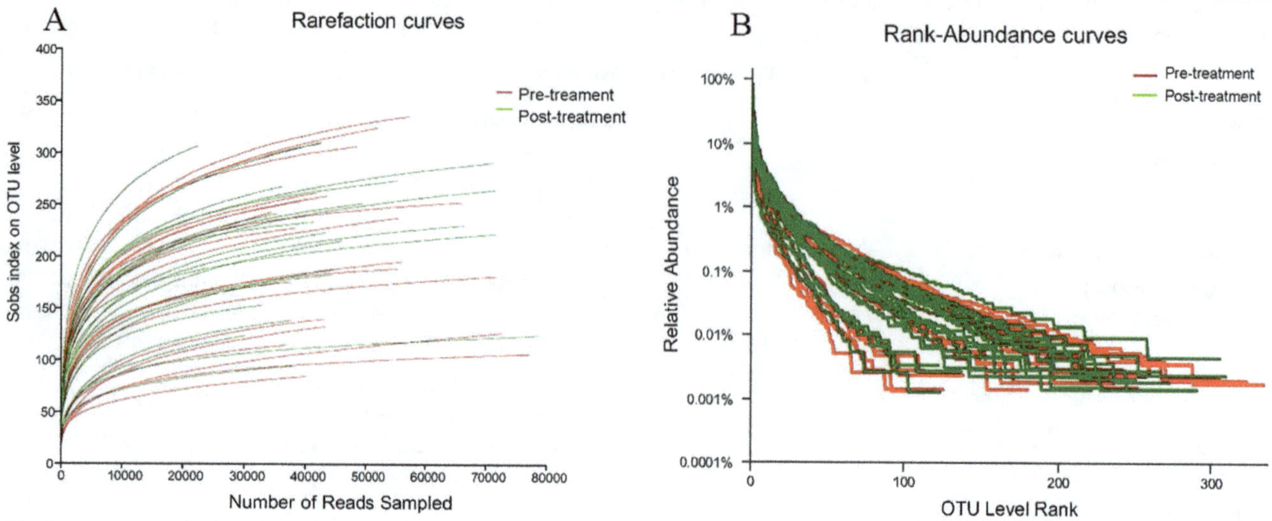

Fig. 1 Sequencing depth of the 42 fecal samples in IBS-D patients before and after Golden bifid treatment. **A** Rarefaction curves. **B** Rank abundance curves

Table 3 Fecal microbiota community indices before and after treatment

Community indices	Pre-treatment (mean)	Pre-treatment (SD[†])	Post-treatment (mean)	Post-treatment (SD)	*P* value
Sobs	214.43	62.752	211.62	75.831	0.8966
Ace	246.15	67.273	245.68	82.401	0.9841
Chao 1	249.03	69.702	240.49	82.558	0.7192
Shannon	3.1523	0.71986	3.0933	0.74728	0.7959
Simpson	0.12578	0.16176	0.12593	0.13854	0.9975
Coverage	0.99913	0.000425	0.99926	0.000341	0.2688

[†] *SD* standard deviation

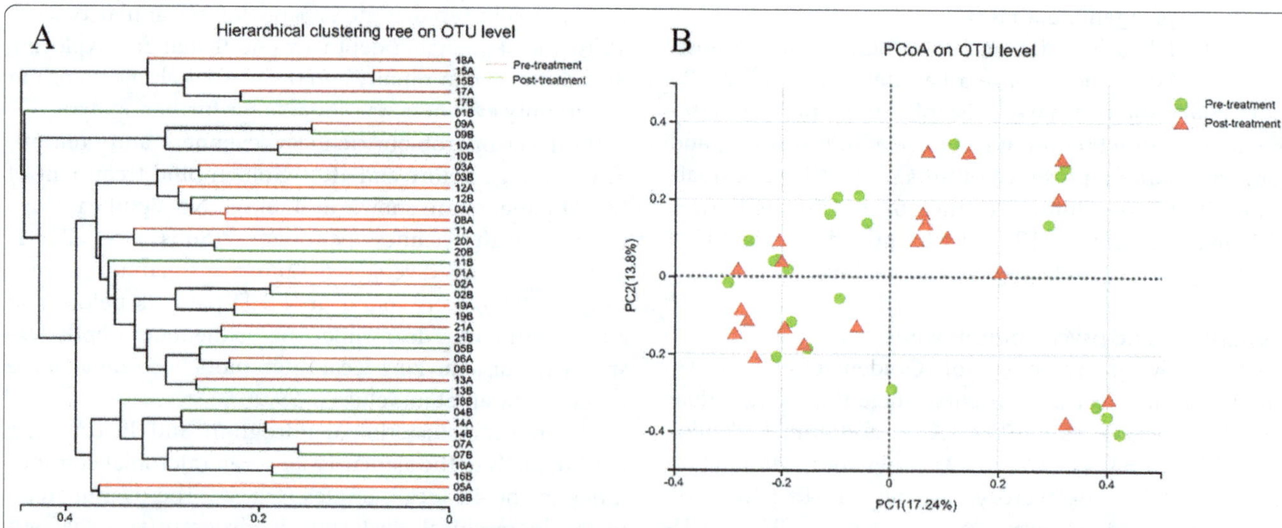

Fig. 2 Structural comparison of fecal microbiota from IBS-D patients before and after Golden bifid treatment. **A** Hierarchical clustering analysis of fecal microbiota in IBS-D patients before and after Golden bifid treatment. Each branch and color on the tree represented one sample and one group (the IBS-D patients before and after Golden bifid treatment), respectively. **B** Principal coordinates analysis (PCoA) of fecal microbiota in IBS-D patients before and after Golden bifid treatment

microbiota from IBS-D patients before and after Golden bifid treatment could not be divided into two different clusters completely (Fig. 2A). Similarly, on the PCoA graph, the fecal microbiota in IBS-D patients before and after treatment could not be separated clearly into two different clusters (Fig. 2B).

RDP classifier was used to analyze the taxonomy of microbiota in the 42 fecal samples. At the phylum level, twelve phyla were found in all fecal samples. As shown in Fig. 3, the composition of fecal microbiota in each sample was different in phylum level (Fig. 3A). There was no significant difference of fecal microbiota at phylum level in IBS-D patients before and after Golden bifid treatment (Fig. 3B).

At the genus levels, 257 genera were found in the 42 fecal samples. *Bacteroides, Blautia, Megamonas, Faecalibacterium* and *Escherichia-shigella* were the most predominant genera in fecal samples from IBS-D patients before and after Golden bifid treatment (Fig. 4). After treatment, the abundance of *Unclassified Lachnospiraceae* and *Dorea* were increased in fecal microbiota of IBS-D patients, while the *Ruminococcaceae NK4A214*

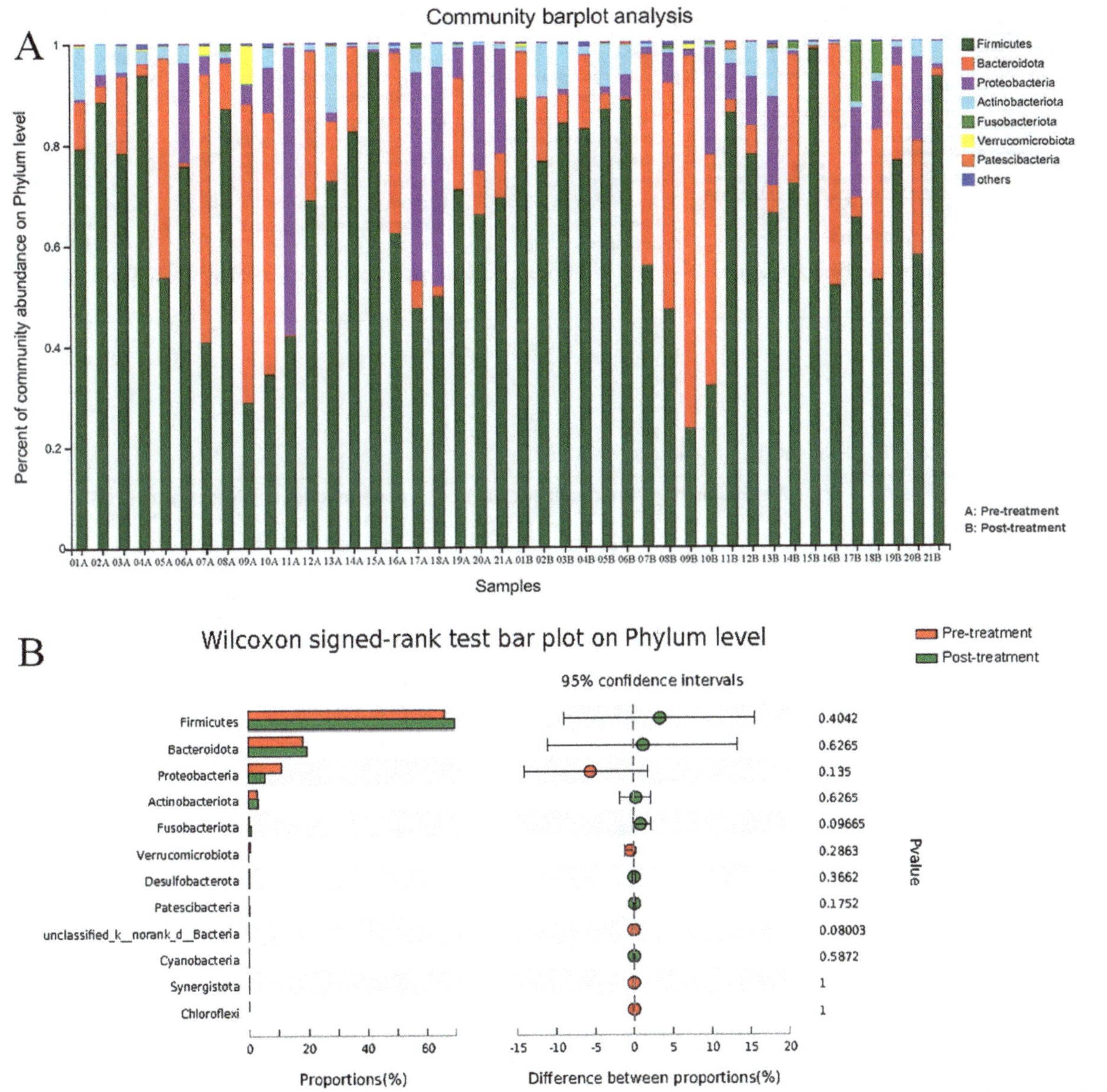

Fig. 3 Characteristics of fecal microbiota at the phylum level. **A** Relative abundance of fecal microbiota at the phylum levels in IBS-D patients before and after Golden bifid treatment. **B** Comparison of relative abundance of fecal microbiota at phylum levels in IBS-D patients before and after Golden bifid treatment

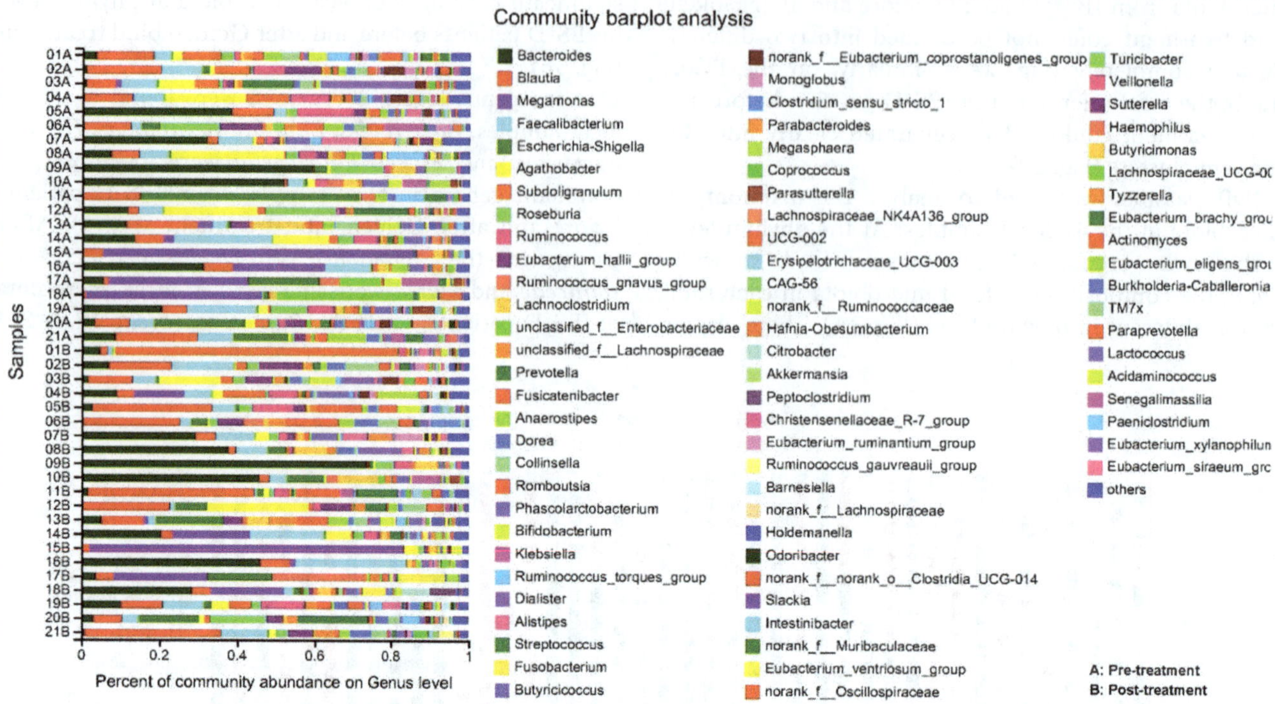

Fig. 4 Characteristics of fecal microbiota at the genus level. Relative abundance of fecal microbiota at the genus levels in IBS-D patients before and after Golden bifid treatment

Table 4 Fecal microbiota in IBS-D patients before and after treatment

Taxon	Pre-treatment (mean)	Pre-treatment (SD[†])	Post-treatment (mean)	Post-treatment (SD)	*P* value
Genus					
Unclassified Lachnospiraceae	1.298	1.024	2.124	1.827	0.02854
Dorea	1.199	1.196	1.88	2.095	0.01987
Ruminococcaceae NK4A214 group	0.146	0.2565	0.09111	0.1912	0.01673
Unclassified Ruminococcaceae	0.1359	0.232	0.05778	0.09483	0.01661
Coriobacteriales Incertae Sedis	0.02911	0.05526	0.006373	0.009627	0.04401
Peptoniphilus	0.002012	0.006217	6.69E-05	0.000307	0.01427
Species					
Bacteroides xylanisolvens Bacteroides	1.588	2.525	2.697	5.52	0.04381
Unclassified Lachnospiraceae	1.298	1.024	2.124	1.827	0.02854
Bacterium Dorea	0.9228	1.063	1.388	1.973	0.0403
Bacterium Butyricicoccus	0.6035	0.9297	0.7092	0.7979	0.04189
Dorea formicigenerans ATCC 27755	0.2761	0.3662	0.4921	0.7504	0.04067
Unclassified Fusobacterium	0.0131	0.02308	0.356	1.197	0.04149
Unclassified NK4A214 group	0.1452	0.2544	0.08982	0.1887	0.01847
Unclassified Ruminococcaceae	0.1359	0.232	0.05778	0.09483	0.01661
Gut metagenome Roseburia	0.03581	0.145	0.01651	0.07418	0.03603
Unclassified Oscillibacter	0.01026	0.01981	0.003806	0.009182	0.01906
Uncultured organism Oribacterium	0.003345	0.003436	0.003265	0.009434	0.03281
Unclassified Bifidobacterium	0	0	0.005316	0.01523	0.03603

[†] *SD* standard deviation

group, unclassified Ruminococcaceae, Coriobacteriales Incertae Sedis and *Peptoniphilus* were decreased ($P < 0.05$) (Table 4, Additional file 1: Fig. S1A). And at the species levels, we found that the abundance of *Bacteroides xylanisolvens Bacteroides, Unclassified Lachnospiraceae, Bacterium Dorea, Bacterium Butyricicoccus, Dorea formicigenerans ATCC 27755, Unclassified Fusobacterium* and *Unclassified Bifidobacterium* were increased in feces, while the *Unclassified NK4A214 group, Unclassified Ruminococcaceae, Gut metagenome Roseburia, Unclassified Oscillibacter* and *Uncultured organism Oribacterium* were decreased ($P < 0.05$) (Table 4, Additional file 1: Fig. S1B).

We found that there were some alterations of microbial community structure in IBS-D patients after Golden bifid treatment at the genus and species level. To explore the potential role of these changes in fecal microbial compositions, we used PICRUSt2 to infer microbial gene content from 16S rRNA gene data and aggregated relative abundance of functional genes into metabolic pathways. We have analyzed the basic metabolism pathways of gut microbiome including carbohydrate metabolism, amino acid metabolism, nucleotide metabolism, energy metabolism, vitamins metabolism and glycan metabolism (Fig. 5). However, no significant differences of these metabolites were found in IBS-D patients before and after treatment.

Adverse events

No deaths and other adverse events occurred during Golden Bifid treatment. Therefore, the treatment of Golden Bifid was well tolerated.

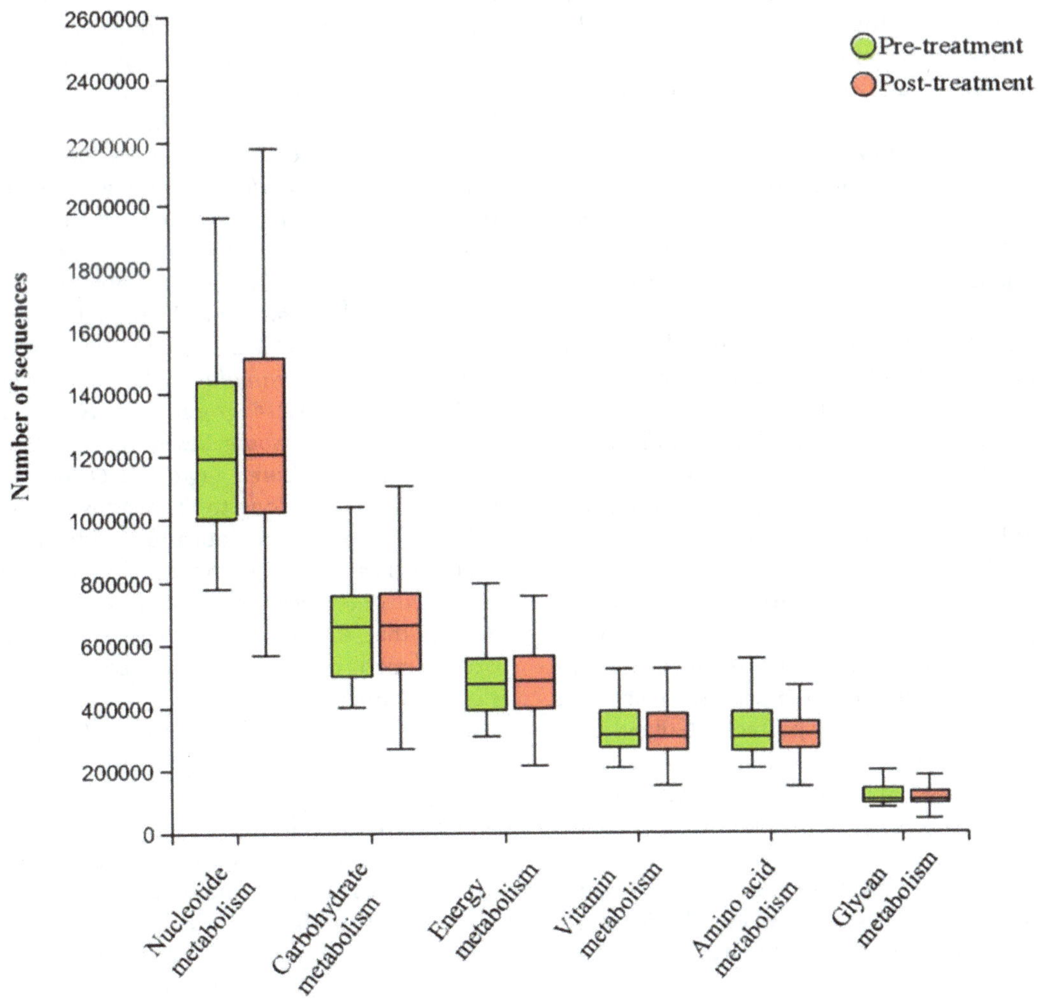

Fig. 5 Basic metabolism pathways of gut microbiome in IBS-D patients before and after Golden bifid treatment

Discussion

In this study, we found that 4-week treatment of Golden bifid could not only alleviate the symptoms of abdominal pain, abdominal distension, diarrhea, defecatory urgency and incomplete evacuation, but also improve the depressive symptoms and modulate the fecal microbiota of IBS-D patients. Thus, we inferred that the Golden bifid might improve the symptoms of IBS-D by intervening gut microbiota.

Many studies have shown that the alterations of gut microbiota might be highly associated with IBS [12, 16]. A systematic review showed that the *Enterobacteriaceae, Lactobacillaceae* and *Bacteroides* were increased, while *uncultured Clostridiales, Faecalibacterium* and *Bifidobacterium* were decreased in IBS patients compared with healthy controls [17]. Therefore, the manipulation of the microbiota and probiotics treatments is becoming therapeutic option for IBS [18] and the effectiveness of probiotics might be different due to the strain and dose-specific [19]. In our study, we found that the GI symptoms including abdominal pain, abdominal distension, diarrhea, defecatory urgency and incomplete evacuation of IBS-D patients were improved significantly after treatment. Hoveyda et al. [20] also showed that probiotics could effectively alleviate the overall symptom score of IBS patients. Although the therapeutic mechanism of Golden bifid is unclear, it might be related to the improvement of intestinal epithelial barrier function, relief of visceral hypersensitivity, inhibition of adhesion pathogenic bacteria and regulation of the immune system. Probiotics intervention could increase the expression of tight junction protein, reduce the levels of interferon and interleukin-4 (IL-4) in colonic mucosa and improve the intestinal barrier function [21], which might relieve the symptom of diarrhea. In addition, *Bifidobacterium longum* alleviated visceral hypersensitivity in rats by enhancing lysozyme production and promoting mucosal repair and result in the relief of abdominal pain [22].

With the development of the viewpoint of brain–gut–microbiota axis, psychological factors are also considered to be a pathogenesis of IBS and abnormalities in gut microbiota can influence changes in psychological health [23]. In this study, we found that the depression scores in IBS-D patients were reduced by probiotic Golden bifid. Similarly, Ma et al. [11] supported that probiotic could improve the mental well-being of IBS and this improvement was possibly mediated by restoration of microbial balance and the brain–gut axis. Probiotics could not only normalize noradrenaline levels in the brainstem region that regulates emotion, but also alter other brain neurotransmitters, such as gamma-aminobutyric acid and serotonin [24, 25], which might be the influencing factors to mental health.

In addition, we observed that a small proportion SIBO could be eradicated in those IBS-D patients with SIBO after Golden bifid treatment, which might imply that Golden bifid could eradicate SIBO by modulating the gut microbiota. Research showed that the abundances of *Lactobacillus* and *Bifidobacterium* in the feces of IBS patients were increased significantly after probiotics intervention [9]. *Bifidobacterium* could increase IgA antibody, provide an immune barrier to mucosal surface, enhance the function of the immune system and ultimately improve the disease resistance of human body [26]. Similarly, the results of 16S rRNA gene-targeted pyrosequencing in our study showed that there were some alterations of fecal microbiota after Golden bifid treatment. At the genus level, the abundance of *Unclassified Lachnospiraceae* and *Dorea* were increased. *Lachnospiraceae* and *Dorea* are genera belonging to Firmicutes and *Lachnospiraceae* produces short-chain fatty acids (SCFAs), especially butyrate, which is not only an important energy source for colonic epithelial cells to maintain normal intestinal barrier function but also a controller in the procedure of intestinal inflammation and the maturation of immune system [27]. At the species level, the abundance of *Bacteroides xylanisolvens Bacteroides, Unclassified Lachnospiraceae, Bacterium Dorea, Bacterium Butyricicoccus, Dorea formicigenerans ATCC 27755, Unclassified Fusobacterium* and *Unclassified Bifidobacterium* were increased after treatment. The *Unclassified Lachnospiraceae, Bacterium Dorea, Bacterium Butyricicoccus* and *Dorea formicigenerans ATCC 27755* are species belonging to Firmicutes phylum. In addition, some decreased bacteria such as *Ruminococcaceae NK4A214 group, unclassified Ruminococcaceae* and *Peptoniphilus* at the genus level, as well as *Unclassified NK4A214 group, Unclassified Ruminococcaceae, Gut metagenome Roseburia, Unclassified Oscillibacter* and *Uncultured organism Oribacterium* at the species level also belong to Firmicutes. It was noticeable that most altered microbiota after Golden bifid treatment belong to Firmicutes. Therefore, although there were no significant differences of Firmicutes after treatment, we thought that the improvement of symptoms in IBS-D patients might be partially attributed to the relative alteration of Firmicutes.

Interestingly, the abundances of *Bifidobacterium Longum, Lactobacillus bulgaricus* and *Streptococcus thermophilus* did not increase after Golden bifid supplementation. Similarly, Martin et al. [28] found that a 6-month probiotic administration did not significantly alter gut microbiota community structure or diversity as compared to placebo, which might indicate that the improved symptoms of IBS-D patients after probiotics supplementation were not only due to the abundance of probiotics itself has altered, but also accompanied by some other notable changes in the internal environment. For example, Zhou et al. [22] have reported that *Bifidobacterium Longum* alleviated visceral hypersensitivity in rats subjected to water avoidance stress (WAS) by enhancing lysozyme production and promoting mucosal repair. In addition, IBS subjects have increased inflammatory cytokines in gut mucosa compared with controls and suggestive of inflammation in IBS [29]. Golden bifid could alleviate or inhibit further inflammation by suppressing the expression of toll-like receptor 4 (TLR4) [30] and *Bifidobacterium infantis 35624* increased the anti-inflammatory interleukin-10 (IL-10)/proinflammatory interleukin-12 (IL-12) ratio [31]. In terms of the metabolism of gut microbiota, no significant differences of carbohydrate metabolism, amino acid metabolism, nucleotide metabolism, energy metabolism, vitamins metabolism and glycan metabolism were found in fecal microbiota before and after Golden bifid treatments in our study. However, Kim et al. [32] found that probiotics could significantly change metabolites including palmitic acid methyl ester (PAME) and 4,6-dihydroxyquinoline, 4-(2-aminophenyl)-2,4-dioxobutanoic acid (DOBA). Another study showed that *Lactobacillus acidophilus NCFM* and *Bifidobacterium lactis Bi-07* supplementation increased levels of glutamate, SCFAs and ketone bodies and decreased levels of choline, creatine and lactate in weaned rats [33]. These results suggest that probiotic supplementation might alleviate IBS by changing the intestinal environment.

There are several limitations in this study. Firstly, due to the lack of placebo group and a relatively small sample size, the conclusion of this study should be drawn cautiously. Secondly, we found that there were some alterations of microbiota in fecal microbiota of IBS-D patients after Golden bifid treatments. And we inferred that these alterations were associated with the improvement of symptoms IBS-D patients, but further experiments are lacking to confirm this conclusion. Thirdly, no significant differences of microbiota metabolism were found in IBS-D patients before and after Golden bifid treatment and more precise method should be adopted to further explore the effects of Golden bifid on microbiota metabolism.

In conclusion, a 4-week treatment of Golden bifid could significantly improve the abdominal pain, abdominal distension, diarrhea, defecatory urgency, incomplete evacuation and depression symptoms of IBS-D patients. Besides it, after Golden bifid treatment, the abundance of some gut bacteria such as *Lachnospiraceae* and *Dorea* have altered in fecal microbiota, which might imply that the Golden bifid could improve IBS-D via microbiota modulation and provide some evidences for the treatments of probiotics in IBS-D. However, the precise strains and mechanisms of probiotic improve the IBS-D are not fully understood and further studies are warranted to define those and provide more evidences for probiotics treatment of IBS.

Abbreviations

IBS: Irritable bowel syndrome; IBS-D: Diarrhea-predominant irritable bowel syndrome; GI: Gastrointestinal; SDS: Self-Rating Depression Scale; SAS: Self-Rating Anxiety Scale; SIBO: Small intestine bacterial overgrowth; FBDs: Functional bowel disorders; LHBT: Lactulose hydrogen breath test; OTUs: Operational taxonomic units; PCoA: Principal coordinates analysis; SCFAs: Short-chain fatty acids.

Acknowledgements

Not applicable.

Author contributions

ML and LSX conceived and designed the study. ML collected the data, conducted the data analysis and drafted the manuscript. LSX, QL and LX reviewed and revised the manuscript. All authors read and approved the final manuscript.

References

1. Xiong LS, Chen MH, Chen HX, Xu AG, Wang WA, Hu PJ. A population-based epidemiologic study of irritable bowel syndrome in South China: stratified randomized study by cluster sampling. Aliment Pharmacol Ther. 2004;19:1217–24.
2. Sperber AD, Dumitrascu D, Fukudo S, et al. The global prevalence of IBS in adults remains elusive due to the heterogeneity of studies: a Rome Foundation working team literature review. Gut. 2017;66:1075–82.
3. Zhang L, Duan L, Liu Y, et al. A meta-analysis of the prevalence and risk factors of irritable bowel syndrome in Chinese community. Zhonghua Nei Ke Za Zhi. 2014;53:969–75.
4. Heitkemper M, Jarrett M, Jun SE. Update on irritable bowel syndrome program of research. J Korean Acad Nurs. 2013;43:579–86.
5. Shanahan F. The colonic microbiota in health and disease. Curr Opin Gastroenterol. 2013;29:49–54.
6. Pickard JM, Zeng MY, Caruso R, Núñez G. Gut microbiota: role in pathogen colonization, immune responses, and inflammatory disease. Immunol Rev. 2017;279:70–89.
7. Piche T. Tight junctions and IBS–the link between epithelial permeability, low-grade inflammation, and symptom generation? Neurogastroenterol Motil. 2014;26:296–302.
8. Mayer EA, Savidge T, Shulman RJ. Brain–gut microbiome interactions and functional bowel disorders. Gastroenterology. 2014;146:1500–12.
9. Sinn DH, Song JH, Kim HJ, et al. Therapeutic effect of *Lactobacillus acidophilus*-SDC 2012, 2013 in patients with irritable bowel syndrome. Dig Dis Sci. 2008;53:2714–8.
10. Guglielmetti S, Mora D, Gschwender M, Popp K. Randomised clinical trial: *Bifidobacterium bifidum* MIMBb75 significantly alleviates irritable bowel syndrome and improves quality of life—a double-blind, placebo-controlled study. Aliment Pharmacol Ther. 2011;33:1123–32.
11. Ma ZF, Yusof N, Hamid N, et al. *Bifidobacterium infantis* M-63 improves mental health in victims with irritable bowel syndrome developed after a major flood disaster. Benef Microbes. 2019;10:111–20.
12. Zhuang X, Tian Z, Li L, Zeng Z, Chen M, Xiong L. Fecal microbiota alterations associated with diarrhea-predominant irritable bowel syndrome. Front Microbiol. 2018;9:1600.
13. Zhuang X, Tian Z, Luo M, Xiong L. Short-course Rifaximin therapy efficacy and lactulose hydrogen breath test in Chinese patients with diarrhea-predominant irritable bowel syndrome. BMC Gastroenterol. 2020;20:187.
14. Zhang Y, Bi YX, Chen J, et al. Association of Peroxiredoxin 1 and brain-derived neurotrophic factor serum levels with depression and anxiety symptoms in patients with irritable bowel syndrome. Gen Hosp Psychiatry. 2021;68:59–64.
15. Langille MG, Zaneveld J, Caporaso JG, et al. Predictive functional profiling of microbial communities using 16S rRNA marker gene sequences. Nat Biotechnol. 2013;31:814–21.

16. Mars R, Frith M, Kashyap PC. Functional gastrointestinal disorders and the microbiome—what is the best strategy for moving microbiome-based therapies for functional gastrointestinal disorders into the clinic? Gastroenterology. 2021;160:538–55.
17. Pittayanon R, Lau JT, Yuan Y, et al. Gut microbiota in patients with irritable bowel syndrome—a systematic review. Gastroenterology. 2019;157:97–108.
18. Distrutti E, Monaldi L, Ricci P, Fiorucci S. Gut microbiota role in irritable bowel syndrome: new therapeutic strategies. World J Gastroenterol. 2016;22:2219–41.
19. Allen AP, Clarke G, Cryan JF, Quigley E, Dinan TG. *Bifidobacterium infantis* 35624 and other probiotics in the management of irritable bowel syndrome. Strain specificity, symptoms, and mechanisms. Curr Med Res Opin. 2017;33:1349–51.
20. Hoveyda N, Heneghan C, Mahtani KR, Perera R, Roberts N, Glasziou P. A systematic review and meta-analysis: probiotics in the treatment of irritable bowel syndrome. BMC Gastroenterol. 2009;9:15.
21. Han X, Lee A, Huang S, Gao J, Spence JR, Owyang C. *Lactobacillus rhamnosus* GG prevents epithelial barrier dysfunction induced by interferon-gamma and fecal supernatants from irritable bowel syndrome patients in human intestinal enteroids and colonoids. Gut Microbes. 2019;10:59–76.
22. Zhou C, Fang X, Xu J, et al. *Bifidobacterium longum* alleviates irritable bowel syndrome-related visceral hypersensitivity and microbiota dysbiosis via Paneth cell regulation. Gut Microbes. 2020;12:1782156.
23. Neufeld KM, Kang N, Bienenstock J, Foster JA. Reduced anxiety-like behavior and central neurochemical change in germ-free mice. Neurogastroenterol Motil. 2011;23:255–64, e119.
24. Desbonnet L, Garrett L, Clarke G, Kiely B, Cryan JF, Dinan TG. Effects of the probiotic *Bifidobacterium infantis* in the maternal separation model of depression. Neuroscience. 2010;170:1179–88.
25. Dinan TG, Stanton C, Cryan JF. Psychobiotics: a novel class of psychotropic. Biol Psychiatry. 2013;74:720–6.
26. Paturi G, Phillips M, Jones M, Kailasapathy K. Immune enhancing effects of *Lactobacillus acidophilus* LAFTI L10 and *Lactobacillus paracasei* LAFTI L26 in mice. Int J Food Microbiol. 2007;115:115–8.
27. Kasahara K, Krautkramer KA, Org E, et al. Interactions between *Roseburia intestinalis* and diet modulate atherogenesis in a murine model. Nat Microbiol. 2018;3:1461–71.
28. Laursen MF, Laursen RP, Larnkjær A, Michaelsen KF, Bahl MI, Licht TR. Administration of two probiotic strains during early childhood does not affect the endogenous gut microbiota composition despite probiotic proliferation. BMC Microbiol. 2017;17:175.
29. Vanner S, Greenwood-Van MB, Mawe G, et al. Fundamentals of neurogastroenterology: basic science. Gastroenterology. 2016;150:1280.
30. Yao P, Tan F, Gao H, Wang L, Yang T, Cheng Y. Effects of probiotics on Toll-like receptor expression in ulcerative colitis rats induced by 2,4,6-trinitro-benzene sulfonic acid. Mol Med Rep. 2017;15:1973–80.
31. O'Mahony L, McCarthy J, Kelly P, et al. *Lactobacillus* and *bifidobacterium* in irritable bowel syndrome: symptom responses and relationship to cytokine profiles. Gastroenterology. 2005;128:541–51.
32. Kim J, Cho K, Kim JS, et al. Probiotic treatment induced change of inflammation related metabolites in IBS-D patients/double-blind, randomized, placebo-controlled trial. Food Sci Biotechnol. 2020;29:837–44.
33. Wang M, Chen Y, Wang Y, et al. Beneficial changes of gut microbiota and metabolism in weaned rats with *Lactobacillus acidophilus* NCFM and *Bifidobacterium lactis* Bi-07 supplementation. J Funct Foods. 2018;48:252–65.

12

A patient with familial Mediterranean fever mimicking diarrhea-dominant irritable bowel syndrome who successfully responded to treatment with colchicine: A case report

Shima Kumei[1], Masatomo Ishioh[2], Yuki Murakami[2], Katsuyoshi Ando[2], Tsukasa Nozu[3] and Toshikatsu Okumura[1,2*]

Abstract

Background: Irritable bowel syndrome is a functional gastrointestinal disease. Visceral hypersensitivity is the most important pathophysiology in irritable bowel syndrome. Currently, diagnosis of irritable bowel syndrome is based on symptoms and exclusion of other organic diseases. Although the diagnosis of irritable bowel syndrome can be made based on the Rome IV criteria, one may speculate that complete exclusion of other organic diseases is not so easy, especially in cases uncontrolled with standard therapies.

Case presentation: We present herein a case of familial Mediterranean fever in a young Japanese patient who had been suffering from an irritable bowel syndrome-like clinical course. A 25-year-old Japanese male had been diagnosed as having diarrhea-predominant irritable bowel syndrome 5 years earlier. Unfortunately, standard therapies failed to improve irritable bowel syndrome symptoms. After careful medical history-taking, we understood that he had also experienced periodic fever since 10 years ago. Although no mutation was identified in the Mediterranean fever gene, not only periodic fever but abdominal symptoms improved completely after colchicine administration. He was therefore diagnosed as having familial Mediterranean fever and that the abdominal symptoms may be related to the disease.

Conclusions: Familial Mediterranean fever should be considered as a cause of irritable bowel syndrome-like symptoms.

Keywords: Familial Mediterranean fever, Irritable bowel syndrome, Colchicine

Background

Irritable bowel syndrome (IBS) is a functional gastrointestinal disease with a high population prevalence [1, 2]. Clinical symptoms of IBS include abdominal pain and stool irregularities, as well as other somatic, visceral, and psychiatric comorbidities [1, 2]. Currently, diagnosis of IBS is based on symptoms and exclusion of other organic diseases. Although a diagnosis of IBS can be made based on the Rome IV criteria [2], one may speculate whether complete exclusion of other organic diseases is not so easy, especially in cases uncontrolled with standard therapies.

Familial Mediterranean fever (FMF) is a genetic autoinflammatory disease characterized by recurrent fever with serosal inflammation [3]. FMF is considered to be rare in Japan, and the clinical features in Japanese tend

*Correspondence: okumurat@asahikawa-med.ac.jp

[2] Division of Metabolism, Systemic Bioscience, Gastroenterology and Hematology/Oncology, Department of Medicine, Asahikawa Medical University, Asahikawa, Japan

Full list of author information is available at the end of the article

to be milder than those observed in the Mediterranean population due to different genotypes of the Mediterranean fever (MEFV) gene [4, 5]. We present herein a case of FMF in a young Japanese patient who had been suffering from an IBS-like clinical course such as chronic severe diarrhea and abdominal pain. In clinical practice, we have experienced patients with an unknown cause of chronic diarrhea. When organic diseases are excluded by clinical tests or images including gastrointestinal endoscopy in patients with chronic diarrhea, we used to make a diagnosis of functional gastrointestinal diseases such as IBS. Based on the present case, we should consider FMF in the differential diagnosis of such patients with chronic diarrhea of unknown cause.

Case report

A 25-year-old Japanese male complained of uncontrollable watery diarrhea over 10 times a day and abdominal pain since 5 years ago. Abdominal pain was mild lower abdominal pain relieving after defecation. There was no convincing aggravating factor for the abdominal pain. He had never had any health problems in the past. There was no particular social, environmental, or family history. His occupation was civil servant. He had never smoked and had drunk socially. Medical examination at the first visit revealed blood pressure of 120/72 mmHg, pulse rate, of 72 times/minutes (regular), and body temperature of 36.2 °C. There were no obvious abdominal and neurological findings, including abdominal tenderness.

He had received esophagogastroduodenoscopy, colonoscopy, and capsule endoscopy in addition to urine and blood examinations, and abdominal imaging such as abdominal computed tomography and magnetic resonance imaging (MRI). However, no abnormal findings had been detected, and he was diagnosed with diarrhea-dominant irritable bowel syndrome (D-IBS) based on the Rome IV criteria. He then received oral medicines including loperamide (1.0 mg/day) for 1 month, albumin tannate (3.0 g/day) for 1 month, or ramosetron hydrochloride (5 μg/day) for 1 month without improvement of his abdominal symptoms prior to his first visit to our department.

He had been introduced to our department because of uncontrollable D-IBS for a long time. Laboratory testing including TSH was normal (Table 1). Whole-body computed tomography reveled no abnormality (Fig. 1A, B). To rule out collagenous colitis, infectious diseases, and celiac disease, colonoscopy including terminal ileum, random biopsies, and culture test of intestinal juice were performed and no macroscopic, pathological abnormality such as collagen band or possible disease-causing bacteria was observed (Fig. 1C, D). After careful medical history-taking, we understood that he had been experienced periodic fever since 10 years ago. Fever is characterized by recurrent (approximately once a month) and self-limited (a couple of days) fever. Figure 2 shows the time course of clinical characteristics. Blood examination on the day of fever revealed high white blood cell (WBC) count (20,400/μL), C-reactive protein

Table 1 Laboratory data at first visit to our department (normal body temperature)

WBC	8800	/μl
Neu	67.4	%
Lymp	25.5	%
Mono	4.4	%
Eos	2.2	%
Baso	0.5	%
RBC	536×10^4	/μl
Hb	16.	g/dl
Plt	25.5×10^4	/μl
TP	7.2	g/dl
Alb	4.7	g/dl
T-Bil	0.4	mg/dl
ChE	434	IU/l
ALP	322	IU/l
AST	28	IU/l
ALT	48	IU/l
LDH	211	IU/l
γGTP	65	IU/l
CK	142	IU/l
AMY	86	IU/l
BUN	10.1	mg/dl
Cre	0.9	mg/dl
UA	6.7	mg/dl
Na	142	mEq/l
K	4.3	mEq/l
Cl	106	mEq/l
Ca	9.5	mEq/l
CRP	< 0.10	mg/dl
Fe	59	μg/dl
UIBC	319	μg/dl
TIBC	378	μg/dl
Ferritin	238.3	ng/dl
HbA1c	5.8	%
T-cho	236	mg/dl
TG	500	mg/dl
FT4	1.31	ng/dl
TSH	2.79	μIU/ml

WBC: white blood cell, RBC: red blood cell, Hb. Hemoglobin, Plt: platelet, TP: total protein, Alb: albumin, T-Bil: total bilirubin, ChE: cholinesterase, ALP: alkaline phosphatase, AST: aspartate aminotransferase, ALT: alanine aminotransferase, LDH: Lactate Dehydrogenase, γGTP: γ-glutamyl transpeptidase, CK: creatine kinase, AMY: amylase, BUN: blood urea nitrogen, Cre: creatinine, UA: uric acid, CRP: c-reactive protein, UIBC: unsaturated iron binding capacity, TIBC: total iron binding capacity, T-cho: total cholesterol, TG: triglyceride, FT4: free thyroxine, TSH: thyroid-stimulating hormone

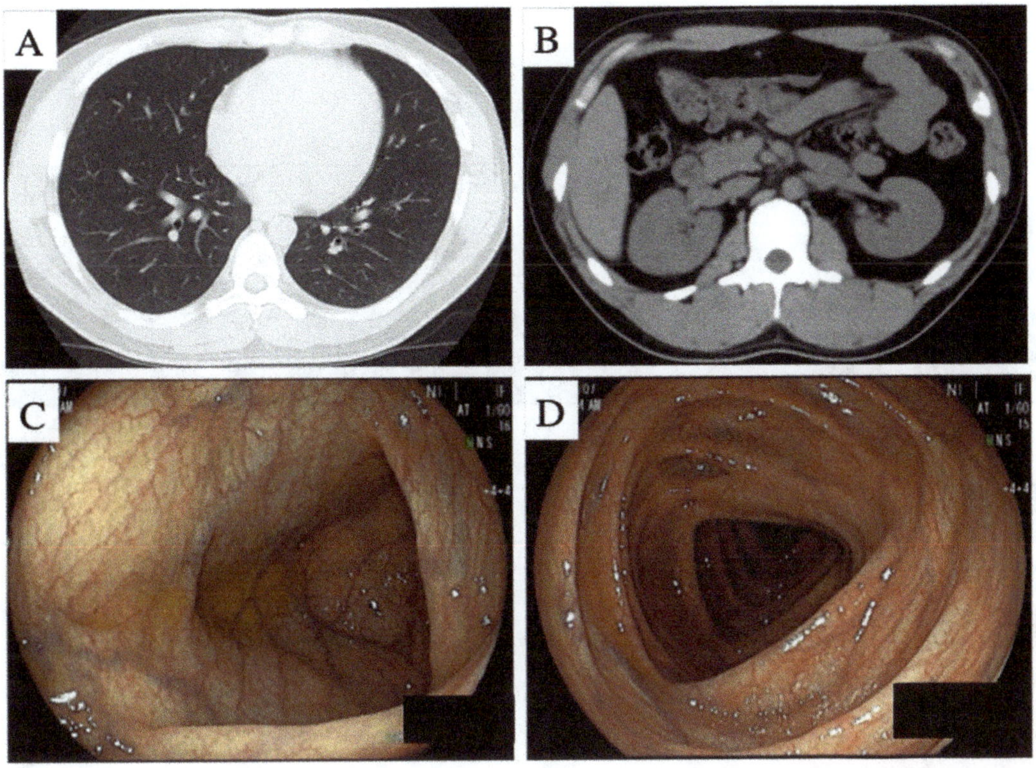

Fig. 1 Clinical images of this case: **A** chest CT scan, **B** abdominal CT scan, **C** colonoscopy for sigmoid colon, and **D** colonoscopy for ascending colon

(CRP) (1.79 mg/dL), and amyloid A protein (169 mg/dL) without anemia. However, during the interval between febrile attacks, his body temperature was normal and the laboratory data of inflammatory reaction were at normal levels. These clinical characteristics suggested a suspicion of familial Mediterranean fever (FMF), although we did not confirm that diarrhea and abdominal pain were associated with FMF. After 12 months since the start of colchicine administration at 0.5 mg/day, the patient has been free of fever. As shown in Fig. 2, not only periodic fever but also abdominal symptoms such as severe diarrhea improved completely after colchicine administration. All exons of the MEFV gene in the patient were sequenced, and no mutation was identified. Based on these findings, we concluded a diagnosis of FMF according to the criteria in Japan [4] in spite of the lack of gene mutation, and that abdominal symptoms may be related to the disease.

Discussion

To our knowledge, there are no reports on the relationship between chronic diarrhea and FMF. The present case suggests that FMF should be considered to be a cause of chronic diarrhea, especially when organic gastrointestinal diseases are excluded.

FMF is characterized by self-limiting fever episodes, usually accompanied by serositis, arthralgia, and arthritis [3]. The diagnosis of FMF is made based on patient history, inflammatory markers, and genetic testing [6]. Several clinical diagnostic criteria sets have been proposed for diagnosis of FMF. The Tel Hashomer criteria, Livneh criteria, and Turkish pediatric criteria all rely on clinical symptoms, family history, and colchicine response [7–9]. In the diagnosis of Japanese patients with FMF, modified Tel Hashmer criteria (Fig. 3) have been suggested [4]. These include: recurrent febrile episodes (three or more episodes lasting 12 h to 3 days with fever $\geq$ 38 °C), and eight minor criteria as shown in Fig. 3. A diagnosis of FMF is determined if the patient exhibits the major criteria and one or more minor criteria. Differential diagnoses include infections, malignancy, and autoinflammatory diseases. In the present case, we diagnosed FMF because of recurrent febrile episodes and a favorable response to colchicine.

With regard to treatment for FMF, there are limited RCTs assessing interventions for patients with FMF in the most recent Cochrane Database [10]. Based on the evidence, daily colchicine may reduce the number of attacks. It has also been described that canakinumab probably reduces the number of attacks, and anakinra or

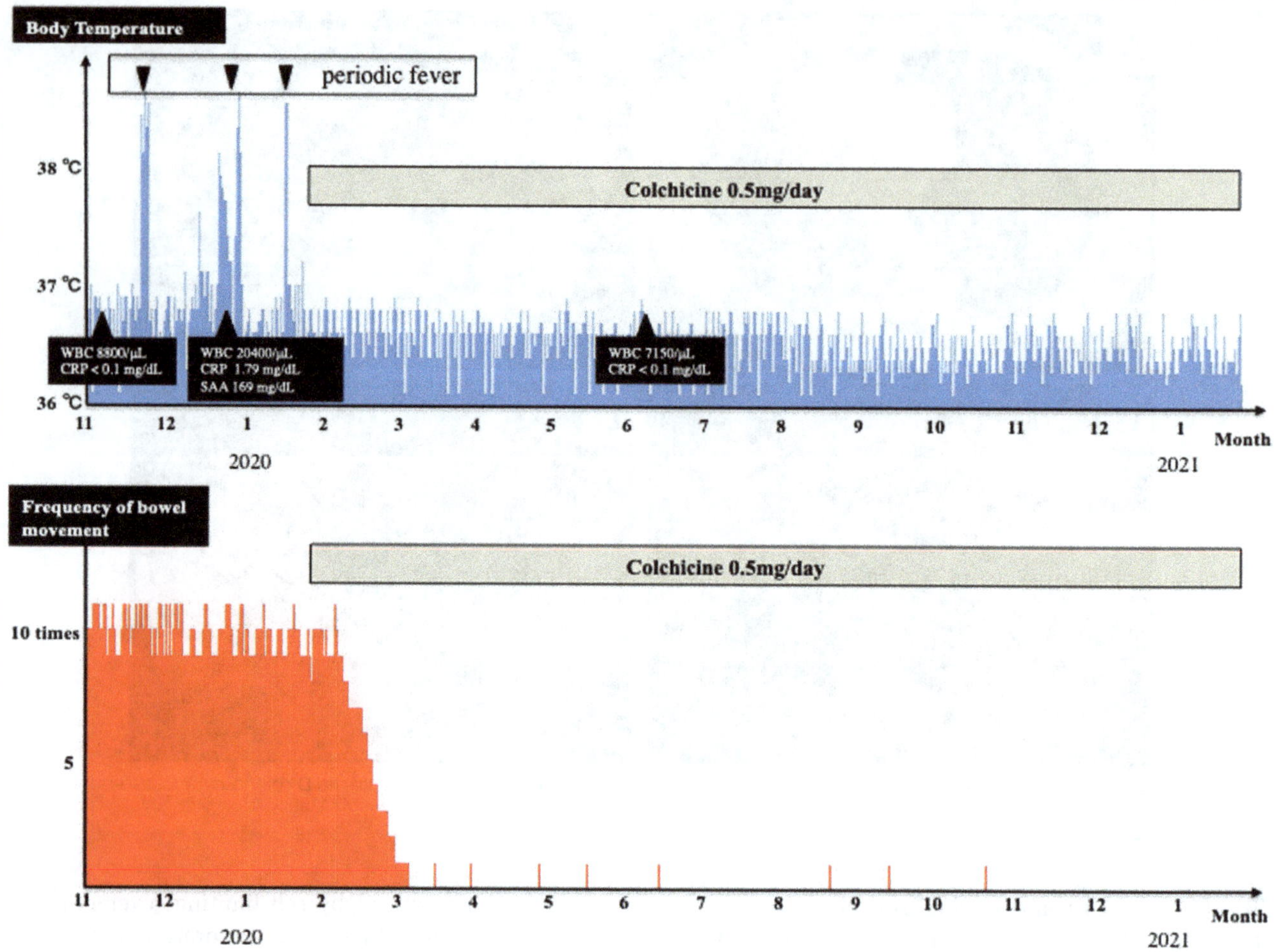

Fig. 2 Time course of clinical characteristics in this case

Diagnostic criteria for familial Mediterranean fever

Major criteria
Recurrent febrile episodes as 3 or more episodes lasting 12 h to 3 days with fever of 38 ℃ or more

Minor criteria
- Abdominal pain due to peritonitis
- Chest pain due to pleuritic Pericarditis
- Monoarthritis of hip, knee or ankle
- Fever alone
- Scrotum pain due to orchitis
- Headache due to aseptic meningitis
- Favourable response to colchicine

A diagnosis of FMF is reached if the patient has 1 major criteria plus 1 or more minor criteria.

Fig. 3 Diagnostic criteria for FMF in Japan [4]

canakinumab probably reduce CRP in colchicine-resistant participants. Thus, further research should be carried out to establish standard therapy for FMF.

With regard to a relationship between FMF and gastrointestinal disorders, accumulating evidence has suggested that some FMF patients exhibit intestinal mucosal lesions resembling inflammatory bowel diseases (IBD) [11, 12]. Uslu *et al.* [13] demonstrated that disease-causing *MEFV* mutations and the FMF disease rate were increased among patients with IBD. This increase was prominent among CD patients. Thus, FMF is considered to be a possible cause in patients with chronic intestinal mucosal lesions. However, in the present case, upper and lower gastrointestinal endoscopy detected no mucosal lesions in the gastrointestinal tract. These findings suggested that chronic diarrhea and abdominal pain came from functional but not organic gastrointestinal diseases such as IBD. Ekinci *et al.* examined a relationship between FMF and functional gastrointestinal disorders [14]. In their report on Turkish people, D-IBS was observed in 3 out of 103 FMF patients (2.9 %) and 2 out of 100 healthy subjects

(2 %), respectively, suggesting that coexistence of FMF and D-IBS was not high in FMF when compared with healthy control. In other words, we suggest that D-IBS was observed incidentally in patients with FMF. In the present case, D-IBS developed from FMF rather than other causes incidentally because colchicine completely prevented not only typical FMF-induced febrile attacks but also severe diarrhea and abdominal pain.

The present case demonstrates that FMF can present IBS-like symptoms without intestinal mucosal lesions. In clinical practice, we do not usually rule in/out FMF when IBS is considered to be a highly possible diagnosis in patients with diarrhea and abdominal pain without any organic abnormality. FMF can be diagnosed even if mutation of MEFV gene is not detected. In Japan, MEFV gene mutation is not detected in approximately 5% of patients with FMF [15]. The present case suggests that patients with FMF may manifest gastrointestinal disease mimicking IBS, because colchicine potently improved not only periodic fever but also gastrointestinal symptoms such as diarrhea and abdominal pain.

Conclusions

FMF should be considered as a cause of IBS-like symptoms, especially in patients diagnosed with IBS who do not respond to conventional IBS treatment.

Abbreviations

IBS: Irritable bowel syndrome; FMF: Familial Mediterranean fever; MEFV: Mediterranean fever; D-IBS: Diarrhea-dominant irritable bowel syndrome; IBD: Inflammatory bowel diseases.

Acknowledgements

The authors thank Dr. Ohhira for English language editing.

Author contributions

SK and TO wrote the manuscript. All authors contributed to data collection. All authors read and approved the final manuscript.

Author details

[1]Department of General Medicine, Asahikawa Medical University, Asahikawa, Japan. [2]Division of Metabolism, Systemic Bioscience, Gastroenterology and Hematology/Oncology, Department of Medicine, Asahikawa Medical University, Asahikawa, Japan. [3]Department of Regional Medicine and Education, Asahikawa Medical University, Asahikawa, Japan.

References

1. Enck P, Aziz Q, Barbara G, *et al.* Irritable bowel syndrome. Nat Rev Dis Primers. 2016;2:16014.
2. Fukudo S, Okumura T, Inamori M, *et al.* Evidence-based clinical practice guidelines for irritable bowel syndrome 2020. J Gastroenterol. 2021;56:193–217.
3. Özen S, Batu ED, Demir S. Familial Mediterranean fever: recent developments in pathogenesis and new recommendations for management. Front Immunol. 2017;8:253.
4. Migita K, Asano T, Sato S, *et al.* Familial Mediterranean fever: overview of pathogenesis, clinical features and management. Immunol Med. 2018;41:55–61.
5. Kishida D, Nakamura A, Yazaki M, *et al.* Genotype-phenotype correlation in Japanese patients with familial Mediterranean fever: differences in genotype and clinical features between Japanese and Mediterranean populations. Arthritis Res Ther. 2014;16:439.
6. Sönmez HE, Batu ED, Özen S. Familial Mediterranean fever: current perspectives. J Inflamm Res. 2016;9:13–20.
7. Livneh A, Langevitz P, Zemer D, *et al.* Criteria for the diagnosis of familial Mediterranean fever. Arthritis Rheum. 1997;40:1879–85.
8. Yalcinkaya F, Ozen S, Ozcakar ZB, *et al.* A new set of criteria for the diagnosis of familial Mediterranean fever in childhood. Rheumatology. 2009;48:95–398.
9. Ozen S, Demirkaya E, Erer B, *et al.* EULAR recommendations for the management of familial Mediterranean fever. Ann Rheum Dis. 2016;75:644–51.
10. Yin X, Tian F, Wu B, Xu T. Interventions for reducing inflammation in familial Mediterranean fever. Cochrane Database Syst Rev. 2022;3:CD010893.
11. Beşer OF, Kasapçopur O, Cokuğraş FC, *et al.* Association of inflammatory bowel disease with familial Mediterranean fever in Turkish children. J Pediatr Gastroenterol Nut. 2013;56:498–502.
12. Saito D, Hibi N, Ozaki R, *et al.* MEFV gene-related enterocolitis account for some cases diagnosed as inflammatory bowel disease unclassified. Digestion. 2020;101:785–93.
13. Uslu N, Yüce A, Demir H, *et al.* The association of inflammatory bowel disease and Mediterranean fever gene (MEFV) mutations in Turkish children. Dig Dis Sci. 2010;55:3488–94.
14. Ekinci RMK, Balcı S, Akay E, *et al.* Frequency of functional gastrointestinal disorders in children with familial Mediterranean fever. Clin Rheumatol. 2019;38:921–6.
15. Migita K, Izumi Y, Jiuchi Y, *et al.* Familial Mediterranean fever is no longer a rare disease in Japan. Arthritis Res Ther. 2016;18:175.

13

Factors affecting the use of herbal products in patients with Irritable Bowel Syndrome and their results: Case–control study

Emin Gemcioglu[1*], Nuray Yılmaz Cakmak[1], Salih Baser[2], Servet Kocaoz[3] and Osman Ersoy[4]

Abstract

Background: Irritable bowel syndrome (IBS) is a functional bowel disease that is characterized by abdominal pain, discomfort, and changes in the frequency and form of stool without any organic pathology. In this study, the factors that affect the herbal treatment choices of IBS patients and their results were investigated.

Methods: Included in the study were 248 IBS patients who were over the age of 18. A questionnaire that comprised 25 questions was applied to the participants. Survey questions were asked to the participants regarding their age, place of birth, gender, educational status, demographic details, social standing, socioeconomic status and job, place of residence, and marital status. In addition, The participants were asked about which IBS symptoms they had, from whom they had received the recommendation for use of herbal products, whether the media had an effect on their selection of herbal products, and whether they had benefited from herbal products.

Results: It was observed that 41.1% of the patients with IBS who participated in the study used herbal medicine, 9.8% of whom used them regularly. It was found that the IBS patients participating in the study made their decision to use herbal products mostly based on the recommendations that they were given by acquaintances (57%) and the media (34%). When the patients were evaluated according to their gender, IBS was found to be more common in unemployed women who had a low level of education, while it was more common in working men ($p=0.015$, $P<0.001$, respectively). The IBS patients who were single used more herbal products that those who were married ($P=0.036$). While the use of herbal herbs and oils was predominant in patients whose recommendation content comprised the media/internet and acquaintances, the herbal treatment content recommended by healthcare professionals consisted of traditional treatments and mixtures ($P=0.012$). It was determined that a higher percentage of those who used herbal treatments lived in city centers when compared to those who did not ($P<0.001$). In addition, it was determined that patients with constipation used herbal products more than those without ($P<0.001$). Among the IBS patients, those who had diarrhea and those who were receiving medical treatment preferred to use significantly less herbal products ($P=0.007$ and $P=0.041$, respectively). It was found that the patients who visited the Gastroenterology Outpatient Clinic mostly used herbal therapy, while those who visited a family doctor used herbal therapy the least ($P=0.029$ and $P<0.001$, respectively).

Conclusion: The IBS patients revealed whose recommendations they followed when purchasing herbal products, which of the products they preferred, and how useful/beneficial they felt that these products were. In this regard, the

*Correspondence: egemcioglu@gmail.com
[1] Department of Internal Medicine, Ankara City Hospital, Ankara 06100, Turkey
Full list of author information is available at the end of the article

addition of training curricula related to herbal treatment for professional healthcare workers will further raise awareness on this topic.

Keywords: Irritable bowel syndrome, Herbal therapy, Audio-visual media

Introduction

Irritable bowel syndrome (IBS) is a functional bowel disease that is characterized by abdominal pain, discomfort, and changes in the frequency and form of stool without any organic pathology. IBS is the most common gastrointestinal system disease in patients who have visited internal and surgical outpatient clinics [1, 2]. Its prevalence is increasing among individuals between the ages of 30 and 50. The disease is twice as common in women than in men worldwide, while this rate is 3 times more in Turkey [3, 4]. High socioeconomic status and modern living conditions have been identified as risks for IBS development [5]. The chronic nature of IBS and the lack of an effective treatment cause a loss of workforce and worsening of the quality of life of patients [6]. IBS physiopathology includes genetic factors, intestinal microbiota, impaired immune system regulation, changes in intestinal permeability, and bowel-brain interaction [7]. Rome IV criteria are used in the diagnosis of IBS [8]. The main goal of treatment is to relieve symptoms. Patients frequently use alternative and complementary treatments due to the chronic nature of the symptoms, inadequate treatment response, and medication side effects in IBS [9]. Complementary and alternative treatments for IBS include hypnosis, acupuncture, cognitive behavioral therapy, yoga, and herbal medicine. Herbal medicine has a therapeutic effect as well as side effects in IBS [9, 10]. Herbal products are usually used uncontrolled and without consulting a doctor or determining the correct dosage. A previous study found that the source of information of patients taking herbal therapy comprised other patients who had the same complaints, the media, the internet, their friends and relatives, spice merchants, and herbalists [11]. In this study, the factors that affect the herbal treatment choices of IBS patients and their results were investigated.

Materials and methods

In this study, patients who applied to the Internal Medicine and Gastroenterology Outpatient Clinic of a tertiary referral hospital, between January and April 2018, were evaluated. Among these patients, those whose clinical situations were in line with the ROME IV criteria were included in the study [8]. Those with malignancy and inflammatory bowel disease, who were pregnant, or had any alarm symptoms (recent onset and rapid exacerbation of complaints, onset of symptoms after the age of 50, weight loss, fever, anemia, bloody defecation, symptoms awakening from sleep at night, family history of gastrointestinal cancer, antibiotics use, and travel history to countries with risk of infection) were excluded from the study. A questionnaire was applied to the patients who were accepted for participation in the study.

Before the questionnaire was administered, the patients were informed about the aim of the study, verbal consent was obtained, and it was stated that they could withdraw from the study at any stage. The questionnaire included questions about the sociodemographic characteristics of the participants, IBS, and herbal therapy.

Statistical analysis

Statistical analysis of the data was performed using IBM SPSS Statistics 25.0 (IBM Corp., Armonk, NY, USA). The compliance of continuous numerical variables to normal distribution was tested using the Kolmogorov–Smirnov test. Among the descriptive statistics, the continuous numerical variables were presented as the mean $\pm$ standard deviation or median [minimum (min) – maximum (max)], while the categorical variables were presented as the frequency and percentage. While the difference between the groups in terms of the mean was evaluated using the student t test, the difference in terms of the median was evaluated using the Mann–Whitney U test. The categorical variables were analyzed using the Pearson chi square test. Unless otherwise stated, $P < 0.05$ was considered as statistically significant.

Results

The number of patients included in the study was 248, and of these, 139 were women (56%) and 109 (44%) were men. The mean age of the patients was 43.6 ± 13.5 years; the mean age of the women was 44.5 ± 13.0 years, while the mean age of the men was 42.4 ± 14 years. Only 41.1% of the patients were receiving herbal treatment, 9.8% of whom were using it regularly. Of the IBS patients, 46% were primary and secondary school graduates, 23.4% were high school graduates, and 20.2% were undergraduates. It was found that IBS was significantly more common in women who had low education than the men with the same educational background ($P = 0.015$). Considering their occupations, IBS was found to be significantly more common in women who did not work than in men who did ($P < 0.001$). Considering their marital status, 74.6% of the patients were married and 25.4% were single.

Table 1 Sociodemographic data of the patients

Sociodemographic characteristics	Frequency (n=248)	Percentage (%)
Gender		
Women	139	56
Men	109	44
Educational status		
Illiterate	13	5.2
Literate	13	5.2
Primary and secondary school graduate	114	46
High-school graduate	58	23.4
Undergraduate	50	20.2
Profession		
Housewife/retired	121	48.8
White-collar	41	16.5
Blue-collar	71	28.6
Student	15	6
Marital status		
Married	185	74.6
Single	63	25.4

Table 2 Complaints of the patients at the time of admission

Complaint	Frequency(n=248)	Percentage (%)
Abdominal pain	166	66.9
Abdominal distention	196	79
Intestinal gas	163	65.7
Nausea	112	45.2
Vomiting	38	15.3
Diarrhea	73	29.4
Constipation	175	70.6
Constipation + diarrhea	58	23.4

Table 3 Symptom duration, outpatient clinic admission, and imaging characteristics of the patients receiving herbal therapy

Variable	Median (min–max)
Symptoms duration	5 (3–43) months
Number of visits to a family doctor	4 (0–12)
Number of visits to a gastroenterology outpatient clinic	1 (0–4)
Number of colonoscopies	1 (0–3)
Number of imagings (ultrasound, CT and MRI)	2 (1–3)

Table 4 Medical treatment and features related to the herbal therapy use of the patients

	Frequency (n=248)	Percentage (%)
How often patients receive medical treatment		
Regularly	4	1.6
Irregularly	216	87.1
Does not receive any	28	11.3
Herbal use		
Using	102	41.1
Not using	146	58.9

It was found that the single patients used significantly more herbal products for IBS ($P=0.036$). The patients were mostly residents of district centers (46%). The sociodemographic data of the patients are given in Table 1. The most common complaints among the patients on admission were abdominal distension (79%), constipation (70.6%), and abdominal pain (66.9%) (Table 2). The mean duration of time that the patients had typical IBS symptoms was 5 months (min: 3, max: 43). The number of outpatient clinic visits and the imaging characteristics are given in Table 3. While 87.1% of the patients did not use the medication that was given to them regularly, 1.6% used it regularly, and 11.3% did not receive any medical treatment (Table 4). Of the patients, 102 were receiving herbal therapy (41.1%), while 146 (58.9%) were not. Those who received herbal therapy mostly preferred a single herb (12.5%) or daily traditional solutions (12.5%), such as mint-lemon and linden. Apart from these, they used vegetable oils (10.1%) and herb mixtures from herbalists (5%), respectively. The patients did not have any detailed information about the ingredients of the mixtures that they bought from most of the spice merchants. In addition, traditional treatments generally vary depending on the society but are known by everyone, such as drinking mint and lemon tea for stomach pain and nausea, using fennel tea for abdominal pain, and using probiotic yogurt that contains olive oil and flaxseed for constipation. Other herbal herbs, concoctions (such as tea mixed with mint, fennel, ginger, chamomile, and cinnamon), and oils are herbal products that are usually prepared by the spice merchants. The information and suggestions that the patients received for the use of herbal therapy were mostly from their neighbors, relatives, and friends (57%). Other sources included the media/internet (34%) and health professionals (9%). While the use of herbal herbs and oils was predominant in patients whose content was the media/internet and acquaintances, the herbal treatment content recommended by healthcare professionals consisted of traditional treatments and mixtures ($P=0.012$). While 23.5% of the patients found the herbal treatment to be ineffective, 22.5% stated that they found it to be weakly effective, and 54% found it to be effective (moderate and very effective). Moreover, 1 patient stated that s/he experienced life-threatening side effects. While 9.8% of the patients used herbal therapy regularly, 47.06% did not (Table 5). There was no significant relationship between the professions of the patients and the herbal therapy that they used ($P=0.774$). There was no significant difference in terms of female and male gender in terms of herbal treatment usage ($P=0.573$). It was found that those who received herbal therapy mostly lived in city centers ($P<0.001$). Those suffering from diarrhea among the IBS patients preferred to use significantly fewer herbal products ($P=0.007$). Patients who received medical treatment used herbal therapy less than the others ($P=0.041$). It was found that the patients who visited the Gastroenterology Outpatient Clinic mostly used herbal therapy, while the patients who visited a family doctor used herbal therapy the least ($P=0.029$, $P<0.001$, respectively) (Table 6). There was no significant relationship between the types of herbal therapies used by the patients and the side effects of these treatments ($P=0.392$) (Table 7). Patients with constipation preferred to use herbal therapy more than the patients without constipation ($P<0.001$) (Table 8).

Table 5 Characteristics of herbal treatment

	Frequency (n=102)	Percentage (%)
Content		
Herbal herbs	31	30.4
Oils	25	24.5
Mixtures	15	14.7
Traditional solution	31	30.4
Recommendation source for herbal use		
Media/internet	35	34
Neighbors/relatives/friend	58	57
Health professionals	9	9
Herbal effect		
No effect	24	23.5
Weak	23	22.5
Medium	26	25.5
Good	22	21.6
Very good	7	6.9
Herbal side effect		
No effect	89	87.2
Weak	8	7.8
Medium	2	2
Strong	2	2
Life-threatening	1	1
Frequency of herbal use		
Regular	10	9.8
Often	44	43.14
Occasionally/rarely	48	47.06

Table 6 Comparison of the patients receiving herbal therapy and those not receiving herbal therapy in terms of symptom duration, outpatient clinic admission and imaging

Variable	Using herbal therapy (n=102) Median (min–max)	Not using herbal therapy (n=146) Median (min–max)	*P* value
Symptom duration	5 (3–43)	5 (3–43)	0.881
Number of visits to a family doctor	3 (0–12)	4 (0–10)	<0.001
Number of visits to a gastroenterology outpatient clinic	1 (0–4)	0 (0–2)	0.029
Number of colonoscopies	1 (0–3)	1 (0–3)	0.811
Number of imagings	2 (1–7)	2 (1–5)	0.159

Discussion

IBS is a chronic functional disorder of the gastrointestinal tract that is characterized by abdominal pain, abdominal distension, diarrhea, and episodes of constipation, and it has a high prevalence and diverse etiology worldwide [9, 12]. The current approach in the treatment of this syndrome is to reduce the symptoms rather than eliminate the underlying causes of the disease. Although there are various pharmacological treatment options, due to the limited effectiveness, high cost, and side effects of these treatments, the use of herbal therapy has become more common worldwide. In the current study, patients who received no medical treatment, lived in city centers, and had a relatively low socioeconomic and cultural levels tended to receive herbal therapy. This study was not a community-based study, and the selection of those who wanted to participate in the survey from the patients who had applied to the outpatient clinics was considered as the reason why the gender difference was not evident in both the frequency of IBS and the use of herbal.

The Chinese herbal products that have been used in East Asia for thousands of years are examples of this treatment [13]. Acupuncture, which is a type of

Table 7 Comparison of the types of herbal therapy and their side effects

Herbal content	No/weak herbal effect n, (%)	Has an herbal effect n, (%)	Total n, (%)	*P* value
Herbal herbs	16, (51.6)	15, (48.4)	31, (100)	0.392
Oils	14, (56)	11, (44)	25, (100)	
Mixtures	6, (40)	9, (60)	15, (100)	
Traditional solution	11, (35.5)	20, (64.5)	31, (100)	

Table 8 Comparison of the patients receiving herbal therapy and those not receiving herbal therapy in terms of their characteristics

Variable	Using herbal therapy n, (%)	Not using herbal therapy n, (%)	Total n, (%)	*P* value
Single	33, (52.4)	30, (47.6)	63, (100)	0.036
Married	69, (37.3)	116, (62.7)	185, (100)	
City center	64, (62.1)	39, (37.9)	103, (100)	< 0.001
District	28, (24.6)	86, (75.4)	114, (100)	
Town/village	10, (32.3)	21, (67.7)	31, (100)	
Women	55, (39.6)	84,(60.4)	139, (100)	0.573
Men	47, (43.1)	62, (56.9)	109, (100)	
Employed	44, (39.3)	68, (60.7)	112, (100)	0.592
Unemployed	58, (42.6)	78, (57.4)	136, (100)	
Receiving medical treatment	96, (43.6)	124, (56.4)	220, (100)	0.041
Not receiving medical treatment	6, (21.4)	22, (78.6)	28, (100)	
Has constipation	86, (49.1)	89, (50.9)	175, (100)	<0.001
Does not have constipation	16, (21.9)	57, (78.1)	73, (100)	

traditional medicine that has been mentioned frequently in the media, can also be used with herbal therapies, and in a study by Yan et al., the administration of herbal therapy together with acupuncture was found to be safe and effective [14]. As it is around the world, some of the patients herein who participated in the study tended to use herbs and traditional methods. Although the herbal therapies used were partially effective with a single use, it has been reported that the combinations created from these products can also be used, and this may be more beneficial [9]. It is also believed that many factors, such as the regular use of these products and the regular maintenance of medical treatment by the patient, affect the benefits obtained from herbal products. It was believed herein that regular treatment and follow-up can have a positive effect on IBS and herbal treatment, as in every disease. These products, which are also popular with IBS patients, have gained vast attention in the written, visual, and verbal media. Although most of the participants in the current study obtained their herbal product recommendations from their neighbors, relatives, and friends, the influence of the media in the selection of herbal products was also quite high. The patients obtained advisory information for these herbal therapies from the media rather than from health professionals. The effect/side effect profile of herbal therapies is not clear, as different herbal therapies may show different effects on patients, and these unpredictable effects have a wide spectrum, from acute renal failure to toxic hepatitis. It is obvious that the information given about these herbal products covered in the media may not be objective, non-commercial, or completely correct [15]. Unfortunately, because of commercial concerns or hearsay information about these products, for which safety and efficacy criteria are not clear, patients may be misled, and these products may cause various side effects or less beneficial effects than expected. A study by Munyaradzi et al. evaluated the effects of advertisements for herbal therapies on African societies and found that the headlines used in media-based advertisements and interesting statements about the product, even if not scientific information, affected the decisions of the patients [16]. It is thought that the herbal products used by IBS patients, which may be beneficial/harmful or have no effect in various situations, may deviate from their purpose due to the biased/unbiased promotion of the media and bilateral relations in daily life. The fact that the majority of patients who participated in the current study did not receive herbal therapy may be a result of these concerns.

Madisch A et al. reported in their study that 54% of primary care physicians were satisfied with the success of spasmolytic treatment, and 75% were satisfied with phyto-therapeutic agents and probiotics [17].

Conclusion

For IBS patients to use herbal products correctly and appropriately, they should be provided unbiased information about these herbal products. Relatives, neighbors, etc. In this regard, the addition of training curricula related to herbal treatment for professional healthcare workers will further raise awareness and it will increase the conscious use of herbal medicine in the treatment of IBS.

Acknowledgements

Thank you to our assistant and specialist doctor friends who have supported our work in the Internal Medicine Clinic.

Authors' contributions
EG, NYC, SB, SK and OE: investigation, project administration, software, visualization, writing-review and editing, methodology. All authors read and approved the final manuscript.

Helsinki declaration
The authors declared that this study is in accordance with the Helsinki Declaration.

Author details
[1]Department of Internal Medicine, Ankara City Hospital, Ankara 06100, Turkey. [2]Department of Internal Medicine, Yıldırım Beyazıt University School of Medicine, Ankara, Turkey. [3]Department of General Surgery, Ankara City Hospital, Ankara, Turkey. [4]Department of Gastroenterology, Yıldırım Beyazıt University School of Medicine, Ankara, Turkey.

References
1. Hungin AP, Whorwell PJ, Tack J, et al. The prevalence, patterns and impact of irritable bowel syndrome: an international survey of 40.000 subjects. Aliment Pharmacol Ther. 2003;17:643–50.
2. Lovell RM, Ford AC. Global prevalence of and risk factors for irritable bowel syndrome: a meta-analysis. Clin Gastroenterol Hepatol. 2012;10:712–21.
3. Brandt LJ, Chey WD, et al. An evidence-based position statement on the management of irritable bowel syndrome: American Collage of Gastroenterology task force on irritable bowel syndrome. Am J Gastroenterol. 2009;104(Suppl 1):S1-35.
4. Houghton LA, Heitkemper M, Crowell MD, et al. Age, gender, and women's health and the patient. Gastroenterology. 2016;150:1332–43.
5. Howell S, Talley NJ, Quine S, Poulton R. The irritable bowel syndrome has origins in the childhood socioeconomic environment. Am J Gastroenterol. 2004;99(8):1572–8. https://doi.org/10.1111/j.1572-0241.2004.40188.x (**PMID: 15307879**).
6. El-Serag HB, Olden K, Bjorkman D. Health-related quality of life among persons with irritable bowel syndrome: a systematic review. Aliment Pharmacol Ther. 2002;16:1171–85.
7. Lacy BE, Chey WD, Lembo AJ. New and emerging treatment options for irritable bowel syndrome. Gastroenterol Hepatol (N Y). 2015;11(4 Suppl 2):1–19.
8. Lacy BE, Mearin F, Chang L, et al. Bowel disorders. Gastroenterology. 2016;150:1393–407.
9. Bahrami HR, Hamedi S, Salari R. Herbal medicines for the management of irritable bowel syndrome: a systematic review. Electron Phys. 2016;8(8):2719–25.
10. Spanier JA, Howden CW, Jones MP. A systematic review of alternative therapies in the irritable bowel syndrome. Arch Intern Med. 2003;163(3):265–74.
11. Ekor M. The growing use of herbal medicines: issues relating to adverse reactions and challenges in monitoring safety. Front Pharmacol. 2014;10(4):177. https://doi.org/10.3389/fphar.2013.00177.
12. Rahimi R, Abdollahi M. Herbal medicines for the management of irritable bowel syndrome: a comprehensive review. World J Gastroenterol. 2012;18(7):589–600. https://doi.org/10.3748/wjg.v18.i7.589.
13. Bi Z, Zheng Y, Yuan J, Bian Z. The efficacy and potential mechanisms of Chinese herbal medicine on irritable bowel syndrome. Curr Pharm Des. 2017;23(34):5163–72. https://doi.org/10.2174/1381612823666170822101606.
14 Yan J, Miao ZW, Lu J, et al. Acupuncture plus Chinese herbal medicine for irritable bowel syndrome with diarrhea: a systematic review and meta-analysis. Evid Based Complement Alternat Med. 2019;2019:7680963. https://doi.org/10.1155/2019/7680963.
15 Peacock M, Badea M, Bruno F, et al. Herbal supplements in the print media: communicating benefits and risks. BMC Complement Altern Med. 2019;19(1):196. https://doi.org/10.1186/s12906-019-2602-9.
16. Munyaradzi M. Ethical quandaries in spiritual healing and herbal medicine: a critical analysis of the morality of traditional medicine advertising in southern African urban societies. Pan Afr Med J. 2011;10:6. https://doi.org/10.4314/pamj.v10i0.72212.
17. Madisch A, Labenz C, Hollenz M, Gross M, Labenz J. Therapiemanagement des reizdarmsyndroms in der hausarztpraxis : probiotika und phytotherapeutika kommen häufig erfolgreich zum einsatz [therapeutic management of irritable bowel syndrome in the family doctor's practice - probiotics and phytotherapeutics are often used successfully]. MMW Fortschr Med. 2020;162(Suppl 5):7–13.

14

Foreign body ingestion mimicking irritable bowel syndrome: A case report

Ioannis D Komninos[1], Ioanna G Tsiligianni[2*]

Abstract

Introduction: Foreign body ingestion is associated with a variety of symptoms and complications, often mimicking various diseases. This case report describes an unusual presentation following foreign body ingestion.

Case presentation: A 56-year-old Greek Caucasian woman presented to a primary care setting, in rural Crete, Greece, with complaints of abdominal pain, cramping and bloating, for the last four months. Alternating constipation and diarrhea was reported. The patient had unknowingly ingested a foreign body that resulted in an irritable bowel syndrome-like presentation.

Conclusions: This case report emphasizes the need for a high index of suspicion from physicians for a wide differential in their approach to abdominal complaints, as well as the importance of an individualized approach to patients in the setting of clinical medicine.

Introduction

Ingestion of foreign bodies is common primarily in children, psychiatric patients, alcoholics, and denture wearing elderly [1,2]. Selivanov *et al.* reported that, in most cases of foreign body ingestion, the most common foreign bodies ingested were coins, bones, food debris, safety pins, and razor blades [3]. Toothpicks and chicken bones were the most common cause of intestinal perforation [3]. In our study our patient unknowingly ingested a foreign body that had a similar shape and texture to a toothpick.

Foreign body ingestion can present without symptoms [4], and in some cases result in a perforation with gastrointestinal bleeding or an obstruction [1,3,5]. Rarely an abscess or an esophagoaortic fistula occurs [6-8]. The foreign body can be found in any location of the gastrointestinal tract or even out of the gastrointestinal tract through a migration process [1,3,5-12]. Foreign bodies, particularly toothpicks, have been reported to mimic renal colic and Crohn's disease [11,13]. To our knowledge, this is the first report of an irritable bowel syndrome (IBS) manifestation caused by the presence of a foreign body in the intestinal tract.

* Correspondence: pdkapa@yahoo.gr
[2]Agia Barbara Primary Health Care Centre, Agia Barbara, Heraklion, Crete, PO 70003, Greece

Case presentation

A 56-year-old Greek Caucasian woman presented to a primary care setting, in rural Crete, Greece complaining of mild lower abdominal pain, cramping and bloating, during the last four months. The pain was located primarily in the left upper quadrant, and often affected the entire abdomen.

Her symptoms gradually worsened over time, with only temporary relief with defecation. She reported that her bowel habits changed approximately one month after the onset of her abdominal symptoms. Alternating constipation and diarrhea was reported, with diarrhea being more predominant. She also reported a sensation of incomplete bowel emptying. A change in the frequency of bowel movements was also reported. She denied any bleeding, fever, or weight loss. She also denied having any aggravating symptoms such as stress and certain foods over the last few months.

Complete physical examination was within normal limits. Vital signs were also within normal limits. Our patient's medical history included hypertension (treated with an angiotensin II receptor antagonist, telmisartan), hypothyroidism (treated with L-thyroxine) and hypercholesterolemia (treated with atorvastatin), as well as some other minor bowel and gastric disorders that were chronic. There were no concerning associated signs or symptoms such as anemia or weight loss that would have

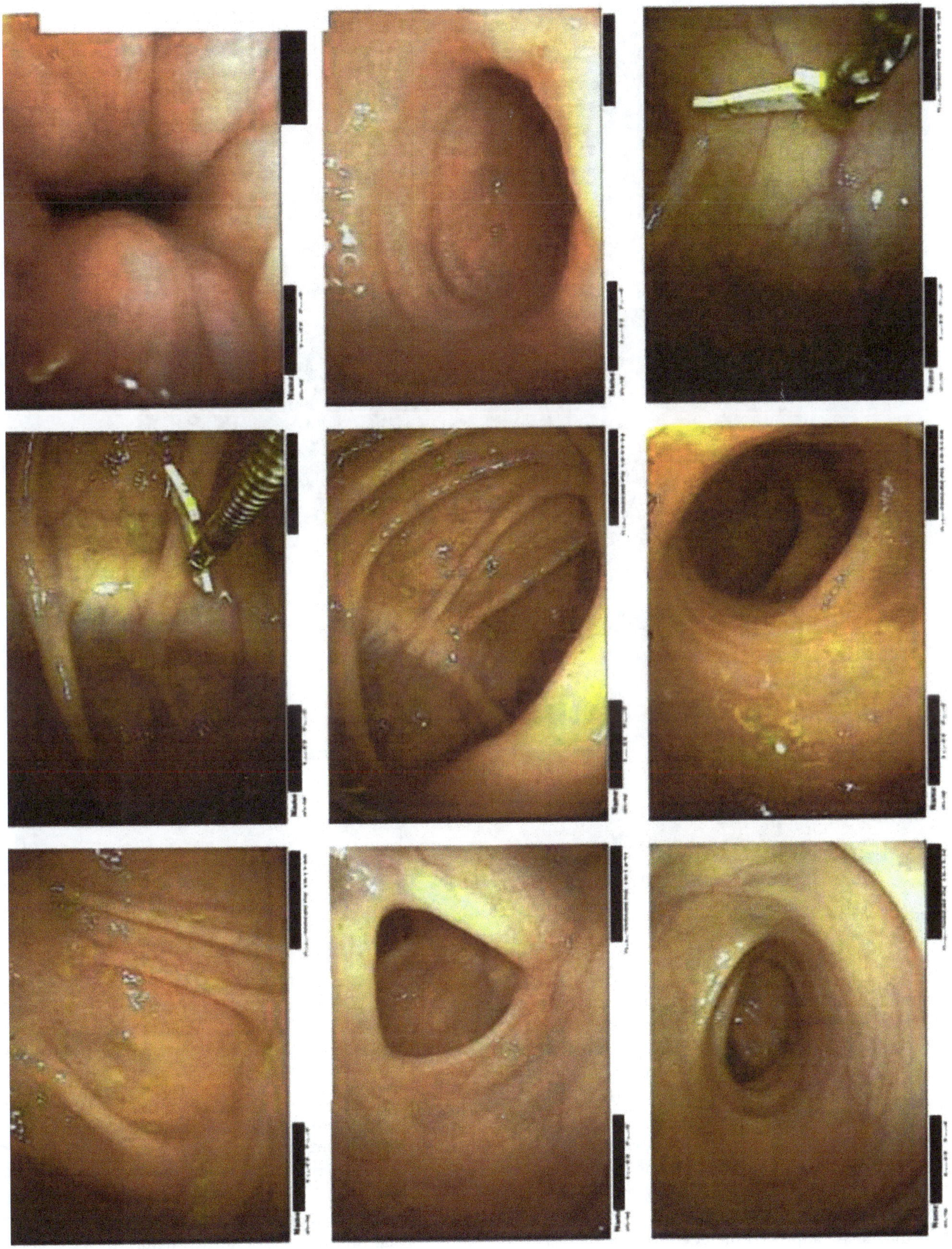

Figure 1 Colonoscopy images showing the foreign body.

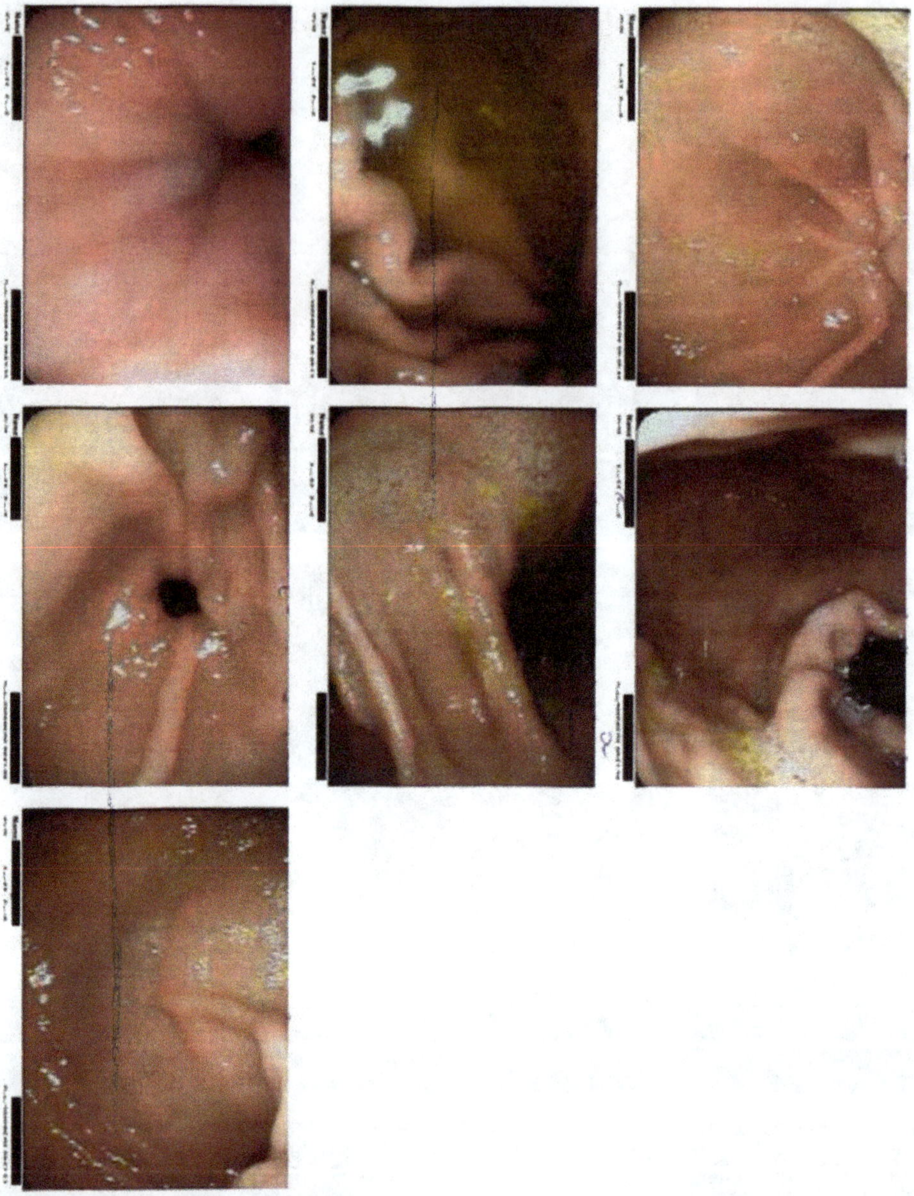

Figure 2 Colonoscopy images showing increased bowel spasticity.

led the family physician to initiate further studies. No abdominal or other surgical operations were reported. The family history for colorectal cancer was negative.

The first impression was that the patient had IBS. General dietary advice according to the National Institute for Health and Clinical Excellence (NICE) guidelines for primary care management of IBS were given (regular meals, avoiding long gaps between eating, adequate and appropriate fluid intake). The patient received also mebeverine hydrochloride 135 mg three times daily for three weeks.

The diagnostic approach included laboratory tests and an abdominal ultrasound control. Laboratory tests results revealed a normal complete blood count, normal erythrocyte sedimentation rate and C-reactive protein, and normal stool studies. Abdominal ultrasound revealed that her gall bladder, biliary tree, pancreas, spleen, and right kidney were all within normal limits. The lower portion of the left kidney was difficult to visual secondary to the presence of a loop of bowel.

Because her symptoms persisted despite treatment, a colonoscopy was ordered. The colonoscopy revealed the following: rectum with first degree hemorrhoids, sigmoid and descending colon with increased spasticity and normal mucosa, and a normal ileum. In the ascending colon a sharp piece of a birthday cake decoration

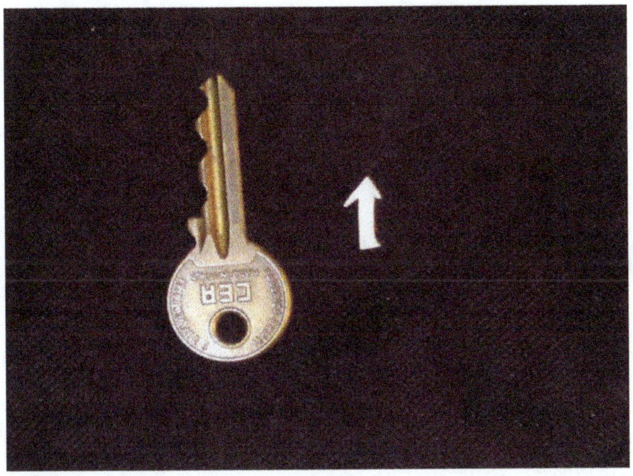

Figure 3 Dimension of the foreign body in comparison with a key.

was found and removed (Figure 1). No necrosis of bowel mucosa or hemorrhage was observed. The increased bowel spasticity that was observed was interpreted by the gastroenterologist who performed the colonoscopy as possibile IBS resulting as a consequence of the foreign body irritation (Figure 2). The dimension of the foreign body is shown in comparison with a key in Figure 3. One week after the removal of the foreign body all symptoms resolved. Our patient was free of symptoms after eight months of follow up.

Discussion

As reported in one large study of 101 cases of foreign body ingestion, patients are usually examined within 48 hours to six days following ingestion [3]. In our case there was a significant delay because our patient was not aware of the foreign body ingestion, and she attributed her symptoms to her previous history of mild gastrointestinal disorders. In our study the foreign body had the shape and texture similar to a toothpick.

The differential diagnoses considering our patient's age and symptoms included several diseases that would manifest with alternating constipation and diarrhea. These diseases include inflammatory bowel disease, irritable bowel disease, malabsorption syndrome, constipation, medication-induced irritation (anti-emetics, codeine), and mineral deficiencies. In this case report our patient presented with symptoms commonly found in IBS. History, physical examination, and laboratory analysis made the diagnosis of IBS more likely, and excluded other diagnoses.

The Rome III diagnostic criteria for IBS [14,15] are: symptoms lasting at least three months, preceded by at least six months of recurrent abdominal pain or discomfort associated with two or more of the following: improvement with defecation and/or; onset associated with a change in frequency of stool and/or; onset associated with a change in form (appearance) of stool.

Our patient met all three criteria, so an IBS diagnosis was thought most likely. Although the NICE guidelines for the diagnosis and management of IBS in the primary care setting does not indicate ultrasound and/or colonoscopy [16], in our case report we made the decision to individualize our patient's workup based on her unique symptoms and presentation and requested a colonoscopy. The American College of Gastroenterology suggests undergoing a colonoscopy every 10 years, beginning at the age of 50, as the preferred colorectal cancer screening strategy [17]. Taking into consideration our patient's age and the ongoing worsening of her symptoms and pain characteristics, we ordered the colonoscopy that ultimately resolved the diagnostic problem. This case report presentation underlines the importance of an individualized approach to patient care. The fact that after the removal of the foreign body the patient remained free of symptoms in an eight month follow-up suggests that the foreign body was responsible for the IBS-like presentation.

Limitations

No biopsies from the left and right colon were taken, therefore other etiologies with similar symptoms such as microscopic colitis (lymphocytic, collagenous) could not be excluded.

Conclusions

This unusual manifestation of IBS-like symptoms as a complication of a foreign body ingestion highlights the need for high index of suspicion from primary care physicians when diagnosing and treating abdominal complaints.

Consent

Written informed consent was obtained from the patient for publication of this case report and any accompanying images. A copy of the written consent is available for review by the journal's Editor-in-Chief.

Acknowledgements
We thank Dr Candida Delgatty for her kind contribution in linguistically checking this manuscript.

Author details
[1]Neapoli Primary Health Care Centre, Neapoli, Crete, PO 72400, Greece. [2]Agia Barbara Primary Health Care Centre, Agia Barbara, Heraklion, Crete, PO 70003, Greece.

Authors' contributions
IK, IT analysed and interpreted the patient's data. IT and IK searched the literature for similar cases, and wrote the manuscript. Both authors read and approved the final manuscript.

References

1. Cheng W, Tam PK: **Foreign-body ingestion in children: experience with 1,265 cases.** *J Pediatr Surg* 1999, **34(10)**:1472-1476.
2. Velitchkov NG, Grigorov GI, Losanoff JE, Kjossev KT: **Ingested foreign bodies of the gastrointestinal tract: retrospective analysis of 542 cases.** *World J Surg* 1996, **20(8)**:1001-1005.
3. Selivanov V, Sheldon GF, Cello JP, Crass RA: **Management of foreign body ingestion.** *Ann Surg* 1984, **199(2)**:187-191.
4. Comman A, Gaetzschmann P, Hanner T, Behrend M: **A case of needle ingestion in a female - laparoscopic retrieval.** *JSLS* 2008, **12(3)**:338-342.
5. Huiping Y, Jian Z, Shixi L: **Esophageal foreign body as a cause of upper gastrointestinal hemorrhage: case report and review of the literature.** *Eur Arch Otorhinolaryngol* 2008, **265(2)**:247-249.
6. Kelly SL, Peters P, Ogg MJ, Li A, Smithers BM: **Successful management of an aortoesophageal fistula caused by a fish bone–case report and review of literature.** *J Cardiothorac Surg* 2009, **4**:21.
7. Drnovsek V, Ruff MB, Riehl PA, Plavsic BM: **Gastrointestinal case of the day. Chronic ileocolocolic intussusception secondary to a mobile cecum and a benign fibrovascular mass.** *Radiographics* 1999, **19(4)**:1102-1104.
8. Dahiya M, Denton JS: **Esophagoaortic perforation by foreign body (coin) causing sudden death in a 3-year-old child.** *Am J Forensic Med Pathol* 1999, **20(2)**:184-188.
9. Tsesmeli NE, Savopoulos CG, Hatzitolios AI, Karamitsos DT: **Public health and potential complications of novel fashion accessories: an unusual foreign body in the upper gastrointestinal tract of an adolescent.** *Cent Eur J Public Health* 2007, **15(4)**:172-174.
10. Renner K, Holzer B, Hochwarter G, Weihsbeck E, Schiessel R: **Needle perforation of the appendix.** *Dig Surg* 2000, **17(4)**:413-414.
11. Li SF, Ender K: **Toothpick injury mimicking renal colic: case report and systematic review.** *J Emerg Med* 2002, **23(1)**:35-38.
12. Liu HJ, Liang CH, Huang B, Xie SF, Wang GY: **Migration of a swallowed toothpick into the liver: the value of multiplanar CT.** *Br J Radiol* 2009, **82(976)**:e79-81.
13. O'Gorman MA, Boyer RS, Jackson WD: **Toothpick foreign body perforation and migration mimicking Crohn's disease in a child.** *J Pediatr Gastroenterol Nutr* 1996, **23(5)**:628-630.
14. [http://www.romecriteria.org/pdfs/RomeCritieraLaunch.pdf].
15. Longstreth GF, Thompson WG, Chey WD, Houghton LA, Mearin F, Spiller RC: **Functional bowel disorders.** *Gastroenterology* 2006, **130(5)**:1480-1491.
16. [http://www.nice.org.uk/nicemedia/pdf/CG61Algorithm.pdf], Updated November 2009.
17. Rex DK, Johnson DA, Anderson JC, Schoenfeld PS, Burke CA, Inadomi JM, American College of Gastroenterology: **American College of Gastroenterology guidelines for colorectal cancer screening 2009.** *Am J Gastroenterol* 2009, **104(3)**:739-750.

Acupuncture for irritable bowel syndrome: Primary care based pragmatic randomised controlled trial

Hugh MacPherson[1*], Helen Tilbrook[1], J Martin Bland[1], Karen Bloor[1], Sally Brabyn[1], Helen Cox[1], Arthur Ricky Kang'ombe[1], Mei-See Man[1], Tracy Stuardi[1], David Torgerson[1], Ian Watt[1] and Peter Whorwell[2]

Abstract

Background: Acupuncture is used by patients as a treatment for irritable bowel syndrome (IBS) but the evidence on effectiveness is limited. The purpose of the study was to evaluate the effectiveness of acupuncture for irritable bowel syndrome in primary care when provided as an adjunct to usual care.

Methods: Design: A two-arm pragmatic randomised controlled trial.
Setting: Primary care in the United Kingdom.
Patients: 233 patients had irritable bowel syndrome with average duration of 13 years and score of at least 100 on the IBS Symptom Severity Score (SSS).
Interventions: 116 patients were offered 10 weekly individualised acupuncture sessions plus usual care, 117 patients continued with usual care alone.
Measurements: Primary outcome was the IBS SSS at three months, with outcome data collected every three months to 12 months.

Results: There was a statistically significant difference between groups at three months favouring acupuncture with a reduction in IBS Symptom Severity Score of −27.43 (95% CI: −48.66 to −6.21, p = 0.012). The number needed to treat for successful treatment (≥50 point reduction in the IBS SSS) was six (95% CI: 3 to 17), based on 49% success in the acupuncture group vs. 31% in the control group, a difference between groups of 18% (95% CI: 6% to 31%). This benefit largely persisted at 6, 9 and 12 months.

Conclusions: Acupuncture for irritable bowel syndrome provided an additional benefit over usual care alone. The magnitude of the effect was sustained over the longer term. Acupuncture should be considered as a treatment option to be offered in primary care alongside other evidenced based treatments.

Trial Registration: Current Controlled Trials ISRCTN08827905

Keywords: Acupuncture, Irritable bowel syndrome, Randomised controlled trial, Primary care

Background

General practitioners [1] and patients [2] have expressed their concerns regarding the adequacy and effectiveness of current treatments for irritable bowel syndrome (IBS). In a UK survey, 5% of patients receiving acupuncture reported having consulted primarily for gastrointestinal complaints, the most common being IBS [3]. However, the evidence on acupuncture for IBS is weak. A Cochrane review of six trials, with a median sample size of 54, found insufficient evidence to determine if acupuncture is an effective treatment for IBS [4]. No evidence of an acupuncture effect beyond placebo was found in two subsequent trials which controlled for non-specific effects [5,6].

Apart from three Chinese-based trials in the Cochrane review, none of the above trials were designed to evaluate the overall effect of acupuncture, *i.e.* an evaluation of the combined specific effect of acupuncture and non-specific effects associated with placebo. Moreover all of

* Correspondence: hugh.macpherson@york.ac.uk
[1]Department of Health Sciences, University of York, York, UK
Full list of author information is available at the end of the article

the trials delivered acupuncture in a way that the intervention was constrained, such that acupuncturists were not delivering acupuncture in a similar way to how they would do so normally in routine care. None of the trials were reported as based in primary care, instead they were reported as based in hospital settings [5-11] or settings were not reported [12,13]. Given this evidence gap, and the uncertainty outlined in the Cochrane review, further investigation of acupuncture for irritable bowel syndrome is merited [4].

In this study we designed an open pragmatic randomised controlled trial, in which we account for both the temporal effects associated with any spontaneous recovery and the effects of regression-to-the-mean, with the aim of capturing the overall impact of acupuncture when provided as a referral option in primary care. Our focus on a primary care setting complements previous studies conducted in secondary care [5-11]. We aimed to provide acupuncture as close as possible to how it would normally be provided in routine care, with the incorporation of explanations and lifestyle advice based on acupuncture theory in a way that is integral to practice [14,15]. This focus on acupuncture as a complex intervention precludes the possibility of a feasible and valid sham to control for all interacting components in a two-arm trial [16,17]. Our design mirrors that used in a trial of acupuncture for chronic low back pain which influenced policy in the UK; the study was central to the decision by the National Institute for Health and Clinical Excellence (NICE) to recommend 10 sessions of acupuncture for persistent low back pain [18].

Based on this rationale, our research therefore aims to provide practical comparative data on acupuncture for irritable bowel syndrome that is relevant to primary care and will be immediately applicable to patients and providers. This design provides the evidence needed to assist policy and decision-makers when considering acupuncture as a referral option for patients with irritable bowel syndrome.

Methods

Design overview

Building on our pilot study (ISRCTN32823720) [19], we conducted a parallel-arm randomised controlled trial to determine the effectiveness of acupuncture plus usual care compared to usual care alone for the treatment of IBS based on a published protocol [20]. We received ethics approval from the York NHS Research Ethics Committee (08/H1311/66) in 2008. A cost-effectiveness analysis is reported separately [21].

Settings and participants

We recruited patients from the databases of five general practices. The GP practices identified potential participants aged 18 or older who had consulted their GP and been diagnosed with IBS, and coded accordingly on the practice database. A letter was sent to all potentially eligible participants, inviting them to complete a baseline questionnaire and consent form and return these to the York Trials Unit. We excluded patients who did not speak English, who had a current diagnosis of haemophilia, hepatitis, HIV, or were receiving cancer care, had had major gastrointestinal surgery in the previous six months, were pregnant, had a history of psychosis or substance abuse, or were receiving acupuncture at the time. Patients were recruited if they provided informed consent and scored 100 or more on the IBS Symptom Severity Score (SSS) [22].

Randomisation

We randomised participants equally to receive either a short course of traditional acupuncture plus usual care or usual care alone. The randomisation sequence was computer generated at the University of York by an independent data manager at the York Trials Unit, and fully concealed from the research and administrative staff who then informed participants of their allocation by telephone and subsequently by letter.

Interventions

Nine professional acupuncturists provided the acupuncture, and all were registered with the British Acupuncture Council with at least three years' post qualification experience, and were working at independent clinics. Their practice style was based on principles of Traditional Chinese Medicine or "TCM". Acupuncturists provided up to 10 sessions of acupuncture, adapted from a previously tested protocol [19], which allowed explanations and life-style advice based on acupuncture theory and clinical judgement [16]. While actual selection of points was individualised for patients and allowed to change over time, there was standardisation of the function of the acupuncture based on the theoretical frameworks used, an approach proposed for maintaining interventional integrity when delivering complex interventions [23].

All patients remained under the care of their general practitioner, and received usual care according to need. We documented usual care, for both NHS and non-NHS treatments, in both groups at three, six, nine and 12 months.

Outcomes and follow-up

Our primary outcome measure was the IBS Symptom Severity Score (IBS SSS). This is scored from 0 to 500 (<75 = no IBS, 75–175 = "mild" case, 175–300 = "moderate" and 300+ = "severe"), and it has been validated for use in IBS patients [22]. Our primary end-point was at three months, with further follow-ups at six, nine and 12 months. We recorded participants' baseline belief in acupuncture, expectations that acupuncture might help their IBS and treatment preferences.

Our secondary outcome measures were the IBS Non-Colonic Symptom Score (which includes lethargy & tiredness, "wind", backache, and other symptoms [24], and SF-12 to evaluate patients' health related quality of life [25]. EQ-5D was the primary outcome for the economic study [26]. Outcomes at follow-up points were sought by postal questionnaire, and where that failed to elicit a response, the main outcome measure was sought by telephone.

Statistical analysis

In our pilot study [19], we calculated that for a 50 point difference on the IBS SSS, and an adjusted standard deviation to be 105 points, we needed to recruit a sample size of 94 patients per arm to have 90% power and a significance level of 0.05. To allow for loss to follow up of a similar proportion as observed in the pilot at three months (13%), our trial required at least 220 patients. In the full-scale trial we used analysis of covariance on an intention-to-treat basis to evaluate changes between groups for the primary outcome of the IBS SSS at three months, while adjusting for baseline scores and general practice. The statistical analysis was conducted using SAS version 9.2 and STATA version 10 using a 2-sided 5% significance level. We took a 50 point improvement [22] or more on the IBS SSS between baseline and three months as a "success" for our number-needed-to-treat analysis. We used similar analyses to explore between-group differences on the IBS SSS at other time points, and on secondary outcome measures. We used linear regression to explore whether expectation, belief and preference were treatment effect modifiers.

Results

Recruitment and follow-up of participants

The trial recruited patients from five general practices (total list size of 53,666) between November 2008 and June 2009. GP practices identified and invited 1,651 potentially eligible patients to participate. Of the 243 patients who responded with baseline documentation to the York Trials Unit, 233 were recruited, see Flow Chart in Figure 1. The average number recruited per general practice was 47 (range 24 to 75).

Baseline characteristics

Patients' mean age at baseline was 44, and 81% were women, see Table 1 for full baseline details. The average duration of their IBS was 13 years. In terms of potential treatment effect modifiers, 56% believed acupuncture worked, 29% expected that acupuncture would help their IBS, 76% had a preference to be allocated to acupuncture, and 39% received their preferred treatment option.

Acupuncture provision within the acupuncture arm of the trial

There were seven female and two male acupuncture practitioners with post-qualification experience ranging from 3 to 25 years (mean 11). Practitioners provided acupuncture for 113 patients, averaging 12 patients each (range 3 to 22), covering 1016 treatments. The reasons for patient non-attendance and discontinuation are provided in Figure 1. Patients received an average of 9 sessions, with 88 patients (76%) receiving the full course, and the average course of treatment was completed within 12 weeks. Sessions were commonly 45 minutes duration and provided at weekly intervals. In Table 2 we provide a summary of the treatment details according to the STRICTA requirements [27] and a full report is published separately [28].

Usual care provision across both arms of the trial

We mapped the provision of usual care in both groups, which was provided or purchased according to need, and found differences in utilisation were minimal (see Additional file 1). For example in the first three months 59/83 (69%) of patients in the acupuncture group consulted at the their GP practice, compared to 72% of patients in the usual care group, with patient consulting on average 2.08 times and 2.25 times respectively, with 68% and 69% of these visits being related to IBS respectively. Over the first three months, 65% of the acupuncture group received prescription medication compared to 61% of the usual care group, with antispasmodics drugs, antidiarrhoeal drugs and laxatives making up a relatively small proportion of this utilisation (Additional file 1). Non-prescription medication was used by 58% in the acupuncture group compared to 60% in the usual care group.

Patient outcomes

Table 3 shows the results from the linear regression model providing IBS Symptom Severity Scores at baseline, 3, 6, 9 and 12 months, as illustrated in Figure 2. The between-group comparison showed a statistically significant reduction in symptoms in those allocated to acupuncture at three months: –27.43 (95% CI: –48.66 to –6.21, $p = 0.012$). The effect size could be described as small to moderate (Cohen's $d = 0.36$). Treatment was assumed "successful" (≥50 points reduction on IBS SSS) in 57/116 (49%) of patients in the acupuncture group and 36/117 (31%) in those receiving usual care alone, a difference of 18% (95% CI: 6% to 31%). The number needed to treat was 6 (95% CI: 3 to 17), which means that for roughly every 6 participants treated with

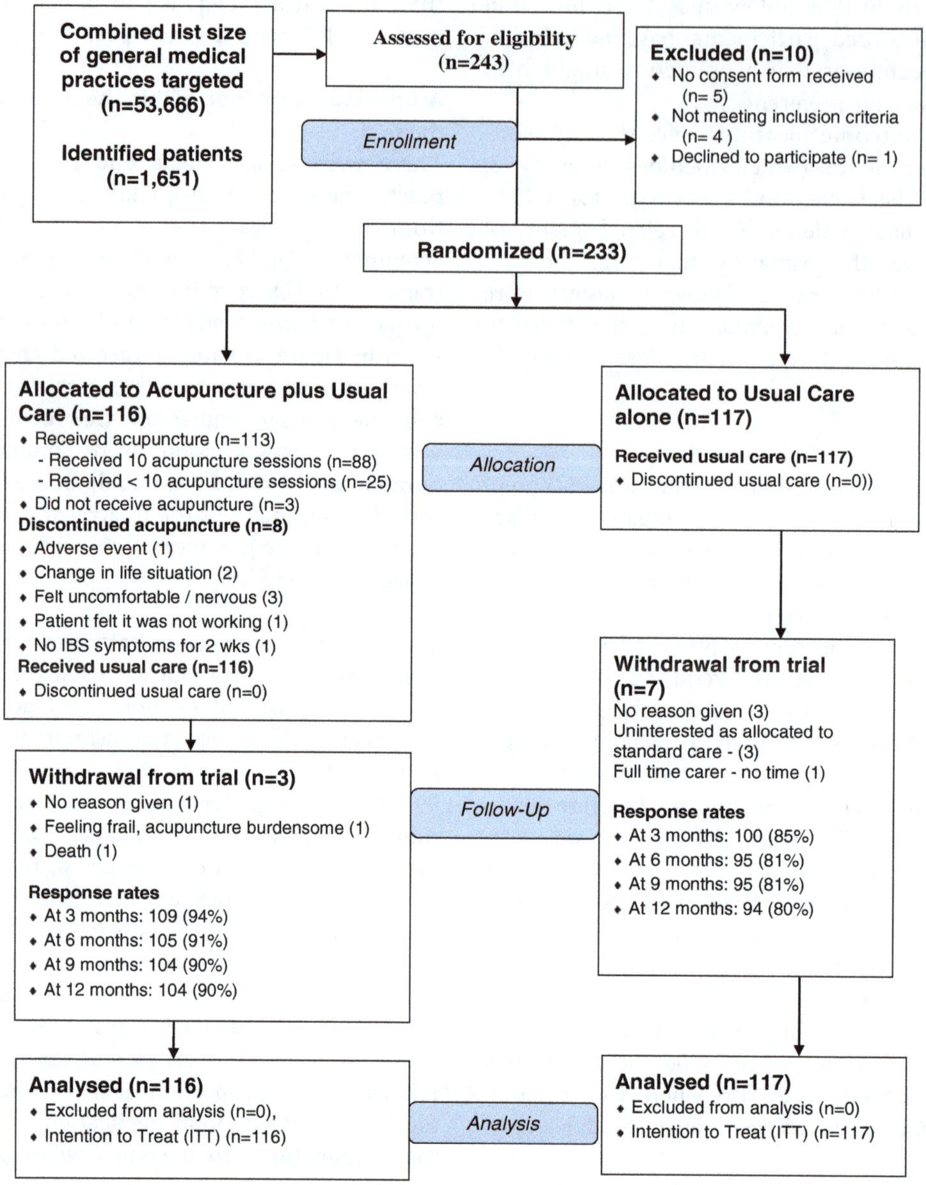

Figure 1 CONSORT flow diagram.

acupuncture, you will see one participant with an improvement equal to or greater than 50 in their baseline IBS SSS score.

The difference on the IBS SSS scores between groups subsequent to 3 months, adjusted for baseline, showed a statistically significant reduction at 6 months [−22.59] and 9 months [−27.0], followed by a near significant reduction at 12 months [−21.33], see Table 3 for confidence intervals. We found that patient expectation and belief were not treatment effect modifiers. Nor was preference, whether on the basis of comparing groups who preferred acupuncture vs. those who didn't mind, or when comparing those who got their preference vs. those who did not. We found a statistically significant reduction favouring the acupuncture group for the IBS Non-Colonic Score only at three months, [−15.24 (95% CI: −29.91 to −0.57)], but no significant differences in the physical and mental component scores on the SF-12 at any time point (see Additional file 2).

Adverse events

No serious adverse events associated with acupuncture were reported by acupuncturists in the logbooks or by patients in follow-up questionnaires. Non-serious adverse events associated with acupuncture were reported by eleven patients: eight experienced pain from the needles (three of the eight also reported nerve pain, bruising or fatigue), one had bruising from the needles, one

Table 1 Baseline patient characteristics

Characteristic	Acupuncture (n = 116)	Usual care (n = 117)	Overall (n = 233)
Age			
Mean (SD)	44.28 (14.31)	42.68 (14.79)	43.47 (14.54)
Median (min to max)	43.81 (21.33 to 78.29)	42.00 (19.51 to 74.47)	42.69 (19.51 to 78.29)
Gender			
Male, n (%)	21 (18.10)	24 (20.51)	45 (19.31)
Education (full time)			
Yes (%)	5 (4.31)	4 (3.42)	9 (3.86)
Work (full time)	**(n = 90)**	**(n = 81)**	**(n = 171)**
Yes (%)	57 (49.14)	63 (53.85)	120 (51.50)
Work (Not full time)	**(n = 54)**	**(n = 51)**	**(n = 105)**
Work part-time	31 (26.72)	19 (16.24)	50 (21.16)
Currently looking for work	1 (0.86)	4 (3.42)	5 (2.15)
Permanently unable to work	4 (3.45)	0 (0.00)	4 (1.72)
Looking after home/family	4 (3.45)	10 (8.55)	14 (6.01)
Retired	11 (9.48)	16 (13.68)	27 (11.59)
Other	3 (2.59)	2 (1.71)	5 (2.15)
Belief: In general, do you think acupuncture can work?			
Yes (%)	61 (52.59)	69 (58.97)	130 (55.79)
No (%)	1 (0.86)	0 (0.00)	1 (0.43)
Don't know (%)	54 (46.55)	48 (41.03)	102 (43.78)
Expectation: Do you think acupuncture may help your IBS?			
Yes (%)	31 (26.72)	37 (31.62)	68 (29.18)
No (%)	1 (0.86)	1 (0.85)	2 (0.86)
Don't know (%)	84 (72.41)	79 (67.52)	163 (69.96)
Preference 1: Which treatment do you prefer?			
Acupuncture (%)	90 (77.59)	88 (75.21)	178 (76.39)
Standard care (%)	0 (0.00)	1 (0.85)	1 (0.43)
Don't mind either (%)	26 (22.41)	28 (23.93)	54 (23.18)
Preference 2: Did you get your treatment preference?			
Got what I preferred (%)	90 (77.59)	1 (0.85)	91 (39.06)
Did not get what I preferred (%)	0 (0.00)	88 (75.21)	88 (37.77)
Did not have preference (%)	26 (22.41)	28 (23.93)	54 (23.18)
Irritable Bowel Syndrome Symptom Severity Score (IBS SSS):			
Mean (SD)	280.00 (81.34)	277.17 (71.50)	278.59 (76.47)

had a slight burn from a moxibustion stick, and one had itchy and swollen skin where one of the needles had been inserted.

Discussion

Summary of main findings

For patients with chronic irritable bowel syndrome, our study showed that acupuncture provided as an adjunct in primary care is associated with a small yet statistically significant clinical reduction in symptoms at three months. This was reflected in 49% of patients in the acupuncture group and 31% in the usual care group improving by more than 50 points in their IBS SSS score, with six being the number-needed-to-treat. This effect was largely sustained through to 12 months. We also found acupuncture for this group of patients had a high level of acceptability, as shown by the willingness by patients to attend for acupuncture once they had commenced treatment, completing on average 9 out of the 10 weekly acupuncture sessions that were available.

Strengths and limitations

This study is the first pragmatic randomised controlled trial of acupuncture for IBS in primary care. The design ensured that we controlled for temporal effects associated

Table 2 Details of the acupuncture treatment in items structured according to the STRICTA [27] reporting guidelines, an official extension to CONSORT

STRICTA item	Details of acupuncture treatment within the trial
1. a) Style	Traditional Chinese Medicine (TCM).
b) Reasoning for treatment provided	Systematic review by Lim [4] and pragmatic design to evaluate acupuncture as provided in routine care.
c) Variation	Individualized treatments using common TCM theoretical frameworks: primarily *zang-fu syndromes* (used with 99% of patients), and also *qi, blood and body fluids, eight principles, five elements*, and *external pathogenic factors.*
2. a) Number of needles per treatment	On average 14 needles were inserted per session (range: 4 – 23) using an average of seven point locations (range 5 to 9).
b) Names	126 different points were used. A common core of points, LI 4, LR 3, ST 36, SP 6, were used in over 50% of treatments.
c) Depth of insertion	Average depth was 1.5 cm (range: 0.2 – 5 cm).
d) Response sought	The response sought varied, most commonly *de qi.*
e) Needle stimulation	Manual.
f) Retention	Average 20 min (range: few seconds to 30 min).
g) Needle type	Most common length was 25 mm (range: 15–40 mm) and diameter 0.20 mm (range: 0.30 to 0.16 mm).
3. a) Number of sessions	Patients were offered 10 sessions and completed an average of 9 sessions.
b) Frequency & duration	Usually once a week over 12 weeks.
4. a) Other components of treatment	Acupuncturists were allowed to use cupping, moxa, brief tui-na, brief acupressure, breathing, and ear seeds. The most commonly used was moxa (used with 13% of patients), brief *tui na* (9%) and brief acupressure (6%). Herbs & magnets were prohibited. Acupuncturists were allowed to provide lifestyle advice as part of the patient's treatment consistent with their routine practice, with a restriction against probiotics. In total 68% of patients received lifestyle advice, most commonly diet (56%), stress reduction and relaxation (24%) and exercise (6%).
b) Setting and context	Provision or treatments in independent clinics. Acupuncturists encouraged to practice as closely as possible as they normally would.
5. Participating acupuncturists	British Acupuncture Council members, with more than three years post-qualification experience. Predominant treatment style: Traditional Chinese Medicine.
6. Control or comparator interventions	Patients in both groups continued to receive their usual care from their general practitioner, as well as over-the-counter treatments according to need. This allowed us to evaluate the impact of acupuncture as an adjunct to usual care. A summary of usual care actually received in both arms are provided in the main text.

with spontaneous recovery and regression-to-mean effects associated with having a minimum cut-off on our IBS SSS scale. The trial had an adequate sample size, and was conducted rigorously at all stages, with unambiguously concealed allocation to prevent subversion of the randomisation. Of the 1,651 potentially eligible patients identified by GP practices that were invited to participate, 243 patients responded, a rate that is typical of trials in primary care that use a database method for recruitment. We used validated outcomes measures, with response rates at 3, 6, 9 and 12 months that were reasonably high, at over 80 per cent in the control group and over 90 per cent in the intervention group. We have documented that there was reasonable equivalence in usual care received in both groups at three months, which leads us to cautiously ascribe any differences between groups to the treatment provided by acupuncturists. We explored the impact of variables that are potentially associated with placebo effects, namely patients' beliefs, expectations and treatment preferences [29], but they were not found to be treatment effect modifiers.

There is likely to be a contribution to the overall benefit we observed due to the additional attention received in the acupuncture group resulting from the contact time with practitioners in the acupuncture arm. We did not control for this bias, which would have required a trial arm with a practitioner-led intervention in order to control for time and attention. The patients in our study were not blind to their group allocation, as would have been the case in a sham-controlled trial. A comparator trial arm with a sham control would have had the limitation that the verum acupuncture would need to be constrained to minimise variability in patient experience between the verum and sham acupuncture arms. There is a trade-off between seeking to know more about the contribution each of the components might (or might not) contribute to any putative benefit and seeking to know more about the impact of acupuncture as a package of care that more closely reflects routine practice. A third trial arm was outside of the scope of our funding support.

Table 3 Results of linear regression models fitted at each separate time point on the IBS Symptom Severity Score

Variable	Baseline Mean (SD)	Month 3 (95% CI)	Month 6 (95% CI)	Month 9 (95% CI)	Month 12 (95% CI)
Primary analysis: IBS Symptom Severity Score					
Acupuncture group	280.00 (81.34)	213.78 (199.31 to 228.25)	201.60 (186.08 to 217.12)	206.40 (190.39 to 222.41)	209.79 (194.56 to 225.03)
Usual care group	277.17 (71.50)	241.21 (225.69 to 256.73)	224.19 (207.91 to 240.48)	233.40 (217.21 to 249.59)	231.12 (214.81 to 247.44)
Between group differences in means (acupuncture-usual care)	-	−27.43 (−48.66 to −6.21)	−22.59 (−45.11 to −0.08)	−27.00 (−49.77 to −4.23)	−21.33 (−43.66 to 1.00)

At each time point, predicted means and their 95% confidence intervals from the fitted model are presented except at baseline where the raw means and their standard deviation are presented.

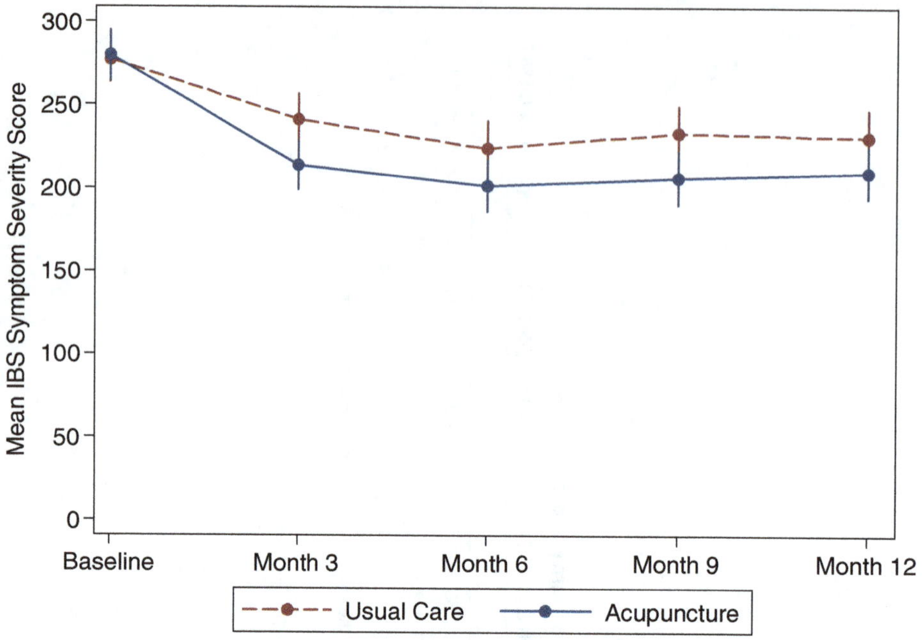

Figure 2 Longitudinal evolution of the mean IBS symptom severity scores against time of follow up by acupuncture and control groups.

The study population was made up of those who have consulted with predominantly "moderate" IBS symptoms in primary care (average IBS SSS score of 279), have experienced these symptoms for an average of 13 years and have not experienced sufficient symptom reduction from their usual care so that they are continuing to seek care. Therefore generalising the results to patients who are consulting their GP for the first time, and who therefore have not experienced usual GP care and its impact on symptoms, must be done with caution. The trial was not powered to determine whether any of the sub-groupings of patients with IBS symptoms (for example based on severity) would have fared better or worse.

Comparison with existing studies

Our study had the longest duration in terms of collecting outcome data through to 12 months after randomisation. By contrast, most other studies have been conducted within hospital based settings, with more narrowly defined populations, smaller sample sizes and shorter term follow-ups [4]. The level of acceptability of acupuncture treatments among patients was high (only three patients out of 116 did not start treatment and 88 (76%) completed their full course of treatment, with an overall average of nine sessions attended out of 10) compared to a trial of cognitive behavioural therapy for IBS in which fewer than half of patients were considered by the therapist to have completed therapy, with 41% either declining therapy or dropping out [30].

Components of acupuncture are drawn from three categories: needling related components; non-needling components that are acupuncture-specific, such as explanations and lifestyle advice; and non-specific components that are generic to the therapeutic encounter, such as the patient-practitioner relationship [31]. Our trial is unique in that it was designed to include the second of these components, as well as the other two. However it was not designed to determine the extent to which each of these components of acupuncture contributed to the overall outcome. To establish a proportional contribution of a component of treatment would require a trial arm with a sham control, for example as has been done recently to explore the impact of the patient-practitioner relationship [10]. In their trial, sham acupuncture needling was used to control for the needling in verum acupuncture arm, which then allowed the impact of a variation in the intensity of patient-practitioner relationship to be measured. By contrast, our focus on acupuncture as a complex intervention with many interacting components meant that a feasible and valid sham control was problematic [16,17].

With regard to placebo effects among patients with IBS, there is some limited evidence from other studies that these effects appear to tail off after three months, according to a study that reviewed 27 randomised controlled trials of treatments for IBS, with individual trials showing no placebo response at 12 months [32]. The results from our trial, in contrast, provide some evidence of a sustained effect at 12 months.

Implications for future research and clinical practice

Our trial focussed on those patients with long term symptoms at recruitment (average 13 years duration) for whom usual GP care was of limited benefit; however, exploring the potential impact of referral to acupuncture soon after an initial diagnosis of IBS would be useful. An appropriately powered study could determine whether any of the sub-groupings of patients with IBS symptoms (for example based on mild, moderate or severe categories) fared better or worse, and also characterize responders and non-responders to acupuncture. A clearer specification of optimal acupuncture treatment for this group of patients would be helpful. In particular it would be useful to determine if more than 10 acupuncture sessions would improve outcomes, as from the graph in Figure 2 the steep improvement of the acupuncture group appears to level off quite abruptly when treatment ceases. To separate out the impact of different components of treatment, a sham controlled trial design similar to that used by Kaptchuk and colleagues [10] could be used to determine whether or not the provision of explanations and life-style advice might (or might not) add to any overall effect, assuming that effects of different treatment components are additive rather than synergistic.

There is a need for a number of effective options for treatment in primary care, given the frustration experienced by some patients with existing treatments [2]. Our results showed that, on average, acupuncture is associated with a small to moderate reduction in symptoms in a population that has had IBS symptoms for many years. If a patient responds at three months, then this benefit is likely on average to be sustained at 12 months. The IBS Symptom Severity Score is now widely used in IBS research and has been translated into many languages. When used in assessing response to treatment, a reduction of 50 points is regarded as clinically significant and, therefore, a reduction of 70 points after 12 months in a group of primary care patients in whom symptoms have been refractory, suggests that this is a treatment option worth considering in such individuals, especially as the beneficial effects seem to be sustained. These data on acupuncture are highly relevant to the primary care context in the UK and have policy implications.

Conclusion

In a rigorously conducted pragmatic randomised controlled trial, we have evaluated the effectiveness of acupuncture as a treatment for irritable bowel syndrome when offered as an adjunct to usual treatment in primary care. Acupuncture was found to significantly improve outcomes at three months, with the number needed to treat being six. We found some evidence of a sustained benefit over the longer term. Acupuncture should be considered as a potential treatment option in primary care alongside other evidence-based treatments.

Abbreviations

IBS: Irritable Bowel Syndrome; NHS: National Health Service; NICE: National Institute for Health & Clinical Excellence; SSS: Symptom Severity Score.

Authors' contributions

HM conceived the study and was the lead applicant and principal investigator for the trial. HT was the lead trial co-coordinator, JMB was a co-applicant for funding and supervising statistician for the trial, KB was a co-applicant for funding and advised on matters relating to health economics and policy, SB was the trial administrator, HC was one of trial coordinators, ARK was the trial statistician and conducted all the clinical analyses, MM contributed as a trial co-ordinator, TS designed aspects of the trial, steered the ethics approval process and collected data on treatments provided, DT was a co-applicant for funding and advised on trial methodology, IW was a co-applicant and advised on matters relating to primary care and adverse events, PW is a consultant gastroenterologist who was a co-applicant and advised on clinical aspects of the trial and made available the primary outcome measure for the trial. All authors have had full access to all of the data (including statistical reports and tables) in the study and can take responsibility for the integrity of the data and the accuracy of the data analysis, and have read and approved the final manuscript.

Authors' information

Helen Tilbrook, Research Fellow, York Trials Unit, Department of Health Sciences, University of York, York, YO10 5DD, UK
Martin Bland, Professor of Health Statistics, Department of Health Sciences, University of York, York, YO10 5DD, UK
Karen Bloor, Senior Research Fellow, Department of Health Sciences, University of York, York, YO10 5DD, UK
Sally Brabyn, Trial Support Officer, Department of Health Sciences, University of York, York, YO10 5DD, UK
Helen Cox, Research Fellow, York Trials Unit, Department of Health Sciences, University of York, York, YO10 5DD, UK
Arthur Ricky Kang'ombe, Biostatistician, York Trials Unit, Department of Health Sciences, University of York, York, YO10 5DD, UK
Mei-See Man, Research Fellow, Department of Health Sciences, University of York, York, YO10 5DD, UK
Tracy Stuardi, PhD Student, Department of Health Sciences, University of York, York, YO10 5DD, UK
David Torgerson, Director of York Trials Unit, Department of Health Sciences, University of York, York, YO10 5DD, UK
Ian Watt, Professor of Primary Care, Hull York Medical School, York, YO10 5DD, UK
Peter Whorwell, Professor of Medicine and Gastroenterology, Wythenshawe Hospital, Manchester M23 9LT, UK.

Acknowledgements

Support for this project came from Dr David Geddes, the Medical Director of the NHS North Yorkshire and York PCT, who was a co-applicant in the bid for funding. Thanks are due to Julie Osborne and Shelagh Grey who contributed to the study as lay representatives. Julie Reynolds contributed her experience of conducting the pilot study, and was a co-applicant for funding and advised on the full-scale trial. Ann Hopton provided additional support in the administration of the trial. We would like to acknowledge Greg Rubin, Professor of General Practice and Primary Care at Durham University, in his role as Chair of the Independent Steering Committee.

Sponsor

The University of York, in its role as sponsor for the study, had no input into study design; in the collection, analysis, and interpretation of data; in the writing of the report; and in the decision to submit the article for publication.

Author details
[1]Department of Health Sciences, University of York, York, UK. [2]Wythenshawe Hospital, Manchester, UK.

References

1. Fisher P, Van Haselen R, Hardy K, Berkovitz S, McCarney R: **Effectiveness gaps: a new concept for evaluating health service and research needs applied to complementary and alternative medicine.** *J Altern Complement Med* 2004, **10**:627–632.
2. Dixon-Woods M, Critchley S: **Medical and lay views of irritable bowel syndrome.** *Fam Pract* 2000, **17**:108–113.
3. MacPherson H, Sinclair-Lian N, Thomas K: **Patients seeking care from acupuncture practitioners in the UK: A national survey.** *Complement Ther Med* 2006, **14**:20–30.
4. Lim B, Manheimer E, Lao L, Ziea E, Wisniewski J, Liu J, Berman B: **Acupuncture for treatment of irritable bowel syndrome.** *Cochrane Database Syst Rev* 2008, doi:10.1002/14651858.CD005111.pub2.
5. Schneider A, Enck P, Streitberger K, Weiland C, Bagheri S, Witte S, Friederich HC, Herzog W, Zipfel S: **Acupuncture treatment in irritable bowel syndrome.** *Gut* 2006, **55**:649–654.
6. Lembo AJ, Conboy L, Kelley JM, Schnyer RS, McManus CA, Quilty MT, Kerr CE, Drossman D, Jacobson EE, Davis RB: **A treatment trial of acupuncture in IBS patients.** *Am J Gastroenterol* 2009, **104**:1489–1497.
7. Fireman Z, Segal A, Kopelman Y, Sternberg A, Carasso R: **Acupuncture treatment for irritable bowel syndrome. A double-blind controlled study.** *Digestion* 2001, **64**:100–103.
8. Forbes A, Jackson S, Walter C, Quraishi S, Jacyna M, Pitcher M: **Acupuncture for irritable bowel syndrome: A blinded placebo-controlled trial.** *World J Gastroenterol* 2005, **11**:4040–4044.
9. Liao YC: **Acupuncture treatment for 132 cases of irritable bowel syndrome.** *Clinical Journal of Acupuncture and Moxibustion* 2000, **16**:13–14.
10. Kaptchuk TJ, Kelley JM, Conboy LA, Davis RB, Kerr CE, Jacobson EE, Kirsch I, Schyner RN, Nam BH, Nguyen LT, *et al*: **Components of placebo effect: randomised controlled trial in patients with irritable bowel syndrome.** *BMJ* 2008, **336**:999–1003.
11. Liu M: **Clinical report of ear acupuncture treatment for functional gastric disorder.** *Shanghai Journal of Acupunctureand Moxibustion* 1995, **14**:247–248.
12. Liu GZ: **Treatment of acupuncture and moxibustion plus psychotherapy for irritable bowel syndrome.** *Chinese Acupuncture and Moxibustion* 1997, **10**:611–612.
13. Lowe C, Depew W, Vanner S: **A placebo-controlled double-blind trial of acupuncture in the treatment of irritable bowel syndrome.** *Gastroenterology* 2000, **118**(4 Suppl 2):A3168.
14. Sherman KJ, Cherkin DC, Eisenberg DM, Erro J, Hrbek A, Deyo RA: **The practice of acupuncture: who are the providers and what do they do?** *Ann Fam Med* 2005, **3**(2):151–158.
15. Hopton AK, Curnoe S, Kanaan M, MacPherson H: **Acupuncture in practice: mapping the providers, the patients and the settings in a national cross-sectional survey.** *BMJ Open* 2012, **2**(1):e000456. Jan 11.
16. MacPherson H, Thomas K: **Self-help advice as a process integral to traditional acupuncture care: implications for trial design.** *Complement Ther Med* 2008, **16**:101–106.
17. Paterson C, Dieppe P: **Characteristic and incidental (placebo) effects in complex interventions such as acupuncture.** *BMJ* 2005, **330**:1202–1205.
18. National Institute for Health and Clinical Excellence: *Low back pain: Early management of persistent non-specific low back pain.* London, UK: NICE Clinical Guideline 88. Developed by the National Collaborating Centre for Primary Care; 2009. http://www.nice.org.uk/nicemedia/live/11887/44343/44343.pdf.
19. Reynolds JA, Bland JM, MacPherson H: **Acupuncture for irritable bowel syndrome an exploratory randomised controlled trial.** *Acupunct Med* 2008, **26**:8–16.
20. MacPherson H, Bland M, Bloor K, Cox H, Geddes D, Kang'ombe A, Reynolds J, Stamuli E, Stuardi T, Tilbrook H, *et al*: **Acupuncture for irritable bowel syndrome: A protocol for a pragmatic randomised controlled trial.** *BMC Gastroenterol* 2010, **10**:63.
21. Stamuli E, Bloor K, MacPherson H, Tilbrook H, Stuardi T, Brabyn S, Torgerson D: **Cost-effectiveness of acupuncture for irritable bowel syndrome: findings from an economic evaluation conducted alongside a pragmatic randomised controlled trial in primary care.** *BMC Gastroenterol* 2012, **12**:138.
22. Francis CY, Morris J, Whorwell PJ: **The irritable bowel severity scoring system: a simple method of monitoring irritable bowel syndrome and its progress.** *Aliment Pharmacol Ther* 1997, **11**:395–402.
23. Hawe P, Shiell A, Riley T: **Complex interventions: how "out of control" can a randomised controlled trial be?** *Br Med J* 2004, **328**:1561–1563.
24. Atkinson W, Sheldon TA, Shaath N, Whorwell PJ: **Food elimination based on IgG antibodies in irritable bowel syndrome: a randomised controlled trial.** *Gut* 2004, **53**:1459–1464.
25. Ware J Jr, Kosinski M, Keller SD: **A 12-Item Short-Form Health Survey: construction of scales and preliminary tests of reliability and validity.** *Med Care* 1996, **34**:220–233.
26. The EuroQol Group: **EuroQol–a new facility for the measurement of health-related quality of life.** *Health Policy* 1990, **16**:199–208.
27. MacPherson H, Altman DG, Hammerschlag R, Youping L, Taixiang W, White A, Moher D: **Revised STandards for Reporting Interventions in Clinical Trials of Acupuncture (STRICTA): extending the CONSORT statement.** *PLoS Med* 2010, **7**:e1000261.
28. Stuardi T, MacPherson H: **Acupuncture for Irritable Bowel Syndrome (ACIBS): The diagnosis and treatment of patients in a pragmatic trial.** *J Altern Complement Med* 2012, in press.
29. Linde K, Witt CM, Streng A, Weidenhammer W, Wagenpfeil S, Brinkhaus B, Willich SN, Melchart D: **The impact of patient expectations on outcomes in four randomized controlled trials of acupuncture in patients with chronic pain.** *Pain* 2007, **128**:264–271.
30. Kennedy T, Jones R, Darnley S, Seed P, Wessely S, Chalder T: **Cognitive behaviour therapy in addition to antispasmodic treatment for irritable bowel syndrome in primary care: randomised controlled trial.** *BMJ* 2005, **331**:435.
31. Langevin HM, Wayne PM, MacPherson H, Schnyer R, Milley RM, Napadow V, Lao L, Park J, Harris RE, Cohen M, *et al*: **Paradoxes in acupuncture research: strategies for moving forward.** *Evid Based Complement Alternat Med* 2011, **2011**:180805.
32. Spiller RC: **Problems and challenges in the design of irritable bowel syndrome clinical trials: experience from published trials.** *Am J Med* 1999, **107**:91S–97S.

Using read codes to identify patients with irritable bowel syndrome in general practice: A database study

Elaine F Harkness[1*], Laura Grant[1], Sarah J O'Brien[2], Carolyn A Chew-Graham[3] and David G Thompson[4]

Abstract

Background: Estimates of the prevalence of irritable bowel syndrome (IBS) vary widely, and a large proportion of patients report having consulted their general practitioner (GP). In patients with new onset gastrointestinal symptoms in primary care it might be possible to predict those at risk of persistent symptoms. However, one of the difficulties is identifying patients within primary care. GPs use a variety of Read Codes to describe patients presenting with IBS. Furthermore, in a qualitative study, exploring GPs' attitudes and approaches to defining patients with IBS, GPs appeared reluctant to add the IBS Read Code to the patient record until more serious conditions were ruled out. Consequently, symptom codes such as 'abdominal pain', 'diarrhoea' or 'constipation' are used. The aim of the current study was to investigate the prevalence of recorded consultations for IBS and to explore the symptom profile of patients with IBS using data from the Salford Integrated Record (SIR).

Methods: This was a database study using the SIR, a local patient sharing record system integrating primary, community and secondary care information. Records were obtained for a cohort of patients with gastrointestinal disorders from January 2002 to December 2011. Prevalence rates, symptom recording, medication prescribing and referral patterns were compared for three patient groups (IBS, abdominal pain (AP) and Inflammatory Bowel Disease (IBD)).

Results: The prevalence of IBS (age standardised rate: 616 per year per 100,000 population) was much lower than expected compared with that reported in the literature. The majority of patients (69%) had no gastrointestinal symptoms recorded in the year prior to their IBS. However a proportion of these (22%) were likely to have been prescribed NICE guideline recommended medications for IBS in that year. The findings for AP and IBD were similar.

Conclusions: Using Read Codes to identify patients with IBS may lead to a large underestimate of the community prevalence. The IBS diagnostic Read Code was rarely applied in practice. There are similarities with many other medically unexplained symptoms which are typically difficult to diagnose in clinical practice.

Keywords: Irritable bowel syndrome, Read Codes, Functional gastrointestinal disorders, Medically unexplained symptoms, Primary care, General practitioners

* Correspondence: Elaine.F.Harkness@manchester.ac.uk
[1]Institute of Inflammation and Repair, Stopford Building, University of Manchester, Oxford Road, Manchester M13 9PL, UK
Full list of author information is available at the end of the article

Background

Irritable Bowel Syndrome (IBS) is a common gastrointestinal condition defined as 'a functional bowel disorder in which abdominal pain or discomfort is associated with defecation or a change in bowel habit, and with features of disordered defecation' [1]. Prevalence estimates for IBS appear to vary widely according to the criteria used, population studied, the mode of study delivery and type of prevalence estimate. Typically estimates range between 2% and 22% in western countries [2]. In the UK, a community survey estimated the prevalence of IBS to be 10.5% with over half of patients having consulted their general practitioner (GP) within the past six months [3].

Medical management of IBS symptoms is empiric usually involving anti-spasmodics, anti-diarrhoeals or laxatives as appropriate to symptoms; and antidepressants, particularly low-dose tricyclic antidepressants [4]. Unfortunately, for some patients medical management is unsatisfactory. For patients with symptoms resistant to conventional medical therapy, current guidelines recommend referral for psychological intervention to cognitive behavioural therapy (CBT) or hypnotherapy [4].

Halder et al. [5] showed that in patients with new onset gastrointestinal symptoms in primary care it might be possible to predict those at risk of persistent symptoms. Thus it might be possible to identify those patients at risk of doing worse and fast-track them to these therapies. This should lead to less distress and lower healthcare utilisation for these patients in the long run. We aimed to test this finding prospectively as a part of a NIHR (National Institute for Health Research) programme of work (RP-PG-0407-10136). However, one of the difficulties encountered in previous work on IBS within primary care is the identification of patients.

GPs use a variety of Read Codes to describe patients presenting with IBS. Furthermore, in a qualitative study to explore GPs attitudes and approaches to defining, diagnosing and managing patients with IBS in primary care we found that, despite recent guidelines from the National Institute for Health and Clinical Excellence (NICE) [4], IBS is still regarded as a diagnosis of exclusion, and GPs are reluctant to add the IBS Read Code to the patient record until more serious conditions are ruled out [6]. As a consequence, symptom codes such as 'abdominal pain', 'diarrhoea' or 'constipation' are Read coded in the patient record. To our knowledge the range of Read Codes used by GPs to define IBS has not previously been investigated. We therefore used a database study to investigate the use of Read Codes in patients with IBS. In addition, two recent systematic reviews have found that the quality of coding of morbidities within primary care varied, and this has been attributed to the distinctiveness of the diagnosis [7,8]. We therefore also wished to explore the differences in coding between a 'functional' and an 'organic' disorder.

Aim

The aim of the current study was to investigate the prevalence of recorded consultations for IBS and to explore the symptom profile of patients with IBS using data from the Salford Integrated Record (SIR). Patients with IBS were our primary group of interest, but we were also interested in how GPs coded patients with other gastrointestinal conditions, to determine whether there were any differences in coding practices across conditions. Patients with abdominal pain (AP) were chosen because it is the main feature of IBS, and must be present with two other symptoms to fulfil a diagnosis of IBS [4]. In addition, we selected patients with IBD because IBD is an organic disorder in which patients present with similar symptoms to IBS and we wished to explore differences in coding practices between a 'functional' and an 'organic' disorder.

Methods

Setting

The setting for this study was Salford Primary Care Organisation, North West of England with an estimated population of 228,992 in 2010 [9].

Population

All patients registered with the 52 General Practices in Salford Primary Care Organisation.

Data collection and coding

The SIR is a local patient sharing record system which integrates primary care, community care and secondary care information into one continuous electronic health record per patient. It is especially important for patients with long-term conditions, who may see many health professionals, saving the patient from having to repeat the same information multiple times. An anonymised dataset is made available for research through the auspices of North West e-Health.

Electronic clinical records from the SIR were obtained for a cohort of patients based on symptom and diagnostic codes for gastrointestinal disorders for the period January 2002 to December 2011. Information was supplied in two separate files: the first contained anonymised patient identifiers, sex and year of birth; the second contained journal entry identifier, anonymised patient identifier, date of journal entry, Read Code description and Read Code. The files were matched on patient identifier, and checked for duplicates and anomalies. Duplicate records and patients under the age of 17 were removed. Read Codes were then coded into a new variable to distinguish between symptom and/or diagnostic codes, medication codes and referral codes.

Analysis

For the study we carried out analysis on three groups. These were patients with:

a) IBS (Read Codes 14CF. and J521. including any subheadings)
b) abdominal pain (Read Codes 196.., 197.. and R090. including any subheadings)
c) Inflammatory Bowel Disease (IBD) (Read Codes J4... (without subheadings), J40.. and J41.. including any subheadings)

For each group of patients we identified an index episode of IBS, abdominal pain or IBD. For each index episode, an index date was created based on the date for that particular journal entry. For each condition we then looked one year pre and post the index date to determine:

i) Symptoms/diagnoses recorded pre and post IBS, abdominal pain and IBD
ii) Medications prescribed pre and post IBS, abdominal pain and IBD
iii) Referrals to gastrointestinal (GI) specialists pre and post IBS, abdominal pain and IBD

The index episode was taken as the first occurrence of IBS, abdominal pain or IBD. The date of this episode was then used to calculate the number of days between the index episode and all corresponding journal entries for the same patient. Where the journal entry date was the same as the index date symptoms/diagnoses were included in the previous year and medications and referrals were included in the year after the index episode. Pre- episode data was based on those with an index episode between 2003 and 2011 (so that only those with a complete year of data available before the index year were included), likewise post-episode data was based on those with an index episode between 2002 and 2010.

We also calculated prevalence estimates based on Salford population data. Population data was obtained from the Office of National Statistics (ONS) website for Salford Primary Care Organisation [9]. Rates were standardised to the Greater Manchester population for 2006. This includes the population of the ten primary care organisations within the Greater Manchester area, which is roughly 2.5 million.

Results

There were 8,444 patients in Salford with an IBS Read Code recorded in the years 2002 to 2011. AP and IBD were Read Coded for 42,490 and 1,510 patients respectively.

IBS and AP were much more common in females, whereas a similar proportion of males and females had IBD (Table 1). The highest proportion of those with IBS, AP or IBD was in those aged 18–39 and declined with age. More patients with IBD were aged 60 or over (26%) compared with those aged 60 or over with IBS (16%) and AP (22%).

Table 1 Demographic information for patients with IBS, AP and IBD, Salford 2002-2011

		IBS		AP		IBD	
		n	%	n	%	n	%
Female		6137	72.7	26071	61.4	755	50.0
Age	18-39	4373	51.8	19662	46.3	629	41.7
	40-59	2703	32.0	13379	31.5	487	32.3
	60+	1368	16.2	9449	22.2	394	26.1

Prevalence estimates

The age standardised rates for IBS, AP and IBD per year per 100,000 population were 616, 3,606 and 139 respectively. Figure 1 shows the age standardised rates per 100,000 population for IBS, AP and IBD by gender in Salford for the years 2002–2011. Rates have been standardised to the Greater Manchester population. The rates for IBD have remained stable across the ten year period for both males and females. IBS shows a similar pattern in males and females with a slight increase in prevalence rates up to 2006 before levelling out over the second half of the ten year period. The rates of AP on the other hand increased considerably in both males and females from 2002 to about 2009, after which they have levelled out for both males and females.

Symptoms pre and post IBS, AP or IBD

Table 2 shows the number of symptoms/diagnoses one year prior to and one year after the index episode of IBS, AP and IBD. The most commonly reported symptoms in the year prior to IBS were AP (19.5%), diarrhoea (6.1%) and bloating (3.8%). However, for most patients

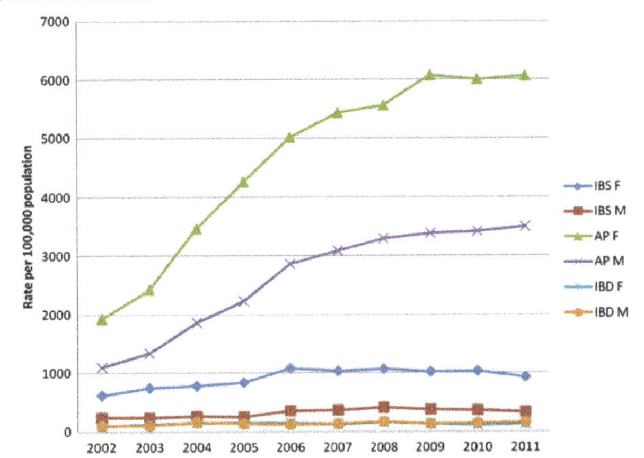

Figure 1 Age standardised rates, Salford 2002–2011.

Table 2 Number (%) of symptoms pre and post IBS, AP and IBD, Salford 2002-2011

	Pre IBS (n = 7728)		Post IBS (n = 7665)		Pre AP (n = 39974)		Post AP (n = 37851)		Pre IBD (n = 1336)		Post IBD (n = 1382)	
Symptoms/diagnoses*	n	%	n	%	n	%	n	%	n	%	n	%
Abdominal pain	1509	19.5	1028	13.4	-	-	8683	22.9	212	15.9	144	10.4
Bloating	291	3.8	137	1.8	411	1.0	374	1.0	8	0.6	7	0.5
Constipation symptom	166	2.1	138	1.8	639	1.6	700	1.8	16	1.2	14	1.0
Change in bowel habit	130	1.7	45	0.6	175	0.4	174	0.5	46	3.4	5	0.4
Diarrhoea symptoms	475	6.1	256	3.3	1046	2.6	972	2.6	158	11.8	74	5.4
Nausea	104	1.3	100	1.3	483	1.2	513	1.4	6	0.4	12	0.9
Vomiting	72	0.9	67	0.9	583	1.5	583	1.5	11	0.8	19	1.4
Diarrhoea & vomiting	47	0.6	43	0.6	202	0.5	192	0.5	12	0.9	6	0.4
Tenesmus	2	0.0	2	0.0	6	0.0	12	0.0	2	0.1	0	0.0
Faeces/motion symptoms	31	0.4	34	0.4	72	0.2	80	0.2	8	0.6	4	0.3
None of the above symptoms	5367	69.4	6062	79.1	36994	92.5	27010	71.4	930	69.6	1143	82.7
1 of the above symptoms	1950	25.2	1380	18.0	2699	6.8	9555	25.2	339	25.4	200	14.5
2 or more of the above symptoms	411	5.3	223	2.9	281	0.7	1286	3.4	67	5.0	39	2.8
Functional constipation	151	2.0	121	1.6	511	1.3	573	1.5	20	1.5	21	1.5
Functional diarrhoea	31	0.4	31	0.4	75	0.2	118	0.3	22	1.6	15	1.1
GI infection	84	1.1	63	0.8	295	0.7	295	0.8	18	1.3	8	0.6
IBS	-	-	1090	14.2	747	1.9	1061	2.8	42	3.1	25	1.8
IBD	33	0.4	40	0.5	128	0.3	204	0.5	-	-	391	28.3

*Symptoms on the same day were coded as pre.

(69.4%) no GI symptoms were recorded in the year prior to their IBS. Likewise in the year after the index episode of IBS most patients did not have any GI symptoms recorded (79.1%), AP was the most commonly recorded symptom (13.4%) and 14% of patients had a further episode of IBS recorded in the year after their index episode. IBD showed a similar pattern to IBS with the majority of patients (69.6%) not having any symptoms recorded in the year prior to their IBD diagnosis. The most commonly reported symptoms were AP (15.9%) and diarrhoea (11.8%). In the year after the index episode of IBD, AP and diarrhoea were still the most commonly reported symptoms but the proportions tended to be lower (10.4% and 5.4% respectively). Almost a third of patients had a further episode of IBD recorded in the year after their index episode.

For patients with AP most patients (92.5%) had no symptoms recorded in the year prior to their index episode of AP. In the year after their index episode, 23% of patients had a further AP episode, and 2.8% of patients had an IBS diagnosis.

The proportion of patients who reported two or more symptoms in the previous year or the year after IBS, AP or IBD was coded in 5% or less in most instances.

Medications pre and post IBS, AP or IBD

Table 3 shows the number of NICE guideline recommended medications for IBS prescribed in the year prior to and after the index episode of IBS, AP and IBD. NICE guideline recommended medications for IBS were prescribed for 31% and 54% of patients in the year prior to and after their index episode of IBS respectively. The increased use of these medications was most marked for antispasmodics which increased from 17% in the year prior to IBS to 44% in the year after. IBS NICE guideline recommended medications were also commonly prescribed in patients with AP and IBD, with about a third of patients being prescribed medications in the year after the index episode of AP or IBD. Prescribing of antispasmodics increased markedly from 5% to 19% in those with AP pre- and post- the index episode. Approximately 10% of patients with IBS, AP or IBD were prescribed selective serotonin reuptake inhibitors (SSRIs), and about 5% tricyclic antidepressants.

Tables 4 and 5 show the number of NICE guideline recommended medications prescribed in the year prior to and year after the index episodes of IBS, AP and IBD for those with and without symptoms respectively. Where GI symptoms were recorded in the year prior to or the year after the index episode, the proportion of patients prescribed NICE guideline recommended medications was higher than in those without symptoms. However, a number of patients still received NICE guideline recommended medications in the year prior to their index episode of IBS (22%), AP (18%) or IBD (20%)

Table 3 Number (%) of medications pre and post IBS, AP and IBD, Salford 2002-2011

	Pre IBS (n = 7728)		Post IBS (n = 7665)		Pre AP (n = 39974)		Post AP (n = 37851)		Pre IBD (n = 1336)		Post IBD (n = 1382)	
Medications†	n	%	n	%	n	%	n	%	n	%	n	%
NICE medications	2395	31.0	4099	53.5	8560	21.4	13871	36.6	389	29.1	442	32.0
Bulking laxatives	288	3.7	629	8.2	754	1.9	1561	4.1	40	3.0	50	3.6
Stimulant laxatives	204	2.6	247	3.2	1106	2.8	1688	4.5	36	2.7	59	4.3
Faecal softeners	0	0.0	0	0.0	0	0.0	0	0.0	0	0.0	0	0.0
Osmotic laxatives	216	2.8	289	3.8	845	2.1	1550	4.1	27	2.0	50	3.6
Antimotility drugs	246	3.2	429	5.6	727	1.8	979	2.6	132	9.9	169	12.2
Antispasmodic drugs	1328	17.2	3397	44.3	1890	4.7	7035	18.6	157	11.8	149	10.8
Tricyclic antidepressants	397	5.1	553	7.2	1924	4.8	2221	5.9	66	4.9	78	5.6
SSRI	808	10.5	957	12.5	3530	8.8	3955	10.4	101	7.6	129	9.3
Other antidepressants	124	1.6	147	1.9	554	1.4	660	1.7	12	0.9	15	1.1

†Medications on the same day were coded as post.

despite not having any symptoms recorded in the year prior to their index episode. In those with IBS approximately 50% of those with no symptoms recorded in the year after their index episode were prescribed NICE guideline recommended medications, compared with about 30% in those with AP or IBD. In those where symptoms had been recorded in the year prior to or after the index episode the proportion prescribed NICE guideline recommended medications was much higher compared to those where no symptoms had been recorded.

Referrals pre and post IBS, AP or IBD

About 4% of patients had a gastrointestinal secondary care referral either in the year prior to or the year after their index episode of IBS (Table 6). This was in contrast to patients with IBD where 9% of patients had a GI referral in the year prior to their index episode and 22% had a GI referral in the year after their index episode. Few patients (0.9%) with AP had a GI referral in the year prior to their index episode. The number of referrals for mental health or lifestyle was low (0.0% to 0.7%) for all three conditions.

Discussion

Summary

This database study demonstrated that the prevalence of IBS in patients who consult, and are recorded by, their GP was low compared with the reported prevalence rates in the literature [2]. Most patients who had an IBS Read Code recorded did not have any gastrointestinal symptoms recorded prior to or after their index date. Likewise the majority of patients with AP or IBD did not have any symptoms recorded prior to or after their index

Table 4 Number (%) of medications pre and post IBS, AP, IBD in those with no symptoms, Salford 2002-2011

	Pre IBS (n = 5367)		Post IBS (n = 6062)		Pre AP (n = 36670)		Post AP (n = 27010)		Pre IBD (n = 930)		Post IBD (n = 1143)	
Medications†	n	%	n	%	n	%	n	%	n	%	n	%
NICE medications	1176	21.9	2974	49.1	6720	18.3	8018	29.7	191	19.9	300	26.2
Bulking laxatives	119	2.2	437	7.2	569	1.6	840	3.1	21	2.2	32	2.8
Stimulant laxatives	77	1.4	129	2.1	795	2.2	896	3.3	19	2.0	33	2.9
Faecal softeners	0	0.0	0	0.0	0	0.0	0	0.0	0	0.0	0	0.0
Osmotic laxatives‡	93	1.7	152	2.5	571	1.6	745	2.8	13	1.4	25	2.2
Antimotility drugs	109	2.0	284	4.7	423	1.2	450	1.7	66	6.9	119	10.4
Antispasmodic drugs	533	9.9	2430	40.1	1414	3.9	3870	14.3	55	5.7	85	7.4
Tricyclic antidepressants	228	4.2	372	6.1	1647	4.5	1364	5.0	46	4.8	52	4.5
SSRI	471	8.8	680	11.2	3061	8.3	2488	9.2	59	6.1	92	8.0
Other antidepressants	55	1.0	84	1.4	472	1.3	383	1.4	8	0.8	10	0.9

†Medications on the same day were coded as post.
‡Excludes lactulose which is not recommended in NICE guidelines.

Table 5 Number (%) of medications pre and post IBS, AP, IBD in those with symptoms, Salford 2002-2011

	Pre IBS (n = 2361)		Post IBS (n = 1603)		Pre AP (n = 3304)		Post AP (n = 10841)		Pre IBD (n = 406)		Post IBD (n = 239)	
Medications[†]	n	%	n	%	n	%	n	%	n	%	n	%
NICE medications	1181	50.0	1103	68.8	1466	44.4	5314	49.0	189	46.6	135	56.5
Bulking laxatives	169	7.2	192	12.0	185	5.6	721	6.7	19	4.7	18	7.5
Stimulant laxatives	127	5.4	118	7.4	311	9.4	792	7.3	17	4.2	26	10.9
Faecal softeners	0	0.0	0	0.0	0	0.0	0	0.0	0	0.0	0	0.0
Osmotic laxatives[‡]	123	5.2	137	8.5	274	8.3	805	7.4	14	3.4	25	10.5
Antimotility drugs	137	5.8	145	9.0	304	9.2	529	4.9	66	16.3	50	20.9
Antispasmodic drugs	795	33.7	967	60.3	476	14.4	3165	29.2	102	25.1	64	26.8
Tricyclic antidepressants	169	7.2	181	11.3	277	8.4	857	7.9	20	4.9	26	10.9
SSRI	337	14.3	277	17.3	469	14.2	1467	13.5	42	10.3	37	15.5
Other antidepressants	69	2.9	63	3.9	82	2.5	277	2.6	4	1.0	5	2.1

[†]Medications on the same day were coded as post.
[‡]Excludes lactulose which is not recommended in NICE guidelines.

date. Antispasmodics were the most commonly prescribed medications for patients with IBS. A significant proportion of patients were prescribed IBS NICE guideline recommended medications in the year prior to their IBS being Read Coded. A small proportion of patients with IBS were referred to GI specialists.

Strengths and limitations

A major advantage of the SIR is the complete linkage between primary care, community care and secondary care datasets, providing a continuous electronic record for each patient in contact with health services in Salford. However, there were certain limitations in using these data for identifying patients with IBS in our study.

We were unable to validate the dataset. Ideally we would have created a cohort of IBS patients from SIR and validated the diagnosis by asking their GPs [10] but this was not possible since the SIR for research is anonymised at both patient and GP level. In addition, a number of computerised systems are available for capturing clinical consultation data in primary care and several different versions of the various operating systems are in use so there may be slight variations at computer operating system level that would have impeded our research.

There are also idiosyncrasies in the Read Code taxonomy, in particular the fact that codes for a lack of existence of a symptom can occur as leaf nodes describing that symptom. For example, the Read Code for "no abdominal pain" (1961.) is included under one of the Read Codes for abdominal pain (196..). However, it seems that GPs might be reluctant to document patients using such negated child node Read Codes as less than 0.1% were found in the data set we used.

Read Codes used to code a consultation are at the discretion of the individual clinician, which means that there can be considerable variation in their use to describe the same set of symptoms in practice (particularly for conditions not incentivised in the Quality Outcomes Framework (QOF)). However, research requires a disciplined approach to data entry and retrieval [11], so that inconsistency in coding potentially presents an important source of information bias.

Recorded prevalence of IBS consultations

This study demonstrates that the recorded prevalence of IBS in patients who consult their GP is low. In the current study, we not only looked at the prevalence of IBS Read Codes in primary care, but the prevalence of AP, the main presenting feature for IBS. Even rates of AP were less than those reported for IBS in the literature. Reassuringly we found similar results using data extracted from Manchester Primary Care Organisation (data not shown) suggesting that the current findings are not an artefact of

Table 6 Number (%) of referrals pre and post IBS, AP and IBD, Salford 2002–2011

	Pre IBS (n = 7728)		Post IBS (n = 7665)		Pre AP (n = 39974)		Post AP (n = 37851)		Pre IBD (n = 1336)		Post IBD (n = 1382)	
Referrals[#]	n	%	n	%	n	%	n	%	n	%	n	%
Gastrointestinal	295	3.8	288	3.8	358	0.9	1230	3.2	123	9.2	303	21.9
Mental health	3	0.0	3	0.0	19	0.0	21	0.1	0	0.0	0	0.0
Lifestyle	24	0.3	24	0.3	79	0.2	99	0.3	6	0.4	9	0.7

[#]Referrals on the same day were coded as post.

the data (Thompson DG, O'Brien S, Kennedy A, Rogers A, Whorwell P, Lovell K, *et al.*: Evaluating and Implementing Better Patient-Orientated Management of Chronic Gastrointestinal Disorders in Primary Care. *Programme Grants Appl Res* 2014, in review).

There are several possible explanations for the lower than expected prevalence of patients consulting with, and recorded as having, IBS.

Firstly, many of the studies estimating the prevalence of IBS have been self-report questionnaire surveys, and may have overestimated the proportion of patients who have been formally diagnosed with IBS, or who seek healthcare for their symptoms. Nevertheless the consultation prevalence for IBS was much lower than expected and the literature suggests that GPs see IBS as a significant problem [12]. Our findings reflect those in rheumatology where large discrepancies have been found in the consultation prevalence of knee pain when comparing primary care records with patient recall [13]. These discrepancies are as a result of 'telescoping' by patients and under recording by GPs, in particular, if patients present with multiple problems or have previously consulted for the same condition [13]. Like knee pain, IBS does not have a definite diagnosis and symptoms fluctuate over time, thus primary care records may only reflect the consultation prevalence of IBS when it forms a major part of the consultation. Moreover, Jordan at el. [13] found that consultation rates increased when the text of the consultation was used in addition to Read Codes alone. Others have also discussed the benefit of narratives during the consultation rather than reducing the clinical encounter to a limited number of codes [14].

Secondly, IBS or GI symptoms, are not included in the Quality Outcomes Framework (QoF), a scheme that incentivises GP practices and rewards them according to how well they care for patients. Consequently, recording IBS is not likely to be a priority for GPs and therefore may be patchy.

Thirdly, GPs appear to be reluctant to code patients for IBS or lower GI symptoms. The IBS diagnosis in primary care appears to be different to, and less exclusive than existing diagnostic criteria [15]. The usefulness of diagnostic criteria is frequently debated in the literature [16-20] and they tend to be of little relevance within primary care, as few GPs are familiar with the criteria and they do not use them to make a diagnosis [17,21,22]. In our qualitative study to investigate how GPs defined, diagnosed and managed patients with IBS, we found that whilst most GPs were aware of the NICE guideline [4] for IBS, few used it to help them make a diagnosis of IBS and add a Read Code to the patient record [6]. Instead they described using an iterative process to exclude sinister symptoms and as a result perhaps not applying a Read Code to the patient record when they first consult.

Fourthly, recorded prevalence depends on the healthcare seeking behaviour of patients. Patients may not consult their GP for IBS for a number of reasons. They may only consult when their symptoms are severe and, consequently, they perhaps feel less able to cope. Indeed, data from our risk assessment study, where patients were recruited either via the consultation or through the use of Read Code searches (and had to have consulted for IBS symptoms in the last three months), suggest that the majority of patients had moderate or severe symptoms (Thompson DG, O'Brien S, Kennedy A, Rogers A, Whorwell P, Lovell K, *et al.*: Evaluating and Implementing Better Patient-Orientated Management of Chronic Gastrointestinal Disorders in Primary Care. *Programme Grants Appl Res* 2014, in review). Evidence suggests that symptom severity may have an influence on health care seeking but that it does explain the majority of the consultation behaviour [23]. Psychological and psychosocial factors have also been implicated in health care seeking behaviours for patients with IBS [24,25]. The present study suggests that a proportion of patients with IBS, AP and IBD were prescribed anti-depressants in the year before and the year after their index episode. However, we cannot infer whether these medications were prescribed for their gastrointestinal symptoms, for related anxiety and/or depression, or for unrelated anxiety and/or depression.

Furthermore, patients may not consult their GP for their IBS because their symptoms are under control through the use of medication or self-management. A relatively large proportion of patients in the current study had no GI symptoms in the year prior to their index episode of IBS but had been prescribed IBS medications, as recommended in the NICE guideline [4]. However, we are unable to say whether these patients had ever been recorded as having IBS prior to the year before their index episode, and whether they had received a repeat prescription from their GP for their symptoms.

Finally, patients may feel there is little that primary care can offer, and therefore learn to live with their symptoms. Stenner et. al. [26] reported that patients felt that doctors were unsympathetic and ignorant about IBS, and often considered IBS 'all being in the mind' of the patient. Others felt GPs were responsible for the worsening of their condition as a result of their ignorance of IBS or 'through the iatrogenic effects of treatment' [26]. Farndale et al. [27] found that IBS patients report alienation from health services for similar reasons. In addition, moderate to high levels of perceived stigma are significantly greater in IBS patients (27%) compared to IBD patients (8%), with the largest difference being for health care providers [28]. It is, therefore, perhaps unsurprising that a proportion of those suffering from the symptoms of IBS do not consult their GP and decide to self-medicate and/or seek alternative therapies. Although alternative therapies are not recommended within the NICE guidance [4] our qualitative study showed that GPs did not discourage their use [6].

IBS and GI symptoms

Our study found that the majority of patients who were coded as having IBS did not have GI symptoms recorded in the year prior to or the year after their index episode. NICE recommends assessment for IBS in patients having any of the following for at least 6 months: abdominal pain or discomfort, bloating or change in bowel habit. Therefore one might expect evidence of this in the recording of symptom codes in the year prior to or after the index episode of IBS. However, this was not the case, despite using symptom codes in order to be as comprehensive as possible and by including other related symptoms, such as nausea and vomiting, tenesmus and faeces/motions. Interestingly though, IBS medications as recommended by NICE were often prescribed in those without recorded symptoms in the year prior to their IBS. GPs in the qualitative study also described making a diagnosis based on the patient response to a trial of medication [6]. This suggests that the use of medication codes may be an alternative approach to identifying patients via symptom or diagnostic Read Codes. GPs must enter a medication on their clinical system in order for a prescription to be issued. However this approach may include patients with other diagnoses as some IBS medications (e.g. laxatives) may also be prescribed for other conditions.

Findings from our qualitative study suggest GPs did not describe difficulties in managing patients with IBS [6]. This is also evident in the current study where a relatively small proportion of patients with IBS had a referral to a GI specialist, compared to those patients with a diagnosis of IBD.

Similarities with other medically unexplained symptoms

Similarities can be seen with other medically unexplained symptoms such as fibromyalgia and chronic fatigue syndrome. For example, Rohrbeck et al. [29] found the recorded annual prevalence of fibromyalgia in primary care to be 8 per 10 000 which is much lower than the estimated general population prevalence of 2%. This implies that the label of fibromyalgia is rarely used within general practice [29]. They also found that fibromyalgia patients are similar to those with overlapping functional syndromes or medically unexplained symptoms [29]. Similarly, in his review of medically unexplained symptoms in primary care, Burton [30] reported that many patients with IBS met the criteria for fibromyalgia and chronic pelvic pain. This overlap with other medically unexplained symptoms, which often appear to share similar psychosocial characteristics, creates further diagnostic complexities.

Conclusions

Our findings suggest that the use of symptom /and or diagnostic Read Codes to identify patients with IBS in primary care is questionable and likely to lead to large underestimates of both the community incidence and prevalence. The discrepancies between the self-reported prevalence rates in the literature and those for consultations within the primary care record, suggest that there may be conflicting priorities between patients and health care professionals, and that database studies, are useful in only identifying the 'tip of the iceberg'.

NIHR disclaimer

This paper presents independent research commissioned by the National Institute for Health Research (NIHR) under its Programme Grants for Applied Research funding scheme (RP-PG-0407-10136). The views expressed in this paper are those of the authors and not necessarily those of the NHS, NIHR or the Department of Health.

Appendix

Tables 7, 8 and 9.

Table 7 Symptoms/diagnoses were defined as any of the following

Symptom/diagnoses	Read codes	Rubric
Irritable bowel syndrome	14CF.	History of IBS
	J521.	IBS
Abdominal pain	196..	Type of gastrointestinal tract pain
	197..	Site of gastrointestinal tract pain
	R090.	[D] Abdominal pain
Bloating	19A..	Abdominal distension symptom
	19B..	Flatulence/wind
	R0734	[D] Bloating
Constipation symptom	19C..	Constipation
Functional constipation	J520.	Constipation - functional
Change in bowel habit	19EA.	Change in bowel habit
	R078.	[D] Change in bowel habit
Diarrhoea	19F..	Diarrhoea symptoms
	19G..	Diarrhoea and vomiting
Functional diarrhoea	J525.	Functional diarrhoea
	J43z.	Chronic diarrhoea
	J4z..	Presumed noninfectious diarrhoea

Table 7 Symptoms/diagnoses were defined as any of the following *(Continued)*

Nausea	198..	Nausea
Vomiting	199..	Vomiting
Diarrhoea and vomiting	19G..	Diarrhoea and vomiting
Tenesmus	19D..	Tenesmus symptom
Faeces/motions symptoms	19E..	Faeces/motions -symptoms
GI infection	A0...	Intestinal infectious diseases
Inflammatory bowel disease	J40..	Crohn's disease
	J41..	Ulcerative colitis or proctitis

Table 8 Medications were defined on the basis of the NICE guidelines [4] and were coded as follows

NICE medications	Read codes	Rubric
Bulk-forming laxatives	ab2..	Isphagula husk
	ab3..	Methylcellulose
	ab4..	Sterculia
Stimulant laxatives	ac5..	Docusate sodium
	ac7..	Senna
	ac8..	Sodium picosulphate
	af1..	Rectal laxatives (Glycerol, biascodyl)
	ac1..	Biascodyl
Faecal softeners	ad1..	Liquid paraffin
Osmotic laxatives	ae4..	Polyethylene glycols
	a12..	Magnesium salts – antacid
	ae2..	Magnesium hydroxide
	ae3..	Magnesium sulphate
	ae7..	Sodium phosphate
Antimotility agents	a81..	Codeine phosphate
	a82..	Diphenoxylate hydrochloride
	a83..	Loperamide: single drug
	a85..	Loperamide: compound preparation
	a842.	Kaolin and morphine mixture
Antispasmodics	a41..	Atrophine sulphate
	a45..	Dicycloverine hydrochloride
	a47..	Hyoscine butylbromide
	a4c..	Propantheline bromide
	a4d..	Alverine citrate
	a4e..	Mebeverine hydrochloride
	a4f..	Peppermint oil
Antidepressants		
Tricyclics and related antidepressants	d71..	Amitripyline
	d91..	Triptafen

Table 8 Medications were defined on the basis of the NICE guidelines [4] and were coded as follows *(Continued)*

	d73..	Clomipramine hydrochloride
	d75..	Dosulephin hydrochloride
	d76..	Doxepin
	d77..	Imipramine hydrochloride
	d79..	Lofepramine
	d7c..	Nortriptyline
	d7f..	Trimipramine
	d7b..	Mianserin hydrochloride
	d7e..	Trazodone hydrochloride
Selective serotonin re-uptake inhibitors (SSRIs)	da9..	Citalopram
	daC..	Escitalopram
Monoamine oxidase inhibitors (MAOIs)	da4..	Fluoxetine hydrochloride
Reversible MAOIs	da3..	Fluvoxamine maleate
	da6..	Paroxetine hydrochloride
	da5..	Sertraline hydrochloride
Other antidepressants	d81..	Phenelzine
	d83..	Isocarboxazid
	d84..	Tranylcypromine
	d85..	Moclobemide
	gde..	Duloxetine
	da1..	Flupentixol
	daB..	Mirtazapine
	daA..	Reboxetine
	da2..	Tryptophan

Table 9 Referrals to specialists or for further for investigation of gastrointestinal symptoms were defined as any of the following

Referral	Read codes	Rubric
Specialist referral	8h48.	Gastroenterological referral
	8h5J.	Referral to colorectal surgeon
	8H5K.	Referral to upper gastrointestinal surgeon
	8HL8.	Gastroenterology DV done
	8HM8.	Listed for gasterenterol admis
	8Hn4.	Fast track referral for suspected colorectal cancer
	8Hn9.	Fast track referral for suspected upper GI cancer
	8HS..	Refer for gastroscopy
	8HS0.	Refer for sigmoidoscopy
	8HU1.	Referral for colonoscopy
	8HU2.	Referral for sigmoidoscopy
	8HVc.	Private referral to colorectal surgeon
	8HVN.	Private referral to gastroenterologist

Authors' contributions

EFH participated in the study design, supervised the data analysis, and led writing the paper. LG participated in data analysis and contributed to writing the paper. SJO'B participated in the study design and contributed to writing the paper. DGT participated in study design and contributed writing the paper. CCG contributed to writing the paper and led on the qualitative study. All authors read and approved the final manuscript.

Acknowledgement

On behalf of the Salford NIHR GI Programme Grant Research Group: Karen Armstrong, David Backhouse, Paula Beech, Peter Bower, Carolyn Chew-Graham, Andrew Clough, Anne Kennedy, Karina Lovell, Jim Nuttall, Sarah O'Brien, Karen Procter, David Reeves, Gerry Richardson, Anne Rogers, David Thompson, and Peter Whorwell.

EFH, LG, DGT and CCG were supported by the University of Manchester, Faculty of Medical & Health Sciences and the Manchester Academic Health Science Centre (MAHSC) at the time of the study.

Author details

[1]Institute of Inflammation and Repair, Stopford Building, University of Manchester, Oxford Road, Manchester M13 9PL, UK. [2]Institute of Infection and Global Health, Leahurst Campus, University of Liverpool, Chester High Road, Neston, South Wirral CH64 7TE, UK. [3]Research Institute, Primary Care and Health Sciences, Keele University, Keele, Staffordshire ST5 5BG, UK. [4]Gastrointestinal Centre, Institute of Inflammation & Repair, University of Manchester, Clinical Sciences Building, Salford Royal NHS Foundation Trust, Stott Lane, Salford M6 8HD, UK.

References

1. Longstreth GF, Thompson WG, Chey WD, Houghton LA, Mearin F, Spiller RC: **Functional bowel disorders.** *Gastroenterology* 2006, **130:**1480–1491.
2. Rey E, Talley NJ: **Irritable bowel syndrome: novel views on the epidemiology and potential risk factors.** *Dig Liver Dis* 2009, **41:**772–780.
3. Wilson S, Roberts L, Roalfe A, Bridge P, Singh S: **Prevalence of irritable bowel syndrome: a community survey.** *Br J Gen Pract* 2004, **54:**495–502.
4. National Institute for Health and Clinical Excellence: *NICE Clinical Guideline 61: Irritable Bowel Syndrome in Adults: Diagnosis and Management of Irritable Bowel Syndrome in Primary Care.* London: National Institute for Health and Clinical Excellence; 2008.
5. Halder S, Macfarlane GJ, Thompson D, O'Brien SJ, Musleh M, McBeth J: **Predictors of persistent gastrointestinal symptoms among new presenters to primary care.** *Eur J Gastroenterol Hepatol* 2010, **22:**296–305.
6. Harkness EF, Harrington V, Hinder S, O'Brien SJ, Thompson DG, Beech P, *et al*: **GP perspectives of irritable bowel syndrome - an accepted illness, but management deviates from guidelines: a qualitative study.** *BMC Fam Pract* 2013, **14:**92.
7. Jordan K, Porcheret M, Croft P: **Quality of morbidity coding in general practice computerized medical records: a systematic review.** *Fam Pract* 2004, **21:**396–412.
8. Khan NF, Harrison SE, Rose PW: **Validity of diagnostic coding within the general practice research database: a systematic review.** *Br J Gen Pract* 2010, **60:**e128–e136.
9. Office for National Statistics: *Primary Care Organisation Population Estimates (Experimental), Mid-2010.* Fareham: Office for National Statistics licensed under the Open Government Licence v.1.0; 2013.
10. Seminara NM, Abuabara K, Shin DB, Langan SM, Kimmel SE, Margolis D, *et al*: **Validity of the health improvement network (THIN) for the study of psoriasis.** *Br J Dermatol* 2011, **164:**602–609.
11. Soler JK, Pringle M: **Research using electronic patient records in general practice: the EGPRN meeting in Bertinoro, Italy, May 2009.** *Eur J Gen Pract* 2010, **16:**186–189.
12. Thompson WG, Heaton KW, Smyth GT, Smyth C: **Irritable bowel syndrome in general practice: prevalence, characteristics, and referral.** *Gut* 2000, **46:**78–82.
13. Jordan K, Jinks C, Croft P: **Health care utilization: measurement using primary care records and patient recall both showed bias.** *J Clin Epidemiol* 2006, **59:**791 797.
14. Walsh SH: **The clinician's perspective on electronic health records and how they can affect patient care.** *BMJ* 2004, **328:**1184–1187.
15. Rubin G, de Wit N, Meineche-Schmidt V, Seifert B, Hall N, Hungin P: **The diagnosis of IBS in primary care: consensus development using nominal group technique.** *Fam Pract* 2006, **23:**687–692.
16. Henderson PK, DiPalma JA: **Diagnosing irritable bowel syndrome: a changing clinical paradigm: [Review].** *Southern Med J* 2011, **104:**195–199.
17. Mearin F, Lacy BE: **Diagnostic criteria in IBS: useful or not?** *Neurogastroenterol Motil* 2012, **24:**791–801.
18. Talley NJ: **Irritable bowel syndrome: definition, diagnosis and epidemiology.** *Baillieres Best Pract Res Clin Gastroenterol* 1999, **13:**371–384.
19. Williams RE, Black CL, Kim HY, Andrews EB, Mangel AW, Buda JJ, *et al*: **Stability of irritable bowel syndrome using a Rome II-based classification.** *Aliment Pharmacol Ther* 2006, **23:**197–205.
20. Yale SH, Musana AK, Kieke A, Hayes J, Glurich I, Chyou PH: **Applying case definition criteria to irritable bowel syndrome.** *Clin Med Res* 2008, **6:**9–16.
21. Lionis C, Olsen-Faresjo A, Anastasiou F, Wallander MA, Johansson S, Faresjo T: **Measuring the frequency of functional gastrointestinal disorders in rural Crete: a need for improving primary care physicians' diagnostic skills.** *Rural Remote Health* 2005, **5:**409.
22. Ford AC, Talley NJ: **Irritable bowel syndrome.** *BMJ* 2012, **345:**e5836.
23. Koloski NA, Talley NJ, Boyce PM: **Predictors of health care seeking for irritable bowel syndrome and nonulcer dyspepsia: a critical review of the literature on symptom and psychosocial factors.** *Am J Gastroenterol* 2001, **96:**1340–1349.
24. Ringstrom G, Abrahamsson H, Strid H, Simren M: **Why do subjects with irritable bowel syndrome seek health care for their symptoms?** *Scand J Gastroenterol* 2007, **42:**1194–1203.
25. Koloski NA, Talley NJ, Boyce PM: **Epidemiology and health care seeking in the functional GI disorders: a population-based study.** *Am J Gastroenterol* 2002, **97:**2290–2299.
26. Stenner PH, Dancey CP, Watts S: **The understanding of their illness amongst people with irritable bowel syndrome: a Q methodological study.** *Soc Sci Med* 2000, **51:**439–452.
27. Farndale R, Roberts L: **Long-term impact of irritable bowel syndrome: a qualitative study.** *Prim Health Care Res Dev* 2011, **12:**52–67.
28. Taft TH, Keefer L, Artz C, Bratten J, Jones MP: **Perceptions of illness stigma in patients with inflammatory bowel disease and irritable bowel syndrome.** *Qual Life Res* 2011, **20:**1391–1399.
29. Rohrbeck J, Jordan K, Croft P: **The frequency and characteristics of chronic widespread pain in general practice: a case–control study.** *Br J Gen Pract* 2007, **57:**109–115.
30. Burton C: **Beyond somatisation: a review of the understanding and treatment of medically unexplained physical symptoms (MUPS).** *Br J Gen Pract* 2003, **53:**231–239.

17

The effect of *Lactobacillus brevis* KB290 against irritable bowel syndrome: A placebo-controlled double-blind crossover trial

Katsumi Murakami[1*], Chizu Habukawa[2], Yukihiro Nobuta[3], Naohiko Moriguchi[1] and Tsukasa Takemura[4]

Abstract

Background: Irritable bowel syndrome (IBS) is a functional disorder of the digestive tract that causes chronic abdominal symptoms. We evaluated the effects of *Lactobacillus brevis* KB290 (KB290), which has been demonstrated to be effective at improving bowel movements and the composition of intestinal microflora, on IBS symptoms.

Methods: We performed a placebo control double-blind cross matched trial. Thirty-five males and females (aged 6 years and above) who had been diagnosed with IBS according to the Rome III criteria were divided into 2 groups, and after a 4-week pre-trial observation period, they were administered test capsules containing KB290 or placebo for 4 weeks (consumption period I). Then, the capsule administration was suspended for 4 weeks in both groups (washout period), before the opposite capsules were administered for a further 4 weeks (consumption period II). Fecal samples were collected on the first day of the pre-consumption observation period, the last day of consumption period I, the last day of the washout period, and the last day of consumption period II. In addition, the subjects' IBS symptoms and quality of life (QOL) and any adverse events that they experienced were evaluated.

Results: No significant difference in IBS symptoms was noted among the various periods. However, the mean QOL scores were improved during the test capsule consumption.
The frequencies of watery and mushy feces were significantly lower in the test capsule consumption period than during the pre-consumption observation period, and the frequency of abdominal pain was significantly reduced in the test capsule consumption period compared with the other periods.
The frequency of the genus *Bifidobacterium* was significantly higher, and that of the genus *Clostridium* was significantly lower, after the test capsule consumption than after the placebo consumption. The frequencies of the genera *Lactobacillus*, *Bacteroides*, and *Enterococcus* were also investigated, but no differences in their frequencies were detected between the placebo and test capsule consumption periods.

Conclusions: Probiotics, the safety of which has been established, are used widely in various foods and can now be purchased readily. The results of the present study suggest that KB290 is useful for early intervention in IBS.

Keywords: Irritable bowel syndrome, *Lactobacillus brevis* KB290, Probiotic

* Correspondence: k-murakami@sakai.med.kindai.ac.jp
[1]Department of Pediatrics, Kinki University Sakai Hospital, 2-7-1 Harayamadai, Minami-ku, Sakai, Osaka 590-0132, Japan
Full list of author information is available at the end of the article

Background

Irritable bowel syndrome (IBS) is a functional disorder of the digestive tract that causes chronic symptoms such as abdominal pain and discomfort and abnormal bowel movements such as diarrhea and constipation but exhibits no organic abnormalities [1]. Its etiology and pathology are yet to be elucidated. However, abnormalities in brain-gut interactions; i.e., excessive stimulation of the digestive tract by the central nervous system during stress; the disturbance of sensory and cognitive mechanisms by disorders of the digestive tract, infection, or inflammation of the digestive tract; and changes in the intestinal microflora have been reported to be involved [2]. This suggests that the symptoms of IBS can be alleviated by restoring the normal intestinal flora and that we need to obtain a greater understanding of intestinal microflora [3]. Analyses of the microflora in IBS patients and healthy individuals have indicated that differences exist between them [4], but no intestinal bacteria that directly trigger the condition have been identified.

Some clinical trials have indicated that probiotics are effective at alleviating IBS symptoms and improving the quality of life (QOL) of IBS patients [5-8]. Also, the mechanism responsible for the beneficial effects of probiotics has not been clarified although improvements in the composition of the intestinal flora and the suppression of intestinal inflammatory reactions have been proposed as possible mechanisms [7,9].

Therefore, in this study we evaluated the effects of *Lactobacillus brevis* KB290 (KB290), which is a plant-derived strain of lactic acid bacillus isolated from *suguki* (a traditional pickle produced in Kyoto) that has been demonstrated to be effective at improving bowel movements and the composition of the intestinal microflora [10-13], on IBS symptoms and examined its effects on intestinal microflora to clarify the mechanism by which it induces the abovementioned improvements.

Methods

Study design

The patients were randomly divided into 2 groups, which were matched in age and gender, according to a computer generated randomized list. After a 4-week pre-trial observation period, they were administered test capsules containing KB290 (freeze-dried KB290 bodies at a dose of $\geq 1.0 \times 1010$ cfu/capsule mixed with corn starch, maltitol syrup, hydroxypropyl methylcellulose, and calcium stearate) or placebo capsules that did not contain KB290 at a rate of 1 capsule/day for 4 weeks (consumption period I). For the next 4 weeks, both groups stopped consuming the capsules (washout period). After the washout period, the groups were administered the opposite capsules to those that they had taken during the 1st consumption period for a further 4 weeks (consumption period II). The study protocol was approved by the ethics committees of the participating institutions (Figure 1).

Determination of the viable KB290 cell count

Counts of viable KB290 cells were obtained during the preparation of the test capsules and after the end of their administration. Then, after carefully weighing out 1.0 g of the powder obtained from 5 capsules, it was serially diluted using 0.1% (w/v) agar dissolved in physiological saline, and a 50 μL suspension was applied to 15 mL plate count agar (PCA) containing bromocresol purple (BCP) (Eiken Chemical). The suspension was cultured at 35°C for 72 hours, and then the number of colonies was counted. Since each capsule contained 0.34 - 0.38 g KB290 (standard content, 0.36 g), the number of living KB290 cells was calculated by assuming the KB290 content per capsule to be 0.34 g.

Patients

Thirty-five males and females (aged 6 years and above) who had been diagnosed with IBS according to the Rome III criteria [14] were selected. We calculated that

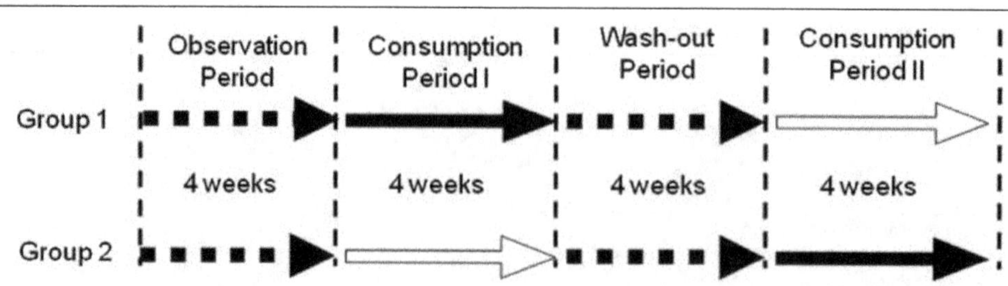

Figure 1 Study design. The subjects were divided into 2 groups, and after a 4-week pre-trial observation period, administered test capsules containing KB290 or placebo capsules not containing KB290 at 1 capsule/day for 4 weeks (consumption period I). Then, the capsule administration was suspended for 4 weeks in both groups (washout period), and the capsules opposite to those administered first were administered for 4 weeks (consumption period II).

in order for our model to possess a power of 80% to detect a difference between the two consumption periods when $\alpha = 0.05$, we would need to analyze 20 patients. In addition, we assumed a worst-case control rate of 67%. Accordingly, we recruited 35 patients for this study. To ensure the safety of the patients and eliminate the effects of factors other than the test capsule on the study outcomes, any patients who had serious disorders other than IBS or allergies to a material contained in the test capsule, had undergone gastrointestinal tract surgery other than appendectomy, had participated in another clinical study within the 3 months prior to the beginning of this study, or who had an infectious disease were excluded. During the patient recruitment, the intentions of the study and its procedures were thoroughly explained to the participants, and written consent to participate in the study was obtained in compliance with the Helsinki Declaration. During the study, the patients were instructed not to eat greater than usual amounts of foods that contained lactic acid bacilli (other than the test capsule).

Any subjects who had been administered antibiotics during the study period, had consumed foods that are known to markedly affect the condition of the bowel, that did not consume the test capsule as instructed, or whose diary entries were defective were excluded from the analysis.

Observation of IBS symptoms

The subjects (or their parents if the subjects could not keep a diary by themselves) kept a daily bowel movements diary during the study. The recorded items were the frequency of bowel movements, fecal properties (amount, color, shape), physical sensations experienced after bowel movement, time required for bowel movements, abdominal symptoms (frequency of attacks of abdominal pain), compliance with the administration schedule, and the consumption of foods that affect the condition of the bowel. Regarding the frequency of bowel movements, the mean weekly number of bowel movements was calculated separately for the pre-consumption observation period, washout period, placebo consumption period, and test capsule consumption period. The volume of feces was recorded in terms of the number of chicken eggs, and the mean value per bowel movement was calculated for each period. Concerning the shape and color of feces and the physical sensations experienced after bowel movement, mean scores were calculated for each period. As for the time required for bowel movements, the mean time of one bowel movement was calculated for each period. The frequency of attacks of abdominal pain was expressed as the mean weekly number for each period.

Analysis of fecal microflora

Fecal samples were collected on the first day of the pre-consumption observation period, the last day of consumption period I, the last day of the washout period, and the last day of consumption period II. Immediately after its discharge, a sample of the targeted feces was suspended in a vessel containing a DNA preservation medium (GCT buffer), the suspension was stored at 4°C until analysis, and the intestinal microflora it contained were analyzed using the terminal restriction fragment length polymorphism (T-RFLP) method [15]. After 16S rRNA had been extracted from the fecal suspension using the Magtration System 12GC automatic nucleic acid extraction machine (Precision System Science), it was reverse transcribed using the universal primer 516F-1510R (Life Technologies Japan) and digested using the restriction enzyme *BslI* (New England Biolabs). The digested cDNA fragments were subjected to capillary electrophoresis using an ABI3100 genetic analyzer (Applied Biosystems), the peak pattern of the DNA fragments obtained by absorptiometry at 260 nm was compared with that of the DNA fragments of the standard, and the bacterial species present in the feces were determined. The percentage areas of the peaks for the genera *Bifidobacterium* and *Clostridium* relative to the total area of all detected peaks were calculated, and the percentage changes in the areas of these peaks were also calculated to analyze the changes induced in the composition of the intestinal microflora by the test food or placebo.

Evaluation of QOL

QOL was evaluated before and after the consumption of the test capsule by assessing the physical activity, emotional problems, social activity, pain, and overall health state of the subjects using a 5-point scale and the Japanese version of the Dartmouth COOP charts [16], and mean scores were calculated for each period.

Evaluation of adverse events

The adverse events that occurred during the study were evaluated on the basis of the subjects' bowel movement diaries and interviews conducted at the end of the study. Abdominal pain and diarrhea, and adverse events that might have been caused by the consumption of the test capsule were recorded, and their frequencies during the test capsule consumption period were compared with those during the other periods.

Statistical analyses

The results for each evaluated item were totaled for each subject for the pre-consumption observation period, washout period, placebo consumption period, and test capsule consumption period and statistically analyzed.

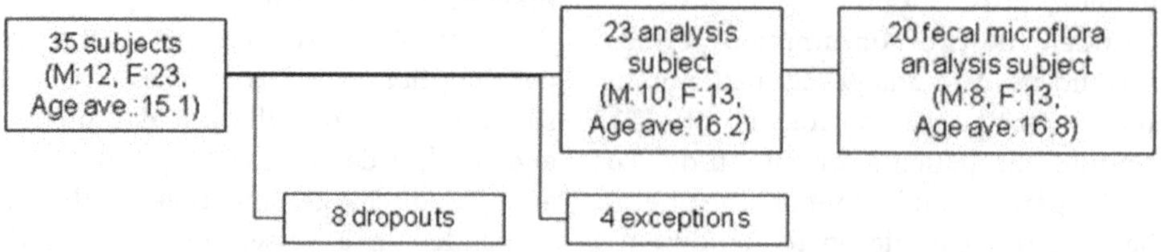

Figure 2 Analysis group. Thirty-five persons who volunteered to participate in the study were interviewed and all were enrolled, because none matched any of the exclusion criteria. Eight of them dropped out during the study, and, from those who completed the study, 23 (10 males and 13 females, mean age 16.2 ± 10.5 years) were selected as an analysis group by excluding 2 with defects in diary entries and 2 in whom the number of days with test capsule consumption was insufficient according to a premeditated procedure. The fecal microflora was analyzed in 20 subjects of the analysis group in whom data could be obtained in all periods.

The frequency of abdominal pain, frequency of bowel movements, fecal properties (volume, shape, color, smell), physical sensations experienced after bowel movement, time required for bowel movements, and frequencies of the genera *Bifidobacterium* and *Clostridium* among the fecal microflora were examined using the paired *t*-test with Bonferroni's correction. The significance of the differences in the QOL score was examined using the Steel-Dwass method. Statistical analyses were performed using the SPSS software (ver15.0, IBM) at a significance level of $p<0.05$.

Results

Number of living KB290 cells

The mean number of living KB290 bacteria in the test capsule was 1.2 ± 0.3×10 [10] cfu/capsule on the day of preparation (December 8, 2008) and 5.5 ± 0.4× 10 [9] and 6.8 ± 0.3×10 [9] cfu/capsule on the last day of test capsule consumption in the first (May 25, 2009) and last (September 5, 2009) subjects, respectively. The mean of these 3 measurements was 8.1 ± 0.4×10 [9] cfu/capsule. Also, no KB290 bacteria were detected in the placebo capsule at any point.

Analysis group

Thirty-five patients were interviewed and enrolled. Eight of them dropped out during the study, and of those who completed the study, four were excluded because of problems with their diary entries or with their compliance with the test or placebo capsule consumption protocol, thus 23 patients (10 males and 13 females, mean age: 16.2 ± 10.5 years) were included in the analysis (Figure 2). The fecal microflora of 20 subjects for whom data were obtained in all periods were analyzed. Three patients were excluded from the fecal microflora analysis because of problems with the fecal collection. No significant differences were noted in any of the examined items between Groups 1 and 2.

IBS symptoms

Table 1 shows our findings regarding the frequency of bowel movements, the volume and color of the subjects' feces, the physical sensations they experienced after bowel movements, and the time they required for bowel movements. No significant difference was noted in any of these items among the various periods.

Figure 3 shows the frequencies of various fecal shapes in each period. No significant difference in the frequency of any fecal shape was detected between the placebo consumption period and the washout period; however, the frequencies of watery and mushy feces were significantly lower in the test capsule consumption period than in the pre-consumption observation period.

Figure 4 shows the frequency of abdominal pain in each period. The frequency of abdominal pain was significantly reduced in the test capsule consumption period compared with the other periods.

Table 1 IBS symptoms

	Observation period	Wash-out period	Consumption period	
			Placebo	KB290
Frequency of bowel movement (times/week)	8.8 ± 3.5	7.8 ± 2.5	7.0 ± 3.8	8.0 ± 3.1
Fecal volume (hen's egg-size)/time	2.0 ± 1.5	1.7 ± 1.1	1.8 ± 1.5	2.1 ± 1.8
Fecal color (score mean value)	3.6 ± 1.5	3.8 ± 1.4	3.6 ± 1.4	3.5 ± 1.8
Feeling of bowel movement (score mean value)	3.2 ± 1.2	3.6 ± 0.8	3.0 ± 1.5	3.8 ± 1.3
Amount of time for bowel movement (minutes/time)	5.5 ± 4.8	5.9 ± 5.1	5.2 ± 5.0	5.3 ± 4.3

Values are expressed as Means ± SD, n = 23.

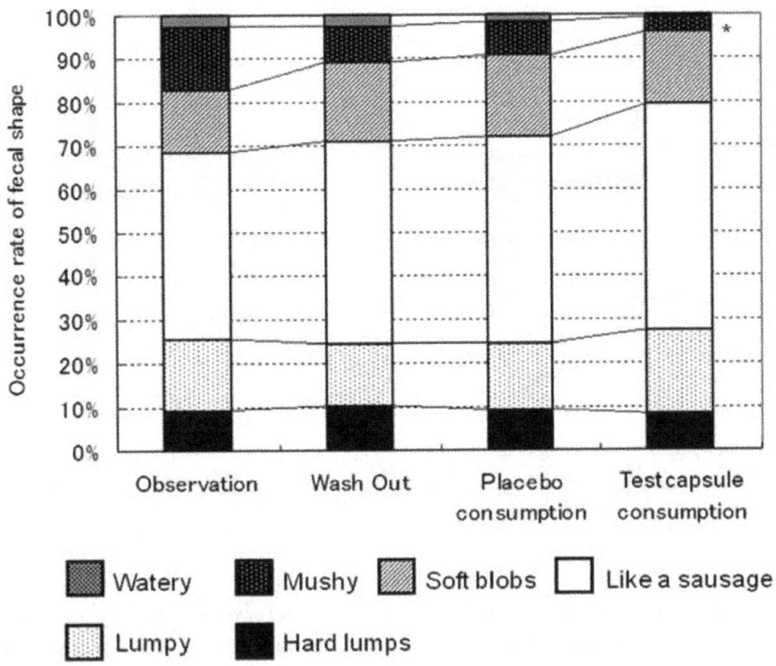

Figure 3 The frequencies of the appearance of various fecal shapes in each period. In the placebo consumption period, no significant difference was noted compared with the washout period, but the frequencies of watery and mushy feces were significantly lower in the test capsule consumption period compared with the pre-consumption observation period.

Intestinal microflora

The frequencies of the genera *Bifidobacterium* and *Clostridium* were assessed by T-RFLP analysis. As a result, we found that the frequency of the genus *Bifidobacterium* was significantly higher, and that of the genus *Clostridium* was significantly lower, after the test capsule consumption than after the placebo consumption (Figure 5). The frequencies of the genera *Lactobacillus (placebo : KB290 = 4.1% : 7.2%)*, *Bacteroides (placebo : KB290 = 33.8% : 34.3%)*, and *Enterobacter (placebo : KB290 = 8.4% : 5.8%)* were also investigated, but no significant differences in their frequencies were detected between the placebo and test capsule consumption periods.

Evaluation of QOL

The Japanese version of the Dartmouth COOP Chart indicates that the lower the score for a QOL item, the fewer problems there are with that item. Table 2 shows the scores for physical activity, emotional problems,

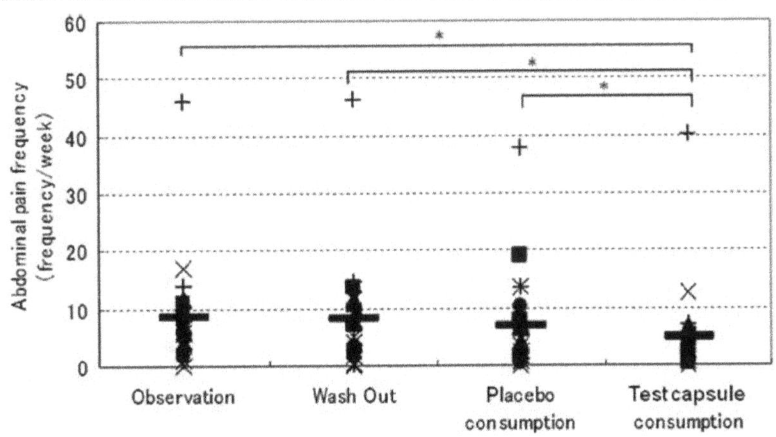

Figure 4 The frequency of abdominal pain in each period. The frequency of abdominal pain was significantly reduced in the test capsule consumption period compared with the other periods.

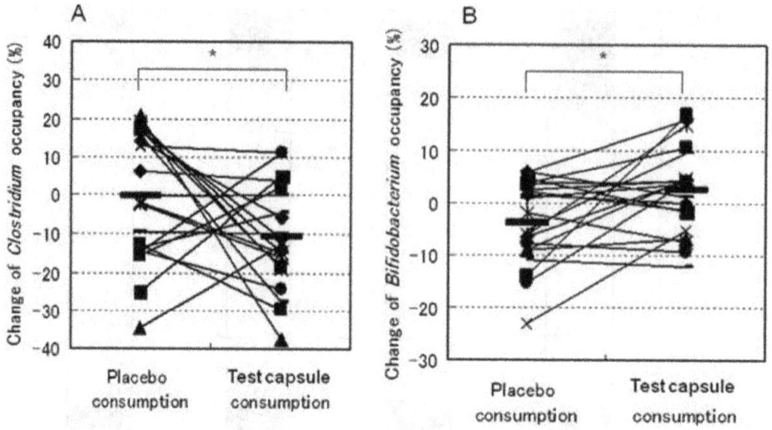

Figure 5 Intestinal microflora. Changes in the percentages of the genera Bifidobacterium and Clostridium were compared by T-RFLP analysis. As a result, the percentage of the genus Bifidobacterium was significantly higher, and that of the genus Clostridium was significantly lower, after test capsule consumption than after placeb consumption.

social activity, pain, and overall health state. While no significant difference was noted in any item among the periods, the mean score for all items was reduced in the test capsule consumption period.

Adverse events

According to the subjects' bowel movement diary entries and interview responses, no adverse events that were suspected to be related to the test capsule were observed during the study other than IBS symptoms, and no increase in the frequency of IBS symptoms such as abdominal pain or diarrhea was noted.

Discussion

We evaluated the effects of KB290 as a probiotic on IBS symptoms and intestinal microflora in IBS patient. As a result, we found that taking KB290 improved the QOL, significantly alleviated their abdominal pain and improved their fecal properties, and significantly changed the composition of their intestinal microflora.

Previous reports have suggested that some probiotics alleviate the symptoms of IBS patients and improve their QOL and the composition of their intestinal microflora [5-8]. The genera *Bifidobacterium* and *Lactobacillus,* and *Enterobacter* and *Clostridium,* have been reported to display lower and higher frequencies, respectively, among the microflora of IBS patients than among those of healthy individuals [17]. In the present study, we focused our analysis on the frequencies of the genera *Bifidobacterium* and *Clostridium,* which have been suggested to be related to IBS symptoms. Previous studies have shown that in healthy individuals with a tendency for constipation the frequencies of the genera *Bifidobacterium* and *Lactobacillus* increase and the frequency of the genus *Enterobacter* decreases after the consumption of KB290. In this study, not only did the frequency of the genus *Bifidobacterium* increase after KB290 intake, but that of the genus *Clostridium* also decreased. However, no increase in the frequency of the genus *Lactobacillus* or decrease in that of the genus *Enterococcus* was detected, probably because of the large inter-individual variations in human intestinal microflora. Human intestinal microflora have been shown to change with age and diet [18-20]. In this study, no dietary restrictions were imposed on the subjects, and this might have been related to the lack of change in the frequencies of these genera after the test capsule consumption.

It is very difficult to obtain a detailed overview of intestinal microflora. For example, studies of intestinal microflora composition almost exclusively rely on the quantitative culturing of microbes from fecal samples. However, recent nucleic acid studies have indicated that the majority of bacteria in a variety of ecosystems are different from those detected in culture [21]. Therefore, only part of the intestinal microflora of IBS patients can be examined by conventional techniques, and abnormalities in intestinal microbes that cause IBS might have been overlooked. Recently, the utility of molecular biological techniques such as RT-PCR analysis, denaturing

Table 2 The scores for physical activity

	Observation Period	Wash-out period	Consumption Period	
			Placebo	KB290
Physical	2.3 ± 0.9	2.5 ± 0.9	2.1 ± 0.9	2.0 ± 0.6
Emotional	2.5 ± 0.7	2.6 ± 0.9	2.5 ± 0.9	2.4 ± 0.7
Social Activities	2.3 ± 0.7	2.4 ± 0.8	2.1 ± 0.7	2.1 ± 0.7
Pain	2.8 ± 0.9	2.8 ± 1.1	2.6 ± 1.0	2.5 ± 0.9
Overall Health	3.0 ± 0.8	3.0 ± 0.8	2.9 ± 0.8	2.8 ± 0.8

Values are expressed as Means ± SD, n = 23.

gradient gel electrophoresis (DGGE), FISH, T-RFLP, and pyrosequencing for analyzing the 98% of intestinal microflora that have so far escaped analysis was evaluated, but no intestinal bacterium that can directly cause IBS has been identified [16,22-25]. In this study, the intestinal microflora were analyzed using the T-RFLP technique, a molecular biological method, but our analysis primarily focused on the genera *Bifidobacterium* and *Clostridium*. In the future, as analytical methods for intestinal microflora are developed, yielding a larger number of reports, intestinal bacterial species that are closely involved in the initiation and exacerbation of IBS might be identified.

A recent study suggested that the intestinal microflora plays an important role in brain-gut interactions [26]. Another report indicated that intestinal microflora affect the central nervous system [27], and changes in host behavior associated with changes in intestinal microflora have been observed in animal experiments [28]. Thus, based on recent findings regarding the functions of microbiota, the "microbiota - gut - brain axis" has been suggested as a new concept that describes the functional relationship that exists among microbiota, the gut, and the brain [29].

It was reported that intestinal inflammation is involved in the pathogenesis of IBS and that probiotics alleviate the symptoms of IBS by normalizing the balance of anti-inflammatory and proinflammatory cytokines. However, we could not determine whether KB290 affects cytokine expression in this study [30].

In this study, KB290 was shown to alleviate IBS symptoms and affect the frequencies of the genera *Bifidobacterium* and *Clostridium* among the constituents of the intestinal microflora, but the mechanism responsible for this could not be clarified. In the future, it will be necessary to more closely analyze the alterations in biomarker levels associated with the changes in intestinal microflora composition and symptom alleviation induced by KB290 intake and to clarify the changes KB290 causes in the composition of the intestinal microflora in greater detail. However, in consideration of the recently clarified role of intestinal microflora in the mechanisms of IBS symptom alleviation and the etiology of the disease, the intake of KB290, a probiotic, is considered to be able to contribute to symptomatic improvement in such patients.

Conclusions

Probiotics, the safety of which has been established, are used widely in various foods and can now be purchased readily. IBS has been reported to occur in children as young as 6, and its symptoms, such as abdominal pain, abdominal distension, and diarrhea, impair the QOL of IBS patients. In addition, as it takes a long time to cure IBS, early therapeutic intervention is important. The results of the present study suggest that KB290 is useful for early intervention in such patients.

Authors' contributions

KM, CH, YN designed the study and conception. KM, CH, NM, TT collected data. KM, YN analysed and interpreted the data. KM, CH prepared the manuscript, with input from KM and CH additionally all authors must approve the final version of the manuscript.

Author details

[1]Department of Pediatrics, Kinki University Sakai Hospital, 2-7-1 Harayamadai, Minami-ku, Sakai, Osaka 590-0132, Japan. [2]Department of Pediatrics, Minami Wakayama Medical Center, 27-1 Takinai-machi, Tanabe-shi, Wakayama 646-0015, Japan. [3]Probiotics Research Group, Nature-Wellness research Department, Research Institute, KAGOME Co., LTD. 17Nishitomiyama, Nasushiobara, Tochigi 329-2762, Japan. [4]Department of Pediatrics, Kinki University Faculty of Medicine, 377-2 ,Onohigashi, Osakasayama-shi, Osaka 589-8511, Japan.

References

1. Longstreth GF, Thompson WG, Chey WD, Houghton LA, Mearin F, Spiller RC: **Functional bowel disorders.** *Gastroenterology* 2006, **130**(5):1480–1491.
2. Naliboff BD, Munakata J, Fullerton S, Gracely RH, Kodner A, Harraf F, Mayer EA: **Evidence for two distinct perceptual alterations in irritable bowel syndrome.** *Gut* 1997, **41**(4):505–512.
3. Pimentel M, Chow EJ, Lin HC: **Eradication of small intestinal bacterial overgrowth reduces symptoms of irritable bowel syndrome.** *Am J Gastroenterol* 2000, **95**(12):3503–3506.
4. Spiller RC: **Postinfectious irritable bowel syndrome.** *Gastroenterology* 2003, **124**(6):1662–1671.
5. Aragon G, Graham DB, Borum M, Doman DB: **Probiotic therapy for Irritable Bowel Syndrome.** *Gastroenterology & Hepatology* 2010, **6**(1):39–44.
6. Bixquert Jimenez M: **Treatment of irritable bowel syndrome with probiotics. An etiopathogenic approach at last?** *Rev Esp Enferm Dig* 2009, **101**(8):553–564.
7. Lee BJ, Bak YT: **Irritable bowel syndrome, gut microbiota and probiotics.** *J Neurogastroenterol Motil* 2011, **17**(3):252–266.
8. Whorwell PJ, Altringer L, Morel J, Bond Y, Charbonneau D, O'Mahony L, Kiely B, Shanahan F, Quigley EM: **Efficacy of an encapsulated probiotic Bifidobacterium infantis 35624 in women with irritable bowel syndrome.** *Am J Gastroenterol* 2006, **101**(7):1581–1590.
9. Lui Y, Fatheree NY, Mangalat N, Rhoads JM: **Human-derived probiotic Lactobacillus reuteri strains differentially reduce intestinal inflammation.** *Am J Physiol Gastrointest Liver Physiol* 2010, **299**:G1087–G1096.
10. Nobuta Y, Inoue T, Suzuki S, Arakawa C, Yakabe T, Ogawa M, Yajima N: **The efficacy and the safety of Lactobacillus brevis KB290 as a human probiotics.** *Inter J Probio Prebio* 2009, **4**(4):263–270.
11. Fukao M, Tomita H, Yakabe T, Nomura T, Ike Y, Yajima N: **Assessment of antibiotic resistance in probiotic strain Lactobacillus brevis KB290.** *J Food Prot* 2009, **72**(9):1923–1929.
12. Yakabe T, Takashima H, Kuwagata M, Fukao M, Kikuchi S, Yajima N: **Teratogenicity and maternal effects of Lactobacillus brevis KB290 in rats and rabbits.** *Food Chem Toxicol* 2011, **49**(4):722–726.
13. Yakabe T, Moore EL, Yokota S, Sui H, Nobuta Y, Fukao M, Palmer H, Yajima N: **Safety assessment of Lactobacillus brevis KB290 as a probiotic strain.** *Food Chem Toxicol* 2009, **47**(10):2450–2453. Epub 2009 Jul 5.
14. Rome Foundation: **Guidelines–Rome III Diagnostic Criteria for Functional Gastrointestinal Disorders.** *J Gastrointestin Liver Dis* 2006, **15**(3):307–312.
15. Nagashima K, Hisada T, Sato M, Mochizuki J: **Application of new primer-enzyme combinations to terminal restriction fragment length polymorphism profiling of bacterial populations in human feces.** *Appl Environ Microbiol* 2003, **69**(2):1251–1262.
16. Hamanishi S, Sekine C, Chin G, Yamaue T, Kagaminori S: **Research on health indicators and QOL of children measured by nutrition, exercise,**

and rest: **QOL. Japanese version of COOP chart for infants.** *Shoni no Eiyo, Undo, Kyuyo kara mita Kenkodo Shihyo to QOL ni kansuru Kenkyu* 2004, :47–50.
17. Madden JA, Hunter JO: **A review of the role of the gut microflora in irritable bowel syndrome and the effects of probiotics.** *Br J Nutr* 2002, **88**(Suppl 1):S67–S72.
18. Mitsuoka T: **Cho-nai kin no sekai.** *Soubunsya* 1984, **1980**:15–20.
19. Midtvedt AC, Carlstedt-Duke B, Midtvedt T: **Establishment of a mucin-degrading intestinal microflora during the first two years of human life.** *J Pediatr Gastroenterol Nutr* 1994, **18**(3):321–326.
20. Hehemann JH, Correc G, Barbeyron T, Helbert W, Czjzek M, Michel G: **Transfer of carbohydrate-active enzymes from marine bacteria to Japanese gut microbiota.** *Nature* 2010, **464**(7290):908–912.
21. Erwin G, Zoetendal Chad T, Collier Satoshi K, Roderick I, Mackie H, Rex G: **Molecular Ecological Analysis of the Gastrointestinal Microbiota: A Review.** *J Nutr* 2004, **134**(2):465–472.
22. Handelsman J: **Metagenomics: application of genomics to uncultured microorganisms.** *Microbiol Mol Biol Rev* 2004, **68**(4):669–685.
23. Tannock GW: **Molecular methods for exploring the intestinal ecosystem.** *Br J Nutr* 2002, **87**(Suppl 2):S199–S201.
24. Apostolou E, Pelto L, Kirjavainen PV, Isolauri E, Salminen SJ, Gibson GR: **Differences in the gut bacterial flora of healthy and milk-hypersensitive adults, as measured by fluorescence in situ hybridization.** *FEMS Immunol Med Microbiol* 2001, **30**(3):217–221.
25. Rousselon N, Delgenès JP, Godon JJ: **A new real time PCR (TaqMan PCR) system for detection of the16S rDNA gene associated with fecal bacteria.** *J Microbiol Methods* 2004, **59**(1):15–22.
26. Diamond B, Huerta PT, Tracey K, Volpe BT: **It takes guts to grow a brain: Increasing evidence of the important role of the intestinal microflora in neuro- and immune-modulatory functions during development and adulthood.** *BioEssays* 2011, **33**(8):588–591.
27. Cryan JF, O'Mahony SM: **The microbiome-gut-brain axis: from bowel to behavior.** *Neurogastroenterol Motil* 2011, **23**(3):187–192.
28. Heijtz RD, Wang S, Anuar F, Qian Y, Björkholm B, Samuelsson A, Hibberd ML, Forssberg H, Pettersson S: **Normal gut microbiota modulates brain development and behavior.** *Proc Natl Acad Sci U S A* 2011, **108**(7):3047–3052.
29. Bercik P, Denou E, Collins J, Jackson W, Lu J, Jury J, Deng Y, Blennerhassett P, Macri J, McCoy KD, Verdu EF, Collins SM: **The intestinal microbiota affect central levels of brain-derived neurotropic factor and behavior in mice.** *Gastroenterology* 2011, **141**(2):599–609.
30. O'Mahony L, McCarthy J, Kelly P, Hurley G, Luo F, Chen K, O'Sullivan GC, Kiely B, Collins JK, Shanahan F, Quigley EM: **Lactobacillus and bifidobacterium in irritable bowel syndrome: symptom responses and relationship to cytokine profiles.** *Gastroenterology* 2005, **128**(3):541–551.

18

Evaluation of the Irritable Bowel Syndrome Quality of Life (IBS-QOL) questionnaire in diarrheal-predominant irritable bowel syndrome patients

David A Andrae[1*], Donald L Patrick[2], Douglas A Drossman[3] and Paul S Covington[1]

Abstract

Background: Diarrhea-predominant irritable bowel syndrome (IBS-d) significantly diminishes the health-related quality of life (HRQOL) of patients. Psychological and social impacts are common with many IBS-d patients reporting comorbid depression, anxiety, decreased intimacy, and lost working days. The Irritable Bowel Syndrome Quality of Life (IBS-QOL) questionnaire is a 34-item instrument developed and validated for measurement of HRQOL in non-subtyped IBS patients. The current paper assesses this previously-validated instrument employing data collected from 754 patients who participated in a randomized clinical trial of a novel treatment, eluxadoline, for IBS-d.

Methods: Psychometric methods common to HRQOL research were employed to evaluate the IBS-QOL. Many of the historical analyses of the IBS-QOL validations were used. Other techniques that extended the original methods were applied where more appropriate for the current dataset. In IBS-d patients, we analyzed the items and substructure of the IBS-QOL via item reduction, factor structure, internal consistency, reproducibility, construct validity, and ability to detect change.

Results: This study supports the IBS-QOL as a psychometrically valid measure. Factor analyses suggested that IBS-specific QOL as measured by the IBS-QOL is a unidimensional construct. Construct validity was further buttressed by significant correlations between IBS-QOL total scores and related measures of IBS-d severity including the historically-relevant Irritable Bowel Syndrome Adequate Relief (IBS-AR) item and the FDA's Clinical Responder definition. The IBS-QOL also showed a significant ability to detect change as evidenced by analysis of treatment effects. A minority of the items, unrelated to the IBS-d, performed less well by the standards set by the original authors.

Conclusions: We established that the IBS-QOL total score is a psychometrically valid measure of HRQOL in IBS-d patients enrolled in this study. Our analyses suggest that the IBS-QOL items demonstrate very good construct validity and ability to detect changes due to treatment effects. Furthermore, our analyses suggest that the IBS-QOL items measure a univariate construct and we believe further modeling of the IBS-QOL from an item response theory (IRT) approach under both non-treatment and treatment conditions would greatly further our understanding as item-based methods could be used to develop a short form.

Keywords: IBS-QOL, Patient-reported Outcomes, Psychometrics, HRQOL, Irritable Bowel Syndrome, Diarrhea, Eluxadoline

* Correspondence: David.Andrae@furiex.com
[1]Furiex Pharmaceuticals, Inc., 3900 Paramount Parkway, Suite 150, Morrisville, NC 27560, USA
Full list of author information is available at the end of the article

Background

Irritable bowel syndrome (IBS) affects an estimated 10-15% of people in western cultures [1]. It is characterized by recurrent abdominal pain and diarrhea [2] and can negatively impact health-related quality of life (HRQOL). IBS subtypes are defined by Rome III and include: diarrhea (IBS-d), constipation (IBS-c), or mixed constipation and diarrhea (IBS-m) [3]. Safe and effective pharmacologic treatments for IBS are limited, with current treatment options including antispasmodics, antidepressants, antidiarrheal agents, and alosetron [4]. Recently, clinical outcome results from a large Phase 2 clinical trial in IBS-d patients of a novel mixed mu-opioid (μ-OR) agonist, delta-opioid (δ-OR) antagonist, eluxadoline, were reported [5]. Additionally, HRQOL instruments were included in the study as secondary outcomes. By subjecting this larger data set to procedures outlined by previous publications [6,7] we plan to confirm the original psychometric validation analyses of the non-subtyped IBS-QOL. More specifically, we hope to assess how the IBS-QOL performs in strictly IBS-d patients.

Historical development and validation of the IBS-QOL

Patrick, et al., describe the steps utilized for item construction to ensure content validity of the IBS-QOL items [6,8] in which a combination of forty IBS-d, IBS-c, and IBS-m patients were interviewed resulting in identification of 117 potential items to describe these patients' IBS. Next, 30 additional patients underwent cognitive debriefing interviews which led to the retention of 45 items from the pool. After review by HRQOL and gastroenterology experts from Europe 41 items were found to be sufficiently content valid for use in the United States, Britain, Germany, Italy, and France. This pilot questionnaire was then mailed to 169 patients who: a) met Rome criteria for IBS, [9] b) were symptomatic at least 2 days/week, and c) were aged 18 to 65; 156 patients responded: 60% IBS-m, 22%, IBS-c, and 19% IBS-d.

Drossman, et al., extended the validation of the IBS-QOL by collecting questionnaires from 156 females with a functional bowel disorder [7]. These patients had moderate to severe symptoms ≥ 2 days/week over 3 months. Patients were assessed the two weeks prior to start of treatment and again after 12 weeks. For abdominal pain, visual analog reports were averaged over the two-week intervals from Week–2 to treatment start and Weeks 11-12.

Drossman, et al., [10] further investigated the IBS-QOL's ability to detect treatment changes. After utilizing pain and treatment satisfaction as anchors for interpreting IBS-QOL total scores from a sample of mostly female IBS patients, the authors concluded that a 14-point improvement in IBS-QOL scoring was clinically meaningful. In the current paper, we will examine the IBS-QOL total score improvement keeping the Drossman, et al., improvement of 14-points as a historical reference point.

Psychometric evaluations utilized in these studies included:

- Item reduction.
- Factor structure analysis employing principal components analysis (PCA) with orthogonal rotation using the varimax method.
- Internal consistency reliability assessed by Cronbach's Coefficient α.
- Reproducibility via comparing the overall IBS-QOL score at Baseline and one week later using the Intraclass Correlation Coefficient (ICC).
- Construct validity determined by correlational analyses for convergence and divergence of IBS-QOL scores with other clinical measures.
- Ability to detect change assessed by statistical comparison of change scores in the IBS-QOL in response to treatment.
- Comparisons among a priori determined responder groups to aid in the interpretation of the IBS-QOL changes in scores due to treatment effects.

Additional file 1 contains the final instrument of 34 items consisting of 8 subscale domains determined by the original work. Previous research has demonstrated that the IBS-QOL is internally consistent, highly reliable, has convergent and divergent validity, and acceptable responsiveness to treatment effects.

Methods

The goal of the current paper is to replicate the original IBS-QOL validation by using similar methodologies as previous efforts but with attention specifically to the IBS-d patient population [6,7]. Psychometric and statistical techniques were applied to 753 patients aged 18-65 years who completed the IBS-QOL at their Baseline visit. Between May 2010 and April 2011, 292 study centers obtained informed consent enrolled 807 patients into the study, with women representing approximately 70% of patients. A list of study investigators appears in Additional file 2. All patients all met the Rome III criteria for IBS-d [2], were compliant with their daily diary during the week prior to randomization, received at least one dose of double-blind study medication, and had at least one post-randomization diary entry. They also had to meet minimal requirements for presence of abdominal pain and stool consistency ratings. Patients were required to complete the electronic diary on 6 of the 7 required days during the week prior to randomization AND on 11 of the 14 required days during the 2 weeks prior to randomization. Patients who were compliant in completing the screening diary on a daily basis on 6 of the 7 required days during the week prior to randomization AND on 11 of the 14 required days during the 2 weeks prior to randomization, had an average of daily worst abdominal pain ratings of 3.0 or greater over the previous week, had a weekly mean Bristol Stool Score of 5.5 or greater over the previous week, and who had not used any rescue medication in the preceding 2 weeks were eligible for participation and immediate randomization into the double blind treatment phase. Conduct of the trial was overseen by Institutional Review Boards and complied with the Declaration of Helsinki. Patients in the trial completed the IBS-QOL, as well as other outcome measures, over 3 months while receiving either placebo or an active dose of eluxadoline (5, 25, 100, or 200 mg) twice daily [5]. HRQOL instruments included the IBS-QOL, Adequate Relief (IBS-AR), and IBS-Symptom Severity Score (IBS-SSS) [11]. These were collected periodically and Dove, et al., detail further the design and conduct of the trial. For the trial data, many of the psychometric assessments were applied to baseline data so that possible treatment effects did not confound the results. Other assessments were made in the presence of treatment effects and these are described below.

Assessments of pretreatment measurements

The potential for item reduction was assessed by applying the item-inclusion criteria from the original validation study [6]. Criteria were applied to the IBS-QOL instrument to see if differences exist between the current large IBS-d sample and the smaller, original, non-subtyped IBS validation sample. The criteria assessed included:

- 50% of patients responded "not at all" and therefore could not improve on the item
- 5% or more missing data
- an item-to-total correlation of <0.4 indicating that the item may be measuring a different latent construct
- pairwise correlations between individual items that exceeded 0.7 indicating redundancies in measurement.

The original factor structure of the IBS-QOL and possible alternative subscale structures were assessed. Several Confirmatory Factor Analysis (CFA) models were fit via maximum likelihood. Diagrams outlining the different conceptual models are included in Additional file 3: Figure S1. The first model corresponds to the original PCA and assumes orthogonal factors adequately measure independent subdomains of IBS-related QOL. The likelihood ratio χ^2, Akaike Information Criterion (AIC), and Schwartz's Bayesian Information Criterion (BIC) were used as indicators of model fit; smaller values are generally considered better. A second, hierarchical CFA was fit which imposed the original structure, but also assumes that the subscales themselves form a generalized factor, [12] presumably, the latent construct of HRQOL in IBS. Hierarchical factor analyses employ a two-step approach; the items are grouped into factors and then the factors are submitted to factor analysis. The third and fourth models fit were confirmatory bi-factor models [13]. The bi-factor approach was employed to refine the strictly hierarchical HRQOL conceptualizations as this method allows for a structure whereby subscales may explain variance not necessarily associated with the general QOL factor. Items were organized into 8 subscales and a general factor with each item having hypothesized relationships to one subscale and the general factor [14]. For example, Item 12 is hypothesized to load onto the Sexual subscale and also the general construct of HRQOL in IBS. The two bi-factor models included: one with orthogonal factors, i.e., in which the model does not allow factors to correlate with one another; and an oblique one in which correlations between factors are allowed. A single factor model in which all items load onto a single factor was also fit for reference to the other CFA models. Such a model imposes a structure in which all items load onto one general factor representing HRQOL in IBS.

Because CFA models involve fitting complex multivariate data, model fit is evaluated by inspecting several fit indices [15]. Numerous fit indices have been suggested, but minimally, a CFA model should be evaluated for fit based on a combination of different indices [16] as each assess different aspects of the model. Indices fit included:

- Goodness of Fit Index (GFI). An analogue to the R2 in regression where higher values are considered better. GFI values of 1.0 indicate perfect fit in that all observed variance is accounted for by the proposed model [17].
- Comparative Fit Index (CFI). This index assesses the amount of variance the model fits above and beyond a null model, i.e., one with no structure [17]. The CFI has a range of 0 to 1 and generally should be above 0.9 for good fit.
- Root Mean Square Error of Approximation (RMSEA). This index assesses the fit of the model according to a noncentral χ^2 distribution that is determined by the degrees of freedom of the model [17]. Values range from 0 to infinity with smaller values being better; less than 0.05 indicates excellent fit, greater than 0.1 indicates poor fit.

- Assessment of the model residuals was also done; good fit is indicated by values between−0.1 and 0.1.

To investigate possible misspecification of any CFA models, an Exploratory Factor Analysis (EFA) of the items was conducted to evaluate what structure would be suggested by the current data sample. EFA imposes no a priori structure to the data [12] and is similar to the approach taken by Patrick, et al. [6].

So-called internal consistency reliability was assessed by computing Coefficient α for the 34-item IBS-QOL total score as well as the Coefficient α-value for all (n-1) combinations, i.e., the so-called α-if-item-deleted, to gauge influence of single items. Values of α above 0.7 indicate a good level of consistency with values above 0.9 being considered excellent. Extremely high values can call into question whether scale items could be eliminated because of redundancy.

Assessments including postbaseline measurements

Consistency of the IBS-QOL total score over time is usually evaluated by correlating responses over repeated measurements. All administrations of the IBS-QOL post Baseline were in the presence of treatment, thus, a traditional ICC would be biased by treatment in the current case. To account for treatment effects and time trajectories on the IBS-QOL total score, reliability was assessed by first estimating variances via a linear model and utilizing the resultant conditional variances to establish reliability. Such an approach has been developed and described in two papers by Laenen, et al. [18,19]. Their reliability measures, R_Λ and R_T, utilize estimated variances from a linear model to calculate reliability over the set of repeated measurements, conditional on the covariates. Thus, in lieu of calculating an ICC, reproducibility was assessed via fitting longitudinal models to the repeated administrations of the IBS-QOL accounting for treatment effect over the treatment period. Details of the approaches are given in Additional file 4.

Construct validity of the IBS-QOL total score was assessed by evaluating it in relation to other clinical outcomes. For the IBS-SSS and EQ-5D, Pearson correlations at Baseline and Week 12 were calculated. Since the scale of the IBS-SSS is opposite to that of the IBS-QOL, a negative correlation between it and the IBS-QOL total score indicates convergence. A positive correlation with the EQ-5D indicates IBS-QOL converging with general HRQOL.

Further, change from Baseline to Week 12 in IBS-QOL total scores were correlated with similar changes from Baseline for IBS-SSS, EQ-5D, and average worst abdominal pain (WAP) [7]. The change score for the WAP variable was calculated as the average of WAP ratings for Weeks 11and12 compared to the average for the two weeks prior to dosing and the average of WAP for Week 12 compared to the average in the week prior to dosing.

Additionally, correlations between the IBS-QOL total score with the IBS-AR and FDA Clinical Responder status were calculated. The IBS-AR is a historically-used global measure of change used for assessing relief in IBS. A single item, "Over the past week have you had adequate relief of your IBS symptoms?" is administered to the patient and they respond either "Yes" or "No." Despite its established value as an endpoint measure for clinical trials dissatisfaction by regulatory agencies with the IBS-AR has led to the desire to develop quantifiable symptom based patient-reported outcome (PRO) measures for IBS [20]. Pending the development of a final IBS PRO, the FDA issued a guidance document in 2012 for drug development in IBS in which they formulated responder analysis definitions based on diary collection of pain and stool consistency ratings. One of the FDA Clinical Responder definitions from the Guidance, utilized by Dove, et al., is also used in the current paper as an additional criterion for assessing the validity of the IBS-QOL total score [5]. The definition is based on a percentage of days a patient has a simultaneous improvement in both pain and stool consistency on the same day—the so-called daily responder definition [21]. Since these outcomes are measured on a dichotomous scale two different biserial correlation approaches were calculated to account for non-continuous variables [22,23]. See Additional file 5 for a full description of the approaches.

The IBS-QOL was previously assessed for responsiveness [7] using Cohen's d statistic [24]. In that analysis, effect sizes for the change in scores from pre-treatment to post-treatment were computed similarly to standardize mean differences by putting changes in scores into standard deviation units. The d statistic originally employed a standard deviation value that was either based on the Baseline pooled data or on the control group only. Both of these methods inherently assume homogeneity of variance, either across time points or across treatment groups. To account for potential heterogeneity of variance across treatment groups and also handle data dependencies due to repeated patient measurements an additional assessment was calculated by estimating a longitudinal model for the change in IBS-QOL total score between Baseline and Week 12 administrations. To visually assess the IBS-QOL total score, the cumulative proportion of patients meeting a certain change from Baseline to Week 12 was also plotted by treatment group and the proportion of patients meeting certain thresholds of improvement for Placebo and Eluxadoline 100 mg treatment groups were compared.

Statistical analyses were performed with R version 3.0, [25] R-package ltm, [26] and SAS® software version 9.3 [27].

Trial registration: ClinicalTrials.gov identifier NCT01130272.

Results

Of the 754 patients included for analysis, 526 were female and 646 were Caucasian. The mean (standard deviation) age was 44.8 (11.93) with Baseline IBS-QOL total scores averaging 53.2 (21.09).

Assessments of pretreatment measurements

For Baseline data, Table 1 displays items that warrant further investigation as they did not meet the original qualitative criteria for inclusion. Of note, while several items displayed relatively high inter-item correlations, two items, 32 and 33, had a majority of patients respond with the, "not at all" category. Item 29, notably, had the opposite problem where many patients responded with the highest category, "a great deal." While not restrictive in the sense that patients cannot improve on this item, such a skewed distribution could cause problems with other items when scoring or modeling is conducted. Such results are also indicative that either a reduced response set is adequate. For example, in our dataset 46.4% patients reported "not at all" for Item 33 ("My bowel problems are affecting my closest relationships"), so simply providing a "yes" versus "no" response set to this item may be adequate for IBS-d patients. Alternatively, the items may not be helpful in measuring the latent construct of interest in IBS-d patients.

Table 2 displays the various fit statistics for the CFA models. Moderately good CFA fits were observed with the exception of the single factor model. In general, models should demonstrate GFI values similar to R^2 in regression and trending above 0.85 or so and CFI—an index that compares the fitted model to a null base model—should be above 0.9. For both these indices, larger values are better. Also, findings from the RMSEA, where smaller values are better, suggest moderately-good fits since results fall between 0.05 and 0.1. Additionally, Table 2 presents both the average residual size and the percentage of residual values that fall outside of the (−0.1, 0.1) interval.

As with the CFA models, the EFA model was fitted for Baseline values of the IBS-QOL. The goal of the EFA was to elucidate any moderate fit of the CFAs to the data. The factor pattern loadings for the EFA solutions are compared with the subscales in Table 3; three of eight original subscales correspond one-to-one with the substructures of the data, i.e., "Body Image", "Food Avoidance", and "Sexual"; the other five factors only approximately fit the original substructure. The most notable departure is with Factor 1, which is a mixture of items from the "Social Reaction", "Relationship", and sporadic items from other subscales.

Coefficient α analysis of the IBS-QOL total score demonstrated a high level of reliability between items of the IBS-QOL [$\alpha = 0.963$, 95% confidence interval (0.959, 0.966)]. Additional file 6: Table S1 lists the full α item analysis. All but Item 32 ("I fear I won't be able to have a bowel Movement") had item-to-total correlations above 0.5. The α-value with Item 32 included is still extraordinarily high without deleting this item, however. In fact, deleting any one item does not reduce the Coefficient α-value by more than

Table 1 Potentially problematic items according to criteria in Patrick, et al. [6]

Item	Reason(s) why item is problematic
6. I feel like I'm losing control of my life because of my bowel problems.	• High item-to-item correlation: $r_{6,7} = 0.732$
	• High item-to-item correlation: $r_{6,10} = 0.702$
7. I feel my life is less enjoyable because of my bowel problems.	• High item-to-item correlation: $r_{7,6} = 0.732$
9. I feel depressed about my bowel problems.	• High item-to-item correlation: $r_{9,10} = 0.707$
10. I feel isolated form others because of my bowel problems.	• High item-to-item correlation: $r_{10,6} = 0.732$
	• High item-to-item correlation: $r_{10,9} = 0.707$
12. Because of my bowel problems, sexual activity is difficult for me.	• High item-to-item correlation: $r_{12,20} = 0.741$
20. My bowel problems reduce my sexual desire.	• High item-to-item correlation: $r_{20,12} = 0.741$
29. It is important to be near a toilet because of my bowel problems.	• High item-to-item correlation: $r_{29,30} = 0.708$
	• Potential ceiling effect: 38.9% of patients reporting, "a great deal"
30. My life revolves around my bowel problems.	• High item-to-item correlation: $r_{30,29} = 0.708$
32. I fear I won't be able to have a bowel movement.	• Floor effect: 72.8% of patients reporting "not at all"
	• Low item-total correlation: $r_{32,Total} = 0.292$
33. My bowel problems are affecting my closest relationships	• Potential floor effect: 46.4% of patients reporting "not at all"

Table 2 Comparison of confirmatory factor model fit statistics

Statistic	Subscales only	Hierarchical	Orthogonal Bi-factor	Oblique Bi-factor	Single factor
χ^2	2441.1	2616.9	2254.9	1923.3	3755.9
(df)	(499)	(519)	(496)	(468)	(527)
AIC	2633.1	2768.9	2452.9	2193.3	3891.9
BIC	3075.7	3119.4	2909.3	2815.7	4205.5
GFI	0.8232	0.8088	0.8346	0.8616	0.7378
CFI	0.877	0.8671	0.8889	0.9073	0.7955
RMSEA	0.072	0.074	0.069	0.066	0.091
(95% CI)	(0.070, 0.075)	(0.071, 0.077)	(0.066, 0.072)	(0.063, 0.069)	(0.089, 0.094)
Average Residual	0.0588	0.062	0.053	0.0448	0.0632
% of Residuals ≥ 0.1 or ≤ −0.1	18.7%	21.2%	16.0%	10.5%	20.0%

Note: χ^2 = Likelihood ratio χ^2; df = χ^2 degrees of freedom; AIC = Akaike's Information Criterion (smaller is better); BIC = Schwartz's Bayesian Information Criterion (smaller is better); GFI = Goodness-of-Fit Index (Acceptable fit > 0.9); CFI = Bentler's Comparative Fit Index (Good fit > 0.9); RMSEA = root-mean-square error of approximation (Very good fit <0.05;Moderate fit between 0.05 and 0.1); CI = confidence interval.

0.003. Further, the average item-to-total correlation was r = 0.642, indicating a high consistency between item responses.

Assessments including postbaseline measurements

The longitudinal model showed that both R_Λ and R_T had very good reliability for the data with $R_\Lambda = 0.89$ and $R_T = 0.76$. By comparison, Patrick, et al., reported an ICC between administrations of 0.86. This indicates the stability of IBS-QOL total scores when treatment and time effects are taken into account as well as consistency with previous assessment.

Correlations between IBS-QOL total score and change scores for IBS-SSS, EQ-5D, 14-day WAP, the 7-day WAP, IBS-AR, and the FDA Clinical Responder values are presented in Table 4. All correlations show statistical significance. Several show moderate to strong linear relationships ($r \geq 0.40$) between other variables and the IBS-QOL total score. Further, all correlations were in the correct direction given the scales of measurement of the variables.

Table 5 displays the analyses of treatment effects detected by the IBS-QOL. Similar patterns of discrimination are observed whether calculations were conducted on the observed changes from baseline or estimated via longitudinal modeling. Additionally, effect sizes based on the pooled standard deviation between groups evaluated for the standard deviation of the Placebo group at Baseline revealed the same pattern with effect size estimates being of similar magnitude. The attenuation of effect sizes relative to Placebo was expected as the standard deviation of the Placebo group at Baseline is expected to be larger. Further, the larger disparity observed in the longitudinal model between pooled- and placebo-based effect size estimates was also expected as the estimate for the pooled standard deviation in the longitudinal model takes repeated measurement information into account.

Figure 1 displays the cumulative proportion of patients meeting a certain change from Baseline by treatment group. Consistent with previous results [5] the higher dose groups demonstrated better improvements in IBS-

Table 3 Comparison between original subscale structure and data-suggested structure

	EFA Model with Varimax Rotation (Eigenvalues)					
Original subscale	**Factor 1**	**Factor 2**	**Factor 3**	**Factor 4**	**Factor 5**	**Factor 6**
	(37.8)	**(3.20)**	**(2.48)**	**(1.76)**	**(1.46)**	**(1.24)**
Dysphoria	13, 16	1, 6, 7, 9, 10	30			
Interference with activity		18	3, 27, 29, 31	22	19	
Body image				5, 21, 25, 26		
Health worry	32			4	15	
Food avoidance					11, 23, 28	
Social reaction	14, 17, 34			2		
Sexual						12, 20
Relationship	8, 24, 33					

Note: Eigenvalues for the extracted factors are in parentheses and higher values represent higher amounts of the variance observed in the data captured by a given factor.

Table 4 Partial correlations between IBS-QOL total score and other clinical measures—controlling for dose level

Variable	Time point	N	Correlation type	Correlation value	p-Value
IBS-SSS	Week 12	427	Pearson	−0.604	<0.0001
	Change from Baseline	383	Pearson	−0.629	<0.0001
EQ-5D	Week 12	694	Pearson	0.581	<0.0001
	Change from Baseline	690	Pearson	0.404	<0.0001
Pain/14-Day	Week 12	550	Pearson	−0.392	<0.0001
	Change from Baseline	549	Pearson	−0.350	<0.0001
Pain/7-Day	Week 12	536	Pearson	−0.397	<0.0001
	Change from Baseline	535	Pearson	−0.357	<0.0001
IBS-AR	Week 12	693	Point Biserial	0.379	<0.0001
			(t-Test)	(10.788)	
			Biserial	0.483	<0.0001
			(t-Test)	(14.523)	
FDA clinical responder definition	Week 12	694	Point Biserial	0.282	<0.0001
			(t-Test)	(7.750)	
			Biserial	0.395	<0.0001
			(t-Test)	(11.316)	

Note: Point biserial and biserial correlation coefficients are evaluated via constructing a t-test.

QOL total score. Table 6 further elucidates the discrimination between Placebo and Eluxadoline 100 mg treatment groups. For this pairwise comparison, higher proportions of Eluxadoline-treated patients were observed for a wide range of improvement levels. Over 80% of placebo patients and over 90% of patients treated with Eluxadoline 100 mg had the same score or higher at Week 12 as compared to Baseline. Furthermore, this approximate 10% difference between these two treatment groups persisted or increased if the criterion was raised all the way up to 30 points of improvement. Interestingly, the 14-point clinically meaningful difference [10] was met by 48% of the placebo patients and over 65% of eluxadoline 100 mg patients and the maximum group difference was observed for a 22 point improvement in which over 25% of placebo patients and over 47% of eluxadoline 100 mg patients responded, respectively, for a group difference of 21.5%.

Discussion

The goal of the current paper was to replicate and expand on the original psychometric assessment of the IBS-QOL when applied to an IBS-d-specific patient set. Our results indicate that male and female IBS-d patients who are highly compliant with daily diary entry and who

Table 5 Analysis of IBS-QOL Responsiveness

	Treatment group	n	Mean change from baseline	Mean difference from placebo	t-Value	Degrees of freedom	p-Value	Effect sizes	
								d_{Pooled}	$d_{Placebo}$
IBS-QOL total score, Observed Data(a)	5 mg	66	19.73	2.02	0.64	189	0.522	0.09	0.09
	25 mg	135	18.75	1.04	0.43	258	0.664	0.05	0.05
	100 mg	130	25.25	7.54	3.10	253	0.002	0.39	0.33
	200 mg	107	25.06	7.35	2.68	230	0.008	0.35	0.32
	Placebo	125	17.70						
IBS-QOL total score, Longitudinal Model(b)	5 mg	105	19.33	2.00	1.09	262	0.279	0.13	0.09
	25 mg	167	18.46	1.13	0.67	324	0.507	0.07	0.05
	100 mg	163	24.53	7.20	4.20	320	<.001	0.47	0.31
	200 mg	160	23.33	6.00	3.64	317	<.001	0.41	0.26
	Placebo	159	17.33						

Note: (a) Effect size estimates based on observed standard deviations (s_{Pooled}, $s_{Placebo}$) (b) Effect size estimates based on estimated standard deviations from a mixed-effects model for IBS-QOL total score with fixed effects of treatment, time, treatment by time interaction, and Baseline IBS-QOL total score and random effects for intercept and time ($\hat{\sigma}_{Pooled}$, $\hat{\sigma}_{Placebo}$).

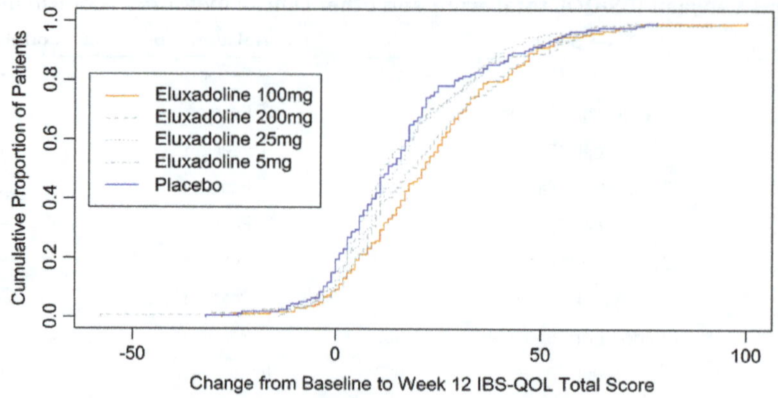

Figure 1 Cumulative proportions of patients meeting a certain change from Baseline to Week 12 in IBS-QOL total scores plotted by treatment group.

have a minimal requirement for pain as well as explicit criteria for diarrhea as defined by the BSS share commonalities with a general population of non-subtyped IBS patients, but that the originally-proposed subscale structure doesn't apply as well as one might anticipate to our patient set. The deviations observed from the original assessment could be attributed to the fact that we evaluated IBS-d patients or due to the much larger sample size employed here. Without such large-scale data on other IBS subtypes, it is difficult to discern the cause of the departures from the original analyses, but in the case that one or both differences are influencing the current results, it is still clear that the IBS-QOL performs well for IBS-d patients.

The item reduction criteria applied to the 34-item version of the IBS-QOL resulted in many items having high bivariate correlations, as defined as $r \geq 0.7$. A possible factor influencing the high correlations between items could be due to priming or order effects, i.e., responses on subsequent items being influenced by earlier-answered items. As the IBS-QOL is a static instrument with only one item order presented to patients, however, testing whether priming influences responses by patients to single items is not possible.

Alternatively, high correlations between items could suggest that the items are measuring a single latent trait. Items 6 ("I feel like I'm losing control of my life because of my bowel problems"), 7 ("I feel my life is less enjoyable because of my bowel problems"), 9 ("I feel depressed about my bowel problems"), and 10 ("I feel isolated from others because of my bowel problems") all showed a fairly high level of correlation with one another. The α-value for the overall sum scale of the IBS-QOL is also very high, suggesting redundancies across these items.

Similarly, Items 12 ("Because of my bowel problems, sexual activity is difficult for me") and 20 ("My bowel problems reduce my sexual desire") exhibited a high correlation with one another ($r = 0.741$) as expected. Both items make up the Sexual subscale and while the language of the two items respectively imply physical and psychological aspects of sexual activity, patient responses tended to suggest that one does not occur without the other.

There were several other pairs of items that exhibited high inter-item correlation values (cf., Table 1). Our results suggest that a possible future research path for the IBS-QOL is to explore whether a shortened version of the IBS-QOL targeted toward IBS-d could be constructed from the current items while maintaining its measurement properties and still being relevant to IBS-d patients. If items have redundancy, then one could

Table 6 Percentages of patients meeting different levels of IBS-QOL total score improvement

Improvement from baseline to Week 12	Placebo	Eluxadoline 100 mg	Difference between treatment groups
0	80.3%	90.6%	10.30%
5	70.4%	80.5%	10.11%
10	57.9%	74.2%	16.32%
15	46.1%	62.9%	16.84%
20	32.2%	52.8%	20.59%
25	21.7%	41.5%	19.80%
30	19.1%	30.8%	11.74%

conceive of an item pool that supplies items to each of slightly different versions of the IBS-QOL. Alternatively, specific cognitive debriefing may also help isolate whether any of these items are truly redundant or if items all closely measure HRQOL in IBS-d and simply represent very closely related aspects of IBS-d-related QOL.

Conversely, in IBS-d patients, a departure from the original validation analyses was not surprising either. For example, 72.8% IBS-d patients answered "Not at all" to Item 32 ("I fear I won't be able to have a bowel movement") at Baseline. This result fits, conceptually, with how patients should answer items that are not geared toward their IBS subset. This item, therefore, could be taken out of a targeted IBS-d instrument or, perhaps, could simply be included with a binary, "yes" versus "no", response instead of the 5-point graded response set.

While some of the results suggested that certain items in the IBS-QOL may be candidates to remove if a reduced-item version were to be sought for IBS-d patients, other results support that the full set of items is relevant and psychometrically sound, consistent with conclusions of previous validation studies of the IBS-QOL. This result is not surprising given the extremely high value of Cronbach's Coefficient α ($\alpha = 0.963$). This is consistent with the interpretation of the bi-factor and EFA models because the common interpretation of Coefficient α analyses is that the items are internally consistent and therefore represent a unidimensional latent construct.

This conclusion is reinforced by a high observed average item-to-total correlation of 0.642. However, one of the limitations here is that modern applications of α analysis stretch interpretation of the statistic beyond its original intent [28]. Coefficient α was intended to substitute alternate forms reliability—in which two equivalent forms of the instrument were to be administered and the results correlated with one another. As most instrument developers do not have the resources to develop two instruments together, Coefficient α was devised as a means of assessing agreement between an instrument and a theoretical one of same length, comprised of items randomly drawn from all possible content valid items. The coefficient, therefore, is laden with assumptions and also is, ostensibly, a lower bound for the theoretical true internal consistency of a measure. Many have criticized the use of α for this and other reasons [29-31]. Further, while an α assessment assumes sum of item responses, the IBS-QOL standardizes responses to a 0-100 scale, so without further study, it is not clear how the scoring algorithm relates back to a simple sum score. Structural equation modeling techniques, e.g., extensions of the CFA models, actually offer the best alternatives to α and other individual indices as they are better equipped to handle multivariate item data [32,33]. However, any positive or negative bias around the α-value of 0.96 would likely still yield acceptable levels of consistency.

In terms of how the items structurally relate to one another at the instrument level, the fact that the oblique bi-factor model fits the data the best, and better than the orthogonal bi-factor model, suggests that the original factor structure is redundant to the total sum score because factors that are allowed to be correlated fit better with the data than hypothetically independent subscales. We do note, however, that more complex CFA models tended to fit better by both standard fit indexes and usual assessment of residuals and that, generally, increasing model complexity provides better fit in most statistical models. While the oblique bi-factor model accounted for a marginal amount of variance (GFI = 0.8616), an acceptable improvement in variance above a null model (CFI = 0.9073) was observed. The RMSEA index imposes a penalty for higher complexity models, thereby allowing us to infer whether the bi-factor models fit better according to other indices based on their complexity. The observed RMSEA value of 0.069, although moderate in size, comparatively supports the oblique bi-factor conceptualization of IBS-d, i.e., that the best of all CFA models fit is on with an overall latent factor supported by the original substructure whilst allowing the substructure factors to correlate with one another. The model fit may have room for improvement as 10.5% of residuals are outside of the preferred limits potentially indicating that some items may not fit well within the proposed structure.

The EFA model supports that there may be pairs or subsets of items of the IBS-QOL that group together more so than with others—an observation that is not surprising given the observed inter-correlations between items. Interestingly, though, the EFA fit did not produce a factor structure in line with the original substructure, suggesting that HRQOL may be qualitatively different for IBS-d as compared to non-subtyped IBS patients as a whole.

Despite the extraction of multiple factors from the analysis, the EFA fit actually further strengthens the interpretation that the IBS-QOL is unidimensional in IBS-d patients. This is because the EFA model has a large first eigenvalue (37.8) as compared to the second (3.8). Eigenvalues of extracted factors measure the amount of variance observed in the items making up that factor. Here the first extracted factor accounts for 79.5% of the total variance in the items. Further, a test of whether the items suggest a structure in which there is at least one common factor to all items was also significant [$\chi^2(561) = 16{,}080.2$, $p < 0.0001$] implying that any structure extracted after that first factor is residual information that could enhance interpretation of the first factor, but one factor would be adequate to interpret the construct under study. This observation indicates that imposing the original factor structure [6] is helping model fit, implying that the original subscale structure of the IBS-QOL seems to be beneficial in accounting for information above and beyond the total sum score. Furthermore, combined with the fit of the orthogonal bi-factor model results, one could conclude for IBS-d patients that the IBS-QOL may be measuring a unidimensional construct, both because of the need to allow factors to correlate and that the original substructure seems only approximately correct.

The CFA and EFA modeling, taken together, suggest that perhaps the best means of assessing the psychometric properties of the IBS-QOL would be to employ Item Response Theory (IRT) methods [34]. IRT approaches estimate a latent construct via a joint model of the individual items. IRT models can also help determine if individual items are performing as intended within the IBS-QOL because relationships between items and the latent trait under study are estimated, directly.

In terms of test-retest reliability, the current analyses demonstrated good levels for the IBS-QOL total score in this regard. Both R_Λ and R_T exceed the traditionally-accepted reliability threshold of around 0.7 and were comparable to the ICC calculated by the original validation study. Both reliability measures employed here are similar to ICCs with slightly different interpretations. R_Λ is the multivariate reliability of the sequence of scores while R_T is the average reliability for the total score over any arbitrary number of administrations. Both will tend to increase for a consistent instrument with more administrations because additional information is being taken into account with each added administration. Therefore, with 3 post-Baseline administrations of the IBS-QOL, we have substantial evidence for good reliability of the total score. Contrastingly, even with less information, e.g., two administrations of the IBS-QOL, we would expect that a reliability level would still be approximately 0.75 by our estimates.

The analysis of IBS-QOL total scores with regard to responsiveness were consistent across effect size definitions for different paired comparisons, with moderate increases in effect sizes seen for higher doses of eluxadoline versus placebo. Interestingly, the pattern of effect size estimates suggest that the 100 mg dose of eluxadoline had the largest impact, the same conclusion as was reached by the analysis of clinical measures [5] as defined in FDA's 2012 IBS Guidance [21]. This conclusion is bolstered by evaluating the cumulative proportions of change from Baseline to Week 12 scores for the IBS-QOL total score with better improvements seen at higher dose levels, specifically 100 and 200 mg. We especially note that within a wide range of improvement levels, the proportion of patients in the eluxadoline 100 mg group meeting given improvements was dramatically higher than those patients receiving placebo. This indicates that the observed treatment effect in the IBS-QOL total score is consistent. Visually, this result is apparent by the wide gap between the placebo and 100 mg eluxadoline lines on Figure 1.

Of note, all treatment groups showed large increases in IBS-QOL total scores at Week 12 as compared to Baseline. Even the Placebo group showed an approximately 17-point increase in total score—higher than the 14-point clinically-significant difference found by Drossman, et al [10]. While further longitudinal study is warranted, we believe that the improvement may be due to natural cycling of disease or due to potential Hawthorne effects, ie, improvements by patients as a result of simply being observed. We do, however, also note that the treatment group differences approximate a dose response that peaks at 100 mg and plateaus with 200 mg. This pattern mimics that of the other outcome measures reported elsewhere [5].

Our analyses suggest that a reduced-form IBS-QOL specific for IBS-d sufferers may improve measurement of IBS-related QOL for these patients. However, further research is necessary to determine which of the items may be ideally suited for a reduced form. We suggest that a better characterization of item-level properties of the IBS-QOL via IRT methodology would be helpful in determining an optimal item configuration.

Conclusions

Much of the original development and validation work on the IBS-QOL items were replicated in the current paper. However, some items do not appear perform ideally for IBS-d patients, either individually or with one another, and a reduced-item set for the IBS-QOL may produce better overall measurement of the IBS-d condition. Despite some indications of improvements that could be made, the current 34-item instrument does work in IBS-d patients; it performs well on the classical set of psychometric assessments and is demonstrated to be: Approximately unidimensional as evidenced by the high first eigenvalue extracted from the EFA model as well as the high Coefficient α value observed among the items; reliable as evidenced by the consistently high R_Λ and R_T values; and correlated with other measures of IBS-d symptoms and outcomes—both new, like the FDA Clinical Responders, and old, i.e., IBS-AR. Combined with good ability to detect change, evidenced by moderately high effect sizes in changes from Baseline to Week 12 and good discrimination of the 100 mg dose versus placebo over a wide range of improvement levels—cf. Figure 1—we believe that the IBS-QOL total score is a psychometrically valid means of assessing QOL in IBS-d patients.

There are indications that the individual items do contain more information than what is expressed in a sum or scaled total score. Thus, directly relating items to the latent construct of IBS-d-specific QOL via IRT modeling should be considered for future research on the IBS-QOL to determine if there are untapped measurement properties within the items. Taken together, the current results suggest the IBS-QOL is a psychometrically sound instrument for patients with diarrhea predominant IBS and the total score is a good, unified measure of HRQOL. Importantly, all of the results together suggest that the IBS-QOL appears to detect the core concepts of IBS-d as well as changes in the disease state. Further, the relatively high observed correlations between the IBS-QOL and other established efficacy measures reinforces the conclusion that the IBS-QOL is not only a reliable, but also a valid and sensitive measure of patients' IBS-d experiences.

Abbreviations

AIC: Akaike Information Criterion; BIC: Bayesian Information Criterion; CFA: Confirmatory factor analysis; CFI: Comparative Fit Index; DF: Degrees of freedom; δ-OR: Delta opioid receptor; EFA: Exploratory factor analysis; FDA: Food and Drug Administration; GFI: Goodness of Fit Index; HRQOL: Health-related quality of life; ICC: Intraclass correlation; IBS: Irritable bowel syndrome; IBS-AR: Irritable Bowel Syndrome Adequate Relief; IBS-c: Irritable bowel syndrome—constipation subtype; IBS-d: Irritable bowel syndrome—diarrheal subtype; IBS-m: Irritable bowel syndrome—mixed subtype; IBS-QOL: Irritable Bowel Syndrome Quality of Life questionnaire; IBS-SSS: Irritable Bowel Syndrome Symptom Severity Score; IRT: Item response theory; μ-OR: Mu opioid receptor; PCA: Principal components analysis; RMSEA: Root mean squared error of approximation; WAP: Worst abdominal pain.

Authors' contributions

DAA contributed to the trial design, conceived the analysis strategy, analyzed the data, and drafted the manuscript. DLP and DAD aided in interpretation of the data and provided critical input to the manuscript development. PSC helped design the clinical trial from which the data were generated, edited and gave significant commentary to the content, and aided in drafting the manuscript. All authors read and approved the final manuscript.

Acknowledgements

The authors would like to thank Randi Gress for administrative support in the production of the manuscript as well as the constructive comments from two anonymous referees.

Author details

[1]Furiex Pharmaceuticals, Inc., 3900 Paramount Parkway, Suite 150, Morrisville, NC 27560, USA. [2]Department of Health Services, University of Washington School of Public Health, Seattle, WA, USA. [3]Drossman Center for the Education and Practice of Biopsychosocial Care LLC, and UNC Center for Functional GI and Motility Disorders, Chapel Hill, NC, USA.

References

1. Lovell R, Ford A: **Global prevalence of and risk factors for irritable bowel syndrome: a meta-analysis.** *Clin Gastroenterol Hepatol* 2012, **10:**712–721.
2. Drossman D: **The functional gastrointestinal disorders and the Rome III process.** *Gastroenterol* 2006, **130:**1377–1390.
3. Drossman D: *Rome III The Functional GI Disorders.* 3rd edition. Lawrence, KS: Allen Press, Inc; 2006.
4. Brandt L, Chey W, Foxx-Orenstein A: **An evidence-based position statement on the management of irritable bowel syndrome.** *Am J Gastroenterol* 2009, **104:**1–35.
5. Dove L, Lembo A, Randall C, Fogel R, Andrae D, Davenport J, McIntyre G, Almenoff J, Covington P: **Eluxadoline benefits patients with irritable bowel syndrome with diarrhea in a phase 2 study.** *Gastroenterology* 2013, **145:**329–338.
6. Patrick D, Drossman D, Frederick I, Dicesare J, Puder K: **Quality of life in persons with irritable bowel syndrome: development and validation of a new measure.** *Dig Dis Sci* 1998, **43:**400–411.
7. Drossman D, Patrick D, Whitehead W, Toner B, Diamant N, Hu Y, Jia H, Bangdiwala S: **Further validation of the IBS-QOL: a disease-specific quality-of-life questionnaire.** *Am J Gastroenterol* 2000, **95:**999–1007.
8. Patrick D, Erickson P: *Health Status and Health Policy: Allocating Resources to Health Care.* New York, NY: Oxford University Press; 1993.
9. Thompson W, Creed F, Drossman D, Heaton K, Mazzacca G: **Functional bowel disorders and functional abdominal pain.** *Gastroenterol Int* 1992, **5:**75–91.
10. Drossman D, Morris CB, Hu Y, Toner BB, Diamant N, Whitehead WE, Dalton CB, Leserman J, Patrick DL, Bangdiwala SI: **Characterization of health related quality of life (HRQOL) for patients with functional bowel disorder (FBD) and its response to treatment.** *Am J Gastroenterol* 2007, **102:**1442–1453.
11. Francis C, Morris J, Whorwell P: **The irritable bowel severity scoring system: a simple method of monitoring irritable bowel syndrome and its progress.** *Aliment Pharmacol Ther* 1997, **11:**395–402.
12. Gorsuch R: *Factor Analysis.* Hillsdale, NJ: Lawrence Earlbaum Associates, Inc; 1983.
13. Holzinger K, Swineford F: **The Bi-factor method.** *Psychometrika* 1937, **2:**41–54.
14. Swineford F: **Some comparisons of the multiple-factor and the bi-factor methods of analysis.** *Psychometrika* 1941, **6:**375–382.
15. Kline R: *Principles and Practice of Structural Equation Modeling.* New York, NY: The Guilford Press; 1998.
16. Schreiber J, Nora A, Stage F, Barlow E, King J: **Reporting structural equation modeling and confirmatory factor analysis results: a review.** *J Educ Res* 2006, **99:**323–338.
17. Bollen K, Curran P: *Latent Curve Models: A Structural Equation Perspective.* Hoboken, NJ: John Wiley & Sons; 2006.
18. Laenen A, Alonso A, Molenberghs G: **A: measure for the reliability of a rating scale based on longitudinal clinical trial data.** *Psychometrika* 2007, **72:**443–448.
19. Laenen A, Alonso A, Molenberghs G, Vangeneugden T: **Reliability of a longitudinal sequence of scale ratings.** *Psychometrika* 2009, **74:**49–64.
20. Spiegel B, Camilleri M, Bolus R, Andresen V, Chey WD, Fehnel S, Mangel A, Talley NJ, Whitehead WE: **Psychometric evaluation of endpoints in IBS randomized controlled trials: a Rome foundation working group report.** *Gastroenterology* 2009, **137:**1944–1953.
21. Food and Drug Administration: **Guidance for industry irritable bowel syndrome–clinical evaluation of drugs for treatment: final guidance.** 2012. http://www.fda.gov/downloads/Drugs/Guidances/UCM205269.pdf.
22. Das Gupta S: **Point biserial correlation and its generalization.** *Psychometrika* 1960, **25:**393–408.
23. Brogden H: **A new coefficient: application to biserial correlation and to estimation of selective efficiency.** *Psychometrika* 1949, **14:**169–182.
24. Cohen J: **A power primer.** *Psychol Bull* 1992, **112:**155–159.
25. R Core Team R: **A language and environment for statistical computing.** 2013. http://www.R-project.org/] R Foundation for Statistical Computing.
26. Rizopoulos D: **Ltm: An R package for latent variable modeling and item response theory analysis.** *J Stat Softw* 2006, **17:**1–25.
27. SAS: *Version 9.3 SAS system for windows.* SAS Institute. http://www.sas.com/.
28. Cronbach L: **Coefficient alpha and the internal structure of tests.** *Psychometrika* 1951, **6:**297–334.
29. Sijtsma K: **On the use, the misuse, and the very limited usefulness of Cronbach's alpha.** *Psychometrika* 2009, **74:**107–120.
30. Green S, Yang Y: **Commentary on coefficient alpha: a cautionary tale.** *Psychometrika* 2009, **74:**121–137.
31. Revelle W, Zinbarg R: **Coefficients alpha, beta, omega, and the GLB: comments on Sijtsma.** *Psychometrika* 2009, **74:**145–154.
32. Bentler P: **Alpha, dimension-free, and model-based internal consistency reliability.** *Psychometrika* 2009, **74:**137–143.

19

A randomised controlled trial of a probiotic 'functional food' in the management of irritable bowel syndrome

Lesley M Roberts[1], Deborah McCahon[1], Roger Holder[1], Sue Wilson[1] and FD Richard Hobbs[2*]

Abstract

Background: Irritable Bowel Syndrome (IBS) is a common condition characterised by pain, distension and altered bowel habit. Evidence suggests functional foods containing probiotics improve gastrointestinal transit, however, data are limited by short follow-up periods and evaluation in selected populations.

Methods: A multi-centre, randomized, double blind, controlled trial to evaluate the effect of a probiotic vs non-probiotic dairy product on symptoms in IBS with a constipation element (IBS – Constipation or IBS – Mixed profile). Set in 13 general practices within central England. Individuals meeting the ROME III criteria for IBS, aged 18–65 completed a pre-study diary. Eligible individuals were randomized to consume dairy 'yoghurt' products which either did or did not contain active probiotics twice daily and to complete a daily diary. Primary outcome was subjective global assessment of symptom relief at week 4. Other outcomes comprised, IBS symptom scores, pain, bloating and flatulence levels, stool frequency, stool consistency, ease of bowel movement and quality of life.

Results: 179 were randomized (91 active, 88 placebo). 76 (43 active, 33 placebo) completed the study. No significant between group differences existed at 4 weeks (57% active vs 53% placebo, reported adequate relief (p = 0.71)). By week 8, 46% active vs 68% placebo reported adequate relief (p = 0.03). This was sustained at week 12.

Conclusions: Significant improvements were reported for most outcomes in all trial participants but improvement did not differ by group. This trial does not provide evidence for effectiveness of a probiotic in IBS, in variance with a body of published literature and review conclusions. Differential drop out may however cloud interpretation of data.

UK Trial registration: ISRCTN78863629

Keywords: Probiotic, Functional food, IBS, RCT

Background

Functional foods are defined as foods which purport to improve health or wellbeing. In 2007 a BMJ editorial called for the closer evaluation of functional foods and recent European Union regulation and directives have formalised the need for such foodstuffs to support claims with robust evidence [1]. Their use by the public has increased considerably, especially in chronic symptomatic disorders with limited treatment options. For example, for the large numbers of individuals suffering symptoms of irritable bowel syndrome (IBS) where conventional treatment is often poorly efficacious, the potential for alternative evidence based therapies is considerable.

IBS, a functional bowel disorder, is a common problem affecting a substantial proportion of the population, with point prevalence estimates ranging from 10-30% [2-10]. It is associated with significantly reduced quality of life [8,11,12] and it is known that many patients seek alternative strategies for symptom relief [13]. One of the simplest and therefore potentially most attractive options to patients is the inclusion of functional foods in the diet, with increasing markets for 'health drinks' in the UK [14] and elsewhere.

Among functional foods, probiotics have gained high interest in recent years since gut microbiota may be involved in gastro-intestinal (GI) functions and alterations

* Correspondence: richard.hobbs@phc.ox.ac.uk
[2]Department of Primary Care Health Sciences, Oxford University, 2nd Floor, 23-38 Hythe Bridge Street, Oxford OX1 2ET, UK
Full list of author information is available at the end of the article

in gut microbiota have been shown in IBS [15,16]. Recent systematic reviews [17-19] of the literature have evaluated the impact of probiotics on IBS. These reviews have highlighted the considerable heterogeneity in study findings and also in outcomes, probiotic combinations and study design. Therefore, despite the number of studies, the evidence base remains poor with data coming largely from small or uncontrolled trials. Overall, within the published literature and systematic reviews [19-22] there is a suggestion that probiotics confer benefit although limitations of available evidence and possibility of publication bias are acknowledged. Larger well-designed studies of probiotics in IBS are therefore required.

A well investigated fermented milk probiotic product, containing a specific *Bifidobacterium* strain (*Bifidobacterium lactis* CNCM I-2494 (previously DN-173 010)) with lactic acid bacteria (*Lactobacillus delbrueckii* subsp. *bulgaricus* and *Streptococcus thermophilus*), has shown beneficial effects on gut functions in several small randomised controlled studies [23-26]. The consumption of this probiotic dairy product (PDP) was associated with shortening of colonic transit time in patients with IBS with predominant constipation (IBSC) together with improvement of abdominal distension and other GI symptoms [24] and modest reduction of GI discomfort in primary care IBS-C patients [25].

This study aimed to compare improvement in subjective assessment of symptom relief, individual symptoms and quality of life over a 12 week period in individuals consuming this commercially available product (Danone, France) and those consuming an inactive identical product. The study focussed on IBS which included constipation as a feature (either constipation predominant or mixed profile), which accounts for approximately 75% of the IBS population, based on preliminary data on the value of probiotics in this sub group [24].

Methods

Design overview

A randomized placebo controlled trial to compare symptom and quality of life in patients with IBS taking a probiotic or non- probiotic fermented dairy product was conducted in primary care practices.

Setting and participants

13 general practices in the Midlands Research Practices Consortium (MidReC) situated within the West Midlands, UK. Patients were identified through searches of electronic patient records for symptomatic individuals with a diagnosis of IBS > 6 months or having received two or more prescriptions in the previous 24 months for anti-spasmodics, bulking agents or laxatives. A confirmatory screening questionnaire based on ROME III criteria [27] was sent to all patients. Lower than anticipated yield, led to administration of the screening questionnaire to all patients aged 18–65 in five of the thirteen practices. No other alterations were made to the study protocol during trial conduct. General practitioners applied discretion to prevent contact with patients considered inappropriate for contact or inclusion, for example individuals known to be in a terminal stage of illness or experiencing acute and severe mental illness.

Study eligibility was assessed from the information provided on the screening questionnaire plus telephone follow-up to verify responses. Individuals were considered eligible for inclusion if they were aged 18–65, met ROME III [27] criteria for a diagnosis of IBS with symptoms being present for > 6 months and reported a constipation element to their symptom profile (either constipation predominant or a mixed symptom profile).

Eligible patients were mailed a symptom diary for completion over the two weeks prior to their randomization appointment. At the baseline recruitment clinic research nurses confirmed eligibility and applied further study exclusions: individuals reporting passing more than 3 soft stools per day in the absence of laxative mediation during the pre-study phase; individuals without problematic symptoms judged by an IBS Symptom Severity Score (IBS-SSS) [28] of <75; individuals with known organic disease or reporting clinical signs of alarm; individuals who were pregnant, breast-feeding or lactose intolerant; individuals with a BMI >35 or <18, as this was deemed suggestive of abnormal diet or function; and those with a recent change of IBS medication (in the preceding month) to reduce likelihood of co-intervention bias.

Randomization and interventions

Blocked randomization lists (1:1 allocation) were produced by the lead statistician (RH) for each general practice site and held centrally. Because of the short shelf-life of dairy products randomised allocation lists were sent to the sponsors for product production prior to randomisation clinics so that two weeks supply of the relevant allocated product was available at the point of randomization. All volunteers gave written informed consent before inclusion in the study.

The test product was a commercially available fermented product containing *Bifidobacterium lactis* (strain number I-2494 in French National Collection of Cultures of Micro-organisms (CNCM, Paris, France; Danone collection number DN-173 010) together with the two classical yoghurt starters, *S. thermophilus* (CNCM strain number I-1630) and *L. bulgaricus* (CNCM strain numbers I-1632 and I-1519). The test product contains 1.25×10^{10} colony forming unit (cfu) of *Bifidobacterium lactis* CNCM I-2494 per cup and 1.2×10^{9} cfu/cup of *S. thermophilus* and *L. bulgaricus*.

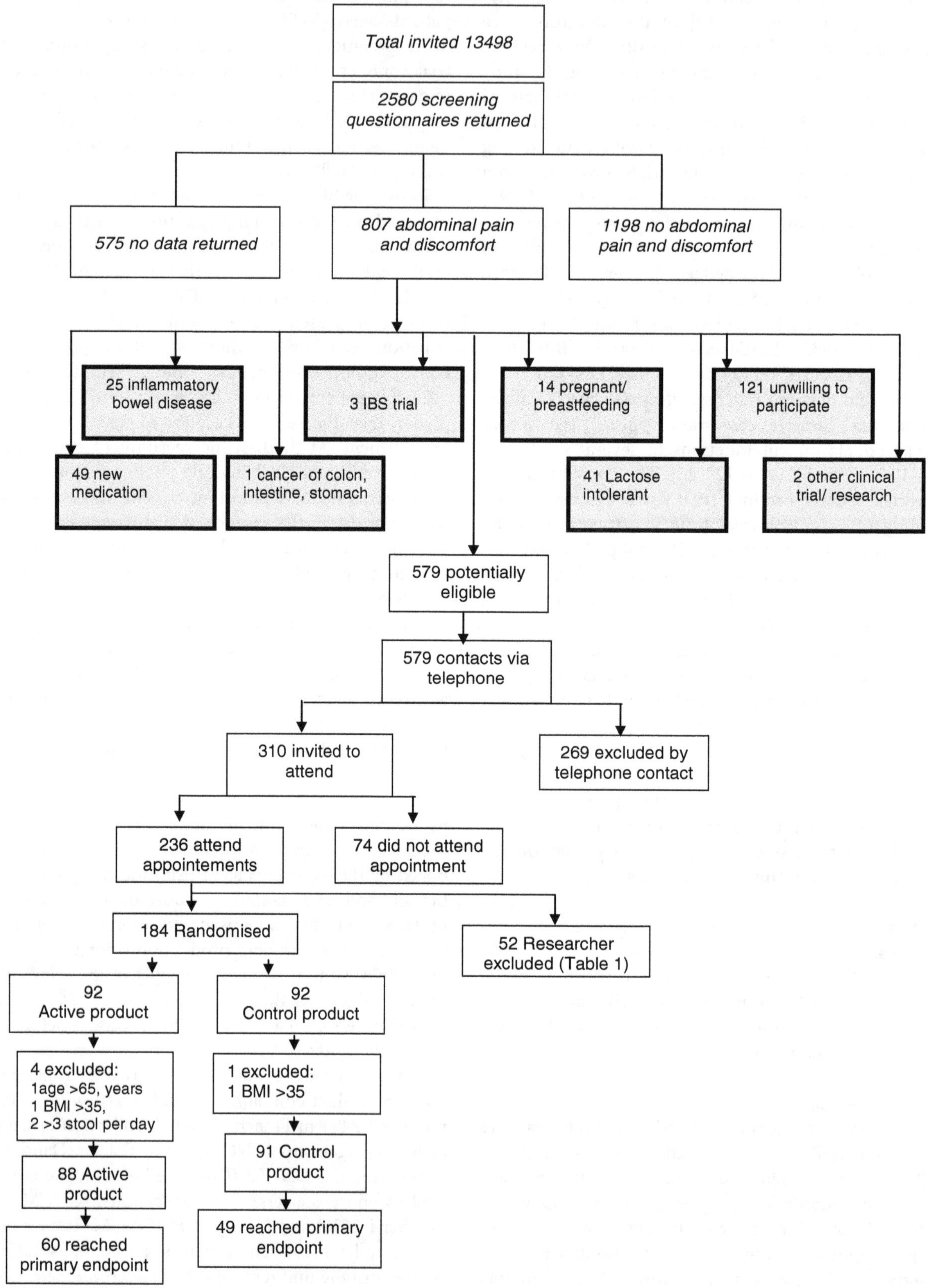

Figure 1 CONSORT diagram of recruitment, randomization & primary endpoint numbers.

Table 1 Exclusions made during randomisation clinics

Exclusion	n = 52 (%)
Average baseline stools frequency >3	14 (27%)
Does not wish to participate	13 (25%)
BMI too high	9 (17%)
Pre study diary not fully completed	3 (6%)
Clinical signs of alarm	3 (6%)
BMI too low	1 (2%)
Anti-psychotic medication in last month	1 (2%)
Lactose intolerance or immunodeficiency	1 (2%)
Organic bowel disease	1 (2%)
2 week holiday during next 4 weeks	1 (2%)
Change of treatment for IBS in last 4 weeks	1 (2%)
History of laxative abuse	1 (2%)
Diet change in last 4 weeks	1 (2%)
IBS SSS less than 75	1 (2%)
General anaesthesia in last month	1 (2%)

The control product was a milk-based non-fermented dairy product without probiotics and with similar lactose content to the test product. Both the test and control products were without flavour. Each pot contained 125 g. Both products were specifically prepared for the study and provided by Danone Research (Palaiseau, France). Nurses, GPs, patients and the research team remained blind to product allocation until all analyses had been completed.

In both groups consumption of the product twice daily was instructed and all patients received a two week supply of the allocated product in the first instance and instructions to collect repeat supplies fortnightly for 12 weeks.

Outcomes and follow-up

All patients returned completed daily diaries at follow-up visits after 4, 8 and 12 weeks. The daily diary assessed stool frequency and consistency (evaluated in accordance with the Bristol stool scale) and bowel movement difficulty (using a 5-point Likert scale which ranged from no difficulty to extreme difficulty). Weekly entries assessed subjective global assessment (SGA) [29,30] of symptom relief ("Do you consider that in the past week you have had adequate relief of your IBS symptoms?") and individual IBS specific symptom assessment of bloating, pain and flatulence (6 point Likert scale ranging from 0 (none) to 5 (very severe)).

Participants completed the Birmingham IBS Symptom Score [31], the IBS SSS [27] and an IBS specific quality of life (QoL) tool [32] at baseline and at weeks 4, 8 and 12. The Birmingham Symptom Score [31] uses 11 questions to assess pain, diarrhoea and constipation, scores range from 0–100 for each dimension with higher scores indicating greater well-being. The IBS –SSS [27] utilises five questions each generating a maximum score of 100 and a total possible score of 500 with higher scores indicating a greater symptom burden. The IBS specific QoL [32] tool evaluates dimensions; dysphoria, interference with activity, body image, health worry, food avoidance, social reaction, sexual and relationship using 34 five point Likert statements. Items are summed to create a total score with higher scores indicating better QoL.

The primary outcome was pre-specified as SGA of symptom relief at week 4 in line with the recent trial evidence on which the study was powered [33] and after discussion with the product manufacturer and sponsor. Comparison of all other outcomes at weeks 4, 8 and 12 between groups formed specified secondary outcome measures.

Statistical analysis

The sample size calculation was based on a previous study [33] demonstrating a 20% between group difference (62% active vs. 42% control) for SGA. Therefore, 107 patients with IBS-C were required in each group to demonstrate a 20% difference between groups in proportions reporting adequate IBS symptoms relief at week 4, with a significance of 5% and 80% power. This was inflated to 240 patients to be divided in two groups of 120 to allow for drop-outs. No stopping guidelines were in place due to the short trial duration and assumed safety of a commercially available product. Data analyses for all outcomes were performed on an intention to treat basis (ITT) and further analyses were undertaken to compare differences in those not deviating from protocol (per protocol). Analyses were performed on available data for each parameter. ANCOVA with primary care centre as a random effect, baseline as a covariate and product as a fixed effect was used to compare the intervention and control groups with respect to all outcomes. Ordinal logistic regression with centre and product as fixed effects was used to explore change within each arm of the study. Analyses were conducted using MINITAB version 14, S Plus version 8 and ML wiN version 2.1 statistical software.

Role of the funding source

The study was funded by Danone Ltd. Contracts including a right to publication of all findings were approved and signed by both parties prior to commencement of the research. The funders contributed to discussion about study design and selection of outcome measures. All subsequent data review was blinded and the analysis was undertaken independently of the funders. The paper was reviewed by the sponsor and an expert nominated by them with some requested changes included in the final version.

Results

In summary, of 13,498 individuals screened by questionnaire, 2580 responded. (Figure 1) Of these, 807 reported

Table 2 Baseline demographic data and symptom scores of participants

	Active product n = 88 Mean (SD)	Control product n = 91 Mean (SD)
Age	44.66 (11.98)	43.71 (12.76)
BMI	26.75 (4.03)	25.85 (3.61)
Percentage		
Male	15	15
Non-smoker	47	56
Light smoker (<10 per day)	8	6
Heavy smoker (>10 per day)	14	18
Former smoker	32	21
White ethnic group	91	86
Other ethnic group combined	9	14
Mental Health	10	1
Score		
IBS-SSS (Max score 500 – higher scores indicating greater symptom burden	258.70 (86.51)	251.73 (76.13)
IBS symptoms (Birmingham Score) (Max score 100 for all dimensions – higher scores represent greater well-being)		
Constipation	47.31 (26.86)	49.08 (25.75)
Diarrhoea	84.58 (15.17)	85.62 (11.72)
Pain	62.50 (19.74)	60.95 (19.62)
Total	68.36 (12.00)	68.90 (11.07)
IBS specific symptoms (Scored 0–5 with greater scores indicating greater symptom burden)		
Pain	2.50 (1.08)	2.50 (1.08)
Bloating	3.13 (1.18)	3.16 (0.97)
Flatulence	3.18 (1.14)	2.88 (1.16)
Composite score	8.80 (2.65)	8.54 (2.50)
Stool frequency (Stools per day)	1.17 (0.93)	1.19 (0.96)
Stool consistency (From Bristol Stool Form)	3.14 (1.64)	3.20 (1.60)
Bowel movement difficulty *(Scored 0–5 with higher scores indicating greater difficulty)*	1.38 (1.19)	1.18 (1.06)
IBS-QoL (Multi-item scale with greater scores indicating better quality of life)		
Dysphoria	66.69 (27.72)	72.94 (23.49)
Activity interference	73.02 (23.06)	73.73 (21.12)
Body image	58.03 (26.07)	60.85 (23.60)
Health worry	56.77 (26.13)	64.65 (24.66)
Food avoidance	58.14 (28.53)	59.34 (30.55)
Social reaction	64.99 (26.08)	73.72 (24.34)
Sexual	75.43 (31.85)	77.75 (26.72)
Relationship	75.43 (24.06)	80.86 (20.25)
Total score	66.45 (22.49)	70.78 (20.08)

the experience of abdominal pain in the preceding 3 months and 579 were deemed potentially eligible. Telephone screening excluded a further 269 individuals, primarily because of a diarrhoea predominant form of IBS, and 310 individuals were issued with a clinic appointment, of which 236 attended. A further 52 were excluded for reasons described in Table 1. One hundred and eighty four individuals were randomized although 5 were subsequently excluded when data quality checks revealed breached exclusion criteria. Eighty eight individuals commenced consumption of the active product and 91 of the control product leading to an ITT population of 179 patients.

Groups were similar with respect to baseline IBS symptom severity scores, demographics, medical history and concomitant disease, with the exception of mental illness with 9 individuals in the active group having a current mental health diagnosis compared to 1 in the control group (Table 2).

Primary outcome

Among the 179 randomized patients, 109 had available data for SGA at week 4 (60 in active group; 49 in control group). There were no between group differences in SGA noted at week 4 with 56.7% of the active group and 53.1% of the control group reporting adequate symptom relief ($p = 0.71$) (Table 3).

Large numbers of withdrawals accrued, with dropout rates of 39% (70/179) at week 4, 48% (86/179) at week 8 and 55% (98/179) at week 12, despite efforts to follow-up all participants. Withdrawal reasons were recorded where provided by participants. Across both groups drop-out was attributable to a range of factors including dislike of product taste, changes in personal circumstances and reported adverse events such as nausea.

At week 8 greater benefit in terms of adequate symptom relief was reported in the control group (68.3% reporting relief versus 46.2%, $p = 0.03$) and this was sustained at week 12 (75.8% versus 45.8%, $p = 0.004$) (Table 3).

Secondary outcomes

During the initial 4 weeks of the trial statistically significant (at the $p < 0.05$ level) improvement from baseline was reported in both groups for the majority of outcomes, including improvements in symptoms scores, bloating, flatulence, ease of bowel movement and quality of life (Table 4). Although both groups reported improvement there was no significant between group difference when

Table 3 Comparison of the proportions reporting adequate symptom relief in intention to treat analyses

Subjective global assessment (SGA)	Active product % (n)	Control product % (n)	Difference between the groups	p value active vs control
Week 4	56.7 (60)	53.1 (49)	3.61	0.707
Week 8	46.2 (52)	68.3 (41)	−22.1	0.027
Week 12	45.8 (48)	75.8 (33)	−29.9	0.004

considering changes in either of the symptom measures used, nor for any individual symptoms or QoL outcomes (Table 4). The improvement from baseline scores demonstrated at week 4 in both groups remained significant for most outcomes at week 8. The absence of a between group difference, however remained constant with both groups demonstrating similar improvements (Table 5).

By week 12, however, change in scores differed significantly between groups for the following outcomes; IBS symptom severity score, IBS symptoms of constipation and associated total score as measured by the Birmingham score, IBS specific symptoms of pain, bloating and associated total score. For all statistically significant outcomes those receiving the control product demonstrated greater improvement than those receiving the active product (Table 5).

Per protocol analyses undertaken at each of the time points (4, 8 and 12 weeks) did not significantly alter the findings reported in the ITT analyses.

Discussion

Summary of main findings

In this double-blind randomized controlled trial of a commercially available probiotic fermented dairy product (yoghurt) containing *bifidobacterium animalis* DN-173010 in

Table 4 Between and within group comparisons at week 4

Study parameter	Active product			Control product			Active versus control
	n	Mean (week 4–baseline) (SD)	p value* (change from baseline)	n	Mean (week 4–baseline) (SD)	p value* (change from baseline)	p value**
IBS-SSS	41	−53.35 (81.98)	<0.002	44	−31.11 (78.57)	0.010	0.233
Birmingham IBS symptom scale							
Constipation	59	9.44 (20.40)	<0.001	49	15.10 (21.59)	<0.001	0.131
Diarrhoea	59	3.88 (12.26)	0.007		2.22 (10.17)	0.106	0.616
Pain	60	7.89 (14.70)	<0.001		11.22 (18.34)	<0.001	0.367
Total score	60	6.10 (10.83)	<0.001		8.28 (11.10)	<0.001	0.251
IBS specific symptoms							
Pain	60	−0.33 (1.19)	0.087	49	−0.61 (1.36)	0.001	0.109
Bloating		−0.66 (1.35)	<0.001	48	−0.68 (1.12)	<0.001	0.432
Flatulence		−0.51 (1.24)	<0.001	49	−0.36 (1.07)	0.0017	0.955
Composite score		−1.48 (3.03)	0.002	49	−1.69 (2.99)	<0.001	0.264
Stool frequency	417	0.07 (0.89)	0.202	341	0.04 (0.85)	0.607	0.648
Stool consistency	341	0.13 (1.20)	0.240	269	0.31 (1.30)	0.007	0.184
Bowel movement difficulty	341	−0.24 (0.97)	0.004	271	−0.28 (0.89)	0.011	0.450
IBS Quality of life							
Dysphoria	60	9.78 (16.89)	<0.001	50	7.53 (15.54)	0.002	0.875
Activity interference	60	5.68 (10.97)	0.003	50	5.07 (13.77)	0.008	0.769
Body image	60	6.63 (16.28)	<0.001	50	8.13 (17.37)	0.004	0.134
Health worry	60	7.92 (15.20)	0.001	50	5.75 (16.17)	0.009	0.958
Food avoidance	60	9.58 (16.01)	0.002	50	4.42 (18.76)	0.078	0.121
Social reaction	60	7.33 (14.23)	0.003	50	4.17 (14.10)	0.029	0.769
Sexual	59	4.24 (15.68)	0.171	48	4.17 (20.36)	0.125	0.853
Relationship	60	7.15 (15.54)	<0.001	50	1.92 (12.43)	0.217	0.139
Total score	60	7.60 (10.88)	<0.001	50	5.69 (12.60)	0.004	0.979

*ANCOVA with centre as a random effect, baseline as a covariate and product as a fixed effect.
**Ordinal logistic regression with centre and product fixed effects.
Stool frequency, consistency and bowel movement difficulty were recorded daily and therefore n represents the number of data items (days) included in analysis for these items.

Table 5 Between and within group comparisons at weeks 8 and 12

Study parameter	A = Active product			C = Control product			A vs C
	n	Mean (week 12–baseline) (SD)	p value* (change from baseline)	n	Mean (week 12–baseline) (SD)	p value* (change from baseline)	p value**
WEEK 8							
IBS-SSS	50	−58.30 (84.96)	<0.001	40	−58.33 (73.37)	<0.001	0.589
Birmingham IBS symptom scale							
Constipation	52	13.78 (24.47)	<0.001	41	17.24 (22.61)	<0.001	0.302
Diarrhoea		4.25 (13.78)	0.210		2.15 (7.71)	0.064	0.907
Pain		11.28 (18.88)	<0.001		13.66 (16.80)	<0.001	0.257
Total score		8.71 (13.09)	<0.001		9.44 (9.75)	<0.001	0.265
IBS specific symptoms							
Pain	53	−0.58 (1.24)	0.012	41	−0.66 (1.43)	0.002	0.292
Bloating	52	−0.80 (1.44)	0.005		−0.85 (1.26)	<0.001	0.408
Flatulence	53	−0.54 (1.28)	0.002	40	−0.50 (1.08)	0.004	0.864
Composite score	52	−1.95 (3.43)	0.003		−1.96 (3.17)	<0.001	0.374
Stool frequency	346	0.07 (0.95)	0.303	276	0.10 (0.05)	0.141	0.828
Stool consistency	290	0.18 (1.17)	0.042	218	0.50 (1.23)	0.001	0.098
Bowel movement difficulty	291	−0.43 (1.01)	<0.001	224	−0.40 (0.78)	<0.001	0.623
IBS Quality of life							
Dysphoria	53	14.66 (19.87)	<0.001	41	9.29 (13.95)	<0.001	0.508
Activity interference		8.20 (14.74)	0.001		6.05 (12.99)	0.001	0.924
Body image		11.95 (15.98)	<0.001		8.54 (13.46)	<0.001	0.735
Health worry		13.29 (17.81)	<0.001		7.62 (15.19)	0.002	0.428
Food avoidance		10.06 (17.63)	<0.001		5.49 (17.84)	0.039	0.372
Social reaction		10.85 (16.18)	<0.001		6.71 (12.21)	<0.001	0.462
Sexual		8.41 (18.31)	0.006		7.05 (16.92)	0.005	0.554
Relationship		7.23 (18.64)	0.015		7.01 (9.88)	<0.001	0.635
Total score		10.95 (13.14)	<0.001		7.52 (10.22)	<0.001	0.483
WEEK 12							
IBS-SSS	43	−61.02 (75.78)	<0.001	33	−97.24 (90.17)	<0.001	0.028
Birmingham IBS symptom scale							
Constipation	48	6.65 (22.56)	0.039	35	17.52 (23.60)	<0.001	0.011
Diarrhoea		3.27 (11.17)	0.048		2.43 (10.60)	0.133	0.889
Pain		10.28 (14.09)	<0.001		15.24 (17.38)	<0.001	<0.107
Total score		6.07 (9.62)	<0.001		10.10 (10.78)	<0.001	<0.022
IBS specific symptoms							
Pain	48	−0.59 (1.24)	0.002	34	−1.04 (1.33)	<0.001	0.016
Bloating	48	−0.58 (1.39)	0.005		−1.35 (1.21)	<0.001	0.006
Flatulence	48	−0.64 (1.04)	0.001		−0.76 (1.23)	<0.001	0.383
Composite score	48	−1.81 (3.03)	<0.001		−3.16 (3.05)	<0.001	0.011
Stool frequency	311	−0.07 (0.75)	0.186	224	0.07 (0.82)	0.464	0.211
Stool consistency	247	0.26 (1.22)	0.045	181	0.31 (0.99)	0.012	0.784
Bowel movement difficulty	246	−0.35 (0.99)	<0.001	180	−0.36 (0.86)	<0.001	0.329
IBS Quality of life							
Dysphoria	48	13.61 (20.12)	<0.001	34	10.83 (10.68)	<0.001	0.933
Activity interference		8.47 (12.31)	<0.001	34	7.09 (8.73)	<0.001	0.806

Table 5 Between and within group comparisons at weeks 8 and 12 *(Continued)*

Body image	11.33 (14.16)	<0.001	34	8.27 (14.08)	0.005	0.857
Health worry	14.15 (21.01)	<0.001	34	9.07 (13.19)	<0.001	0.634
Food avoidance	8.16 (20.45)	0.008	34	8.58 (13.37)	<0.001	0.687
Social reaction	9.64 (17.15)	<0.001	34	9.38 (8.74)	<0.001	0.660
Sexual	8.07 (21.34)	0.031	32	10.55 (16.53)	<0.001	0.382
Relationship	7.03 (15.81)	0.002	34	5.51 (9.22)	<0.001	0.751
Total score	10.43 (12.92)	<0.001	34	8.83 (6.12)	<0.001	0.810

*ANCOVA with centre as a random effect, baseline as a covariate and product as a fixed effect.
**Ordinal logistic regression with centre and product fixed effects.
Stool frequency, consistency and bowel movement difficulty were recorded daily and therefore n represents the number of data items (days) included in analysis for these items.

community based IBS patients with a constipation element, both the inactive (control) and active product groups demonstrated significant improvement across a range of symptom and quality of life outcomes. Improvement was maintained throughout the 12-week period of observation. Reductions in symptoms were, however, reported at similar levels in both groups when assessed in weeks 4 and 8. At week 12 there was the suggestion of a benefit of the control product over the active formulation but this is likely to be attributable to differential drop-outs between groups.

The sustained and large improvement observed in both groups suggests there may be benefit from regular consumption of a dairy product but does not suggest any additional benefit of the addition of a probiotic to such products. If such a benefit is accrued the mechanism through which this works is unclear and product effect, regularisation of eating habits and increased fluid intake are all possible explanations. The fact that benefits were also accrued by control participants supports these potential mechanisms of effect. In the absence of a non-intervention group this effect cannot be confirmed but the substantial effect size is worthy of further consideration and exploration of sub-groups in which greatest benefit is accrued would be advisable. In this study there was the suggestion that drop-out may be related to baseline symptom severity with those remaining in the study having greater baseline symptom severity scores than those withdrawing (IBS SSS 264.15 versus 238.09, p = 0.04). This could suggest greater benefit was accrued by those with more severe symptoms encouraging continued participation or may reflect and greater motivation to pursue therapy in this group.

Study strengths and limitations

This primary care based RCT is one of the largest trials of probiotics in IBS to date and one of the only functional food trials to be conducted outside small hospital populations. The main study limitation was not reaching the target recruitment of 240 patients between the two arms, with only 179 recruited of whom 109 provided data for the primary outcome. The failure to meet the trial target recruitment was due to a contractually fixed end date for the trial and the 109 participants providing 4 week data reduced study power to 47%. However, at study close the trial showed futility of continuance given the observed lack of treatment benefit. A post-hoc re-estimate of sample size, based on observed difference in the study primary outcome (proportions 0.57 versus 0.53), indicated 2477 patients would have been required in each arm to demonstrate a statistically significant treatment effect.

The observed imbalance in the randomization numbers was due to the study requirement to randomize eligible patients prior to the baseline visit (to enable product manufacture) and there was differential clinic attendance by chance. Since the study power was reduced through a high level of drop-outs and differential drop-out, it therefore remains a possibility that an effect of the active product was missed. The high drop-out rate highlights the difficulty of conducting functional food trials but does call into question the acceptability of such interventions to patients over even short periods.

Comparison with existing literature

This study focused only on individuals who had a constipation element to their IBS since earlier data suggested this might be the population who might obtain most benefit from consumption of a probiotic: prior trials [34-36] have suggested that daily consumption of fermented milk products containing Bifidobacterium animalis DN-173 010 improves transit and alleviates bloating in individuals with low stool frequency. However the heterogeneous nature of the cohort recruited (some with a constipation predominant form of IBS and others with a mixed profile) may further mask an effect which would be demonstrated in a more homogeneous IBS constipation predominant patient group. Despite screening to ensure all participants were symptomatic at baseline and with a constipation feature to their IBS, the mean number of stools passed daily at baseline was greater than one and the mean stool consistency was 3 on the Bristol Stool Form Scale which equates to only a slightly drier than average stool suggesting this cohort did not comprise those with more significant forms of constipation. Recruitment of participants with a more extreme manifestation of constipation may have more closely replicated the small hospital populations in previous trials where modest benefits of probiotics were observed. However, given the dominance of small positive trials in the literature, it is also possible that the literature in this area is subject to publication bias. This highlights the importance of establishing the efficacy of treatments across the wide range of IBS phenotypes if they are to be made widely available. If functional foods are to be advocated for a common disorder like IBS it is important to have clear indications as to the symptoms most likely to accrue benefit. This study importantly illustrates that data from the presumed more persistent and extreme IBS phenotypes seen in hospitals cannot routinely be extrapolated to the general population.

The interest in the use of functional foods is demonstrated by the large numbers of reviews conducted in recent years [20,21,37-41]. Despite this major body of review evidence, the trial evidence upon which it is based remains limited. This carefully conducted double blind randomized 12 week study assessing a wider range of outcomes in a general population of IBS with a constipation element, did not reproduce these earlier hospital based findings. Explanations for this may be attributable to differences in participant groups, outcomes and follow-up. However this study best reflects current practice for the majority of patients with IBS who might consider probiotic milk products to try to reduce symptoms.

Implication for future research or clinical practice

Clinicians advising patients with IBS managed in the community featuring a constipation element may wish to suggest the inclusion of a fermented dairy product, given that significant improvements were reported for most outcomes in all trial participants. The requirement of such products to contain a probiotic is not supported by this study.

Further research is required to consider the mechanism via which improvement in symptoms may be effected in trials of this nature through consideration of dietary habits and fluid intake. Such work will ensure the most accurate dietary advice can be provided to patients.

Conclusions

Significant improvements were reported for most outcomes in all trial participants but improvement did not differ by intervention or placebo group. This trial therefore does not provide evidence for effectiveness of a probiotic in IBS, in variance with much published literature and review conclusions.

Competing interests

All authors declare that:

1. DM and RH salary or supervision costs were funded in part from a research grant received from Danone Ltd for the conduct of this study. Payments received were exclusively used by the University of Birmingham to offset the salary costs of these individuals for their time on the study. All surpluses were retained by the University.
2. All authors confirm no other relationship with Danone Ltd.
3. A publication clause was included within the contract between Danone Ltd and the University of Birmingham permitting publication of all findings after Danone had 2 months notice to comment on the final draft.
4. All authors confirm their spouses, partners and children have no financial relationships which may be relevant to the submitted work.
5. All authors confirm that they have no non-financial interest that may be relevant to the submitted work.

Authors' contributions

The study was designed by LR, SW and FDRH following an approach from Danone Ltd. LR and DM undertook management of the study, including overseeing data collection and management and quality assurance. RH undertook all analyses. All authors contributed to data interpretation. LR wrote the first draft of this paper and all authors were responsible for subsequent critical revision of the manuscript. FDRH is the guarantor and corresponding author for this paper. All authors read and approved the final manuscript.

Acknowledgments

The authors would like to thank the patients and GPs that participated and also the general practice staff that facilitated collection of data.

Author details

[1]Primary Care Clinical Sciences, School of Health and Population Sciences, University of Birmingham, Edgbaston, Birmingham B15 2TT, UK. [2]Department of Primary Care Health Sciences, Oxford University, 2nd Floor, 23-38 Hythe Bridge Street, Oxford OX1 2ET, UK.

References

1. de Jong N, Klungel OH, Verhagen H, *et al*: **Functional foods: the case for closer evaluation.** *BMJ* 2007, **334**(7602):1037–1039.
2. Talley NJ, Gabriel SE, Harmsen WS, *et al*: **Medical costs in community subjects with irritable bowel syndrome.** *Gastroenterology* 1995, **109**(6):1736–1741.
3. Kennedy TM, Jones RH, Hungin AP, *et al*: **Irritable bowel syndrome, gastro-oesophageal reflux, and bronchial hyper-responsiveness in the general population.** *Gut* 1998, **43**(6):770–774.
4. Thompson WG, Heaton KW, Smyth GT, *et al*: **Irritable bowel syndrome in general practice: prevalence, characteristics, and referral.** *Gut* 2000, **46**(1):78–82.
5. Agreus L, Svardsudd K, Nyren O, *et al*: **Irritable bowel syndrome and dyspepsia in the general population: overlap and lack of stability over time.** *Gastroenterology* 1995, **109**(3):671–680.
6. Wilson S, Roberts L, Roalfe A, *et al*: **Prevalence of irritable bowel syndrome: a community survey.** *Br J Gen Pract* 2004, **54**(504):495–502.
7. Drossman DA, Li Z, Andruzzi E, *et al*: **U.S. householder survey of functional gastrointestinal disorders. Prevalence, sociodemography, and health impact.** *Dig Dis Sci* 1993, **38**(9):1569–1580.
8. Hungin AP, Whorwell PJ, Tack J, *et al*: **The prevalence, patterns and impact of irritable bowel syndrome: an international survey of 40,000 subjects.** *Aliment Pharmacol Ther* 2003, **17**(5):643–650.
9. Jones R, Lydeard S: **Irritable bowel syndrome in the general population.** *BMJ* 1992, **304**(6819):87–90.
10. Posserud I, Ersryd A, Simren M: **Functional findings in irritable bowel syndrome.** *World J Gastroenterol* 2006, **12**(18):2830–2838.
11. O'Keefe EA, Talley NJ, Zinsmeister AR, *et al*: **Bowel disorders impair functional status and quality of life in the elderly: a population-based study.** *J Gerontol A Biol Sci Med Sci* 1995, **50**(4):M184–M189.
12. Farndale R, Roberts LM: **Long-term impact of irritable bowel syndrome: a qualitative study.** *Primary Health Care Research & Development* 2011, **12**:52–67.
13. Harris LR, Roberts L: **Treatments for irritable bowel syndrome: patients' attitudes and acceptability.** *BMC Complement Altern Med* 2008, **8**:65.

14. Leatherhead Food International: *The international market for functional foods. Market report leaflet.* 2006.
15. Salonen A, de Vos WM, Palva A: **Gastrointestinal microbiota in irritable bowel syndrome: present state and perspectives.** *Microbiology* 2010, **156**:3205–3215.
16. Quigley EM: **Therapies aimed at the gut microbiota and inflammation: antibiotics, prebiotics, probiotics, synbiotics, anti-inflammatory therapies.** *Gastroenterol Clin North Am* 2011, **40**:207–222.
17. Moayyedi P, Ford AC, Talley NJ, *et al*: **The efficacy of probiotics in the treatment of irritable bowel syndrome: a systematic review.** *Gut* 2010, **59**:325–332.
18. Hoveyda N, Heneghan C, Mahatani KR, *et al*: **A systematic review and meta-analysis: probiotics in the treatment of irritable bowel syndrome.** *BMC Gastroenterol* 2009, **9**:15.
19. Montrose DC, Floch MH: **Probiotics used in human studies.** *J Clin Gastroenterol* 2005, **39**(6):469–484.
20. Floch MH: **Use of diet and probiotic therapy in the irritable bowel syndrome: analysis of the literature.** *J Clin Gastroenterol* 2005, **39**(5 Suppl):S243–S246.
21. Krammer HJ, Schlieger F, Harder H, *et al*: **Probiotics as therapeutic agents in irritable bowel syndrome.** *Z Gastroenterol* 2005, **43**(5):467–471.
22. Young P, Cash BD: **Probiotic use in irritable bowel syndrome.** *Curr Gastroenterol Rep* 2006, **8**(4):321–326.
23. Guyonnet D, Schlumberger A, Mhamdi L, *et al*: **Fermented milk containing Bifidobacterium lactis DN-173 010 improves gastrointestinal well-being and digestive symptoms in women reporting minor digestive symptoms. A randomised, double-blind, parallel, controlled study.** *Br J Nut* 2009, **102**:1654–1662.
24. Agrawal A, Houghton LA, Morris J, *et al*: **Clinical trial: the effects of a fermented milk product containing Bifidobacterium lactis DN-173-010 on abdominal distension and gastrointestinal transit in irritable bowel syndrome with constipation.** *Aliment Pharmacol Ther* 2009, **29**:104–114.
25. Guyonnet D, Chassany O, Ducrotté P, *et al*: **Effect of a fermented milk containing Bifidobacterium animalis DN-173 010 on the health-related quality of life and symptoms in irritable bowel syndrome in adults in primary care: a multicentre, randomized, double-blind, controlled trial.** *Aliment Pharmacol Ther* 2007, **26**:475–486.
26. Marteau P, Cuillerier E, Meance S, *et al*: **Bifidobacterium animalis strain DN-173 010 shortens the colonic transit time in healthy women: a double-blind, randomized, controlled study.** *Aliment Pharmacol Ther* 2002, **16**(3):587–593.
27. Drossman DA, Corazziari E, Delvaux M, *et al*: *Rome III. The functional gastrointestinal disorders.* 3rd edition. Virginia, USA: Degnon Associates; 2006.
28. Francis CY, Morris J, Whorwell PJ: **The irritable bowel severity scoring system: a simple method of monitoring irritable bowel syndrome and its progress.** *Aliment Pharmacol Ther* 1997, **11**(2):395–402.
29. Irvine EJ, Whitehead WE, Chey WD, *et al*: **Design of treatment trials for functional gastrointestinal disorders.** *Gastroenterology* 2006, **130**(5):1538–1551.
30. Mangel AW: **Personal view: adequate relief as a primary endpoint in irritable bowel syndrome.** *Aliment Pharmacol Ther* 2006, **23**(7):879–881.
31. Roalfe A, Roberts L, Wilson S: **Evaluation of an IBS-specific symptom questionnaire.** *BMC Gastroenterol* 2008, **8**:30.
32. Patrick DL, Drossman DA, Frederick IO, *et al*: **Quality of life in persons with irritable bowel syndrome: development and validation of a new measure.** *Dig Dis Sci* 1998, **43**(2):400–411.
33. Whorwell PJ, Altringer L, Morel J, *et al*: **Efficacy of an Encapsulated Probiotic Bifidobacterium infantis 35624 in Women with Irritable Bowel Syndrome.** *Am J Gstroenterol* 2006, **101**:1581–1590.
34. Méance S, Cayuela C, Turchet P, *et al*: **A fermented milk with a *Bifidobacterium* probiotic strain DN-173 010 shortened oro-fecal gut transit time in elderly.** *Microb Ecol Health Dis* 2001, **13**:217–222.
35. Méance S, Cayuela C, Turchet P, *et al*: **Recent advances in the use of functional foods: effects of the commercial fermented milk with *Bifidobacterium animalis* strain DN-173 010 and yoghurt strains on gut transit time in the elderly.** *Microb Ecol Health Dis* 2003, **15**:15–22.
36. Bouvier M, Méance S, Bouley C, *et al*: **Effects of consumption of a milk fermented by a probiotic *Bifidobacterium animalis* (strain DN-173 010) on colonic transit times in healthy humans.** *Bioscience Microflora* 2001, **20**:43–48.
37. Camilleri M: **Probiotics and irritable bowel syndrome: rationale, putative mechanisms, and evidence of clinical efficacy.** *J Clin Gastroenterol* 2006, **40**(3):264–269.
38. Faber SM: **Are probiotics useful in irritable bowel syndrome?** *J Clin Gastroenterol* 2003, **37**(1):93–94.
39. Madden JA, Hunter JO: **A review of the role of the gut microflora in irritable bowel syndrome and the effects of probiotics.** *Br J Nutr* 2002, **88**(Suppl 1):S67–S72.
40. Quigley EM, Flourie B: **Probiotics and irritable bowel syndrome: a rationale for their use and an assessment of the evidence to date.** *Neurogastroenterol Motil* 2007, **19**(3):166–172.
41. Quigley EM: **The use of probiotics in functional bowel disease.** *Gastroenterol Clin North Am* 2005, **34**(3):533–545.

Parasites in Mexican patients with irritable bowel syndrome: A case-control study

Maria Elena Ramirez-Miranda[1], Rosaura Hernandez-Castellanos[1], Eduardo Lopez-Escamilla[1], David Moncada[1], Alfredo Rodriguez-Magallan[2], Carlos Pagaza-Melero[2], Alberto Gonzalez-Angulo[1], Ana Flisser[3], Simon Kawa-Karasik[1], Pablo Maravilla[1*]

Abstract

One hundred and fifteen patients with symptoms suggestive of irritable bowel syndrome (IBS) according to Rome III criteria and 209 patients with gastrointestinal symptoms different from IBS (control) were identified through medical records from the Gastroenterology Clinic of the "Dr. Manuel Gea Gonzalez General Hospital" from January 2008 to March 2010. No statistical differences in IBS data as compared with control groups were observed except in bloating, that was more frequent in the IBS group ($P = 0.043$). Although the pathogenicity of specific intestinal protozoa could not be demonstrated due to lack of association with the development of gastrointestinal symptoms, *Blastocystis spp*, in the IBS group, exhibited a trend of association to diarrhoea (odds ratio = 2.73, 95% confidence interval = 0.84-8.80, $P = 0.053$), while having any parasite and diarrhoea was significant (odds ratio = 3.38, 95% confidence interval = 1.33-8.57, $P = 0.008$). The association between *Blastocystis* and diarrhoea in IBS patients although not conclusive is an interesting finding; nonetheless more extensive case-controlled studies are required to clearly define the role of some "non-pathogenic" parasites in intestinal disease and IBS.

Findings

In recent times, some common "non-pathogenic" parasites such as *Blastocystis hominis* and *Diantamoeba fragilis* have been associated with abdominal pain, bloating, and alteration of bowel habits resembling irritable bowel syndrome (IBS) [1,2]. IBS is a functional bowel disorder in which abdominal pain or discomfort is associated with defecation disorders [3]. IBS is a frequent disease in clinical practice, representing 12% of all diagnoses obtained in general medical visits and 25% to 50% of all gastroenterology consultations [3,4]. The objective of the present study was to determine the role of intestinal protozoa among IBS patients and to analyze the clinical course of the disease.

Individuals who had attended the gastroenterology clinic of the "Dr. Manuel Gea Gonzalez General Hospital" between January 2008 and March 2010 were identified from the database of medical records. The study was reviewed and approved by the Ethical and Research Committee of the hospital. Cases were defined as patients with symptoms of IBS according to the Rome III criteria. Such symptoms would consist of recurrent abdominal pain or uncomfortable sensation at least 3 days per month in the last 3 months associated with 2 or more of the following: i) improvement with defecation, ii) onset associated with a change in frequency of stool release, iii) onset associated with a change in form or appearance of stools [3]. The control group consisted of individuals without diagnosis of IBS but with other physiological alterations and gastrointestinal symptoms i.e., polypus, diabetes, haemorrhoids, ulcerative colitis, etc. Coprological studies were performed using Faust's technique with three faecal samples [5,6]. Descriptive statistics were expressed as mean and standard deviation (SD). Variables were analyzed by χ^2 tests for categorical variables; odds ratio and confidence interval were also obtained. Data analysis was performed with SSPS Version 15.0 for Windows (SPSS Institute, Chicago, IL).

A total of 253 female and 112 male patient records were analyzed during the two-year study period. The mean age was 52 (SD = 15) years; all patients resided in urban areas. Table 1 shows the results and a statistical analysis of clinical signs and symptoms and parasites in

* Correspondence: maravillap@yahoo.com
[1]Dr. Manuel Gea Gonzalez General Hospital, Mexico, DF 14080, Mexico
Full list of author information is available at the end of the article

Table 1 Demographic, clinical characteristics and parasites in IBS patients and in the control group

Characteristic	Frequency		
	IBS group	Control group	*P* value
Age at diagnosis, years	51 ± 15	53 ± 15	0.482
Female/male, n	91/24	162/47	0.736
Clinical symptoms, %			
Abdominal pain	81.7	85.6	0.355
Bloating	84.3	74.6	0.043
Constipation	65.2	60.3	0.381
Diarrhoea	26.1	28.2	0.679
Flatulence	12.2	10.0	0.555
Diarrhoea-Constipation	8.7	5.3	0.229
Parasites found, %			
Any parasite	22.6	19.6	0.524
Blastocystis spp	15.7	12.0	0.348
Endolimax nana	8.7	6.7	0.511
Entamoeba histolytica/dispar	2.6	2.9	0.890
Giardia lamblia	1.7	1.4	0.831
Co-infection with 2 parasites	6.0	3.4	0.246

the IBS vs. the control group. No statistical differences in both groups were observed except in bloating, that was more frequent in IBS patients (P = 0.043). In both groups, abdominal pain and constipation were in general the predominant symptoms (84% and 62% respectively) and *Blastocystis, Endolimax nana and Entamoeba histolytica/dispar* were the most frequent parasites (21%, 13%, and 7% respectively). Group analysis showed a significant association between having any parasite and diarrhoea in IBS patients, while *Blastocystis* exhibited a trend of association with diarrhoea in the same group (Table 2). In all the parasitized patients, stool was examined before treatment with the drug nitazoxanide according to Diaz *et al.* [7].

Table 2 Association between having any protozoan parasite or *Blastocystis* and diarrhoea

Group (n)	Variable	OR*	95%IC‡	χ^2	*P* value
IBS group (115)	Any parasite/ Diarrhoea	3.38	1.33-8.57	7.02	0.008
	Blastocystis/ Diarrhoea	2.73	0.84-8.80	3.74	0.053
Control group (209)	Any parasite/ Diarrhoea	0.783	0.36-1.72	0.37	0.542
	Blastocystis/ Diarrhoea	0.781	0.29-2.06	0.25	0.617
All participants (324)	Any parasite/ Diarrhoea	1.39	0.77-2.48	1.22	0.269
	Blastocystis/ Diarrhoea	1.33	0.62-2.8	0.64	0.420

*OR, Odds ratio; ‡95%IC, 95% Confidence interval.

There are no previous clear reports about association between IBS and parasites in Latin American patients. Our results show that the overall prevalence of intestinal protozoa in Mexican IBS patients was 23% (*Blastocystis spp* in 16%, *E. nana* in 9% and *E. histolytica/dispar* in 3%), these findings suggest an association between IBS and *Blastocystis*. A prior study by Yamamoto-Furusho and Torijano-Carrera [8] explored the prevalence of intestinal protozoa in Mexican patients from urban areas with ulcerative colitis and found a prevalence of 24% for intestinal protozoa (*Blastocystis spp* 10%, *E. nana* 9% and *E. histolytica* 5%); in the present study and in Yamamoto-Furusho's one, *Blastocystis* was the most frequent parasite, in spite of the fact that in both studies different diagnostic techniques (trichrome-staining and concentration by flotation, respectively) were used. Yakoob *et al.* [9] demonstrated that faecal carriage of *B. hominis* occurred more frequently in Pakistani patients with IBS (46%) than the control group (7%). In contrast, Tungtrongchitr *et al.* [10] found no association between faecal carriage of *Blastocystis* and IBS in Thailand participants.

According to some researchers [5,11], *Blastocystis* is currently the main dominant parasite found in human stool samples; it may have displaced other protozoa due the reluctance of physicians to treat the infection, as symptoms are self-limiting, and its pathogenicity has been considered as controversial. An additional factor leading to *Blastocystis*' dominance may be that this microorganism has developed resistance to antiparasitic drugs which treat pathogenic protozoa. Following conventional treatment, intestinal empty niches may be easily colonized by *Blastocystis spp.* Finally, similar to other intestinal protozoa, the presence of deficient hygienic habits and lack of health education programs increase the prevalence of this parasite.

Studies into the clinical significance of *Blastocystis* may be influenced by the sensitivity of detection methods. Conventionally, it is detected using standardized clinical coprological methods, which are also used to detect other enteric parasites [12]. Faecal concentration, direct smears and staining have been used by several authors to detect the presence of *Blastocystis*, although those methods have been shown to have a low sensitivity [11,12], Recently, amplification of specific DNA directly from faeces provides a significantly higher sensitivity than concentration techniques and is 100% specific [12,13], although this molecular technique is not commonly available in developing countries.

The pathophysiology of IBS remains elusive because no mechanism is unique to, or characteristic of IBS. There are no firm recommendations about the extent and type of testing required to exclude other pathologies in this disease; investigation of stool for ova, cysts and parasites is generally recommended when diarrhoea is the major manifestation of IBS, but the role that protozoan parasites may play in this complex disease has not been fully investigated [1,3,14]. Furthermore, prior studies had found that IBS patients exhibit certain genetic polymorphisms related to IL-10, TNF-alpha, IL-4, and serotonin [15,16]; thus, we can hypothesize that when patients with certain cytokine gene polymorphisms are infected with *Blastocystis*, they are more likely to develop diarrhoea. Although our results showed a trend of association between this parasite and diarrhoea in IBS patients, more extensive case-control studies that include parasitological molecular diagnostic techniques and genetic profiles of pro-inflammatory cytokines are required to clearly define the potential role of "non-pathogenic" intestinal parasites.

Abbreviations

IBS: Irritable Bowel Syndrome; CPS: Coproparasitoscopic studies; SD: Standard deviation.

Acknowledgements

To anonymous reviewer for his/her excellent critical comments; this work was supported by Grant Conacyt 69589.

Author details

[1]Dr. Manuel Gea Gonzalez General Hospital, Mexico, DF 14080, Mexico. [2]Hospital Juarez de Mexico, Mexico, DF 07760, Mexico. [3]Departamento de Microbiologia y Parasitologia, Facultad de Medicina, Universidad Nacional Autonoma de Mexico, Mexico DF 04510, Mexico.

Authors' contributions

MERM, RHC and AGA attended patients in the gastroenterology clinic of the "Dr. Manuel Gea Gonzalez General Hospital" and collected data. ELE and DM performed CPS. ARM, CPM, AF and SKK participated in the discussion. MERM and PM formulated the idea and PM performed the statistical analysis. All authors contributed in writing the manuscript.

References

1. Stark D, van Hal S, Marriott D, Ellis J, Harkness J: **Irritable bowel syndrome: a review on the role of intestinal protozoa and the importance of their detection and diagnosis.** *Int J Parasitol* 2007, **37**:11-20.
2. Yakoob J, Jafri W, Beg MA, Abbas Z, Naz S, Islam M, Khan R: ***Blastocystis hominis*** **and** ***Dientamoeba fragilis*** **in patients fulfilling irritable bowel syndrome criteria.** *Parasitol Res* 2010, **107**:679-684.
3. Longstreth GF, Thompson WG, Chey WD, Houghton LA, Mearin F, Spiller RC: **Functional bowel disorders.** *Gastroenterology* 2006, **130**:1480-1491.
4. Leyva-Jimenez R, Olvera-Torres P, Alvarez-Cordova MM, Alcantar-Saldivar EL: **Irritable bowel syndrome in adults attending to medical offices at UMF.** *Rev Med Inst Mex Seguro Soc* 2006, **44**:473-479.
5. Rodriguez E, Mateos B, Gonzalez JC, Aguilar YM, Elsa Alarcon, Mendoza AA, Mier M, Mora MA, Bernal R: **Transicion parasitaria a** ***Blastocystis hominis*** **en niños de la zona centro del estado de Guerrero, Mexico.** *Parasitol Latinoam* 2008, **63**:20-28.
6. Guimarães S, Sogayar MI: ***Blastocystis hominis*****: occurrence in children and staff members of municipal day-care centers from Botucatu, Sáo Paulo State, Brazil.** *Mem Inst Oswaldo Cruz* 1993, **88**:427-429.
7. Diaz E, Mondragon J, Ramirez E, Bernal R: **Epidemiology and control of intestinal parasites with nitazoxanide in children in Mexico.** *Am J Trop Med Hyg* 2003, **68**:384-385.
8. Yamamoto-Furusho JK, Torijano-Carrera E: **Intestinal protozoa infections among patients with ulcerative colitis: prevalence and impact on clinical disease course.** *Digestion* 2010, **82**:18-23.
9. Yakoob J, Jafri W, Jafri N, Khan R, Islam M, Beg MA, Zaman V: **Irritable bowel syndrome: in search of an etiology: role of** ***Blastocystis hominis.*** *Am J Trop Med Hyg* 2004, **70**:383-385.
10. Tungtrongchitr A, Manatsathit S, Kositchaiwat C, Ongrotchanakun J, Munkong N, Chinabutr P, Leelakusolvong S, Chaicumpa W: ***Blastocystis hominis*** **infection in irritable bowel syndrome patients.** *Southeast Asian J Trop Med Public Health* 2004, **35**:705-710.
11. Tan KS: **New insights on classification, identification, and clinical relevance of** ***Blastocystis spp.*** *Clin Microbiol Rev* 2008, **21**:639-665.
12. Stensvold CR, Nielsen HV, Mølbak K, Smith HV: **Pursuing the clinical significance of** ***Blastocystis*****–diagnostic limitations.** *Trends Parasitol* 2009, **25**:23-29.
13. Stensvold R, Brillowska-Dabrowska A, Nielsen HV, Arendrup MC: **Detection of** ***Blastocystis hominis*** **in unpreserved stool specimens by using polymerase chain reaction.** *J Parasitol* 2006, **92**:1081-1087.
14. Boorom KF, Smith H, Nimri L, Viscogliosi E, Spanakos G, Parkar U, Li LH, Zhou XN, Ok UZ, Leelayoova S, Jones MS: **Oh my aching gut: irritable bowel syndrome,** ***Blastocystis,*** **and asymptomatic infection.** *Parasit Vectors* 2008, **1**:40.
15. van der Veek PP, van den Berg M, de Kroon YE, Verspaget HW, Masclee AA: **Role of tumor necrosis factor-alpha and interleukin-10 gene polymorphisms in irritable bowel syndrome.** *Am J Gastroenterol* 2005, **100**:2510-2516.
16. Barkhordari E, Rezaei N, Mahmoudi M, Larki P, Ahmadi-Ashtiani HR, Ansaripour B, Alighardashi M, Bashashati M, Amirzargar AA, Ebrahimi-Daryani N: **T-helper 1, T-helper 2, and T-regulatory cytokines gene polymorphisms in irritable bowel syndrome.** *Inflammation* 2010, **33**:281-286.

21

The impact of irritable bowel syndrome on health-related quality of life in women with polycystic ovary syndrome

Fatemeh Bazarganipour[1], Seyed-Abdolvahab Taghavi[2], Zatollah Asemi[3], Helen Allan[4], Zahra Khashavi[5], Tahereh Safarzadeh[6], Shamsi Pourchangiz[6], Fatemeh Zare[6], Samaneh Ghasemi[6], Zivar Karimi[6] and Maryam Azizi Kutenaee[7*]

Abstract

Background: The objectives of this study were to compare the prevalence and quality of life (QOL) of irritable bowel syndrome (IBS) in women with polycystic ovary syndrome (PCOS) compared with healthy women.

Methods: This was a case-control study of 201 women recruited at an infertility clinic in Iran. The control group were healthy women (n = 100) and the comparison group, women with PCOS (n = 101). Data were collected by clinical Rome III criteria to determine the IBS, Bristol scale for stool consistency and IBS QOL.

Results: The reporting of IBS symptoms were higher in PCOS (20.7%) than control group (11%) ($P = 0.05$). The IBS QOL score in the IBS + PCOS group was lower than other groups (IBS+ non PCOS, non IBS + PCOS, non IBS+ non PCOS; scores in food avoidance and worries about health domains were significant ($P < 0.01$).

Conclusions: We conclude that having PCOS and an increased level of LH/FSH tends to cause IBS symptoms. IBS + PCOS women experience significant impaired quality of life scores particularly in relation to worries about health and food avoidance. These results offer further insights into IBS in PCOS women and their functional status and wellbeing.

Keywords: Polycystic ovary syndrome, Irritable bowel syndrome, Quality of life

Introduction

Irritable bowel syndrome (IBS) is one of the most common disorders of the digestive system, with a 10–20% incidence globally [1]. People with IBS have sensitive intestines and suffer from intestinal muscle spasms in response to food, gas, and stress. These spasms can lead to abdominal cramps and pains, changes in bowel function, bloating, diarrhoea, and constipation [2]. Patients with IBS also experience higher rates of absence from work, disruption of interpersonal relations, including a reluctance to have sexual intercourse. IBS can prevent patients from attending social gatherings and travelling for fear of experiencing symptoms in public. Many studies have reported a lower level of the quality of life (QOL) for these patients than the general population [3–6].

Although studies have shown that the prevalence of IBS in women is twice that of men generally, it was believed that this disorder was lower in women with PCOS compared to healthy women. However a recent study reported an increased prevalence of IBS in women with PCOS compared to healthy women [7]. Polycystic ovarian syndrome (PCOS) is a common chronic endocrine disease which affects 5–10% of women of reproductive age. It is characterized by chronic anovulation, with

* Correspondence: maryamazizikut86@gmail.com
[7]Fertility and Infertility Research Center, Hormozgan University of Medical Sciences, Bandar Abbas, Iran
Full list of author information is available at the end of the article

clinical or laboratory signs of hyperandrogenism [8]. Obesity is prevalent in women with PCOS due to elevated androgen levels [9]. However, there is no detailed description of the relationship between IBS and women with PCOS symptoms in relation to raised androgen levels and raised body mass index (BMI) [7].

These factors influenced the decision to investigate the prevalence of IBS in women with PCOS compared to healthy women and to compare QOL in a group of women with PCOS and healthy women.

Methods

Design and data collection

This was a case-control study of women with PCOS who attended an infertility clinic at a hospital in Hormozgan Province, Iran from May to September 2014. This clinic is the only referral center for infertility in the province. The sample size (201) was calculated using Mathur, et al., (2010) information. Women with a confirmed diagnosis of PCOS (n = 300) were invited to participate in the study as a case comparison group. After explaining the study objectives and obtaining written consent from each woman, final participants were randomly allocated to the PCOS (n = 101); a control group of healthy women whose partners had a diagnosis of male infertility (n = 100) were approached in the same way. Inclusion criteria were include being 15–40 years of age [10–17]; married; absence of non-classic adrenal hyperplasia, thyroid dysfunction, hyperprolactinemia; non-smoking; absence of following warning signs that rejected IBS included extreme weight loss over the past few months, fever, nocturnal symptoms, severe chronic constipation, diarrhea, frequent vomiting, progressive dysphasia, a history of travel to areas of parasitic infections, family history of colon cancer, inflammatory bowel disease; not having cough (bronchitis) during the last 3 months; no problems in speaking or listening; Iranian; not taking any prescription medication (except allergy medications and occasional pain medications) for at least 3 months before entering the study; having two of the following Rotterdam diagnostic criteria:

1) Polycystic ovaries visualized on ultrasound scan (presence of 12 follicles or more in one or both ovaries and/or increased ovarian volume i.e., > 10 ml),
2) Clinical signs of hyperandrogenism (hirsutism score based on hirsutism score greater than 7 or obvious acne),
3) having an interval between menstrual periods > 35 days and/or amenorrhea, defined as the absence of vaginal bleeding for at least 6 months (i.e. 199 days).

The women were requested to complete the study measures in clinic.

Measures

1. Menstrual history: all women were asked for the interval between menstrual periods during the preceding 12 months; results were categorized to < 21 days, 21–34 days, 35–60 days (oligomenorrhea), > 199 days (amenorrhea) and variable.
2. BMI: weight and height were calculated by weight/height squared [kg/m2] in all women.
3. Body hair: Clinical assessment of hirsutism in all women was determined using the Ferriman-Gallwey Scoring System (F/G score). Nine body sites (the upper lip, chin, chest, upper back, lower back, upper abdomen, lower abdomen, arm, and thigh) were graded from 0 (no terminal hair) to 4 (severe hirsutism). Scores can range from zero to 36. A score of seven or above was considered positive for hirsutism [18].
4. Acne: the Global Acne Grading System (GAGS) was used to determine acne in all women. The GAGS assesses six locations on the face and chest/upper back, calculating surface area, distribution, and density of pilosebaceous units of lesions. Each of the six locations is graded separately on a scale 0-to-4, with the most severe lesion within that location determining the local score. The global score is a summation of all local scores [19].
5. Socio-demographic status: The study used years of formal education as a measure of socioeconomic status, categorized into five levels: no education, first level (1 to 5 years), second level (6–9 years), third level (10–12 years) and fourth level (more than 12 years). Donyavi et al., (2011) show that education is a good proxy measure for socioeconomic status for Iranians.
6. Laboratory measures: An overnight or 8 h fasting venous blood sample was obtained from each patient. Follicle-stimulating hormone (FSH) and Luteinizing hormone (LH) were assessed in all participants by ELIZA (DRG Instruments GmbH, Marburg, Germany).
7. ROME III diagnostic criteria: since IBS has no structural disorder or biochemical signs, the diagnosis is based on clinical signs. The ROME III criteria for the diagnosis of IBS (2006) includes intermittent abdominal pain on at least 3 days of the month in the last 3 months with at least two of the following three criteria combined: (i) abdominal pain or discomfort improves with defecation, (ii) abdominal pain or discomfort starts with a change in frequency of defecation, (iii) abdominal pain or discomfort start with a change in stool consistency (appearance). It should be noted that the above criteria must be present in the last 3 months before

the diagnosis, as well as at least last 6 months from the onset of symptoms. The validity and reliability of these tools are approved in Iran [20].

8. IBS-QOL questionnaire was designed by Patrick, et al., (1998) and contains 34 items with a five degree Likert scale. There are eight domains: dysphoria, relationships, sexual concern, health worry, social reaction, body image, food avoidance, and interference with activity. Scores were between 0 to 100; a higher score in this tool represents a worse quality of life [21]. The validity and reliability of these tools are approved in Iran.

9. Bristol scale stool consistency: Bristol stool form scale is a medical aid designed to classify the form of human feces into seven categories including type 1: Separate hard lumps, like nuts (hard to pass); type 2: sausage-shaped, but lumpy; type 3: like a sausage but with cracks on its surface; type 4: like a sausage or snake, smooth and soft; type 5: soft blobs with clear cut edges (passed easily); type 6: fluffy pieces with ragged edges, a mushy stool; type 7: watery, no solid pieces, entirely liquid. Types one and two indicate constipation, with three and four being the ideal stools (especially the latter), as they are easy to defecate while not containing excess liquid, and five, six and seven tending towards diarrhea [22].

Statistical analysis

Data were presented as mean ± Standard Deviation (SD) and frequency (percent) for quantitative and qualitative variables, respectively. Pearson Chi square test was used to compare demographic variables in the two groups. Ordinal demographic variables were compared between the two groups using the Mann-Whitney U test. Independent samples t-test was used to compare the means of in two groups.

Results

The study sample

Over a period of 6 months, 201 women were recruited to the study. The socioeconomic and clinical characteristics of patients are presented in Table 1. There was a significant difference between the two groups in terms of PCOS related features (such as acne, hirsutism and menstrual pattern and LH/FSH ratio) ($P < 0.001$).

IBS subtype & stool frequency

IBS cases in women with PCOS was 29.7% and the control group 11% ($P < 0.01$). The highest number of PCOS women placed in subtype of IBS – Constipation (20.8). According to Bristol stool consistency scale, women were in 2 rd and 3rd rank (sausage-shaped, but lumpy; and like a sausage but with cracks on its surface, respectively) that matches with IBS-Constipation relatively (Table 2).

Table 1 Socio-demographic & clinical characteristics in patients

	PCOS (n = 101)	Control (n = 100)	P value
Age (year)	28 ± 4.92	29.68 ± 5.36	0.02
Education (year)	11.74 ± 3.53	10.77 ± 3.84	0.06
BMI	25.52 ± 4.70	24.53 ± 3.88	0.1
Occupation			
Occupied	18	19	0.82
Housewife	83	81	
Parity	0.16 ± 0.42	0.15 ± 0.35	0.74
Menstruation			
< 21	2 (1.98)	2 (2)	< 0.001
21–35	34 (33.66)	79 (79)	
35–60	17 (16.83)	6 (6)	
> 3 month	7 (6.93)	1 (1)	
Variable	41 (40.59)	12 (12)	
Hirsutism score	3.35 ± 3.15	0.58 ± 1.39	< 0.001
Acne score	4.20 ± 5.01	1.76 ± 3.8	< 0.001
LH/FSH	1.88 ± 1.52	0.93 ± 1.21	< 0.001

Comparison of sum scores of IBSQOL

There was significant difference in QOL scores between two groups ($P < 0.001$) mainly in food avoidance and worries about health (Table 3). In other word, in PCOS

Table 2 IBS subtype and bristol scale stool consistency in patients

	PCOS (n = 101)	Control (n = 100)	P value
IBS subtype			
No IBS	71 (70.3)	89 (89)	0.002
IBS-C	21 (20.8)	5 (5)	
IBS-D	4 (4)	2 (2)	
IBS-M	5 (5)	4 (4)	
Bristol scale stool consistency			
0	71 (70.3)	89 (89)	< 0.001
1	4 (4)	2 (2)	
2	7 (6.9)	3 (3)	
3	10 (9.9)	3 (3)	
4	5 (5)	1 (1)	
5	2 (2)	1 (1)	
6	2 (2)	1 (1)	
7	–	–	

Table 3 comparison the IBS-QOL scores in patients

	PCOS ($n = 101$)		Control ($n = 100$)		*P* value[b]
	IBS	No IBS	IBS	No IBS	
Overall	60.71 ± 13.30	99.46 ± 2.98	74.13 ± 20.92	98.40 ± 6.02	< 0.001
P value[a]	< 0.001		< 0.001		
Dysphoria	61.30 ± 13.94	99.64 ± 2.96	75.94 ± 2.77	99.39 ± 6.04	< 0.001
P value	< 0.001		< 0.001		
Interference with activity	60.83 ± 12.96	99.64 ± 2.96	74.02 ± 20.70	98.35 ± 6.16	< 0.001
P value	< 0.001		< 0.001		
Relationship	61.38 ± 12.58	99.64 ± 2.96	75 ± 23.27	98.04 ± 6	< 0.001
P value	< 0.001		< 0.001		
Sexual	61.66 ± 14.28	99.64 ± 2.96	76.13 ± 12.97	98.31 ± 6.30	< 0.001
P value	< 0.001		< 0.001		
Health worry	60.05 ± 13.79	99.64 ± 2.98	73.48 ± 21.02	98.59 ± 5.78	< 0.001
P value	< 0.001		< 0.001		
Food avoidance	59.72 ± 13.80	99.64 ± 2.96	70.45 ± 21.20	98.31 ± 6.30	< 0.001
P value	< 0.001		< 0.001		
Social reaction	61.85 ± 13.36	99.64 ± 2.96	75 ± 21.83	98.52 ± 5.80	< 0.001
P value	< 0.001		< 0.001		
Body image	61.66 ± 13.90	99.64 ± 2.96	73.29 ± 20.17	98.31 ± 6.30	< 0.001
P value	< 0.001		< 0.001		

[a]Between IBS and no IBS in PCOS / control groups, separately
[b]Between PCOS and control groups with IBS

patients the lowest scores of QOL were belong to IBS subgroup. Similarly, in control group the lowest scores of QOL were belong to IBS subgroup. Moreover, the IBS+ PCOS patients had lower QOL scores than IBS+ non PCOS patients.

Discussion

In this study, IBS cases in patients with PCOS (29.7%) by using Rome III criteria is higher than the values reported in the general population. Mathur et al. (2010) have also reported the IBS prevalence 41.7% by criteria Rome I in women with PCOS. Several studies in Iran have also reported the prevalence of IBS in different populations. The prevalence of IBS in Iranian blood donors was 5.6% [23]. The prevalence of IBS in 18,180 people in five cities in Tehran province was estimated to be about 1% by employing Rome III criteria [24]. Several issues may contribute to such the wide range reported in these studies which use different diagnostic criteria for IBS. Rome III is less restrictive then Rome II which demands patients to report their symptoms over longer periods. Compared to Rome III, a higher number of patients self diagnose with IBS using Rome II. Therefore, it's seemed that the prevalence estimated by Rome III is lower than Rome II and I [25]. proposes using Rome III criteria in studies. Moreover, the role of socioeconomic status and cultural differences should be taken into account. Ho et al., 1998 suggested that the IBS in the urban group more than rural probably because the urban group reported a significantly greater influence of stress than the rural group. It is believed that the prevalence of IBS is less in developing countries (like Iran) compared to western countries [26, 27].

Increased levels of ovarian hormones decrease gastrointestinal transit [28]. Therefore women with IBS report the symptoms related to constipation more than men, except at the time of menstruation when hormone levels have reduced [29]. In the present study, the majority of patients with PCOS (20.8%) have IBS dominant constipation (IBS-C). It seems the cause of this variant of IBS is due to the high levels of hormones in PCOS which interference with bowel function. However, if only the hyper-androgenic condition is involved in the increased risk of IBS, it might be expected that IBS cases in the PCOS group should be less than the control groups.

Stress can affect the gastrointestinal function, so that the start and the severity of the symptoms of IBS are related to acute and chronic stress. Therefore, patients with IBS have hyperactivity to stress (excessive response of limbic system to the stress) [30]. A history of adverse life events and stress cause changes in the hypothalamic–pituitary–adrenal axis response to stress and inappropriate signaling of Corticotropin-releasing hormone as the most important factor in the increased prevalence of IBS [31]. Previous studies have reported that women with PCOS have more anxiety and stress which may cause a higher prevalence of IBS in these patients [32]. In addition to PCOS, an increase in the amount of LH/FSH was also an important predictor variable of IBS. In women with PCOS, the LH/FSH ratio was higher and it seems that an increase the perceived stress by patients may lead to increased sensitivity of the hypothalamic–pituitary–adrenal axis and LH and consequently a higher prevalence of IBS in these patients. Use of gonadotropin releasing hormone analogue leuprolide acetate which dramatically decreases LH which would be improves of chronic abdominal pain in women [33]..

IBS has a strong effect on the quality of life in women are diagnosed with it as it imposes substantial social and economic costs due to the need for medical care and absenteeism at work. One study in Iran investigated the economic burden of IBS and showed the cost of IBS in Iran about 2.8 million dollars and this is of great significant for Iranian population [34].

There are no specific biomarkers to assess the condition of patients with IBS. Thus there needs to be increased attention to the non-pathological markers in evaluating the impact of IBS as a chronic disease on well being, daily functioning and QOL. According Frank et al., 2002) patients with IBS have poor QOL compared to the general population; the same authors emphasize that IBS has a greater negative impact on QOL than asthma, gastroesophageal reflux disease (GERD) or migraine headaches. In the present study, QOL in women with IBS in both groups was significantly lower than in women without IBS. In both groups, worries about health and food avoidance were the areas of QOL most affected by IBS. Sung Kim et al. (2010) reported that the most affected areas were dysphonia, worries about health and the food avoidance [35]. These findings suggests that in our patients like Korean female with IBS, IBS patients suffer more from anxiety about their disease than impairment of social activity or relationship by bowel symptom.

Studies on women with PCOS using an IBS specific QOL tools have not been found identified in the literature; our study is the first to use IBS specific QOL measures in women with PCOS compared to healthy women. Studies using SF36 [36] and WHOQOL [37] to measure QOL minimize the influence of gastrointestinal symptoms on general QOL. Specific QOL tools associated with IBS have been designed and validated and include specific areas associated with QOL most affected by IBS.

Limitations

There are some limitations in our study. The study population is from a limited region of Iran and is not be representative of the general population either in Iran or other countries. Moreover, there are unmeasured covariates that may play an important role in the association between IBS and PCOS, for example, psychological history; that IBS was self-indentified may be another limitation.

Conclusion

As the results of this study show, having PCOS and an increased level of LH/FSH might cause IBS. IBS + PCOS patients experience significant effects on QOL particularly in relation to worries about health and food avoidance. These data offer insights for clinicians into IBS in women with PCOS and their functional status and wellbeing.

Abbreviations

QOL: Quality of life; IBS : Irritable bowel syndrome; PCOS: Polycystic ovary syndrome; BMI: Body mass index; GAGS: Global Acne Grading System; FSH: Follicle-stimulating hormone; LH: Luteinizing hormone

Acknowledgements

Not Applicable.

Authors' contributions

FB and MA contributed in conception, design and drafting of the manuscript. FB,SAT,ZA,HA,SKH,TS,SHP,FZ,SGH,Zk and MA contributed in data collection. FB,SAT and MA contributed in manuscript drafting. All authors approved the final version for submission. FB oversaw the study.

Author details

Social Determinants of Health Research Center, Yasuj University of Medical Sciences, Yasuj, Iran. [2]Medicinal Plants Research Center, Yasuj University of Medical Sciences, Yasuj, Iran. [3]Research Center for Biochemistry and Nutrition in Metabolic Diseases, Institute for Basic Sciences, Kashan University of Medical Sciences, Kashan, IR, Iran. [4]Centre for Critical Research in Nursing & Midwifery, School of Health & Education, Middlesex University, London, UK. Infertility Clinic, Omeleila Hospital, Bandar Abbas, Hormozgan, Iran. [6]Student Research Committee, Hormozgan University of Medical Sciences, Bandar Abbas, Iran. [7]Fertility and Infertility Research Center, Hormozgan University of Medical Sciences, Bandar Abbas, Iran.

References

1. Agrawal A, Whorwell PJ. Irritable bowel syndrome: diagnosis and management. BMJ (Clinical research ed). 2006;332(7536):280–3 Epub 2006/02/04.
2. Brandt LJ, Chey WD, Foxx-Orenstein AE, Schiller LR, Schoenfeld PS, Spiegel BM, et al. An evidence-based position statement on the management of irritable bowel syndrome. Am J Gastroenterol. 2009;104(Suppl 1):S1–35 Epub 2009/06/19.
3. Lea R, Whorwell PJ. Quality of life in irritable bowel syndrome. PharmacoEconomics. 2001;19(6):643–53 Epub 2001/07/18.
4. Brun-Strang C, Dapoigny M, Lafuma A, Wainsten JP, Fagnani F. Irritable bowel syndrome in France: quality of life, medical management, and costs: the Encoli study. Eur J Gastroenterol Hepatol. 2007;19(12):1097–103 Epub 2007/11/14.
5. Wilson A, Longstreth GF, Knight K, Wong J, Wade S, Chiou CF, et al. Quality of life in managed care patients with irritable bowel syndrome. Manag Care Interface. 2004;17(2):24–8 34. Epub 2004/03/25.
6. Frank L, Kleinman L, Rentz A, Ciesla G, Kim JJ, Zacker C. Health-related quality of life associated with irritable bowel syndrome: comparison with other chronic diseases. Clin Ther. 2002;24(4):675–89 discussion 4. Epub 2002/05/23.

7. Mathur R, Ko A, Hwang LJ, Low K, Azziz R, Pimentel M. Polycystic ovary syndrome is associated with an increased prevalence of irritable bowel syndrome. Dig Dis Sci. 2010;55(4):1085–9.
8. Mason H, Colao A, Blume-Peytavi U, Rice S, Qureshi A, Pellatt L, et al. Polycystic ovary syndrome (PCOS) trilogy: a translational and clinical review. Clin Endocrinol. 2008;69(6):831–44 Epub 2008/07/12.
9. Douchi T, Yamamoto S, Oki T, Maruta K, Kuwahata R, Nagata Y. Serum androgen levels and muscle mass in women with polycystic ovary syndrome. Obstet Gynecol. 1999;94(3):337–40 Epub 1999/09/03.
10. Bazarganipour F, Ziaei S, Montazeri A, Foroozanfard F, Kazemnejad A, Faghihzadeh S. Sexual functioning among married Iranian women with polycystic ovary syndrome. Int J Fertil Steril. 2014;8(3):273–80 Epub 2014 Nov 1.
11. Bazarganipour F, Ziaei S, Montazeri A, Foroozanfard F, Faghihzadeh S. Iranian version of modified polycystic ovary syndrome health-related quality of life questionnaire: discriminant and convergent validity. Iran J Reprod Med. 2013;11(9):753–60.
12. Bazarganipour F, Ziaei S, Montazeri A, Foroozanfard F, Faghihzadeh S. Health-related quality of life and its relationship with clinical symptoms among Iranian patients with polycystic ovarian syndrome. Iran J Reprod Med. 2013;11(5):371–8.
13. Bazarganipour F, Ziaei S, Montazeri A, Foroozanfard F, Kazemnejad A, Faghihzadeh S. Body image satisfaction and self-esteem status among the patients with polycystic ovary syndrome. Iran J Reprod Med. 2013;11(10): 829–36.
14. Bazarganipour F, Ziaei S, Montazeri A, Foroozanfard F, Kazemnejad A, Faghihzadeh S. Health-related quality of life in patients with polycystic ovary syndrome (PCOS): a model-based study of predictive factors. J Sex Med. 2014;11(4):1023–32. https://doi.org/10.1111/jsm.12405 Epub 2013 Dec 6.
15. Bazarganipour F, Ziaei S, Montazeri A, Foroozanfard F, Kazemnejad A, Faghihzadeh S. Psychological investigation in patients with polycystic ovary syndrome. Health Qual Life Outcomes. 2013;11:141. https://doi.org/10.1186/477-7525-11-141.
16. Bazarganipour F, Ziaei S, Montazeri A, Foroozanfard F, Kazemnejad A, Faghihzadeh S. Predictive factors of health-related quality of life in patients with polycystic ovary syndrome: a structural equation modeling approach. Fertil Steril. 2013;100(5):1389–96. https://doi.org/10.1016/j.fertnstert.2013.06.043 Epub Jul 25.
17. Bazarganipour F, Ziaei S, Montazeri A, Faghihzadeh S, Frozanfard F. Psychometric properties of the Iranian version of modified polycystic ovary syndrome health-related quality-of-life questionnaire. Hum Reprod. 2012; 27(9):2729–36. https://doi.org/10.1093/humrep/des199 Epub 2012 Jun 26.
18. Ferriman D, Gallwey JD. Clinical assessment of body hair growth in women. J Clin Endocrinol Metab. 1961;21:1440–7 Epub 1961/11/01.
19. Lever WF, Schaumburg-Lever G. Acne vulgaris. Histopatbology of the Skin. 7th edn Philadelphia. JB Lippincott. 1990;218:9.
20. Drossman DA, Dumitrascu DL. Rome III: New standard for functional gastrointestinal disorders. J Gastrointestinal Liver Dis. 2006;15(3):237–41 Epub 2006/10/03.
21. Patrick DL, Drossman DA. Re: Groll et al.--Comparison of IBS-36 and IBS-QOL instruments. Am J Gastroenterol. 2002;97(12):3204 author reply –5. Epub 2002/12/21.
22. Lewis SJ, Heaton KW. Stool form scale as a useful guide to intestinal transit time. Scand J Gastroenterol. 1997;32(9):920–4 Epub 1997/09/23.
23. Hatami K, Pourshams A, Azimi K, Sarrafi M, Mehrabani M, Mostajabi P, et al. Dyspepsia, gastroesophageal reflux disease and irritable bowel syndrome among blood donors. Govaresh. 2003;8(4):138–46.
24. Sorouri M, Pourhoseingholi MA, Vahedi M, Safaee A, Moghimi-Dehkordi B, Pourhoseingholi A, et al. Functional bowel disorders in Iranian population using Rome III criteria. Saudi J Gastroenterol. 2010;16(3):154–60 Epub 2010/07/10.
25. Shen L, Kong H, Hou X. Prevalence of irritable bowel syndrome and its relationship with psychological stress status in Chinese university students. J Gastroenterol Hepatol. 2009;24(12):1885–90 Epub 2009/09/29.
26. Danivat D, Tankeyoon M, Sriratanaban A. Prevalence of irritable bowel syndrome in a non-Western population. British Medical J (Clinical research ed). 1988;296(6638):1710 Epub 1988/06/18.
27. Ho KY, Kang JY, Seow A. Prevalence of gastrointestinal symptoms in a multiracial Asian population, with particular reference to reflux-type symptoms. Am J Gastroenterol. 1998;93(10):1816 22 Epub 1998/10/15.
28. Heitkemper M, Jarrett M, Bond EF, Chang L. Impact of sex and gender on irritable bowel syndrome. Biological Res Nurs. 2003;5(1):56–65 Epub 2003/07/31.
29. Lee OY, Mayer EA, Schmulson M, Chang L, Naliboff B. Gender-related differences in IBS symptoms. Am J Gastroenterol. 2001;96(7):2184–93.
30. Chang L, Heitkemper MM. Gender differences in irritable bowel syndrome. Gastroenterology. 2002;123(5):1686–701.
31. Whitehead WE, Crowell MD, Robinson JC, Heller BR, Schuster MM. Effects of stressful life events on bowel symptoms: subjects with irritable bowel syndrome compared with subjects without bowel dysfunction. Gut. 1992; 33(6):825–30 Epub 1992/06/01.
32. Himelein MJ, Thatcher SS. Polycystic ovary syndrome and mental health: a review. Obstet Gynecol Surv. 2006;61(11):723–32 Epub 2006/10/19.
33. Palomba S, Orio F Jr, Manguso F, Russo T, Falbo A, Lombardi G, et al. Leuprolide acetate treatment with and without coadministration of tibolone in premenopausal women with menstrual cycle-related irritable bowel syndrome. Fertil Steril. 2005;83(4):1012–20 Epub 2005/04/12.
34. Roshandel D, Rezailashkajani M, Shafaee S, Zali MR. A cost analysis of functional bowel disorders in Iran. Int J Color Dis. 2007;22(7):791–9 Epub 2006/10/26.
35. Kim YS, Choi SC, Park JM, Choi CH, Lee DH, Son HJ, et al. The effect of tegaserod on symptoms and quality of life in korean women with irritable bowel syndrome with constipation. J Neurogastroenterol Motil. 2010;16(1): 61–70 Epub 2010/06/11.
36. Icks A, Haastert B, Enck P, Rathmann W, Giani G. Health-related quality of life in subjects with functional bowel disorders in Germany. Zeitschrift fur Gastroenterologie. 2002;40(10):863–7 Epub 2002/11/19.
37. Jamali R, Biglari M. The comparison of WHOQOL-BREF with disease specific heath related quality of life questionnaire in irritable bowel syndrome. Acta medica Iranica. 2015;53(11):717–24 Epub 2016/01/21.

22

Multi-omics profiles of the intestinal microbiome in irritable bowel syndrome and its bowel habit subtypes

Jonathan P. Jacobs[1,2,3*], Venu Lagishetty[1], Megan C. Hauer[1], Jennifer S. Labus[1,2], Tien S. Dong[1,3], Ryan Toma[4], Momchilo Vuyisich[4], Bruce D. Naliboff[1,2], Jeffrey M. Lackner[5], Arpana Gupta[1,2], Kirsten Tillisch[1,2,6] and Emeran A. Mayer[1,2*]

Abstract

Background Irritable bowel syndrome (IBS) is a common gastrointestinal disorder that is thought to involve alterations in the gut microbiome, but robust microbial signatures have been challenging to identify. As prior studies have primarily focused on composition, we hypothesized that multi-omics assessment of microbial function incorporating both metatranscriptomics and metabolomics would further delineate microbial profiles of IBS and its subtypes.

Methods Fecal samples were collected from a racially/ethnically diverse cohort of 495 subjects, including 318 IBS patients and 177 healthy controls, for analysis by 16S rRNA gene sequencing ($n = 486$), metatranscriptomics ($n = 327$), and untargeted metabolomics ($n = 368$). Differentially abundant microbes, predicted genes, transcripts, and metabolites in IBS were identified by multivariate models incorporating age, sex, race/ethnicity, BMI, diet, and HAD-Anxiety. Inter-omic functional relationships were assessed by transcript/gene ratios and microbial metabolic modeling. Differential features were used to construct random forests classifiers.

Results IBS was associated with global alterations in microbiome composition by 16S rRNA sequencing and metatranscriptomics, and in microbiome function by predicted metagenomics, metatranscriptomics, and metabolomics. After adjusting for age, sex, race/ethnicity, BMI, diet, and anxiety, IBS was associated with differential abundance of bacterial taxa such as *Bacteroides dorei*; metabolites including increased tyramine and decreased gentisate and hydrocinnamate; and transcripts related to fructooligosaccharide and polyol utilization. IBS further showed transcriptional upregulation of enzymes involved in fructose and glucan metabolism as well as the succinate pathway of carbohydrate fermentation. A multi-omics classifier for IBS had significantly higher accuracy (AUC 0.82) than classifiers using individual datasets. Diarrhea-predominant IBS (IBS-D) demonstrated shifts in the metatranscriptome and metabolome including increased bile acids, polyamines, succinate pathway intermediates (malate, fumarate), and transcripts involved in fructose, mannose, and polyol metabolism compared to constipation-predominant IBS (IBS-C). A classifier incorporating metabolites and gene-normalized transcripts differentiated IBS-D from IBS-C with high accuracy (AUC 0.86).

*Correspondence:
Jonathan P. Jacobs
JJacobs@mednet.ucla.edu
Emeran A. Mayer
emayer@ucla.edu
Full list of author information is available at the end of the article

Conclusions IBS is characterized by a multi-omics microbial signature indicating increased capacity to utilize fermentable carbohydrates—consistent with the clinical benefit of diets restricting this energy source—that also includes multiple previously unrecognized metabolites and metabolic pathways. These findings support the need for integrative assessment of microbial function to investigate the microbiome in IBS and identify novel microbiome-related therapeutic targets.

Keywords: Irritable bowel syndrome, Bowel habit subtypes, Microbiome, Multi-omics, Metatranscriptomics, Metabolomics, Biomarkers

Introduction

Irritable bowel syndrome (IBS) is the most common gastrointestinal disorder, affecting 10–15% of the USA population [1]. IBS is currently defined by symptom criteria, including recurrent abdominal pain associated with altered bowel habits in the absence of detectable anatomic, inflammatory, or biochemical pathology [2]. There has been considerable interest in the role of the gut microbiome in IBS. This is supported by the development of IBS symptoms following gastrointestinal infections in some patients, the relationship of IBS symptomatology with diet, and effects of GI microbiota on intestinal motility and visceral sensitivity [3]. Moreover, microbiota transfer from IBS patients into rodents has been reported to confer alterations in intestinal transit and visceral sensitivity to recipient animals [4, 5].

Despite a strong scientific rationale and gastrointestinal symptom improvements following interventions believed to act via the microbiome including rifaximin and FODMAPS diet, existing human microbiome association studies have shown mixed results. Large studies of microbiome composition by 16S rRNA gene sequencing or shotgun metagenomics have in some cases shown minimal diversity change and taxonomic associations with IBS, while others have reported reduced diversity and taxonomic shifts that were not consistent across studies [6–10]. Recent studies have shifted to focus on functional characterization of the microbiome by shotgun metagenomics, which assesses functional potential by microbial gene content, or metabolomics, which assesses products of bacterial metabolism detected in feces [7, 11–16]. While these studies have reported significant shifts in gene content and metabolites, the specific features have not been consistent across studies. Overall, no robust compositional or functional microbiome signature has emerged for IBS diagnosis, unlike other gastrointestinal conditions such as inflammatory bowel disease [17]. This likely reflects variability in clinical definitions of IBS, demographic heterogeneity across studies, confounding factors that influence the microbiome, differences among phenotypic subsets of IBS (with some studies arguing that only certain bowel habit subtypes show differences compared to controls), and challenges of inferring bacterial metabolism from bacterial gene content or fecal metabolite measurements alone.

To provide further insight into the functional properties of gut microbes in IBS, we assembled a diverse, well-phenotyped cross-sectional cohort of 318 IBS patients and 177 healthy controls for multi-omics analysis of the gut microbiome. This encompassed compositional assessment by 16S rRNA gene sequencing and functional assessment by a combination of metatranscriptomics and fecal metabolomics. We found that IBS could be robustly distinguished from healthy controls by a functional signature derived from differential bacterial transcripts and microbiome-associated metabolites after adjusting for multiple covariates influencing the microbiome, and that IBS bowel habit subtypes were similarly distinguished by multi-omics functional signatures.

Methods

Participants

Two hundred seventy-five IBS patients and 177 healthy controls were recruited from the Los Angeles area by community advertisement and an additional 43 IBS patients were recruited from the Buffalo area for a study of cognitive behavioral therapy [18]. IBS patients were eligible if they were over age 18 and diagnosed with IBS via Rome III criteria [19]. Potential participants were excluded if they had accompanying organic GI disease that could contribute to presenting IBS symptoms, malignancy in the past 5 years, body mass index (BMI) greater than 35, reported a gastrointestinal infection within 2 weeks before evaluation, or used a gut-sensitive antibiotic during the 12 weeks prior to evaluation. Participants were asked to provide a fecal sample and complete demographic and medical questionnaires. Dietary pattern was assessed using our previously validated dietary pattern form [20]. Psychological and symptom instruments included Hospital Anxiety and Depression (HAD), State-Trait Anxiety Inventory (STAI), Visceral Sensitivity Index (VSI)—a measure of gastrointestinal symptom-specific anxiety, and Pennebaker Inventory of Limbic Languidness (PILL)—an assessment of frequency of stress-sensitive somatic complaints. The IBS Symptom Severity Scale (IBS-SSS) was used to measure IBS symptom severity including pain, distention, bowel dysfunction, and quality of life [21]. This study was approved by the Institutional Review Boards at UCLA and the University at Buffalo.

Fresh frozen fecal sample collection

Participants were provided with home stool collection kits and asked to store their stool samples in a freezer immediately after collection until they could either be dropped off to a study coordinator or picked up by a courier service within 24–48 h of collection. Study coordinators then transferred samples to lab freezers for long-term storage at − 80°C. Frozen fecal samples were later ground into a coarse powder by mortar and pestle under liquid nitrogen then aliquoted.

Fecal 16S rRNA gene sequencing

DNA extraction by bead beating and amplification of the V4 hypervariable region of the 16S rRNA gene were performed according to our published protocol [22, 23]. Sequencing libraries underwent 2 × 150 or 2 × 250 sequencing on Illumina HiSeq 2500 to a mean depth of 67,801 merged sequences per sample. Samples in each of two sequencing batches (292 and 195 samples) were separately processed using the DADA2 R package to generate tables of denoised amplicon sequence variants (ASVs) which were then merged [24]. Taxonomy was assigned to the 11,429 ASVs using the SILVA 138.1 database. The final ASV table was inputted into PICRUSt2 to predict abundances of bacterial gene families annotated as KEGG orthologs (KOs) based on nearest reference genomes to 16S sequences [25, 26].

Fecal metatranscriptomics

Fecal aliquots were sent to Viome Life Sciences, Inc., for RNA extraction, metatranscriptomics sequencing, and annotation as previously described [27]. In brief, RNA extraction by bead beading was performed, DNA degraded by DNase, and 16S/23S ribosomal RNA depleted by subtractive hybridization. Sequencing libraries were prepared from the resulting RNA and underwent 150 × 2 paired-end sequencing on Illumina NovaSeq. Taxonomy was assigned by aligning sequencing reads to a precomputed database of unique k-mers; 898 taxa were identified, including bacteria, fungi, viruses, and bacteriophages. Functional annotation was performed by aligning sequencing reads to the integrated gene catalog from the MetaHIT consortium then mapping these genes to the KEGG database; 5896 distinct transcripts annotated as KOs were identified [28].

Fecal metabolomics

Fecal aliquots were shipped to Metabolon, Inc., for analysis on their global HD4 metabolomics platform. Samples were run in three batches; the largest contained 250 samples and additional batches included 75 and 43 samples. Compounds were identified by comparison of spectral features to Metabolon's proprietary library, which includes MS/MS spectral data on more than 3300 purified standards. Within each batch, features were retained that were detected in over 30% of samples. Imputation of missing data was performed separately for each batch using a k-nearest neighbor algorithm (kNN, k = 10) as previously described for Metabolon datasets [29]. The three batches were then combined using reference-based ComBat implemented in the sva package in R with the largest batch used as a reference and IBS vs. HC as a covariate; only the 601 metabolites with greater than 30% detection rate in all three batches were retained [30–32]. Metabolomics data subsequently underwent log2 transformation and normalization by the vsn2 package in R prior to downstream analyses [33].

Alpha and beta diversity analyses

Microbial alpha diversity was assessed on unfiltered 16S data (rarefied to 10,000 sequences/sample) and metatranscriptomics taxonomy data using the Shannon index of richness and evenness calculated with the phyloseq package in R [34]. Significance was assessed by the Mann-Whitney U test and multivariate ANOVA using the aov function in R with sex, age, race, BMI, diet category, and HAD-Anxiety as covariates. Beta diversity analysis was performed on all five datasets including 16S composition, predicted metagenome, metatranscriptome taxonomy, metatranscriptome KO, and metabolome. Bray-Curtis dissimilarity was applied for all datasets except metabolomics, for which Euclidean distance was used since it is not a compositional dataset. In each case, datasets were filtered to remove features present in less than 10% of samples, leaving 228 ASVs, 5370 predicted genes, 269 metatranscriptomics taxa, 3837 transcripts, and 601 metabolites. Constrained ordination of these distance matrices was performed using distance-based redundancy analysis (dbRDA) implemented with the capscale function of vegan in R [35]. Models for dbRDA included sex, age, race/ethnicity (African-American, Asian, Hispanic, non-Hispanic white, multiracial), BMI, diet category (standard, restrictive, other), HAD-Anxiety, batch (sequencing or metabolomics), and IBS group. Missing HAD and dietary pattern data were imputed by kNN using the VIM package in R for use as covariates in these and other multivariate models. Visualization of categorical and continuous variables on the first two constrained axes of dbRDA ordination was performed using the envfit function of vegan. The significance of differences in beta diversity was assessed using permutational multivariate analysis of variance (PERMANOVA) implemented with the adonis2 function of vegan with 10,000 permutations

[36]. Univariate models included IBS group or one of the covariates and batch (sequencing or metabolomics); multivariate models also included sex, age, race, BMI, diet category, and HAD-Anxiety. Adonis2 was run by "margin," which calculates the marginal R^2 for each variable after adjusting for the other variables in the model (i.e., running separate models for each variable in which it is ordered last).

Differential abundance testing

Differentially abundant microbes, genes, transcripts, and metabolites were identified using multivariate general linear models implemented in MaAsLin2 [37]. Sequencing data underwent total sum scaling to generate relative abundances which were log-transformed prior to model fitting. Normalized, log-transformed metabolomics data did not undergo further transformation. All datasets were filtered to retain features present in > 10% of samples. *P* alues were adjusted for multiple hypothesis testing by the Benjamini-Hochberg method to generate *q* values. Significance was set at $q < 0.25$ for all analyses as is recommended for MaAsLin2 [37]. Functional annotations were made using KEGG pathway assignments and metabolite categories provided by Metabolon.

Inter-omic comparisons

Global comparison of datasets was performed by applying the Mantel test to distance matrices of Bray-Curtis dissimilarity (or Euclidean distance for metabolomics) using vegan in R. The resulting Mantel r was calculated using Spearman correlation, with significance determined by 10,000 permutations. Visualization of global similarities across datasets was performed by rotating then superimposing one dbRDA ordination onto another using Procrustes in vegan.

Comparison of RNA vs. DNA taxonomic representation was performed at the genus level to maximize matching of taxa between the metatranscriptome and 16S data given the limitations of taxonomic resolution with 16S rRNA gene sequencing. For each genus, ratios of relative abundances were calculated for samples in which there was non-zero abundance in both the 16S and metatranscriptomics data; if a genus was not detected in one dataset, no ratio was calculated. The same strategy was used to calculate RNA/DNA ratios comparing transcript relative abundances to predicted gene relative abundances. RNA/DNA ratios for genera and KOs were only further analyzed if the features were detected in > 25% of both DNA and RNA samples. Log-transformed ratios were analyzed by multivariate general linear models in MaAsLin2 to identify statistically significant differences ($q < 0.25$) between IBS and HC in RNA/DNA ratios after adjusting for covariates. This approach has previously been applied to simulated and real fecal datasets and shown to be suitable for differential expression analysis [38]. Missing values were dropped for model fitting in MaAsLin2 and imputed by kNN for input into random forests classifiers.

Pathway enrichment analysis for differentially expressed KOs was performed using Gene Set Enrichment Analysis (GSEA) software [39]. *q* values were used to rank KOs by their strength of association with IBS or IBS bowel habits, and KO assignments to KEGG pathways were inputted as gene sets. Significance was calculated using the classic enrichment statistic, 10,000 permutations, and a threshold of $p < 0.05$.

Identification of metabolites associated with microbial metabolism

Metabolic modeling was performed using MIMOSA2 to estimate the community-wide metabolic output of the metatranscriptome and predicted metagenome as summarized by Community-wide Metabolic Potential (CMP) scores [40, 41]. The scores are a surrogate for the relative capacity of the metagenome or metatranscriptome to produce or deplete the metabolite. MIMOSA2 performs regression of CMP scores for each metabolite with measured levels of that metabolite to identify a subset of metabolites with significant positive association with microbial metabolic potential. The recommended threshold of $p < 0.10$ was used.

Random forests classifiers

Datasets were divided 60%/40% into training and test sets with equivalent proportion of IBS subjects (or BH subtypes) and random forests classifiers were constructed using the caret R package [42]. Differentially abundant features were inputted into the classifiers. Contribution of each feature to classifier accuracy was assessed by variable importance scores, which represent the decrease in classifier accuracy when that variable is permuted. Features were retained in the final model if they had an importance score > 2 in the initial model iteration using training data. The accuracy of the resulting classifiers was determined by calculating the area under the receiver operating characteristic curve (AUC) using test data. Significance of differences in classifier performance was assessed using the bootstrap method of roc.test in the pROC R package.

Results

IBS is associated with shifts in microbial taxa, transcripts, and metabolites

Four hundred ninety-five subjects, including 318 IBS patients and 177 healthy controls (HC), provided fecal samples and completed demographic, dietary, and psychological questionnaires (Table 1). IBS patients and HC did not differ by age (median 30 vs. 29 years old) but a higher proportion of IBS subjects were females (77% vs. 60%). The cohort was racially diverse, with 56% of subjects belonging to a racial/ethnic minority group in the USA. The IBS subjects and HC showed different racial/ethnic composition, with the IBS group having increased proportion of non-Hispanic whites and corresponding reduced proportions of other racial/ethnic groups. There was no statistically significant difference in educational attainment between the two groups, with the majority of subjects being college graduates. Dietary patterns were grouped into one of three categories using a paradigm recently established by our group for IBS studies: standard diet, restrictive diet (which includes gluten-free, lactose-free, and FODMAPS diets), and other (representing dietary patterns considered exclusionary but not in one of the IBS-associated restrictive dietary patterns) [20]. Consistent with our prior findings, IBS patients had increased frequency of restrictive diets—specifically, gluten-free and lactose-free diets (15% vs. 3% and 13% vs. 4%, respectively)—and a corresponding reduction in the frequency of a Standard or Modified American diet (Additional file 1: Table S1). Participants also completed psychological questionnaires including the HAD and STAI, which together measure depression, current anxiety, and trait anxiety, respectively. All three instruments showed elevated scores in IBS compared to HC. As anticipated, IBS patients showed markedly higher scores for visceral sensitivity (VSI) and stress-sensitive somatic complaints (PILL). Approximately equal numbers of IBS patients were diarrhea-predominant (IBS-D, 38%) and constipation-predominant (IBS-C, 35%), and most had moderate (IBS-SSS of 175–300, 49%) or severe (IBS-SSS of 301–500, 27%) symptom severity.

Table 1 Cohort demographics

	HC ($N = 177$)	IBS ($N = 318$)	*P* value
Samples			
16S rRNA sequencing	174	312	
Metatranscriptomics	119	208	
Metabolomics	139	229	
Gender			
Male	40%	23%	**0.00013**
Female	60%	77%	
Age	30 (23–38)	29 (23–41)	0.57
BMI	26.9 (23.4–30.2)	23.4 (21.0–26.0)	$\mathbf{3 \times 10^{-12}}$
Race/ethnicity			
Non-Hispanic white	31%	52%	**0.00016**
Hispanic	25%	20%	
African-American	12%	7%	
Asian	21%	14%	
Multiracial	10%	7%	
Education			
Some high school	1%	1%	0.12
High school grad	7%	6%	
Some college	28%	39%	
College grad	33%	24%	
Any postgrad	31%	30%	
Diet			
Standard	79%	55%	**0.0005**
Restrictive	8%	30%	
Other	13%	15%	
HAD-Anxiety	3 (1–6)	7 (4–10)	$\mathbf{8 \times 10^{-14}}$
HAD-Depression	1 (0–3)	2 (1–5)	$\mathbf{7 \times 10^{-6}}$
STAI Trait Anxiety	32 (26–38)	37 (27–44)	**0.0055**
PILL	4 (2–7)	16 (11–22)	$\mathbf{< 2 \times 10^{-16}}$
VSI	2 (0–8)	40 (28–54)	$\mathbf{< 2 \times 10^{-16}}$
Bowel habit subtype			
IBS-D		38%	
IBS-C		35%	
IBS-M		17%	
IBS-U		9%	
IBS-SSS		241 (184–312)	

Values shown as median (interquartile range); *p* values calculated by the Mann-Whitney *U* test (numerical traits) or Fisher's exact test (categorical traits)

Fecal samples underwent analysis by 16S rRNA gene sequencing ($n = 486$), metatranscriptomics sequencing ($n = 327$), and untargeted global metabolomics ($n = 368$). Microbial composition was assessed by 16S rRNA gene abundances and by taxonomic assignment of sequenced transcripts, which reflects composition weighted by transcriptional activity. Alpha diversity (i.e., within-sample diversity) was compared between IBS and HC using the Shannon index of richness and evenness. Both compositional datasets showed no significant difference in Shannon index by non-parametric tests and multivariate linear models (Fig. 1A). In contrast, beta diversity analysis (i.e., diversity across samples) using Bray-Curtis dissimilarity demonstrated statistically significant differences in composition by 16S rRNA profiles and metatranscriptomics taxonomy between IBS and HC (Fig. 1B). Many covariates were also found to be significantly associated with microbial composition in one or both datasets, including age, sex, race, BMI, dietary category, HAD-Anxiety, and HAD-Depression. Given the strong correlation between anxiety and depression and the greater differential between IBS and HC in HAD-Anxiety, this was selected as a covariate to represent the association of mood with the microbiome. In multivariate analyses adjusting for these covariates, IBS remained significantly associated with microbial composition by 16S rRNA and

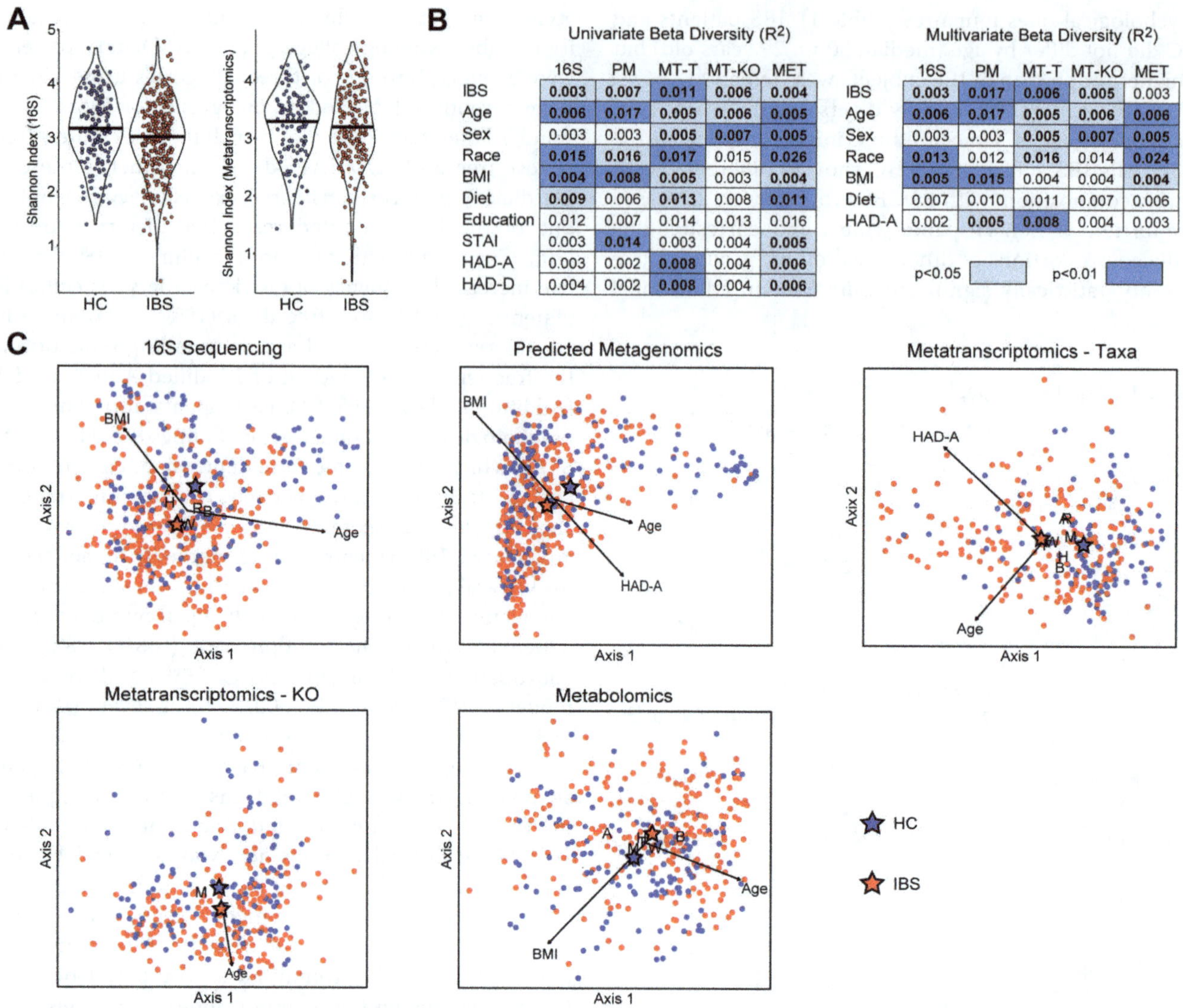

Fig. 1 IBS is associated with global alterations in microbiome composition and function. **A** The Shannon index of microbial richness and evenness in fecal samples from IBS subjects and healthy controls (HC) is shown for 16S rRNA sequencing and metatranscriptomics data. **B** Beta diversity was assessed by Bray-Curtis dissimilarity for 16S rRNA sequence data, predicted metagenomics (PM), metatranscriptomics taxonomy (MT-T), and KEGG orthology transcript annotations (MT-KO). Euclidean distance was used for normalized metabolomics data (MET). Contribution of clinical and demographic traits to variation in these five datasets was determined by R^2 calculated from univariate (left) and multivariate (right) PERMANOVA. R^2 in the multivariate model reflects the remaining explained variance after accounting for the other variables. All PERMANOVA analyses included batch (sequencing or metabolomics) as a covariate. Significance of differences was calculated by permutation and is denoted by color. (**C**) Distance-based redundancy analysis (dbRDA) was performed to visualize variation in beta diversity related to IBS status, age, sex, race/ethnicity, BMI, dietary category, and HAD-Anxiety (HAD-A). IBS group and statistically significant categorical variables are denoted by letters or symbols indicating the centroid for each category. Statistically significant continuous variables are shown as arrows originating from the centroid of all samples, with length proportional to strength of association. F = female, M = male, A = Asian, B = African-American, H = Hispanic, W = non-Hispanic white, R = multiracial

metatranscriptomics sequencing, as did several of the covariates including age and race (Fig. 1B, C).

Multivariate general linear models were then used to identify microbial taxa that significantly differed in IBS compared to HC after adjusting for covariates identified by beta diversity analysis as influencing the microbiome including age, sex, race, BMI, diet, and HAD-Anxiety. IBS was found to be characterized by increased abundance of *Alistipes ihumii*, *Bacteroides dorei*, *Actinomyces odontolyticus*, and multiple members of the Firmicutes phylum such as *Intestinibacter bartlettii* and *Roumboutsia ilealis* (Fig. 2A). IBS showed reduced abundance of *Facealibacterium prausnitzii* and *Bacteroides thetaiotamicron*. When assessing the taxonomic

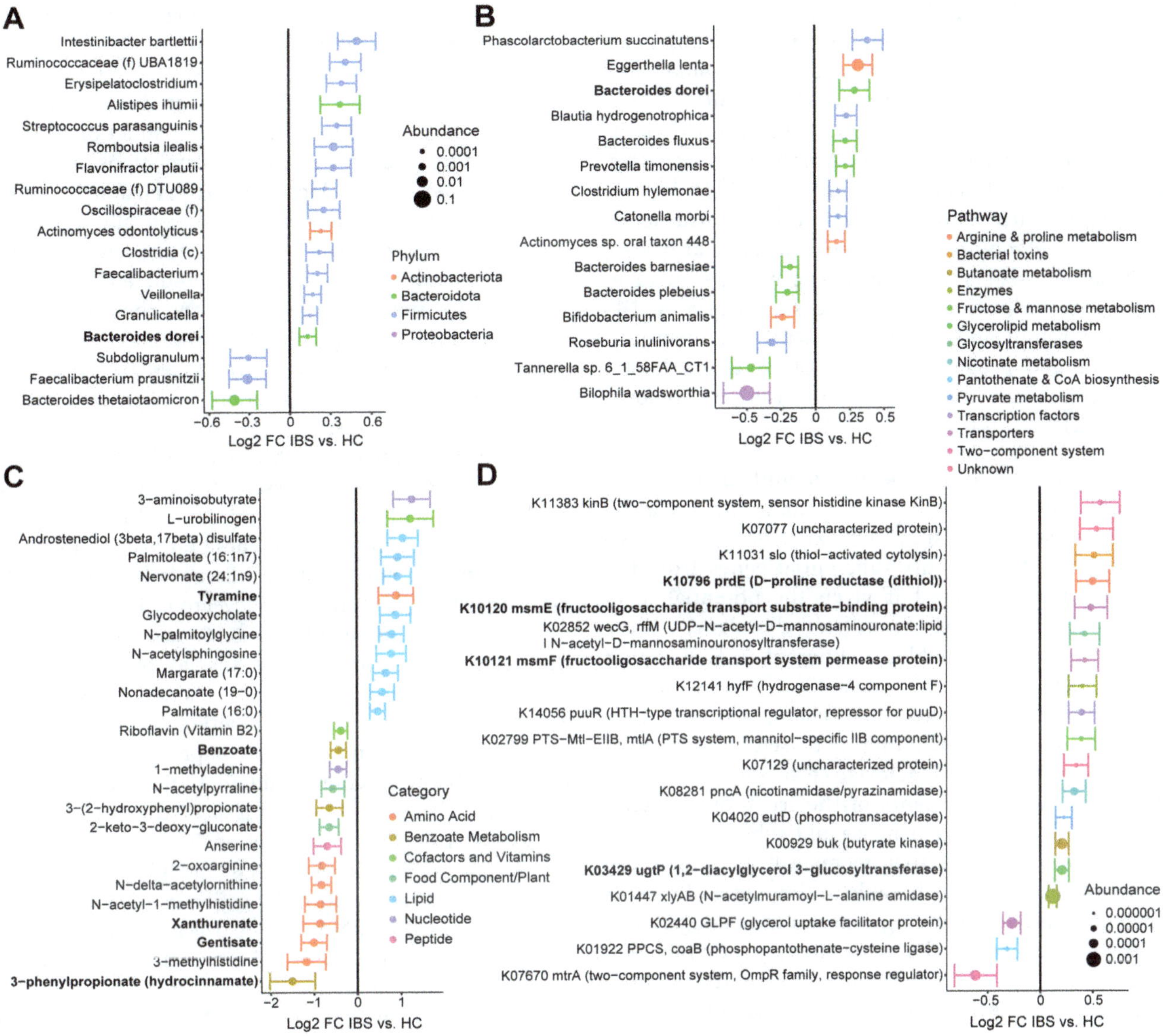

Fig. 2 IBS is characterized by altered abundances of bacterial taxa, metabolites, and transcripts, including for genes involved in fructooligosaccharide utilization. **A, B** Differentially abundant bacterial taxa ($q < 0.25$) between IBS subjects and HC were identified in multivariate models adjusting for batch, age, sex, race/ethnicity, BMI, dietary category, and HAD-A. Results are shown for **A** 16S rRNA sequence data ($n = 486$) and **B** metatranscriptomics data ($n = 327$), with bold indicating the single overlapping taxon (*B. dorei*). Effect size is represented as log2 of the fold change (FC). Color indicates phylum and dot size is proportional to taxon abundance. Bars indicate standard error of log2 fold change estimates. **C** Differentially abundant fecal metabolites ($q < 0.25$ in multivariate models) detected by global untargeted metabolomics ($n = 368$) are shown, with color representing functional category. Bold indicates metabolites that were associated with microbial community metabolic potential by MIMOSA2. **D** Differentially abundant bacterial transcripts, annotated by KEGG KO number, gene symbol, and gene name. Transcripts for genes that were also differentially abundant in the predicted metagenome are shown in bold. Dot size is proportional to transcript relative abundance and color represents KEGG pathway annotation (legend above the plot)

profiles of the metatranscriptome, only *B. dorei* showed concordant change with the 16S sequencing findings (Fig. 2B). Bacteria with increased transcript abundance in IBS included *Eggerthella lenta*, two *Bacteroides* species (*B. dorei* and *B. fluxus*), *Phascolarctobacterium succinatutens*, *Blautia hydrogenotrophica*, *Prevotella timonsensis*, *Clostridium hylemonae*, *Catonella morbi*, and an unidentified *Actinomyces* species. IBS showed decreased transcript abundance of *Bilophila wadsworthia*, *Roseburia inulinivorans*, *Bifidobacterium animals*, and two *Bacteroides* species (*B. plebeius* and *B. barnesiae*).

Microbial function was assessed by bacterial transcript abundances (annotated by KEGG orthology

(KO)), bacterial gene abundances predicted from 16S rRNA compositional data using phylogenetically-nearest reference genomes (predicted metagenome), and metabolite levels. IBS status was significantly associated with variation in beta diversity of all three datasets in univariate analyses (Fig. 1B). Among the covariates, age, sex, race, BMI, dietary category, and HAD-Anxiety were significantly associated with the metatranscriptome and metabolome; age, race, and BMI also were significantly associated with the predicted metagenome. After adjustment for these six covariates, IBS remained significantly associated with the metatranscriptome and predicted metagenome but no longer had a significant association with the metabolome (Fig. 1B, C).

Differential abundance testing identified 16 bacterial transcripts with increased abundance in IBS and 3 with decreased abundance (Fig. 2D). Similar analysis was performed to identify differential genes from the predicted metagenome, but given the potential inaccuracies at the KO level of predicted abundances, these were used only to highlight differential KOs found in the metatranscriptomics data [25]. A total of four transcripts showed concordant changes in the predicted metagenome, including increased abundance of D-proline reductase, 1-2-diacylglycerol 3-glucosyltransferase, and two components of the fructooligosaccharide transport system (permease and substrate-binding protein). This suggests that increased levels of these transcripts could be attributable to differences in abundance of their corresponding genes in the metagenome. Other notable shifts in the metatranscriptome included increased abundance of butyrate kinase and the phosphotransferase system for uptake of mannitol (a fermentable polyol).

While IBS was not associated with significant global change in the metabolome after adjusting for covariates, IBS showed statistically significant increases in 12 metabolites (Fig. 2C). Nine of these were classified as lipids including free fatty acids such as palmitate and margarate, a bile acid (glycodeoxycholate), and N-acetylsphingosine. The other elevated metabolites included L-urobilinogen (a product of bacterial metabolism of biliruben), 3-aminoisobutyrate, and tyramine. There were 14 metabolites with reduced levels in IBS, which included 6 amino acid derivatives (e.g., 3-methylhistidine, N-acetyl-1-methylhistidine, gentisate, xanthurenate), anserine (a dipeptide that includes 3-methylhistidine), benzoate as well as two related metabolites (3-(2-hydroxyphenol)propionate and hydrocinnamate), and riboflavin.

Inter-omic analyses reveal consistent metabolic shifts across datasets that differentiate IBS from HC

Given that all five datasets demonstrated alterations in IBS compared to HC, we then assessed whether there were conserved compositional and functional shifts across multiple data types. Global correlations of datasets were assessed by the Mantel test. All pairwise combinations of the five datasets showed statistically significant positive correlation, with the greatest association (other than 16S and the metagenome predicted from 16S) observed for metatranscriptomics and the metabolome (Additional file 1: Figure S1). These significant associations across datasets were visualized by Procrustes, which highlighted the separation of IBS from HC in superimposed datasets.

We further investigated three categories of inter-omic association. First, we assessed the ratio of microbial abundances in the metatranscriptome (RNA) to those from 16S sequencing (DNA). These ratios broadly represent transcriptional activity of microbes [43]. This analysis was performed at the genus level to facilitate matching of taxonomic assignments from 16S sequencing (which does not consistently achieve species resolution) with those from metatranscriptomics. Consistent with prior reports, transcriptional representation of microbes could differ by orders of magnitude compared to their abundance in the metagenome, differentiating microbes that are transcriptionally active from those that are quiescent (Fig. 3A). The most transcriptionally active genus was *Veillonella* (median RNA/DNA 89 in HC and 114 in IBS) and the least transcriptionally active genus was *Faecalibacterium* (median RNA/DNA 0.074 in HC and 0.087 in IBS). Comparing IBS to HC, the two groups were found to have similar patterns of microbial transcriptional activity at the genus level (Fig. 3B). No taxa showed a statistically significant difference between IBS and HC.

Second, we calculated gene-normalized transcript abundances using the ratio of transcript abundances (RNA) to predicted gene abundances (DNA) for differential gene expression analysis. This approach provides an assessment of transcriptional upregulation or downregulation, which is not possible with transcript abundances alone as these reflect a combination of gene abundance as well as transcriptional regulation. Transcripts were found to have a wide range of ratios relative to genes, from less than 0.1 to over 1000 (Fig. 3C). While RNA/DNA ratios were highly correlated between IBS and HC, 182 KOs were found to be differentially regulated between IBS and HC after adjusting for covariates (Fig. 3D, Additional file 1: Table S2). To identify consistent functional shifts among gene-normalized transcript abundances, pathway enrichment analysis was performed. This demonstrated that the pathways of citrate cycle, fructose and

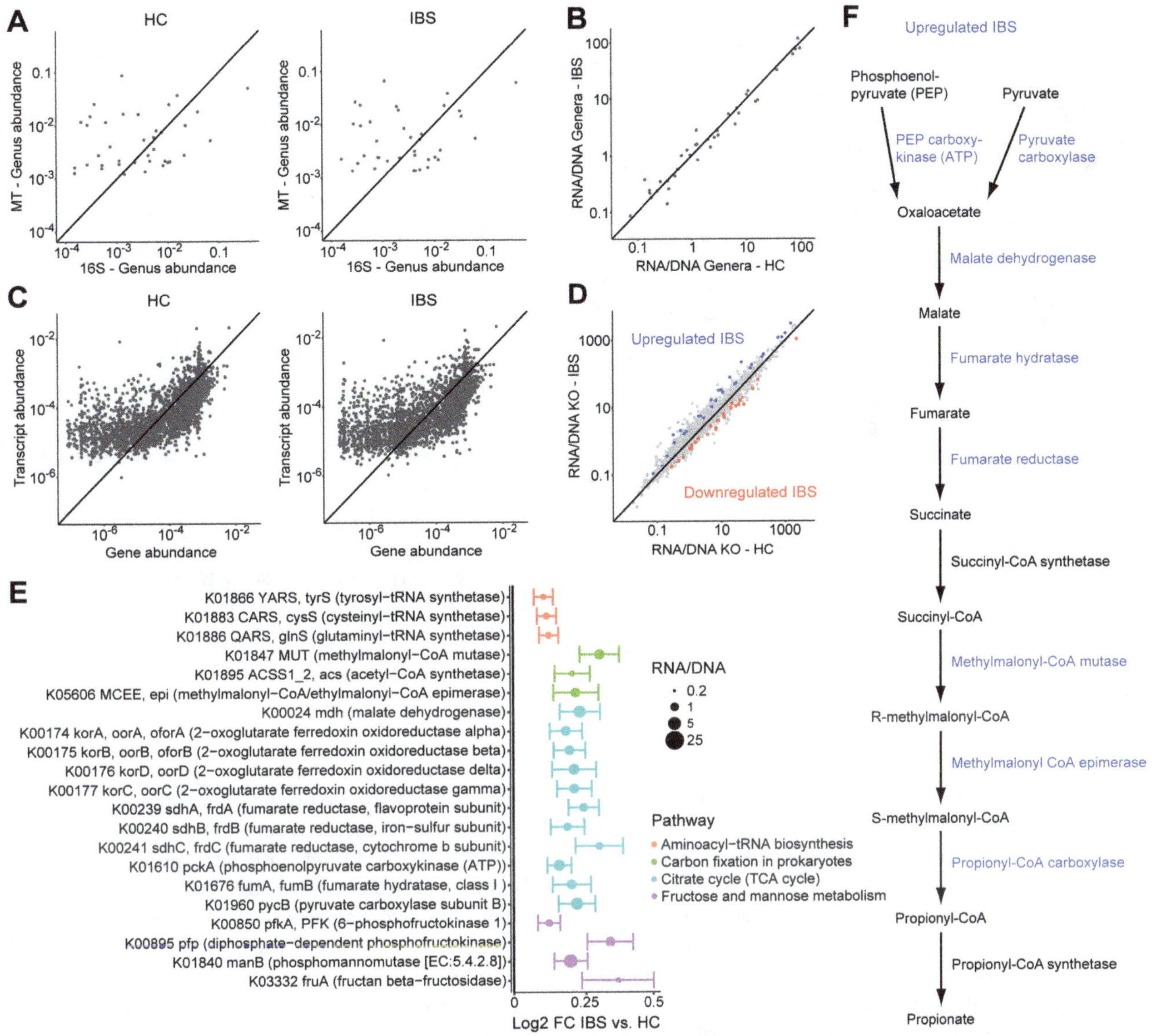

Fig. 3 Inter-omic comparison of bacterial taxonomy and function demonstrated upregulation in IBS of transcripts involved in the succinate pathway of carbohydrate fermentation. **A** Scatterplots depicting median relative abundances of genera in 16S rRNA sequence data and in the metatranscriptome for the 322 subjects with both data types available. **B** Median ratios of genus abundances in the metatranscriptome (RNA) vs. 16S data (DNA) are plotted for IBS subjects and HC. **C** Scatterplots of median gene abundances in the predicted metagenome compared to median transcript abundances. **D** Median transcript/gene abundance ratios are plotted for IBS subjects and HC. Transcripts that were significantly upregulated or downregulated in IBS compared to HC (adjusting for batch, age, sex, race/ethnicity, BMI, dietary category, and HAD-A) are colored. **E** Pathways that were significantly enriched in differentially regulated transcripts were identified. Significant transcripts within these pathways (represented by dot color) are shown, with dot size proportional to RNA/DNA ratio. Bars indicate standard error of log2 fold change estimates. **F** Succinate pathway of carbohydrate fermentation. Enzymes transcriptionally upregulated in IBS are colored blue

mannose metabolism, carbon fixation in prokaryotes, and aminoacyl-tRNA biosynthesis were enriched in differentially regulated transcripts (Fig. 3E). Within these pathways, 21 differential transcripts were highlighted which were all upregulated in IBS. This included multiple key enzymes in the citric acid cycle including pyruvate carboxylase, phosphoenolpyruvate carboxylase, succinate dehydrogenase, fumarate hydratase, and malate dehydrogenase. The carbon fixation pathway transcripts included acetyl-CoA synthetase as well as methylmalonyl-CoA mutase and methylmalonyl-CoA epimerase (which are involved in the production of the short chain fatty acid, propionate) [44]. Taken together, the transcripts in these two pathways encompass nearly

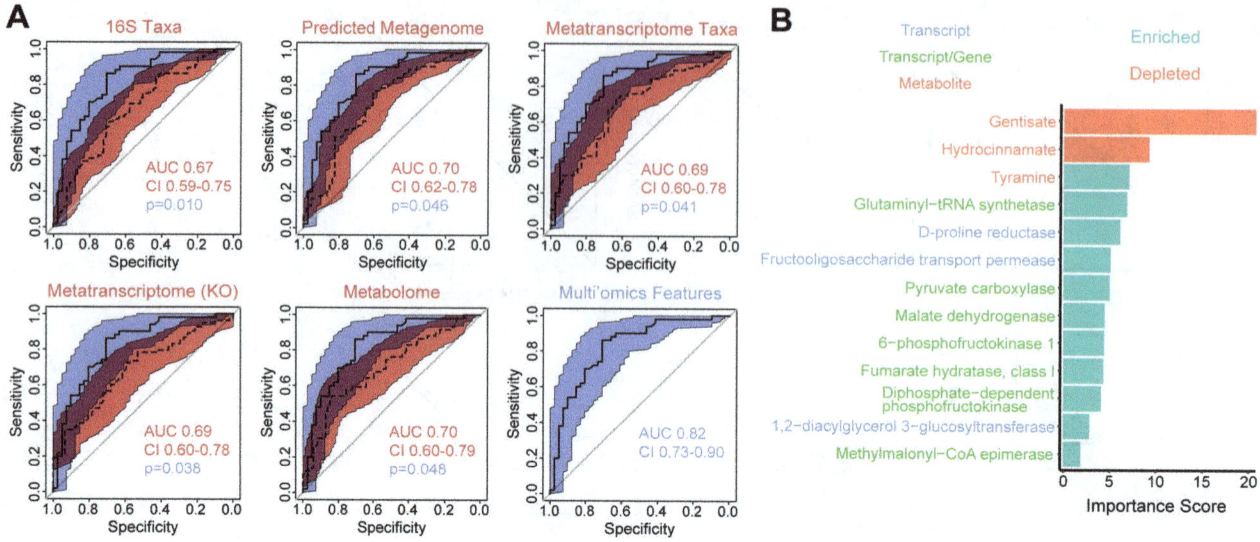

Fig. 4 Multi-omics microbiome classifier for IBS showed increased accuracy compared to classifiers using single datasets. **A** ROC curves for random forest classifiers constructed from differentially abundant features in each of the five datasets (colored in red) are compared to the ROC curve for a multi-omics classifier (colored in blue). The multi-omics classifier was constructed from transcripts that were differentially abundant in both the metatranscriptome and predicted metagenome, significantly upregulated transcripts in enriched pathways, and differentially abundant metabolites associated with microbial community metabolic potential. All classifiers were trained on 60% of the dataset and tested on the remaining 40% of samples ($n = 230$ with all three data types). Colored areas indicate the 95% confidence intervals of the ROC curves. *P* values for the AUC of single dataset classifiers compared to the multi-omics classifier were calculated by bootstrapping. **B** Importance scores are shown for features included in the multi-omics classifier, colored by feature type. Bar color indicates whether each feature shown was enriched or depleted in IBS subjects compared to HC

all of the enzymes in the succinate pathway for carbohydrate fermentation to propionate (Fig. 3F) [45]. There were also three transcripts for subunits of the 2-oxoglutarate ferredoxin oxidoreductase, which fixes carbon in the reductive tricarboxylic acid cycle by adding CO_2 to succinyl-CoA to generate 2-oxoglutarate. The fructose- and mannose-related metabolism transcripts included fructan beta-fructosidase (breakdown of fructans such as inulin), 6-phosphofructokinase 1 (entry of fructose into the glycolytic pathway), diphosphate-dependent phosphofructokinase, and phosphomannomutase. Three tRNA synthetases (glutaminyl, cysteinyl, tryosyl) were also upregulated, though with low magnitude of effect compared to the other transcripts.

Third, we identified fecal metabolites that were likely influenced by microbial metabolism by modeling microbial metabolic potential from metatranscriptomics and predicted metagenomics. Using this strategy, 5 differential metabolites were associated with the microbiome (Additional file 1: Figure S2). Of these, only one metabolite had increased levels in IBS–tyramine, which was associated with metabolic potential from the metatranscriptome. Of the four decreased metabolites, hydrocinnamate was found to be significantly associated with microbial metabolic potential by both metatranscriptomics and predicted metagenomics. Benzoate and gentisate were associated with the predicted metagenome and xanthurenate with the metatranscriptome.

These three sets of inter-omic analyses yielded a group of features associated with IBS based upon analyses incorporating two datasets. This included differentially abundant gene-normalized transcripts in enriched pathways, transcripts that were differentially abundant in both the metatranscriptome and predicted metagenome, and differentially abundant metabolites that were associated with microbial metabolic potential. Using these multi-omics features, a random forests classifier was trained to differentiate IBS from HC that had AUC of 0.82. This performance was statistically significantly superior to classifiers constructed using microbial features from single datasets, which achieved AUC of 0.67–0.70 (Fig. 4). The three microbial features that contributed most to this classifier were metabolites: gentisate, hydrocinnamate, and tyramine. The other ten features in the classifier included three transcripts related to fructooligosaccharide metabolism (diphosphate-dependent phosphofructokinase, 6-phosphofructokinase 1, fructooligosaccharide transport permease protein), three transcripts in the citric acid cycle (pyruvate carboxylase, malate dehydrogenase, fumarate hydratase), glutaminyl-tRNA synthetase, D-proline reductase, 1,2-diacylglycerol 3-glucosyltransferase, and methylmalonyl-CoA epimerase.

Bacterial transcripts and metabolites differentiate IBS bowel habit subtypes

Having identified robust microbial profiles differentiating IBS from HC, we then assessed the relationship of microbial composition and function to phenotypes within IBS. Bowel habit subtypes were significantly associated with metatranscriptomics KOs and metabolomics but not with microbiome composition or the predicted metagenome (Fig. 5). Visceral sensitivity (VSI), general physical symptom perception (PILL), and IBS-specific symptom severity (IBS-SSS) were not significantly associated with either global microbiome composition or function by transcripts, predicted genes, and metabolites.

To further delineate microbial functional features that were associated with IBS bowel habit subtype, we focused on comparison of the diarrhea-predominant (IBS-D) and constipation-predominant IBS-C) subtypes. These are the two most numerous BH subtypes and show more consistent BH patterns compared to the remaining two subtypes (IBS-mixed, IBS-M; IBS-unspecified, IBS-U). Differential abundance testing further supported the absence of a clear taxonomic signature of IBS-D vs. IBS-C, as only 2 taxa were significantly different by 16S sequencing and 4 taxa by metatranscriptomics with no overlap between the two datasets (Additional file 1: Figure S3A). In contrast, metatranscriptomics functional assessment demonstrated 54 differential transcripts belonging to diverse pathways, included 51 increased in IBS-D (Additional file 1: Figure S3B). Among these, many were associated with fructose and mannose metabolism pathway, including L-iditol 2-dehydrogenase (polyol dehydrogenase), three components of the mannose-specific phosphotransferase system, and L-fucose/D-arabinose isomerase (which produces ribulose). There was also enrichment of transcripts involved in D-glutamate synthesis (glutamate synthase and glutamate racemase) and ethanolamine utilization. None of these overlapped with differential predicted gene abundances.

Inter-omic analysis was then performed of gene-normalized transcript abundances to assess transcriptional regulation patterns in IBS-D vs. IBS-C. IBS-D was associated with significant shifts in 140 transcript RNA/DNA ratios, of which 128 were upregulated in IBS-D (Fig. 6, Additional file 1: Table S3). Pathway analysis demonstrated 10 pathways enriched for differentially abundant transcripts, including fructose and mannose metabolism,

A

p<0.05 (light shading) p<0.01 (dark shading)

	16S	PM-KO	MT-T	MT-KO	MET
BH	0.008	0.009	0.006	**0.025**	**0.016**
VSI	0.003	0.002	0.006	0.006	0.004
PILL	0.002	0.004	0.006	0.006	0.005
IBS-SSS	0.003	0.006	0.004	0.007	0.003
Age	**0.008**	**0.025**	**0.008**	0.007	**0.008**
Sex	0.003	0.001	**0.008**	0.007	**0.006**
Race	**0.017**	**0.021**	0.022	0.019	**0.029**
BMI	0.004	0.004	0.005	0.004	**0.007**
Diet	0.011	0.017	0.014	0.014	0.009
HAD-A	0.003	0.001	0.006	0.004	0.004

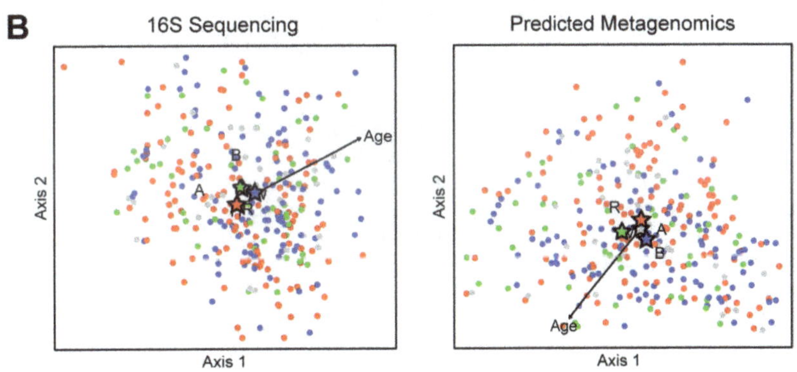

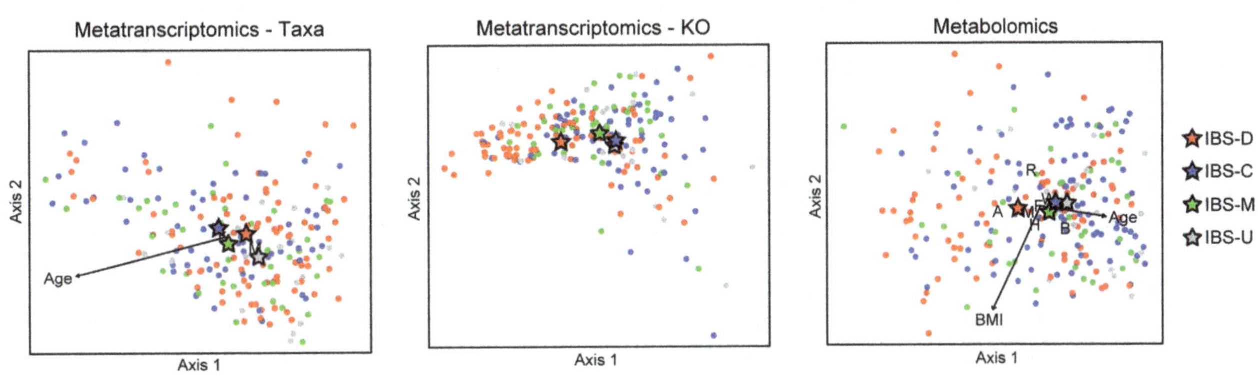

Fig. 5 IBS bowel habit (BH) subtypes have distinct functional profiles by metatranscriptomics and metabolomics. **A** Multivariate PERMONOVA models were used to assess the association of phenotypes within IBS including BH subtype, visceral sensitivity (VSI), general physical symptom perception (PILL), and IBS severity (IBS-SSS) with the five datasets, adjusting for batch, age, sex, race/ethnicity, BMI, dietary category, and HAD-A. **B** DbRDA plots for each of the five datasets visualizing differences in beta diversity related to BH subtype and significant categorical or continuous covariates. F = female, M = male, A = Asian, B = African-American, H = Hispanic, W = non-Hispanic white, R = multiracial

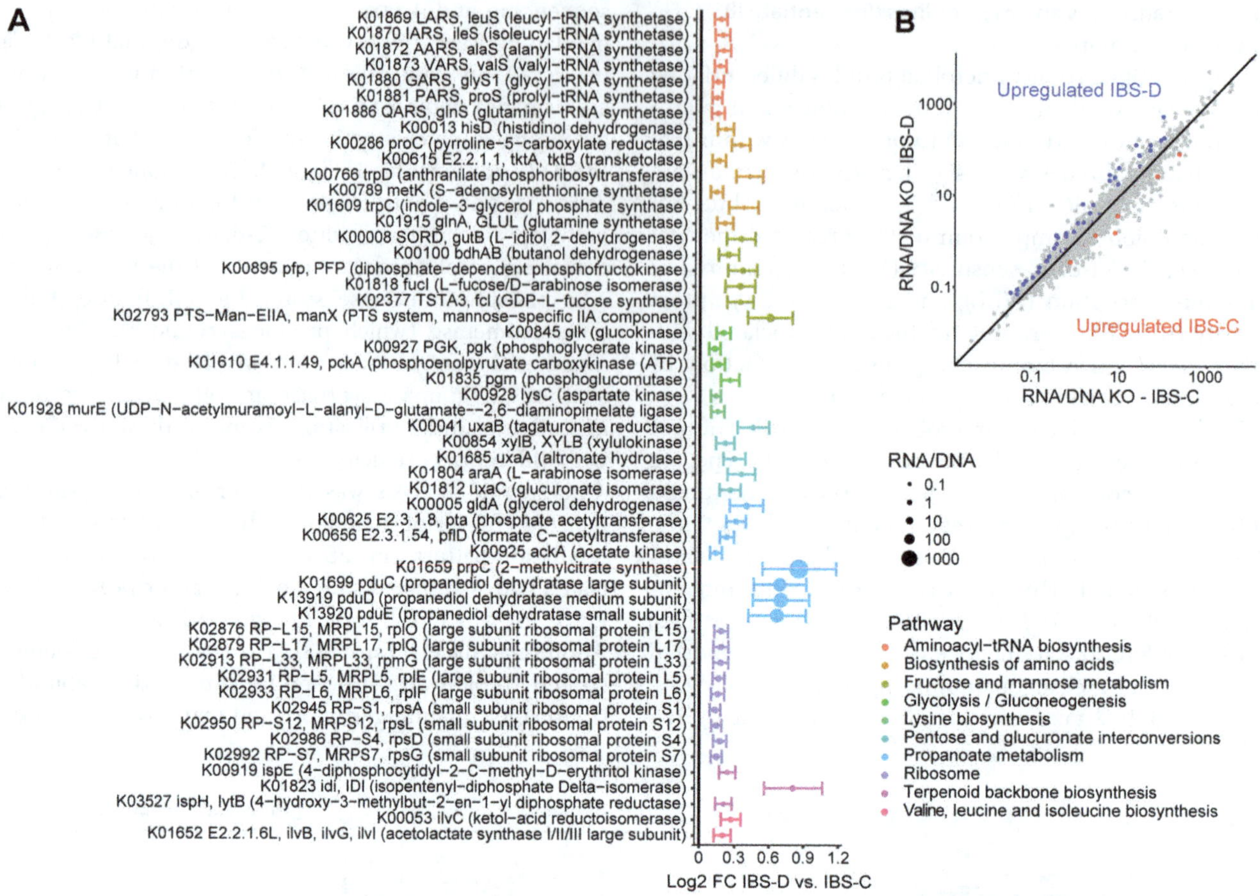

Fig. 6 IBS-D is characterized by transcriptional upregulation relative to IBS-C of genes involved in proponoate metabolism, terpenoid biosynthesis, fructose and mannose metabolism, and glycolysis. **A** Pathways that were significantly enriched in transcripts differentially regulated in IBS-D vs. IBS-C were identified. Significant transcripts within these pathways ($q < 0.25$ adjusting for batch, age, sex, race/ethnicity, BMI, dietary category, and HAD-A) are shown, with color denoting pathway and dot size proportional to RNA/DNA ratio. Bars indicate standard error of log2 fold change estimates. **B** Transcript/gene abundance ratios are plotted for the 205 IBS-D and IBS-C subjects with both data types available. Transcripts that were significantly upregulated or downregulated in IBS-D compared to IBS-C are colored

propanoate metabolism, aminoacyl-tRNA biosynthesis, terpenoid biosynthesis, and pentose and glucuronate interconversions. The most significantly upregulated transcripts were involved in proprionate metabolism, including 2-methylcitrate synthase, three subunits of propanediol dehydratase, and glycerol dehydrogenase. Upregulated fructose and mannose metabolism-related transcripts included those that had been enriched in the metatranscriptome without consideration of gene abundance (mannose phosphotransferases, L-iditol 2-dehydrogenase, L-fucose/D-arabinose isomerase) as well as others including diphosphate-dependent phosphofructokinase, GDP-L-fucose synthase, and butanol dehydrogenase.

Consistent with the functional shifts in the microbiome in IBS-D vs. IBS-C, there were 46 differentially abundant metabolites (Additional file 1: Figure S3C). This included increased levels of two bile acids (cholate and isoursodeoxycholate), polyamine products of amino acid fermentation (cadaverine, N-acetyl-cadaverine, N-acetylputrescine), carbohydrates (mannose, glucose, ribulose, glucuronate, ribose), intermediates in the citric acid cycle (malate, fumarate), and nucleotides (hypoxanthine, thymidine, 2'-deoxycytidine). IBS-D had decreased levels of fatty acids (myristate, palmitate, stearate), food components (carotene diol, phytanate, digalacturonic acid), phenylacetate, and the bacterial metabolites P-cresol and enterolactone. Of these metabolites, fumarate and hypoxanthine were significantly associated with microbial metabolic potential by both the metatranscriptome and predicted metagenome; glucose and nicotinate were associated with the metatranscriptome; and cholate, cadaverine, glucuronate, thymidine, and phenylacetate were associated with the predicted metagenome (Additional file 1: Figure S2).

We then assessed the ability of differential transcripts, metabolites, and multi-omics features (gene-normalized transcript abundances and differential metabolites with significant association with microbial metabolic potential) to differentiate IBS-D from IBS-C. The multi-omics classifier had the highest performance with AUC 0.86, which was significantly greater than that of the predicted metagenome, which only had AUC of 0.65 (Fig. 7A). Classifiers constructed from metatranscriptomics KOs and metabolites each had AUC 0.79, which was not significantly different from the multi-omics classifier. Random forests classifiers were not constructed using microbial composition (16S or metatranscriptomics taxonomy) given the lack of differentially abundant taxa. Transcripts in the metatranscriptomics classifier included ethanolamine utilization proteins, propanediol dehydratase, sodium/proline symporter, and N-acetylglucosamine phosphotransferase (Fig. 7B). The metabolomics classifier incorporated all three differential products of amino acid fermentation (cadaverine, N-acetyl-cadaverine, N-acetylputrescine), malate, fatty acids (mytristate and 2-palmitoylglycerol), and digalacturonic acid (a product of pectin breakdown) (Fig. 7C). The features contributing to the multi-omics classifier included fumarate and transcripts in pathways for fructose and mannose metabolism (diphosphate-dependent phosphofructokinase, GDP-L-fucose synthase), terpenoid biosynthesis (isopentenyl-diphosphate delta-isomerase, 4-hydroxy-3-methylbut-2-en-1-yl diphosphate reductase, 4-diphosphocytidyl-2-c-methyl-d-erythritol kinase), pentose and glucuronate interconversions (L-arabinose isomerase), and propionate metabolism (2-methylcitrate synthase, glycerol dehydrogenase) (Fig. 7D).

Discussion

In this study, we present the results of the first large-scale metatranscriptomics analysis of a well-phenotyped IBS cohort and one of the two largest IBS cross-sectional global metabolomics studies to-date [15]. In combination with 16S rRNA sequencing data and predicted metagenomics, five datasets were analyzed to provide a comprehensive multi-omics assessment of microbial composition and function. Each dataset included microbial features that were significantly associated with IBS status but could only achieve modest accuracy in classification algorithms. Using multi-omics features that

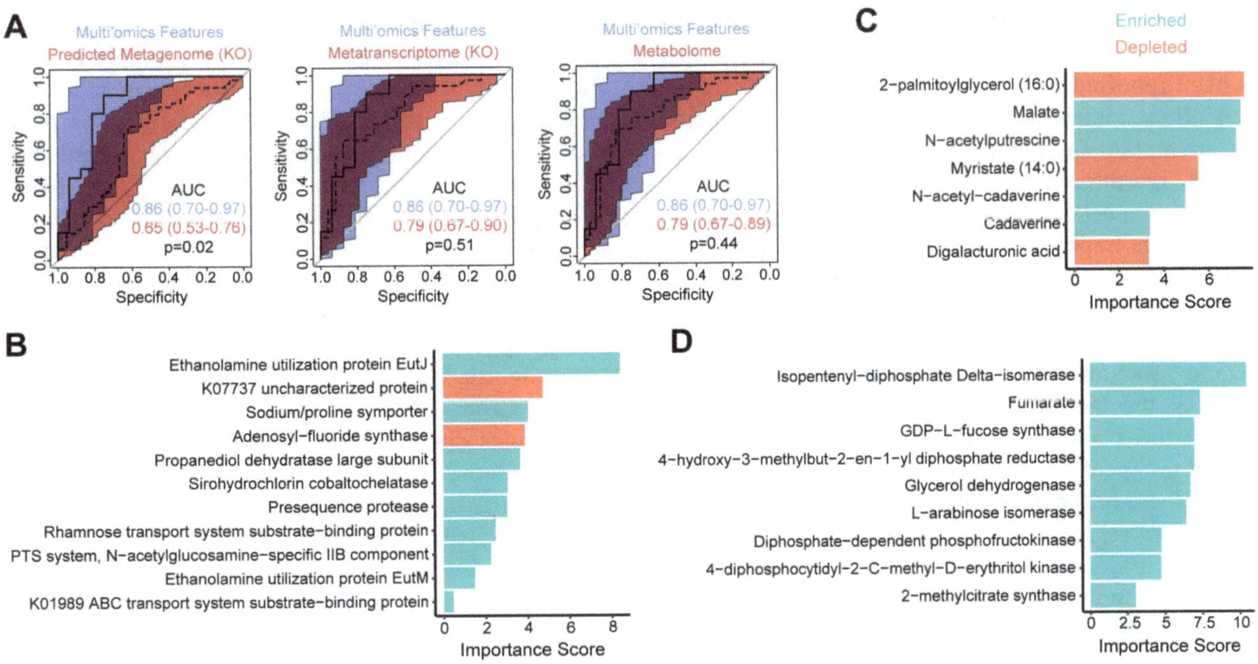

Fig. 7 Metabolites, transcripts, and transcript/gene ratios can differentiate IBS-D from IBS-C with high accuracy. **A** ROC curves for random forest classifiers constructed from differentially abundant predicted genes, transcripts, and metabolites (colored in red) are compared to the ROC curve for a multi-omics classifier (colored in blue). The multi-omics classifier was constructed from significantly upregulated transcripts (by RNA/DNA ratio) in enriched pathways and differential metabolites associated with microbial community metabolic potential. All classifiers were trained on 60% of the dataset and tested on the remaining 40% of samples ($n = 126$ with all three data types). Colored areas indicate the 95% confidence intervals of the ROC curves. *P* values were calculated by bootstrapping. **B–D** Importance scores are shown for features included in the **B** metatranscriptomics, **C** metabolomics, and **D** multi-omics classifiers, with bar color denoting features that were enriched or depleted in IBS-D

incorporated information from two related datasets (e.g., metatranscriptome KOs and predicted KO gene abundances, metabolites, and metatranscriptome metabolic potential), an accurate classifier for IBS vs. HC could be achieved. This supports that IBS is characterized by a distinct microbial functional state across a large cohort representative of the racial/ethnic diversity in the USA.

Compositional shifts in the microbiome of IBS compared to HC were observed based on both 16S relative abundances and transcriptional representation. A consistent finding in both 16S and metatranscriptomics data was increased *Bacteroides dorei*, which has not been previously reported in IBS. Both datasets also showed increased levels of *Actinomyces* spp., which is consistent with a large shotgun metagenomics study describing enrichment of multiple *Actinomyces* spp. including *A. odontolyticus* as seen here [7]. Additional species level microbial shifts detected by 16S sequencing or metatranscriptomics that have been previously noted in large shotgun metagenomics studies include increased *Streptococcus* species (*S. parasanguinis*), *Eggerthella lenta*, and *Blautia hydrogenotrophica* as well as reduced *Faecalibacterium prausnitzii*, *Bacteroides thetaiotaomicron*, and *Bilophila wadsworthia* [11, 16, 23]. Other taxonomic shifts observed in this study have not been previously reported and many taxa that were reported in prior studies were not significant in our study. We also did not observe reduced alpha diversity in IBS, which has been reported in some prior studies but not others [6–9]. These differences could reflect multiple factors that differentiated our study including racial/ethnic composition, recruitment of subjects from the community rather than specialty clinics, and differences in analytical approach. Importantly, this study differed from many prior ones in using multivariate strategies to adjust for a wide range of covariates differing between IBS and HC that could confound analyses [7, 11, 13–16].

Among the functional microbial features associated with IBS, the largest contribution to the multi-omics IBS signature came from three microbiome-related fecal metabolites: gentisate, hydrocinnamate, and tyramine. None of these or the other differentially abundant metabolites in IBS vs. HC have been previously implicated in IBS, possibly due to differences in metabolomics pipelines across studies which affect the specific metabolites that are detected and validated [13–15]. Gentisate, the most strongly predictive metabolite, is an intermediate in bacterial aerobic metabolism of aromatic compounds including hydroxybenzoates [46]. It has been reported to be undetectable in the serum of germ-free mice and strongly induced by bacterial colonization [47]. Gentisate inhibits fibroblast growth factor signaling to reduce tumor growth and associated angiogenesis [48]. It is unclear whether the decreased levels in IBS have any functional consequences for intestinal fibroblast growth factor signaling, which plays important roles in epithelial homeostasis and bile acid regulation [49]. Hydrocinnamate (3-phenylpropionate) is produced by microbial metabolism of polyphenols and serum levels of hydrocinnamate are positively associated with microbial alpha diversity [50–52]. IBS feces also showed reduced levels of benzoate and another member of the benzoate class, 3-(2-hydroxyphenol)propionate, which can also be derived from bacterial metabolism of polyphenols [53, 54]. These changes may reflect altered microbial metabolic activity or reduced polyphenol intake by IBS patients that was not captured by assessment of global dietary patterns. Tyramine is a biogenic amine that signals through trace amine-associated receptors. Bacteria can synthesize tyramine from tyrosine, and fecal tyramine levels are greatly increased by microbial colonization of germ-free mice and modulated by diet [55–57]. Tyramine induces intestinal contraction, mesenteric vasodilation, serotonin release by enterochromaffin cells, and inflammatory response by intestinal epithelial cells and macrophages, potential mechanisms by which it may promote symptoms in IBS [58–60]. Among the other differentially abundant metabolites, IBS was notably characterized by increased levels of many lipids including the bile acid glycodeoxycholate—which was previously reported to be elevated in IBS—and multiple free fatty acids [61]. Interestingly, IBS-D showed reduced free fatty acids compared to IBS-C. The increased levels of free fatty acids particularly in IBS-C may reflect increased delivery to the colon from dietary intake, altered intestinal epithelial lipid metabolism, or bacterial fatty acid metabolism. Gut microbes are thought to be unable to utilize fatty acids for energy harvest but are capable of synthesizing free fatty acids and using exogenous fatty acids for phospholipid biosynthesis [62, 63].

Despite the many metabolite associations with IBS and the strong contribution of three metabolites to the multi-omics classifier, the metabolomics only classifier had a modest AUC of 0.7 similar to what was reported in the two largest previously published fecal metabolomics studies [15, 16]. This supports that metabolic end product measurements need to be considered in the context of bacterial transcriptional profiles to accurately characterize the microbial metabolic state in IBS. We found that IBS was characterized by upregulation of transcripts involved in bacterial uptake and breakdown of fructooligosaccharides, polyols, and glucans. We further identified upregulation of bacterial enzymes involved in the succinate pathway of carbohydrate fermentation, which culminates in the production of propionate [45]. This increased capacity for carbohydrate utilization by the

IBS microbiota is consistent with a prior large shotgun metagenomics study reporting increased carbohydrate degradation and fermentation pathways in IBS [7]. Moreover, a recent shotgun metagenomics reported that carbohydrate-metabolism associated genes (CAZy) were associated with symptom severity in IBS, further supporting a role for bacterial carbohydrate metabolism in IBS pathophysiology [64]. Preferential utilization of the succinate pathway in IBS for carbohydrate fermentation is supported by a meta-analysis of fecal short chain fatty acids (SCFAs) in IBS demonstrating increased proportion of propionate relative to other SCFAs [65]. Taken together, our findings and those of others support that gut microbes in IBS patients have increased capacity to utilize certain fermentable carbohydrates. Reliance of IBS-associated bacteria on this energy source may explain the clinical association of fermentable carbohydrates with IBS symptoms and clinical improvement with the FODMAPS diet, which restricts dietary intake of fermentable oligosaccharides, disaccharides, monosaccharides, and polyols [66]. It is important to note that there was low prevalence of FODMAPS diet in our IBS cohort (2%) and that IBS populations with greater prevalence of FODMAPS diet may not show the same transcriptional profile.

In addition to identifying metabolic features of IBS, we further found that IBS BH subtypes were robustly distinguished by functional microbial profiles. IBS-D was characterized by increased cholate and isoursodeoxycholate, which is consistent with prior studies reporting increased levels of cholate in IBS-D compared to IBS-C and bile acid malabsorption in IBS-D [14, 16]. Bile acids are known to induce diarrhea by triggering colonic chloride secretion, supporting direct involvement in the bowel habit phenotype of IBS-D [67]. Besides these bile acid shifts, IBS-D was characterized by upregulation of multiple metabolic pathways for bacterial energy harvest including transcripts involved in fructose, mannose, and polyol metabolism. This increased machinery for carbohydrate utilization corresponded to increased levels of multiple monosaccharides including mannose, glucose, ribulose, and ribose. IBS-D also had increased levels of intermediates of the succinate pathway of carbohydrate fermentation including fumarate and malate (succinate showed a non-significant increase and other intermediates were not detected), suggesting increased flux through this pathway compared to IBS-C. IBS-D also showed transcriptional upregulation of components of an alternative fermentation pathway to generate propionate via the 1,2-propanediol pathway. This included upregulation of three components of propanediol dehydratase as well as glycerol dehydrogenase, which participates in the generation of propanediol from monosaccharides [45]. Beyond carbohydrate metabolism, IBS-D also demonstrated evidence of increased amino acid catabolism based upon higher levels of several polyamines including cadaverine, N-acetylcadaverine, and N-acetylputrescine. Cadaverine and putrescine are products of arginine and lysine fermentation, respectively, which can further undergo N-acylation by gut microbes [68, 69]. Our findings are consistent with a prior study reporting elevated putrescine in IBS-D compared to IBS-C [13]. In addition, IBS-D demonstrated increased levels of three ethanolamine utilization proteins. Ethanolamine is released from breakdown of the membrane phospholipid phosphatidylethanolamine and has been reported to be metabolized primarily by enteric bacteria with pathogenic potential [70]. Overall, gut microbes in IBS-D demonstrate a profile consistent with increased utilization of multiple energy sources. It is unclear if these metabolic shifts promote symptoms in IBS-D or reflect adaptation of gut microbes to altered GI motility and secretion in IBS-D [71]. Of note, metabolites reported in other studies to differentiate IBS bowel habit subtypes such as tryptamine were not differentially abundant in this study, potentially reflecting the previously noted differences in study population and analytic strategy [14].

The strengths of this study include the large cohort size, inclusion of diverse racial/ethnic groups, extensive clinical phenotyping of IBS and control subjects, adjustment for relevant covariates in all analyses, and integration for the first time of metatranscriptomics and metabolomics to assess functional profiles in IBS. However, we acknowledge some limitations. Controls differed from IBS subjects in important parameters including sex, BMI, race/ethnicity, and diet. While considerable effort was made to account for these covariates, we cannot exclude residual effects of confounding. This study had a cross-sectional design, which may provide a less accurate assessment of complex microbial compositional and functional relationships compared to longitudinal studies [14]. Diet was assessed by a dietary pattern questionnaire, but this may not capture nutrient differences such as in polyphenol intake that may underlie observed microbial profiles. In addition, bacterial gene content was predicted from 16S rRNA gene sequencing rather than directly assessed by shotgun metagenomics. While predicted abundances of individual genes were not used directly as differential features for IBS or its BH subtypes, they were incorporated into gene-normalized transcriptional analyses. Predictions made using PICRUSt2 have been reported to have Spearman correlation of between 0.79 and 0.88 with shotgun metagenomics data, supporting that they are robust overall [25]. However, given the potential inaccuracies of gene abundance prediction, further studies incorporating shotgun metagenomics are required to confirm the findings of gene-normalized transcriptional analyses. Finally, the global metabolomics pipeline used for this study does not detect SCFAs, so we were unable to assess whether transcript patterns were associated with altered fecal levels of SCFAs.

Conclusions

IBS is characterized by both compositional changes and robust shifts in microbial function that emerge from multi-omics integration of bacterial transcriptional patterns and fecal metabolite levels. The metabolic signature of IBS supports the utilization of multiple fermentable carbohydrates through the succinate pathway. This is consistent with the efficacy of interventions such as FODMAPS diet that exclude such energy sources. Additional novel metabolic pathways and metabolites such as tyramine were also identified. Further investigation of these pathways could elucidate mechanisms by which gut microbes contribute to IBS pathophysiology and inform our understanding of current microbiome-directed therapeutic strategies for IBS. Moreover, IBS BH subtypes showed strong functional differentiation, implying a critical role for microbial metabolic activity in dictating the bowel habit alterations seen in IBS. Our findings support the need for integrative assessment of microbial function incorporating both metabolomics and metatranscriptomics in IBS microbiome studies to identify relevant pathways that impact symptom generation and could represent novel mechanistic targets for microbiome-directed interventions.

Supplementary Information

Additional file 1: Figure S1. Significant associations were seen across all pairwise combinations of datasets. (A) Procrustes analysis was used to superimpose dbRDA ordinations of the indicated pairs of datasets. IBS and HC samples are denoted by color. (B) Mantel test of association for all pairwise combinations of datasets. All were significant, with color indicating level of significance. **Figure S2.** Metabolites that were differentially abundant in IBS vs. HC or IBS-D vs. IBS-C and were associated with the gut microbiome by metabolic modeling. (A) Metabolites that were associated with the community metabolic potential (CMP) scores derived from predicted bacterial gene content are shown. Metabolomics and predicted metagenomics data were available for 361 subjects. Each sample is plotted by its CMP score and the log2 of the normalized metabolite level. The dashed lines represent linear regression of metabolite levels with CMP scores and the number in the upper right of each plot indicates the R^2. (B) Metabolites that were associated with CMP scores derived from the metatranscriptome. Metabolomics and metatranscriptomics data were available for 234 subjects. **Figure S3.** IBS-D is differentiated from IBS-C by diverse functional shifts including increased polyamines, bile acids, glutamate synthesis, and ethanolamine utilization. (A) Differentially abundant taxa (q<0.25) in 16S sequencing (n=312) and metatranscriptomics (n=208) datasets adjusting for batch, age, sex, race/ethnicity, BMI, dietary category, and HAD-A. Effect size is shown as the log2 fold change (FC) of IBS-D compared to IBS-C. Dot size is proportional to abundance and color represents phylum. Bars indicate standard error of log2 fold change estimates. (B) Differentially abundant transcripts in IBS-D vs. IBS-C, colored by pathway with dot size proportional to abundance. (C) Metabolites that significantly differed in IBS-D vs. IBS-C by global metabolomics (n=229), colored by functional category. **Table S1.** Dietary patterns. **Table S2.** Differentially regulated transcripts in IBS vs. HC. **Table S3.** Differentially regulated transcripts in IBS-D vs. IBS-C.

Additional file 2.

Additional file 3.

Additional file 4.

Acknowledgements

We thank Cathy Liu and Shamir King for their support of various aspects of this study.

Authors' contributions

Study concept and design—JPJ, EAM; acquisition of data—VL, MH, JSL, TSD, RT, MV, BDN, JML, AG, KT; analysis and interpretation of data—JPJ, EAM; drafting of the manuscript—JPJ, EAM; critical revision of the manuscript—all authors; statistical analysis—JPJ; obtained funding—JSL, JML, AG, KT, EAM; study supervision—EAM. All authors read and approved the final manuscript.

Author details

[1]Vatche and Tamar Manoukian Division of Digestive Diseases, Department of Medicine, David Geffen School of Medicine, University of California Los Angeles, Los Angeles, CA, USA. [2]G. Oppenheimer Center for Neurobiology of Stress and Resilience, David Geffen School of Medicine, University of California Los Angeles, Los Angeles, CA, USA. [3]Division of Gastroenterology, Hepatology and Parenteral Nutrition, VA Greater Los Angeles Healthcare System, Los Angeles, CA, USA. [4]Viome Life Sciences, Bellevue, WA, USA. [5]Division of Behavioral Medicine, Department of Medicine, Jacobs School of Medicine, University at Buffalo, SUNY, Buffalo, NY, USA. [6] Integrative Medicine, VA Greater Los Angeles Healthcare System, Los Angeles, CA, USA.

References

1. Chey WD, Kurlander J, Eswaran S. Irritable bowel syndrome: a clinical review. *JAMA*. 2015;313(9):949–58.
2. Hellstrom PM, Benno P. The Rome IV: irritable bowel syndrome - a functional disorder. *Best Pract Res Clin Gastroenterol*. 2019;40-41:101634.
3. Bhattarai Y, Muniz Pedrogo DA, Kashyap PC. Irritable bowel syndrome: a gut microbiota-related disorder? *Am J Physiol Gastrointest Liver Physiol*. 2017;312(1):G52–62.
4. De Palma G, Lynch MD, Lu J, Dang VT, Deng Y, Jury J, et al. Transplantation of fecal microbiota from patients with irritable bowel syndrome alters gut function and behavior in recipient mice. Sci Transl Med. 2017;9(379):eaaf6397.
5. Crouzet L, Gaultier E, Del'Homme C, Cartier C, Delmas E, Dapoigny M, et al. The hypersensitivity to colonic distension of IBS patients can be transferred to rats through their fecal microbiota. *Neurogastroenterol Motil*. 2013;25(4):e272–82.
6. Tap J, Derrien M, Tornblom H, Brazeilles R, Cools-Portier S, Dore J, et al. Identification of an intestinal microbiota signature associated with severity of irritable bowel syndrome. *Gastroenterology*. 2017;152(1):111–123 e118.
7. Vich Vila A, Imhann F, Collij V, Jankipersadsing SA, Gurry T, Mujagic Z, et al. Gut microbiota composition and functional changes in inflammatory bowel disease and irritable bowel syndrome. Sci Transl Med. 2018;10(472):eaap8914.
8. Hugerth LW, Andreasson A, Talley NJ, Forsberg AM, Kjellstrom L, Schmidt PT, et al. No distinct microbiome signature of irritable bowel syndrome found in a Swedish random population. *Gut*. 2020;69(6):1076–84.
9. Pittayanon R, Lau JT, Yuan Y, Leontiadis GI, Tse F, Surette M, et al. Gut Microbiota in Patients With Irritable Bowel Syndrome-A Systematic Review. *Gastroenterology*. 2019;157(1):97–108.
10. Labus JS, Hollister EB, Jacobs J, Kirbach K, Oezguen N, Gupta A, et al. Differences in gut microbial composition correlate with regional brain volumes in irritable bowel syndrome. *Microbiome*. 2017;5(1):49.

11. Phan J, Nair D, Jain S, Montagne T, Flores DV, Nguyen A, et al. Alterations in gut microbiome composition and function in irritable bowel syndrome and increased probiotic abundance with daily supplementation. *mSystems*. 2021;6(6):e0121521.
12. Bennet SM, Keshteli AH, Bercik P, Madsen KL, Reed D, Vanner SJ. Application of metabolomics to the study of irritable bowel syndrome. *Neurogastroenterol Motil*. 2020;32(6):e13884.
13. Ahluwalia B, Iribarren C, Magnusson MK, Sundin J, Clevers E, Savolainen O, et al. A distinct faecal microbiota and metabolite profile linked to bowel habits in patients with irritable bowel syndrome. Cells. 2021;10(6):1459.
14. Mars RAT, Yang Y, Ward T, Houtti M, Priya S, Lekatz HR, et al. Longitudinal multi-omics reveals subset-specific mechanisms underlying irritable bowel syndrome. *Cell*. 2020;182(6):1460–1473 e1417.
15. Han L, Zhao L, Zhou Y, Yang C, Xiong T, Lu L, et al. Altered metabolome and microbiome features provide clues in understanding irritable bowel syndrome and depression comorbidity. ISME J. 2021;16(4):983-96.
16. Jeffery IB, Das A, O'Herlihy E, Coughlan S, Cisek K, Moore M, et al. Differences in fecal microbiomes and metabolomes of people with vs without irritable bowel syndrome and bile acid malabsorption. *Gastroenterology*. 2020;158(4):1016–1028 e1018.
17. Mars RAT, Frith M, Kashyap PC. Functional gastrointestinal disorders and the microbiome-what is the best strategy for moving microbiome-based therapies for functional gastrointestinal disorders into the clinic? *Gastroenterology*. 2021;160(2):538–55.
18. Jacobs JP, Gupta A, Bhatt RR, Brawer J, Gao K, Tillisch K, et al. Cognitive behavioral therapy for irritable bowel syndrome induces bidirectional alterations in the brain-gut-microbiome axis associated with gastrointestinal symptom improvement. *Microbiome*. 2021;9(1):236.
19. Drossman DA. The functional gastrointestinal disorders and the Rome III process. *Gastroenterology*. 2006;130(5):1377–90.
20. Lenhart A, Dong T, Joshi S, Jaffe N, Choo C, Liu C, et al. Effect of exclusion diets on symptom severity and the gut microbiota in patients with irritable bowel syndrome. *Clin Gastroenterol Hepatol*. 2022;20(3):e465–83.
21. Francis CY, Morris J, Whorwell PJ. The irritable bowel severity scoring system: a simple method of monitoring irritable bowel syndrome and its progress. *Aliment Pharmacol Ther*. 1997;11(2):395–402.
22. Tong M, Jacobs JP, McHardy IH, Braun J. Sampling of intestinal microbiota and targeted amplification of bacterial 16S rRNA genes for microbial ecologic analysis. *Curr Protoc Immunol*. 2014;107:7–41.
23. Jacobs JP, Goudarzi M, Singh N, Tong M, McHardy IH, Ruegger P, et al. A disease-associated microbial and metabolomics state in relatives of pediatric inflammatory bowel disease patients. *Cell Mol Gastroenterol Hepatol*. 2016;2(6):750–66.
24. Callahan BJ, McMurdie PJ, Rosen MJ, Han AW, Johnson AJ, Holmes SP. DADA2: high-resolution sample inference from Illumina amplicon data. *Nat Methods*. 2016;13(7):581–3.
25. Douglas GM, Maffei VJ, Zaneveld JR, Yurgel SN, Brown JR, Taylor CM, et al. PICRUSt2 for prediction of metagenome functions. *Nat Biotechnol*. 2020;38(6):685–8.
26. Kanehisa M, Goto S. KEGG: kyoto encyclopedia of genes and genomes. *Nucleic Acids Res*. 2000;28(1):27–30.
27. Hatch A, Horne J, Toma R, Twibell BL, Somerville KM, Pelle B, et al. A robust metatranscriptomic technology for population-scale studies of diet, gut microbiome, and human health. *Int J Genomics*. 2019;2019:1718741.
28. Li J, Jia H, Cai X, Zhong H, Feng Q, Sunagawa S, et al. An integrated catalog of reference genes in the human gut microbiome. *Nat Biotechnol*. 2014;32(8):834–41.
29. Do KT, Wahl S, Raffler J, Molnos S, Laimighofer M, Adamski J, et al. Characterization of missing values in untargeted MS-based metabolomics data and evaluation of missing data handling strategies. *Metabolomics*. 2018;14(10):128.
30. Johnson WE, Li C, Rabinovic A. Adjusting batch effects in microarray expression data using empirical Bayes methods. *Biostatistics*. 2007;8(1):118–27.
31. Zhang Y, Jenkins DF, Manimaran S, Johnson WE. Alternative empirical Bayes models for adjusting for batch effects in genomic studies. *BMC Bioinformatics*. 2018;19(1):262.
32. Han W, Li L. Evaluating and minimizing batch effects in metabolomics. *Mass Spectrom Rev*. 2022;41(3):421–42.
33. Li B, Tang J, Yang Q, Cui X, Li S, Chen S, et al. Performance evaluation and online realization of data-driven normalization methods used in LC/MS based untargeted metabolomics analysis. *Sci Rep*. 2016;6:38881.
34. McMurdie PJ, Holmes S. phyloseq: an R package for reproducible interactive analysis and graphics of microbiome census data. *PLoS One*. 2013;8(4):e61217.
35. Legendre P, Anderson MJ. Distance-based redundancy analysis: testing multispecies responses in multifactorial ecological experiments. *Ecological Monographs*. 1999;69(1):1–24.
36. Anderson MJ. A new method for non-parametric multivariate analysis of variance. *Austral Ecol*. 2001;26(1):32–46.
37. Mallick H, Rahnavard A, McIver LJ, Ma S, Zhang Y, Nguyen LH, et al. Multivariable association discovery in population-scale meta-omics studies. *PLoS Comput Biol*. 2021;17(11):e1009442.
38. Zhang Y, Thompson KN, Huttenhower C, Franzosa EA. Statistical approaches for differential expression analysis in metatranscriptomics. *Bioinformatics*. 2021;37(Suppl_1):i34–41.
39. Subramanian A, Tamayo P, Mootha VK, Mukherjee S, Ebert BL, Gillette MA, et al. Gene set enrichment analysis: a knowledge-based approach for interpreting genome-wide expression profiles. *Proc Natl Acad Sci U S A*. 2005;102(43):15545–50.
40. Manor O, Borenstein E. Systematic characterization and analysis of the taxonomic drivers of functional shifts in the human microbiome. *Cell Host Microbe*. 2017;21(2):254–67.
41. Noecker CE, Eng A, Borenstein E. MIMOSA2: a metabolic network-based tool for inferring mechanism-supported relationships in microbiome-metabolome data. *BioRxiv*. 2021. https://doi.org/10.1101/2021.09.14.459910v1.
42. Breiman L, et al. *Mach Learn*. 2001;45(1):5–32.
43. Franzosa EA, Morgan XC, Segata N, Waldron L, Reyes J, Earl AM, et al. Relating the metatranscriptome and metagenome of the human gut. *Proc Natl Acad Sci U S A*. 2014;111(22):E2329–38.
44. Gonzalez-Garcia RA, McCubbin T, Wille A, Plan M, Nielsen LK, Marcellin E. Awakening sleeping beauty: production of propionic acid in Escherichia coli through the sbm operon requires the activity of a methylmalonyl-CoA epimerase. *Microb Cell Fact*. 2017;16(1):121.
45. Louis P, Flint HJ. Formation of propionate and butyrate by the human colonic microbiota. *Environ Microbiol*. 2017;19(1):29–41.
46. Adams MA, Singh VK, Keller BO, Jia Z. Structural and biochemical characterization of gentisate 1,2-dioxygenase from Escherichia coli O157:H7. *Mol Microbiol*. 2006;61(6):1469–84.
47. Cheema MU, Pluznick JL. Gut microbiota plays a central role to modulate the plasma and fecal metabolomes in response to angiotensin II. *Hypertension*. 2019;74(1):184–93.
48. Fernandez IS, Cuevas P, Angulo J, Lopez-Navajas P, Canales-Mayordomo A, Gonzalez-Corrochano R, et al. Gentisic acid, a compound associated with plant defense and a metabolite of aspirin, heads a new class of in vivo fibroblast growth factor inhibitors. *J Biol Chem*. 2010;285(15):11714–29.
49. Danopoulos S, Schlieve CR, Grikscheit TC, Al Alam D. Fibroblast growth factors in the gastrointestinal tract: twists and turns. *Dev Dyn*. 2017;246(4):344–52.
50. Parkar SG, Trower TM, Stevenson DE. Fecal microbial metabolism of polyphenols and its effects on human gut microbiota. *Anaerobe*. 2013;23:12–9.
51. Pallister T, Jackson MA, Martin TC, Zierer J, Jennings A, Mohney RP, et al. Hippurate as a metabolomic marker of gut microbiome diversity: Modulation by diet and relationship to metabolic syndrome. *Sci Rep*. 2017;7(1):13670.
52. Wilmanski T, Rappaport N, Earls JC, Magis AT, Manor O, Lovejoy J, et al. Blood metabolome predicts gut microbiome alpha-diversity in humans. *Nat Biotechnol*. 2019;37(10):1217–28.
53. Gonthier MP, Verny MA, Besson C, Remesy C, Scalbert A. Chlorogenic acid bioavailability largely depends on its metabolism by the gut microflora in rats. *J Nutr*. 2003;133(6):1853–9.
54. Jacobi JL, Yang B, Li X, Menze AK, Laurentz SM, Janle EM, et al. Impacts on sirtuin function and bioavailability of the dietary bioactive compound dihydrocoumarin. *PLoS One*. 2016;11(2):e0149207.
55. Lai Y, Liu CW, Yang Y, Hsiao YC, Ru H, Lu K. High-coverage metabolomics uncovers microbiota-driven biochemical landscape of interorgan transport and gut-brain communication in mice. *Nat Commun*. 2021;12(1):6000.
56. Bonnin-Jusserand M, Grandvalet C, Rieu A, Weidmann S, Alexandre H. Tyrosine-containing peptides are precursors of tyramine produced by Lactobacillus plantarum strain IR BL0076 isolated from wine. *BMC Microbiol*. 2012;12:199.

57. Fujisaka S, Avila-Pacheco J, Soto M, Kostic A, Dreyfuss JM, Pan H, et al. Diet, genetics, and the gut microbiome drive dynamic changes in plasma metabolites. *Cell Rep.* 2018;22(11):3072–86.
58. Broadley KJ, Akhtar Anwar M, Herbert AA, Fehler M, Jones EM, Davies WE, et al. Effects of dietary amines on the gut and its vasculature. *Br J Nutr.* 2009;101(11):1645–52.
59. Yano JM, Yu K, Donaldson GP, Shastri GG, Ann P, Ma L, et al. Indigenous bacteria from the gut microbiota regulate host serotonin biosynthesis. *Cell.* 2015;161(2):264–76.
60. Bugda Gwilt K, Gonzalez DP, Olliffe N, Oller H, Hoffing R, Puzan M, et al. Actions of trace amines in the brain-gut-microbiome axis via trace amine-associated receptor-1 (TAAR1). *Cell Mol Neurobiol.* 2020;40(2):191–201.
61. Kamp KJ, Cain KC, Utleg A, Burr RL, Raftery D, Luna RA, et al. Bile acids and microbiome among individuals with irritable bowel syndrome and healthy volunteers. *Biol Res Nurs.* 2021;23(1):65–74.
62. Candido FG, Valente FX, Grzeskowiak LM, Moreira APB, Rocha D, Alfenas RCG. Impact of dietary fat on gut microbiota and low-grade systemic inflammation: mechanisms and clinical implications on obesity. *Int J Food Sci Nutr.* 2018;69(2):125–43.
63. Yao J, Rock CO. Exogenous fatty acid metabolism in bacteria. *Biochimie.* 2017;141:30–9.
64. Tap J, Storsrud S, Le Neve B, Cotillard A, Pons N, Dore J, et al. Diet and gut microbiome interactions of relevance for symptoms in irritable bowel syndrome. *Microbiome.* 2021;9(1):74.
65. Sun Q, Jia Q, Song L, Duan L. Alterations in fecal short-chain fatty acids in patients with irritable bowel syndrome: a systematic review and meta-analysis. *Medicine.* 2019;98(7):e14513.
66. Chey WD, Keefer L, Whelan K, Gibson PR. Behavioral and diet therapies in integrated care for patients with irritable bowel syndrome. *Gastroenterology.* 2021;160(1):47–62.
67. Keely SJ, Barrett KE. Intestinal secretory mechanisms and diarrhea. *Am J Physiol Gastrointest Liver Physiol.* 2022;322(4):G405–20.
68. Murray KE, Shaw KJ, Adams RF, Conway PL. Presence of N-acyl and acetoxy derivatives of putrescine and cadaverine in the human gut. *Gut.* 1993;34(4):489–93.
69. Oliphant K, Allen-Vercoe E. Macronutrient metabolism by the human gut microbiome: major fermentation by-products and their impact on host health. *Microbiome.* 2019;7(1):91.
70. Kaval KG, Garsin DA. Ethanolamine utilization in bacteria. mBio. 2018;9(1):e00066-18.
71. Midenfjord I, Polster A, Sjovall H, Friberg P, Tornblom H, Simren M. Associations among neurophysiology measures in irritable bowel syndrome (IBS) and their relevance for IBS symptoms. *Sci Rep.* 2020;10(1):9794.

23

Effects of personality traits on the manifestations of irritable bowel syndrome

Jun Tayama[1], Naoki Nakaya[2], Toyohiro Hamaguchi[3], Tadaaki Tomiie[4], Masae Shinozaki[5], Tatsuo Saigo[1], Susumu Shirabe[1] and Shin Fukudo[5*]

Abstract

Objective: Previous studies have reported that patients with irritable bowel syndrome (IBS) show high neuroticism. However, the precise association between the IBS subtypes and the degree of neuroticism in younger populations is largely unknown. We tested our hypothesis that subjects with diarrhea-predominant IBS may have a higher degree of neuroticism than subjects without IBS or those with other subtypes of IBS. We also verified the additional hypothesis that the severity of neuroticism might be correlated with the severity of IBS in younger populations.

Methods: We conducted a cross-sectional survey of 557 university students, ranging in age from 18 to 21 years. Presence/ absence of IBS and determination of the IBS subtype was by the Rome II Modular Questionnaire, while the severity of IBS was determined by the IBS severity index (IBS-SI). The degree of neuroticism was evaluated using the Maudsely Personality Inventory (MPI). The presence/absence of psychological distress was measured with the K6 scale.

Results: Neuroticism scores in the subjects with diarrhea-predominant IBS were significantly higher than those in the non-IBS subjects or subjects with constipation-predominant IBS. The neuroticism scores were significantly correlated with the IBS-SI scores in all subjects with IBS.

Conclusion: These results suggest that neuroticism is involved in the pathophysiology of IBS in young subjects, especially in that of the diarrhea-predominant subtype.

Keywords: Personality, Irritable bowel syndrome, Depression, Neuroticism, Brain- gut interactions

Introduction

Irritable bowel syndrome (IBS) is a functional gastrointestinal disorder not associated with major organic diseases [1,2]. The characteristic pathophysiological features of IBS are dysmotility of the lower gastrointestinal tract [3], visceral hypersensitivity [4], and psychological abnormalities [5]. A previous study focusing on the psychological abnormalities in IBS reported that the gastrointestinal symptoms of IBS worsened with aggravation of the psychological state and that they improved with recovery of the psychological state [5]. Several epidemiologic studies have revealed that the prevalence rates of depression and anxiety are higher in IBS patients than those in healthy persons [6-8]. In a study that examined the depressive symptoms in 80 IBS patients and 21 healthy persons aged 21 years to 65 years old, the average scores for depression were higher in the group with constipation-predominant IBS (C-IBS) and the IBS group with alternating diarrhea and constipation (A-IBS) than in the healthy persons; however, no significant difference in the score for depression was seen between the subjects with diarrhea-predominant IBS (D-IBS) and healthy persons [9].

Among the several known personality traits, neuroticism has been suggested as a risk factor for the development of IBS [10-13]. In the study conducted in 41 IBS patients and 2000 healthy persons aged 41 to 49 years old by Palmer et al. using [10] Eysenck's index (Maudsely Personality Inventory: MPI), the average score for neuroticism was higher in the IBS patients than that in healthy persons. In a study performed in 60 IBS patients (average age ± standard deviation: 29 ± 7) and 55 healthy persons (average age ±

* Correspondence: sfukudo@med.tohoku.ac.jp
[5]Department of Behavioral Medicine, Tohoku University Graduate School of Medicine, Tohoku, Japan
Full list of author information is available at the end of the article

standard deviation: 27 ± 7) using the Minnesota Multiphasic Personality Inventory (MMPI-2), Mousavinasab et al. [11] reported a higher average score for hypochondriasis in the IBS patients than that in the healthy persons. Farman et al. [12] showed that the average score for neuroticism in an evaluation conducted using the NEO Five-Factor Inventory (NEO-FFI) was significantly higher in the C-IBS group (33 patients) than the scores in the groups with other subtypes of IBS (71 with D-IBS patients and 46 A-IBS patients). In the study conducted by Tanum et al. [14] in 56 patients with functional gastrointestinal disorders (FGIDs), including 31 IBS patients and 55 age-matched healthy persons (age range: 18–70 years old), the average score for neuroticism on the NEO Personality Inventory (NEO-PI) was higher in the FGID patients than that in the healthy persons. Thus, neuroticism may indeed play some role in the pathophysiology of IBS.

In an epidemiologic survey of 10,000 Japanese adults aged over 20 years old, the prevalence rate of IBS in persons aged 20–29 years, as diagnosed based on the ROME-III criteria, was 14% among males and 22% among females [15]. In persons aged 30 years or over, the prevalence rate of IBS decreased gradually with increasing age [15]. In an investigation of 1,087 Japanese college students with an average age of 20 years (SD ± 2), the prevalence rate of IBS, as diagnosed based on the ROME-III criteria, was 19% overall, 17% in males, and 20% in females [16]. The above reports suggest that the prevalence of IBS may be higher in college students as compared with that in older age groups, which warrants further analysis.

Despite the earlier studies mentioned above, there is no evidence yet to show that neuroticism is a risk factor for the onset of any subtype of IBS in young patients. Also, no study has been performed yet to determine the relationship between the severity of neuroticism and the severity of IBS among subjects with IBS. Investigation of the relationship between the severity of neuroticism and the severity of IBS in subjects with each subtype of IBS may clarify the physiological relationship between neuroticism and the development of gastrointestinal symptoms. Neuroticism has been linked to the development of mood and anxiety disorders [17,18]. Anxiety has been shown to play a role in patients with diarrhea-predominant IBS [19]. Therefore, neuroticism may be closely related to the development of D-IBS. In this research, we attempted to verify the following two hypotheses in university students, who represent the young population.

1) In the young population, subjects with diarrhea-predominant IBS show a higher degree of neuroticism than subjects not suffering from IBS or subjects with other IBS subtypes.
2) In the young population, the neuroticism score is correlated with the severity of IBS.

Method

Subjects

We conducted a cross-sectional study of 655 university students, ranging in age from 18 years to 21 years. Of the 655 subjects, 11 refused to provide consent for the use of their data for research/participation in this study, and 87 did not respond to the questionnaire. We therefore analyzed the data of the remaining 557 persons who answered all the items of the questionnaire (Figure 1). Of these 557 subjects, 143 (26%) were diagnosed as having IBS based on responses to the IBS screening questionnaire described below.

Measurements

The Rome II Modular Questionnaire (RIIMQ)

Rome II criteria, described below, are widely used for the diagnosis of IBS [20]: at least 12 weeks, which need not be consecutive, during the preceding 12 months during which the patient suffered from abdominal discomfort or pain satisfying the following three features: (1) relieved by defecation, (2) onset associated with a change in the stool frequency, and/or (3) onset associated with a change in the form (appearance) of the stool. The following symptoms cumulatively support the diagnosis and subtyping of IBS: (a) fewer than 3 bowel movements a week; (b) more than 3 bowel movements a day; (c) hard or lumpy stools; (d) loose (mushy) or watery stools; (e) straining during a bowel movement; (f) urgency (having to rush to have a bowel movement); (g) feeling of incomplete evacuation; (h) passage of mucus; (i) bloating or feeling of abdominal distension. D-IBS is defined by one or more of b, d or f and none of a, c or e, or 2 or more of b, d, or f and one of a or e. C-IBS is defined by one or more of a, c, or e and none of b, d or f, or 2 or more of a, c, or e and one of b, d or f. IBS patients not fulfilling the aforementioned criteria for D-IBS or C-IBS were defined as having A-IBS in this study. RIIMQ has been reported as a reliable tool for epidemiological surveys [21]. The Japanese version of the RIIMQ is a questionnaire that is used for both diagnosis of IBS and for determination of the subtype of IBS [22].

IBS severity

The Japanese version [22] of the IBS severity index (IBS-SI) [23] was used in this study to assess the severity of the lower gastrointestinal symptoms and the degree of impairment of the quality of life by the IBS. This instrument is composed of five items, with the possible total score in the range of 0 to 500. The IBS-SI scores the

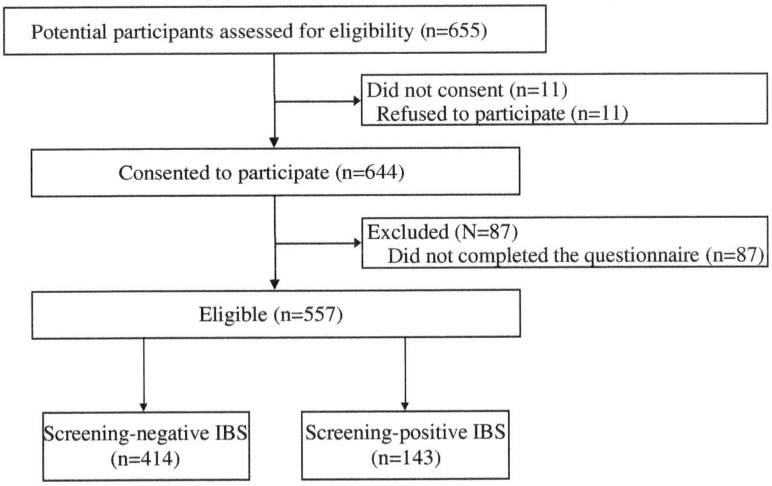

Figure 1 Study flow. Of 655 subjects, 11 did not provide consent for participation, and 87 did not respond to the questionnaire. We analyzed the data of the remaining 557 persons who answered all the items of the questionnaire.

severity of the abdominal pain, abdominal distension, bowel movements, and the quality of life.

Psychological distress

The six-item K6 [24] was used in this study to evaluate the presence/absence of psychological distress in the subjects. The K6 has been developed to identify persons who are at a risk of developing mental states such as depression and anxiety [25]. The K6 total score can range from 0 to 24, and patients with scores of 13 or greater are categorized as suffering from psychological distress.

Personality

The Maudsely Personality Inventory (MPI) [26] is a measure used to assess personality in two dimensions, namely, neuroticism and extroversion/introversion. It is composed of 80 items calling for a yes/no response; Extroversion (E): 24-items; Neuroticism (N): 24-items; Lie (L): 20-items; Filler items: 12-items.

Procedure

The questionnaire survey was given during an academic session in the classroom. First, we explained the research content and provided both a written and verbal explanation about the intended use of the data. In addition, we explained that persons not providing consent for participation in the study would not be placed at any disadvantage whatsoever. We only included the data of those students who agreed to cooperate with the research for the analysis in this study.

Data analysis

Data are presented as means ± standard deviation (SD). An unpaired *t*-test was used to compare any two groups. Correlation coefficients were calculated by determination of the Pearson's correlation coefficients. Chi-square test was used to evaluate differences in percentages. One-way ANOVA was performed to compare data between groups. One-way ANOVA was performed for between group comparisons. SPSS, version 18.0, was used for the statistical analyses.

Results

The demographic data of the study subjects and the reference values in healthy persons established in a previous study are shown in Table 1 [16,27-31]. Males comprised 59% of all subjects (95% confidence interval (CI), 55 to 63%). The mean (±SD) age of the subjects was 19 (±1) years. The prevalences of D-IBS, C-IBS and A-IBS in the study population were 4% (95% CI, 3 to 6), 9% (95% CI, 7 to 12) and 12% (95% CI, 10 to 15), respectively. In addition, the prevalence of psychological distress in the overall study population was 7% (95% CI, 5 to 9), consistent with the finding of a previous study [30].

The scores for each of the evaluated items in the IBS group and non-IBS group are shown in Table 2. The proportion of males/females in the non-IBS group was 64%/36%, and that in the IBS group was 48%/52%, with a significant difference in the proportion of males/females between the two groups (p = 0.0001). Scores on the IBS-SI in the IBS group (53.9 ± 50.2) were significantly higher than those in the non-IBS group (27.3 ± 39.8, p = 0.0001). Scores on K6 in the IBS group (6.7 ± 5.0) were also significantly higher than those in the non-

Table 1 Demographic data and reference values

Variables	All subjects (n = 557) (95% CI)	Reference value (general population (95% CI))	
Sex (male (%))	59 (55–63)	47 (36–45)	Sugaya and Nomura[16]
Age	19 ± 1 (19–19)	-	-
IBS+ (%)[a]	26 (22–30)	14 (12–15)	Kubo M, et al. [27]
D-IBS (%)[b]	4 (3–6)	4 (–)	Kubo M, et al. [27]
C-IBS (%)[c]	9 (7–12)	3 (–)	Kubo M, et al. [27]
A-IBS (%)[d]	12 (10–15)	3 (–)	Kubo M, et al. [27]
IBS-SI	34.1 ± 44.2 (30.4-37.8)	30 (–)[g]	Tana C, et al. [28]
K6[e,f]	5.4 ± 4.5 (5.0-5.7)	3.6 ± 3.9 (–)	Sakurai K, et al. [29]
Persons with psychological distress (%)[g]	7 (5–9)	7 (7–7)	Kuriyama S, et al. [30]
MPI	-	-	-
Extroversion	27.2 ± 10.3 (26.3-28.0)	27. 2 ± 7.0 (–)	Iwawaki, S et al. [31]
Neuroticism	21.6 ± 10.7 (20.7-22.5)	21.6 ± 7.9 (–)	Iwawaki, S et al. [31]
Lie score	13.4 ± 5.8 (12.9-13.8)	13.4 ± 5.1 (–)	Iwawaki, S et al. [31]

Data are expressed as mean ± standard deviation. CI, confidence interval.
[a-e,g] The numerical values represent the percentage of the total number of participants, namely, IBS patients plus healthy persons.
[f]Persons with a score of ≥13 points (out of a total 24 points) on the K6 were defined as experiencing psychological distress.
The data (score) represent median values.

IBS group (4.9 ± 4.2, p = 0.0001). The differences in the scores on the IBS-SI and K6 were seen even after adjustment for the sex distribution (p = 0.0001 for all). The percentage of persons with psychological distress was significantly higher in the IBS group than that in the non-IBS group (11% vs. 5%, p = 0.0081).

The scores for each of the evaluated items in the non-IBS group and the groups with each subtype of IBS are shown in Table 2. The main effects were seen in the scores on the IBS-SI (F (3,553) = 14.1, p = 0.0001) and K6 (F (3,553) = 3.6, p = 0.0001), as calculated by ANOVA. The percentage of persons with psychological distress was 13% in the D-IBS group, 6% in the C-IBS group, and 15% in the A-IBS group, and significant differences among the three groups were revealed by the chi-square test (χ^2 = 10.5, p = 0.0146). Scores on the IBS-SI in all of the D-IBS (47.9 ± 39.5, p = 0.0109), C-IBS (51.6 ± 56.0, p = 0.0002) and A-IBS (57.6 ± 49.3, p = 0.0001) groups were significantly higher than the score in the non-IBS group (27.3 ± 39.8). Scores on K6 in the D-IBS group (8.3 ± 5.1, p = 0.0001) and the A-IBS group (7.1 ± 5.4, p = 0.0001) were significantly higher

Table 2 Difference between non-IBS group and IBS subgroups in the personality scales

Variables	Non-IBS group (n = 414)	IBS group (n = 143)	IBS subgroup			p value[c]
			D-IBS (n = 24)	C-IBS (n = 50)	A-IBS (n = 69)	
Sex (male (%))	64	48 §	58	32	55	p = 0.0001
Age	19 ± 1	19 ± 1	19 ± 1	19 ± 1	19 ± 1	p = 0.1479
IBS-SI	27.3 ± 39.8	53.9 ± 50.2 †	47.9 ± 39.5 **	51.6 ± 56.0 **	57.6 ± 49.3 **	p = 0.0001
K6[a]	4.9 ± 4.2	6.7 ± 5.0 †	8.3 ± 5.1 **	5.5 ± 4.0	7.1 ± 5.4 **	p = 0.0001
Persons with psychological distress (%)[b]	5	11 §	13	6	15	p = 0.0001
EPI	-	-	-	-	-	-
Extroversion	27.6 ± 10.2	25.8 ± 10.4	25.3 ± 10.8	27.1 ± 9.2	25.1 ± 11.2 *	p = 0.2228
Neuroticism	21.4 ± 10.8	22.4 ± 10.4	26.0 ± 9.4 * ¶	20.5 ± 11.5	22.5 ± 9.6	p = 0.1430
Lie score	13.3 ± 5.7	13.4 ± 6.0	12.4 ± 5.8	14.1 ± 6.6	13.3 ± 5.7	p = 0.6855

[a]Persons with scores of ≥13 points (out of a total 24 points) on the K6 were defined as experiencing psychological distress.
[b]Values are the percentages of the total number of participants (i.e., IBS group plus non-IBS group).
[c]One-way ANOVA was performed using the data from the non-IBS group, and the groups with the diarrhea-type, constipation-type and alternating-type IBS.
†p < 0.01 vs. non-IBS group; *p < 0.05 and **p < 0.01 vs. non-IBS group, unpaired *t*-test.
§p< 0.01 vs. non-IBS group, chi square test.
¶p < 0.05 vs. C-IBS group, unpaired *t*-test.

than the score in the non-IBS group (4.9 ± 4.2). Scores for extroversion as assessed by the MPI in the A-IBS group were significantly lower than those in the non-IBS group (25.1 ± 11.2 vs. 27.6 ± 10.2, p = 0.0305). Scores of neuroticism in the D-IBS group (26.0 ± 9.4) were significantly higher than those in the non-IBS group (21.4 ± 10.8, p = 0.0182). Furthermore, the scores for neuroticism in the D-IBS (26.0 ± 9.4) were significantly higher than those in the C-IBS group (20.5 ± 11.5, p = 0.0183). The differences in the scores on the IBS-SI and K6, and in the scores for extroversion, and neuroticism, between the two groups were seen even after adjustment for the sex distribution (p = 0.0001 for all).

A significant correlation was observed between the scores for neuroticism and the IBS-SI scores in all the subjects (p = 0.0001), as shown in Figure 2. A significant correlation was observed between the degree of neuroticism and the IBS-SI score in the D-IBS patients (r = 0.21, p = 0.0001), as shown in Figure 3. The corresponding correlation was r = 0.12 ($p < 0.01$) in the C-IBS group, r = 0.09 ($p < 0.05$) in the A-IBS group, and r = 0.15 ($p < 0.01$) in the non-IBS group, both representing only weak correlations. There was no significant correlation between the scores for extroversion and the IBS-SI scores.

Discussion

The results of our cross-sectional study performed in a young population of university freshmen revealed higher degrees of neuroticism in patients with D-IBS, diagnosed based on the ROME criteria, than in subjects not suffering from IBS and those diagnosed as having C-IBS. Therefore, hypothesis 1 was supported. Furthermore, the correlation between the degree of neuroticism and the severity of IBS also supported hypothesis 2.

A previous report indicated that among patients with IBS, the severity of neuroticism was higher in patients with C-IBS than that in patients with other subtypes of IBS [12]. However in this study, in contrast to the aforementioned report, the neuroticism score was higher only in the D-IBS group as compared with that in the non-IBS group. According to another previous study, while the scores for depressive mood were higher in the C-IBS and A-IBS groups than the score in healthy people, the scores did not differ significantly between the D-IBS group and healthy persons [9]. Furthermore, a survey of 1,087 Japanese college students revealed no differences in the average scores for depressive mood between patients with D-IBS or C-IBS and healthy persons [16]. Although Sugaya and Nomura reported that males comprised 64% of the D-IBS group but only 22% of the C-IBS group in their series [16], males in this study accounted for 58% and 32% of the patients in the D-IBS and C-IBS groups, respectively. It has been reported that, among Japanese adults, the prevalence of psychological distress, as judged by K6, is higher in females than in males [30], and that the prevalence rate of IBS is higher in females than in males [32]. Based on the higher percentage of females in the D-IBS group in this study, such a result may have been output in this study.

The following reason is speculated to explain the correlation between the neuroticism scores and the scores on IBS-SI in the D-IBS group in this study. Neuroticism in patients with depression has been reported to increase

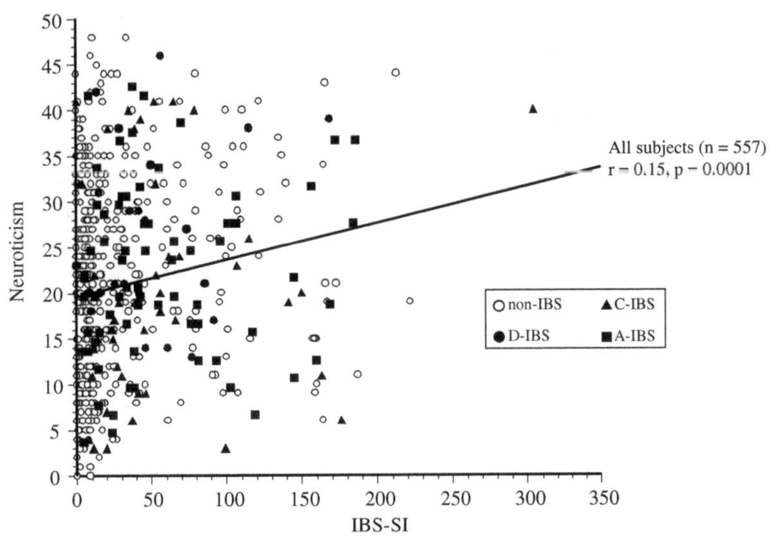

Figure 2 Correlation between neuroticism and the total score of the IBS severity index in the study population. A significant correlation was observed between the score for neuroticism and the IBS-SI score in all the subjects (r = 0.15, p = 0.0001). The corresponding correlation was r = 0.12 (p = 0.0001) in the C-IBS group and r = 0.09 (p = 0.0440) in the A-IBS group, both representing weak correlations. There was no significant correlation between the scores for extroversion and the IBS-SI scores.

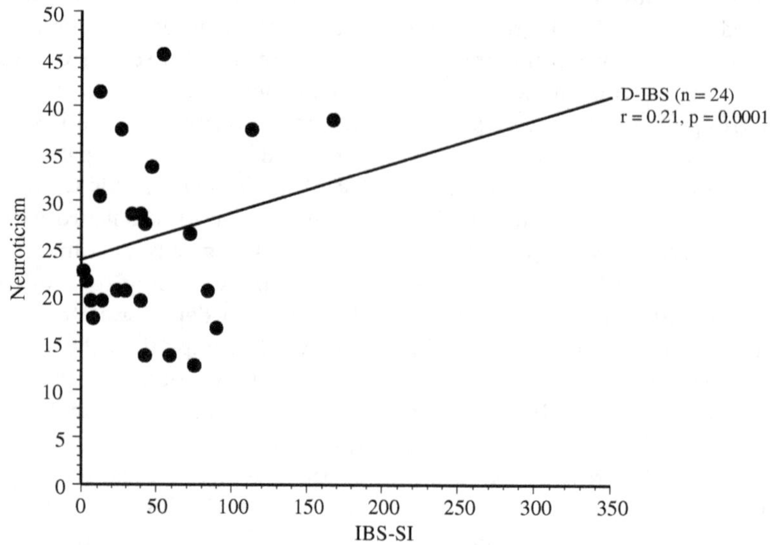

Figure 3 Correlation between the score for neuroticism and the total score of the IBS-SI in the D-IBS subjects. A significant correlation was observed between the scores for neuroticism and the IBS-SI scores in the D-IBS subjects (r = 0.21, p = 0.0001).

the score for depressive mood [33,34]. In patients with depression, the hypothalamic-pituitary-adrenocortical (HPA) axis is reported to be activated [35-37]. Therefore, the HPA-axis is assumed to also be activated in subjects with a high severity of neuroticism. In animal experiments, corticotropin-releasing hormone (CRH) has been reported to increase the fecal pellet output and exaggerate colonic motility [38]. A previous study reported HPA hyperactivity in adults with a high degree of neuroticism [39]. In IBS patients, exogenous CRH administration aggravates the brain-gut axis [40] and administration of CRH antagonists normalizes the axis [41]. Therefore, a high degree of neuroticism may aggravate the symptom of diarrhea by worsening the depressive mood and enhancing the activity of the HPA-axis, especially in younger age groups. Furthermore, in this study, subjects were categorized as having/not having IBS based on the results of a questionnaire, and not by a physician. Thus, the rate of IBS identified in this study may be an overestimate as compared with the potential diagnosis rate by a physician. If the prevalence rate of IBS found in this study were indeed higher than the potential prevalence rate determined based on a physician's diagnosis, it is possible that our results may include the data of persons with relatively minor symptoms. Therefore, if the study were conducted only with patients with physician-diagnosed IBS, the relationship between psychological traits and the severity of IBS may have become more apparent, and the relationship may have been underestimated in this study.

In this study, no difference in the neuroticism score was observed between the subjects with and without IBS. By contrast, in some earlier studies, higher neuroticism scores have been reported in patients with IBS than in subjects without IBS [10,11]. A possible major reason for the absence of any significant difference in the neuroticism score between subjects with and without IBS in our study was that the subjects were all freshmen college students. The frequency of major depression has been reported to increase with age [42]. Neuroticism in patients with depression has been reported to raise the score for depressive mood [33,34]. Therefore, the lack of increased score for neuroticism in the IBS subjects overall, and of a correlation between the degree of neuroticism and the severity of IBS in the overall subject population in this study may suggest a subliminal role of neuroticism in IBS pathophysiology. Moreover, the hypothesis of involvement of neuroticism in the development of IBS may have originated from the relationship between the degree of neuroticism and that of the D-IBS phenotype in the younger generation.

The strength of this study is that it examined the involvement of neuroticism in college students with each subtype of IBS, and it was the first study to do so in college students. There are three limitations to this study. First, this research targeted only one university. The prevalence rates of IBS differ by culture [43,44]. The target university is located in a medium-sized city on the island of Kyushu in western Japan. Therefore, it is unknown whether the results can be extrapolated to Japanese university students in general. Second, since this study is a cross-sectional study, it could not be judged how the presence/degree of neuroticism influenced the severity of diarrhea in the subjects. Therefore, prospective studies are required. Third, although we evaluated psychological distress in the subjects using K6 in this study, we did not sufficiently evaluate the prevalence of depression. The lack of adequate evaluation of depression in the present study might limit the interpretation of the obtained results.

In conclusion, in a young study population in Japan, patients with D-IBS showed higher degrees of neuroticism as compared to subjects not suffering from IBS and subjects with C-IBS. Furthermore, the degree of neuroticism was correlated with the severity of IBS in the young subjects. This suggests that neuroticism may be involved in the onset and aggravation of IBS, and therapeutic approaches for D-IBS should take this finding into consideration.

Abbreviations

IBS: Irritable bowel syndrome; C-IBS: Constipation-predominant IBS; D-IBS: Diarrhea-predominant IBS; A-IBS: IBS with alternating diarrhea and constipation; SD: Standard deviation; CI: Confidence interval.

Authors' contributions

JT designed and coordinated the study; NN, TH, TT, and MS provided the information about the psychological variables; TS supported the analysis of the data; MH, SS, and SF supported the interpretation of the data. All authors have read and approved the final manuscript.

Acknowledgments

The authors would like to express their appreciation to the participants of this study. This study was supported by the Center for Health and Community Medicine, Nagasaki University.

Author details

[1]Center for Health and Community Medicine, Nagasaki University, Nagasaki, Japan. [2]Department of Preventive Medicine and Epidemiology, Tohoku Medical Megabank Organization, Tohoku University, Tohoku, Japan. [3]Department of Occupational Therapy, School of Health and Social Services, Saitama Prefectural University, Saitama, Japan. [4]School of Psychological Science, Health Sciences University of Hokkaido, Hokkaido, Japan. [5]Department of Behavioral Medicine, Tohoku University Graduate School of Medicine, Tohoku, Japan.

References

1. Mayer EA, Raybould HE: **Role of visceral afferent mechanism in functional bowel disorders.** *Gastroenterology* 1990, **99:**1688–1704.
2. Sagami Y, Shimada Y, Tayama J, Nomura T, Satake M, Endo Y, Shoji T, Karahashi K, Hongo M, Fukudo S: **Effect of a corticotropin-releasing hormone receptor antagonist on colonic sensory and motor function in patients with irritable bowel syndrome.** *Gut* 2004, **53:**958–964.
3. Drossman DA, Sandler RS, McKee DC, Levity AJ: **Bowel Patterns among subjects not seeking health care.** *Gastroenterology* 1982, **83:**529–532.
4. Richie J: **Pain from distension of the pervic colon by inflating a balloon in the irritable bowel syndrome.** *Gut* 1973, **14:**125–132.
5. Whitehead WE, Schuster MM: **Irritable bowel syndrome: definition of the syndrome and relation to other disorder.** In *Gastrointestinal disorders: behavioral and physiological basis for treatment.* New York: Academic; 1985:155–177.
6. Osterberg E, Blomquist L, Krakau I, Weinryb RM, Asberg M, Hultcrantz R: **A population study on irritable bowel syndrome and mental health.** *Scand J Gastroenterol* 2000, **35:**264–268.
7. Whitehead WE, Palsson O, Jones KR: **Systematic review of the comorbidity of irritable bowel syndrome with other disorders: what are the causes and implications?** *Gastroenterology* 2002, **122:**1140–1156.
8. Ladep NG, Obindo TJ, Audu MD, Okeke EN, Malu AO: **Depression in patients with irritable bowel syndrome in Jos, Nigeria.** *World J Gastroenterol* 2006, **12:**7844–7847.
9. Eriksson EM, Andrén KI, Eriksson HT, Kurlberg GK: **Irritable bowel syndrome subtypes differ in body awareness, psychological symptoms and biochemical stress markers.** *World J Gastroenterol* 2008, **14:**4889–4896.
10. Palmer RL, Stonehill E, Crisp AH, Waller SL, Misiewicz JJ: **Psychological characteristics of patients with the irritable bowel syndrome.** *Postgrad Med J* 1974, **50:**416–419.
11. Mousavinasab SM, Gorganinezhad-Moshiri M, Saberifirouzi M, Dehbozorgi G, Mehrabani D: **Personality characteristics and irritable bowel syndrome in Shiraz, southern Iran.** *Saudi J Gastroenterol* 2007, **13:**168–171.
12. Farnam A, Somi MH, Sarami F, Farhang S, Yasrebinia S: **Personality factors and profiles in variants of irritable bowel syndrome.** *World J Gastroenterol* 2007, **13:**6414–6418.
13. Farnam A, Somi MH, Sarami F, Farhang S: **Five personality dimensions in patients with irritable bowel syndrome.** *Neuropsychiatr Dis Treat* 2008, **4:**959–962.
14. Tanum L, Malt UF: **Personality and physical symptoms in nonpsychiatric patients with functional gastrointestinal disorder.** *J Psychosom Res* 2001, **50:**139–146.
15. Miwa H: **Prevalence of irritable bowel syndrome in Japan: Internet survey using Rome III criteria.** *Patient Prefer Adherence* 2008, **2:**143–147.
16. Sugaya N, Nomura S: **Relationship between cognitive appraisals of symptoms and negative mood for subtypes of irritable bowel syndrome.** *BioPsychoSocial Medicine* 2008, **2:**9. doi:10.1186/1751-0759-2-9.
17. Batterham PJ, Glozier N, Christensen H: **Sleep disturbance, personality and the onset of depression and anxiety: Prospective cohort study.** *Aust N Z J Psychiatry* 2012, doi:10.1177/0004867412457997.
18. Haas BW, Omura K, Constable RT, Canli T: **Emotional conflict and neuroticism: personality-dependent activation in the amygdala and subgenual anterior cingulate.** *Behav Neurosci* 2007, **121:**249–256.
19. Singh RK, Pandey HP, Singh RH: **Correlation of serotonin and monoamine oxidase levels with anxiety level in diarrhea-predominant irritable bowel syndrome.** *Indian J Gastroenterol* 2003, **22:**88–90.
20. Thompson WG, Longstreth GF, Drossman DA, Heaton KW, Irvine EJ, Müller-Lissner SA: **Functional bowel disorders and functional abdominal pain.** *Gut* 1999, **45**(Suppl 2):II43–II47.
21. Drossman DA, Talley NJ, Whitehead WE, Thompson WE, Corazziari E: **Research diagnostic questions for functional gastrointestinal disorders: Rome II Modular Questionnaire: Investigator and Respondent Forms.** In *Rome II The Functional Gastrointestinal Disorders.* 2nd edition. Edited by Drossman DA, Corazziari E, Talley NJ, Thompson WG, Whitehead WE. Boston: McLean: Degnon Associates; 2000:669–688.
22. Shinozaki M, Kanazawa M, Sagami Y, Endo Y, Hongo M, Drossman DA, *et al*: **Validation of the Japanese version of the Rome II modular questionnaire and irritable bowel syndrome severity index.** *J Gastroenterol* 2006, **41:**491–494.
23. Francis CY, Morris J, Whorwell PJ: **The irritable bowel severity scoring system: a simple method of monitoring irritable bowel syndrome and its progress.** *Aliment Pharmacol Ther* 1997, **11:**395–402.
24. Kessler RC, Andrews G, Colpe LJ, Hiripi E, Mroczek DK, Normand SL, Walters EE, Zaslavsky AM: **Short screening scales to monitor population prevalences and trends in non-specific psychological distress.** *Psychol Med* 2002, **32:**959–976.
25. Furukawa TA, Kessler RC, Slade T, Andrews G: **The performance of the K6 and K10 screening scales for psychological distress in the Australian National Survey of Mental Health and Well-Being.** *Psychol Med* 2003, **33:**357–362.
26. Jensen AR: **The Maudsley Personality Inventory.** *Acta Psychol* 1958, **14:**314–325.
27. Kubo M, Fujiwara Y, Shiba M, Kohata Y, Yamagami H, Tanigawa T, Watanabe K, Watanabe T, Tominaga K, Arakawa T: **Differences between risk factors among irritable bowel syndrome subtypes in Japanese adults.** *Neurogastroenterol Motil* 2011, **23:**249–254.
28. Tana C, Umesaki Y, Imaoka A, Handa T, Kanazawa M, Fukudo S: **Altered profiles of intestinal microbiota and organic acids may be the origin of symptoms in irritable bowel syndrome.** *Neurogastroenterol Motil* 2010, **22:**512–519.
29. Sakurai K, Nishi A, Kondo K, Yanagida K, Kawakami N: **Screening performance of K6/K10 and other screening instruments for mood and anxiety disorders in Japan.** *Psychiatry Clin Neurosci* 2011, **65:**434–441.
30. Kuriyama S, Nakaya N, Ohmori-Matsuda K, Shimazu T, Kikuchi N, Kakizaki M, Sone T, Sato F, Nagai M, Sugawara Y, Akhter M, Higashiguchi M, Fukuchi N, Takahashi H, Hozawa A, Tsuji I: **Factors Associated With Psychological Distress in a Community-Dwelling Japanese Population: The Ohsaki Cohort 2006 Study.** *J Epidemiol* 2009, **19:**294–302.
31. Iwawaki S, Oyama T, Sugiyama Y, Kikuchi M, Komatsu R: **Development and validation of the Japanese version of the MPI (Maudsley Personality Inventory).** *Jpn Psychol Res* 1970, **12:**176–183.

32. Chang L, Heitkemper MM: **Gender Differences in Irritable Bowel Syndrome.** *Gastroenterology* 2002, **123:**1686–1701.
33. Barnhofer T, Chittka T: **Cognitive reactivity mediates the relationship between neuroticism and depression.** *Behav Res Ther* 2010, **48:**275–281.
34. Brown TA, Rosellini AJ: **The direct and interactive effects of neuroticism and life stress on the severity and longitudinal course of depressive symptoms.** *J Abnorm Psychol* 2011, **120:**844–856.
35. Nemeroff CB, Widerlöv E, Bissette G, Walléus H, Karlsson I, Eklund K, Kilts CD, Loosen PT, Vale W: **Elevated concentrations of CSF corticotropin-releasing factor-like immunoreactivity in depressed patients.** *Science* 1984, **226:**1342–1344.
36. Rubin RT, Phillips JJ, Sadow TF, McCracken JT: **Adrenal gland volume in major depression. Increase during the depressive episode and decrease with successful treatment.** *Arch Gen Psychiatry* 1995, **52:**213–218.
37. MacMaster FP, Kusumakar V: **MRI study of the pituitary gland in adolescent depression.** *J Psychiatr Res* 2004, **38:**231–236.
38. Mönnikes H, Schmidt BG, Taché Y: **Psychological stress-induced accelerated colonic transit in rats involves hypothalamic corticotrophin-releasing factor.** *Gastroenterology* 1993, **104:**716–723.
39. Tyrka AR, Mello AF, Mello MF, Gagne GG, Grover KE, Anderson GM, Price LH, Carpenter LL: **Temperament and hypothalamic-pituitary-adrenal axis function in healthy adults.** *Psychoneuroendocrinology* 2006, **31:**1036–1345.
40. Fukudo S, Nomura T, Hongo M: **Impact of corticotropin-releasing hormone on gastrointestinal motility and adrenocorticotropic hormone in normal controls and patients with irritable bowel syndrome.** *Gut* 1998, **42:**845–849.
41. Tayama J, Sagami Y, Shimada Y, Hongo M, Fukudo S: **Effect of alpha-helical CRH on quantitative electroencephalogram in patients with irritable bowel syndrome.** *Neurogastroenterol Motil* 2007, **19:**471–483.
42. Weissman MM, Bland RC, Canino GJ, Faravelli C, Greenwald S, Hwu HG, Joyce PR, Karam EG, Lee CK, Lellouch J, Lépine JP, Newman SC, Rubio-Stipec M, Wells JE, Wickramaratne PJ, Wittchen H, Yeh EK: **Cross-national epidemiology of major depression and bipolar disorder.** *JAMA* 1996, **276:**293–299.
43. Gwee KA: **Irritable bowel syndrome in developing countries – disorder of civilization or colonization?** *Neurogastroenterol Motil* 2005, **17:**317–324.
44. Gwee KA, Lu CL, Ghoshal UC: **Epidemiology of irritable bowel syndrome in Asia: something old, something new, something borrowed.** *J Gastroenterol Hepatol* 2009, **24:**1601–1607.

Gut-directed hypnotherapy in children with irritable bowel syndrome or functional abdominal pain (syndrome): A randomized controlled trial on self exercises at home using CD versus individual therapy by qualified therapists

Juliette MTM Rutten[1*], Arine M Vlieger[2], Carla Frankenhuis[1], Elvira K George[3], Michael Groeneweg[4], Obbe F Norbruis[5], Walther Tjon a Ten[6], Herbert Van Wering[7], Marcel GW Dijkgraaf[8], Maruschka P Merkus[8] and Marc A Benninga[1]

Abstract

Background: Irritable bowel syndrome (IBS) and functional abdominal pain (syndrome) (FAP(S)) are common pediatric disorders, characterized by chronic or recurrent abdominal pain. Treatment is challenging, especially in children with persisting symptoms. Gut-directed hypnotherapy (HT) performed by a therapist has been shown to be effective in these children, but is still unavailable to many children due to costs, a lack of qualified child-hypnotherapists and because it requires a significant investment of time by child and parent(s). Home-based hypnotherapy by means of exercises on CD has been shown effective as well, and has potential benefits, such as lower costs and less time investment. The aim of this randomized controlled trial (RCT) is to compare cost-effectiveness of individual HT performed by a qualified therapist with HT by means of CD recorded self-exercises at home in children with IBS or FAP(S).

Methods/Design: 260 children, aged 8-18 years with IBS or FAP(S) according to Rome III criteria are included in this currently conducted RCT with a follow-up period of one year. Children are randomized to either 6 sessions of individual HT given by a qualified therapist over a 3-month period or HT through self-exercises at home with CD for 3 months. The primary outcome is the proportion of patients in which treatment is successful at the end of treatment and after one year follow-up. Treatment success is defined as at least 50% reduction in both abdominal pain frequency and intensity scores. Secondary outcomes include adequate relief, cost-effectiveness and effects of both therapies on depression and anxiety scores, somatization scores, QoL, pain beliefs and coping strategies.

Discussion: If the effectiveness of home-based HT with CD is comparable to, or only slightly lower, than HT by a therapist, this treatment may become an attractive form of therapy in children with IBS or FAP(S), because of its low costs and direct availability.

Trial registration: Dutch Trial Register number NTR2725 (date of registration: 1 February 2011)

Keywords: Irritable bowel syndrome (IBS), Functional abdominal pain (FAP), Functional abdominal pain syndrome (FAPS), Hypnotherapy, Children, Pediatrics, Hypnosis, Randomized controlled trial (RCT), Functional gastrointestinal disorders

* Correspondence: j.m.rutten@amc.nl
[1]Department of Pediatric Gastroenterology, Emma Children's Hospital/Academic Medical Center, PO Box 22700, 1100 DD Amsterdam, The Netherlands
Full list of author information is available at the end of the article

Background

Irritable bowel syndrome (IBS) and functional abdominal pain (syndrome) (FAP(S)) are functional gastrointestinal disorders (FGIDs) that are characterized by chronic or recurrent abdominal pain in absence of an underlying organic disorder causing the symptoms [1]. These disorders affect approximately 20% of children in Western countries and are also prevalent in Asian countries such as Sri Lanka and China, affecting 12,5 to 20% of school-aged children [2-4]. Altered bowel movements and/or relief of abdominal pain after defecation are present in children with IBS, while defecation pattern is normal in children with FAP(S) [1].

Quality of life (QoL) is significantly impaired in most children with IBS or FAP(S): QoL scores are lower compared to healthy peers and comparable to children with inflammatory bowel diseases [5]. Children with IBS or FAP(S) have an increased risk for anxiety and/or depression and have high rates of school absenteeism [6,7]. Health care costs associated with these FGIDs are considerable. Diagnostic workup for a child with IBS or FAP(S) in the United States costs approximately 6000 dollar. The exact costs of treatment of these children are not known, but are also likely to be significant since treatment of adult patients with IBS costs more than $20 billion per year [8,9].

Pathophysiological mechanisms causing IBS and FAP(S) are not fully clarified to this date, but these FGIDs are thought to be a result of a complex interplay of multiple genetic, psychosocial and physiological factors [10]. Standard medical treatment of IBS and FAP(S) consists of a combination of dietary advice, education and pharmacological therapy, such as pain medication, laxatives, antidiarrheal medication and antispasmodics [11,12]. Despite these treatments, a significant part of children with IBS or FAP(S) continues to experience symptoms, even into adulthood [13].

In the last 30 years, multiple trials have demonstrated that gut-directed hypnotherapy (HT) is an effective therapy in patients with IBS [14-25]. In gut-directed HT, a hypnotic state is induced and a patient is guided to respond to suggestions towards control and normalization of gut functioning, stress reduction and ego-strengthening [26]. Adult IBS-trials have shown that patients receiving HT report significantly lower levels of abdominal pain and symptom scores compared to patients receiving various control treatments. In addition, these effects of gut-directed HT were shown to be long lasting, up to seven years after treatment [20-22]. Gut-directed HT by a therapist has also been studied in children with IBS or FAP(S) and, in accordance with results of adult studies, these trials show HT to be highly effective compared to standard care [23-25] with persisting positive effects after a period of approximately five years [27]. Although these trials show that gut-directed HT is a valuable therapeutic option, especially in children with persisting symptoms, it is still unavailable to many children with IBS or FAP(S), because gut-directed HT performed by a therapist is costly and frequently not reimbursed by health insurance companies. In addition, the number of well-trained child-hypnotherapists is very limited in most countries and the treatment requires a significant investment of both children and parent(s), since visits to the hypnotherapist may cause work and school absences. Van Tilburg et al. studied the efficacy of home-based HT using self-exercises on compact disc (CD) and showed that approximately two thirds of children receiving this home based treatment responded well with >50% reduction in abdominal pain scores [28]. Potential benefits of this treatment at home include that it is less time consuming and less costly compared to HT with a therapist.

Therefore, the primary aim of this study is to compare efficacy of individual HT performed by a qualified therapist with HT by means of CD recorded self-exercises at home in children with IBS or FAP(S). Secondary aims include adequate relief, the cost-effectiveness, effects on depression and anxiety scores, somatization scores, QoL, pain beliefs and coping strategies.

Methods/Design

Study design and population

A randomized controlled trial (RCT) with 1 year follow-up is currently conducted to evaluate the efficacy of individual HT performed by a qualified therapist versus HT at home with self-exercises on CD in children with IBS or FAP(S). This study has been designed in line with the methodological recommendations established by the Rome II consensus on 'Design of treatment trials for gastrointestinal disorders' [29]. Nine hospitals throughout the Netherlands participate in this RCT. Children are recruited at the outpatient clinic of the department of pediatric gastroenterology of the academic medical centers in Amsterdam and Maastricht and at the outpatient clinic of the departments of pediatrics of the Medical Center Alkmaar, the Flevo Hospital Almere, the Amphia Hospital Breda, St. Antonius Hospital Nieuwegein, the Maasstad Hospital in Rotterdam, the Maxima Medical Center Veldhoven and the Isala Clinics Zwolle. This RCT has been reviewed and approved by the medical ethics committees of all participating hospitals and has been registered in the Dutch Trial Register number NTR2725. It is granted by the Netherlands Organization for Health Research and Development, ZonMW.

A total of 260 children aged 8-18 years diagnosed with IBS, FAP or FAPS according to the Rome III criteria are included in this RCT [1]. Before inclusion, all patients undergo routine laboratory testing to exclude underlying organic disorders: complete blood cell count, C-reactive protein, alanine transaminase (ALT), aspartate aminotransferase (AST), glutamyltransferase (GGT), creatinine, total bilirubin, amylase, celiac screening (anti-transglutaminase antibodies and IgA), urinalysis, stool parasite analysis and *H pylori* antigens in stool. The need for further diagnostic testing is left to the discretion of the treating physician.

Verbal and written information about the study is given by the pediatrician/pediatric gastroenterologist and patients are asked to participate in this RCT if all criteria are met. Subsequently, verbal and written informed consent is obtained from the child and/or both parents. If the child or parent(s) decide not to participate in this RCT, the reason(s) for not participating are documented, if they want to reveal these.

Inclusion and exclusion criteria

Inclusion criteria
(1) Diagnosis of irritable bowel syndrome (IBS) or functional abdominal pain (syndrome) (FAP(S)) according to Rome III criteria [1]
(2) Age 8-18 years at inclusion
Exclusion criteria
(1) Concomitant organic gastrointestinal disease
(2) Treatment by another health care professional for abdominal pain symptoms
(3) Previous hypnotherapy
(4) Mental retardation
(5) Insufficient knowledge of the Dutch language

After obtaining informed consent, children are randomly allocated using a computerized random-number generator for concealment, to either individual hypnotherapy given by a qualified therapist or home-based therapy with hypnotherapy exercises on CD. Randomization is performed on a 1:1 basis with varying block sizes of 2, 4 and 6. Stratification is based on the including hospital and school level (primary/secondary school).

Interventions

The HT protocol used in this RCT is based on the Manchester protocol for gut-directed HT adapted for children [30] and is comparable to the treatment protocol used in a previous RCT on gut-directed HT in the Netherlands [24]. Hypnotherapy consists of exercises on general relaxation, control of abdominal pain and gut functioning and ego-strengthening suggestions. Several scripts for the exercises used in this RCT are based on scripts used in the van Tilburg et al. trial [28]. Given the nature of HT, blinding of patients and health care professionals involved in the treatment of the participants is not possible.

Individual hypnotherapy by a therapist

Individual HT consists of six sessions of 50-60 minutes over a period of three months and is carried out by 11 hypnotherapists affiliated to the recruiting hospitals. All participating hypnotherapists are qualified and have many years of experience in performing HT in children. They have been trained in working with the treatment protocol and instructed to use the same scripts that are used in the CD group, but are allowed to adapt contents and order of these scripts to the child's interests and specific issues that may come up during therapy. The same protocol is used for children of all ages, but the language used is adapted to the child's developmental age.

In the first HT session, therapists take a full history. Furthermore, it is explained to both child and parent(s) what hypnotherapy is and how it can help in reducing chronic abdominal pain.

Also, children and parent(s) are instructed not to talk about the pain anymore. In the same session, an exercise on breathing and progressive relaxation is introduced in which children imagine floating on a big cloud. Positive suggestions for decreasing discomfort are given, such as making their hands warm and to place both hands on their belly, imagining the warmth spreading through their abdomen. In the second session, the exercise on progressive relaxation is repeated. Furthermore, an exercise focusing on reduction of anxiety and stress is introduced ('the favorite place exercise'). In session three, an exercise on ego-strengthening is introduced ('the rainbow planet exercise' for children attending primary school; 'the air balloon exercise' for children in secondary school). In this hypnosis exercise children choose colors from the rainbow for different needs, for example health, tranquility, courage or confidence. During the fourth session the 'beach without worries exercise' is introduced, in which children are encouraged to release stress and again, ego-strengthening suggestions are made. In the fifth session, children do 'the slide exercise' in which children visualize sitting on a slide. Suggestions on reduction of anxiety and stress and ego-strengthening suggestions are given as well as visualizations of a well working digestive system with food sliding through the bowel in a comfortable way. In the last session, evaluation of the previous three months will take place. In addition, remaining issues related to the abdominal pain may be addressed and previous exercises are repeated, depending on the needs of the individual patient. Children are advised to keep practicing the HT exercises at home on a regular basis. After the first HT-session all children in the HT-group receive a CD containing standard scripts of all exercises used and they are instructed to listen to the exercises or to practice self-hypnosis on a daily basis. Furthermore, they are encouraged to practice the breathing exercise a few times a day.

Hypnotherapy through self-exercises on CD

Children assigned to the CD-group are visited at home by a specially trained research nurse. During this visit the research nurse explains the nature of HT and the exercises to the child and parent(s) and children receive the CD together with an instruction leaflet. In addition, children and parent(s) are instructed not to talk about the abdominal pain anymore. Children are asked to do the first exercise of the CD during this visit, to check whether the child understands the given instructions. The previous trial on home-based treatment has demonstrated that this method is very easy to understand and use [28]. The CD contains five standard scripts of the hypnosis exercises, which are identical to the exercises used by the hypnotherapists. These exercises consist of one exercise on breathing and progressive relaxation and four visualization exercises: 'the favorite place exercise', 'the rainbow planet/air balloon exercise' (depending on developmental age), 'the beach without worries exercise' and 'the slide exercise'). Two separate CDs are used to make sure that the language used is adapted to the child's developmental age: one CD for children visiting primary school and one CD for children visiting secondary school. Prior to this RCT, the CD has been tested by three children with chronic abdominal pain and no changes were required. Children are instructed to listen to the hypnosis exercises at least five times a week over a period of three months. Furthermore, they are encouraged to practice the breathing exercise a few times a day. The frequency of listening to the CD will be recorded by the participants in their instruction leaflet. The research nurse will make phone calls to the children after 4 and 8 weeks of treatment to stimulate treatment compliance.

Co-interventions

All children participating in this RCT are seen by their pediatrician or pediatric gastroenterologist after three months of HT to evaluate the effects of HT and to provide standard medical care if considered necessary. In addition, children will also visit their physician after 6 months of follow up if necessary.

Outcomes

Outcomes are measured at baseline (T0), after 3 months of therapy (T1) and at 6 and 12 months follow-up after the end of therapy (T2, T3).

Outcomes are recorded by patients and/or parents at home. At inclusion, a questionnaire on demographics and clinical features is filled out by the treating physician. An overview of the assessments made in this RCT is shown in Table 1.

1. Abdominal pain

The main goal of treatment in IBS/FAP(S) patients is a reduction in levels of abdominal pain.

Abdominal pain is assessed with a diary, in which children record the frequency and intensity of abdominal pain episodes on seven consecutive days [14,24,27,31]. *Pain frequency* is recorded in minutes of abdominal pain per day and is scored as 0 when there was no pain, 1 if children experience 1-30 minutes of pain, 2 for 31-120 minutes of pain and 3 if abdominal pain lasts more than 120 minutes. A pain frequency score (PFS) is subsequently calculated by summing the scores of the seven days, giving a maximum PFS of 21 [24,27,31]. *Pain intensity* is scored using an affective facial scale with faces ranging from showing no pain at all (face A) to the most severe pain (face I). Scores on the facial scale are transported to a daily 0-3 score. No abdominal pain is scored as 0, faces A-C are scored as 1, faces D-F score 2 and faces G-I score as 3. Again, scores of seven days are totaled giving a pain intensity score (PIS), with a maximum of 21 [24,27,31].

The primary outcomes in this RCT are the proportion of patients in which treatment is successful at the end of treatment and the proportion of successfully treated patients after 1 year follow-up. Treatment success is defined as at least 50% reduction in both abdominal pain frequency and intensity scores.

2. Hypnotic susceptibility

Hypnotic susceptibility is defined as a generalized tendency to respond to hypnosis and hypnotic suggestions [32] and is assessed using a Dutch translation of the Stanford hypnotic clinical scale for children [33]. It is administered by the treating hypnotherapist in children assigned to the HT-group and by the research nurse in children assessed to the CD-group. The Stanford hypnotic clinical scale for children consists of seven items. Scores are based on assessment of the child's behavior and experiences which are verbally reported to the therapist/research nurse. Scores on this scale range from 0 to 7 and higher scores represent higher hypnotic susceptibility.

3. Treatment expectations

Expectations about the response to treatment are assessed for the child, mother and father separately. Child and parents are asked whether they expect the child to improve with treatment and this question is scored on a 11-point scale (0 = not at all; 10 = complete recovery). It is also assessed whether they have a (strong) preference for HT with a therapist or home-based with CD.

4. Depression and anxiety

Table 1 Overview of outcomes

Outcome	Instrument	T0	4 wks	8 wks	T1	T2	T3
Abdominal pain	Abdominal pain dairies	X	X	X	X	X	X
Hypnotic susceptibility	Stanford hypnotic clinical scale for children	X					
Treatment expectations	Self-designed questionnaire for child and parents	X					
Depression and anxiety	Revised Anxiety and Depression Scale-short version (RCADS-25)	X			X	X	X
Somatization	Children's Somatization Inventory (CSI)	X			X	X	X
Health related quality of life	KIDSCREEN-52	X			X	X	X
Pain beliefs	Pain Beliefs Questionnaire (PBQ)	X			X	X	X
Coping strategies	Children's Coping Strategies Checklist-revision 1 (CCSC-R1)	X			X	X	X
Cost-effectiveness/cost-utility	Health Utility Index Mark 3 (HUI-3) & costs-questionnaire	X			X	X	X
Adequate relief	Binary question on adequate relief				X	X	X

The short version of the Revised Anxiety and Depression Scale (RCADS-25) is a valid and reliable instrument for the Dutch population to assess symptoms of depression and anxiety [34]. It contains five subscales measuring symptoms of generalized anxiety disorders, separation anxiety disorder, social phobia, panic disorder and major depressive disorder. Each subscale consists of five items, which are scored on a 0 to 3 scale (0 = never; 3 = always). A total score on anxiety is calculated by summing scores on the four individual anxiety scales.

5. Somatization

Child somatization scores are assessed using the Dutch version of the Children's Somatization Inventory (CSI), which has been shown to be a reliable and valid self-report instrument in children and adolescents [35]. It contains 35 items on the extent to which children experienced somatic symptoms in the previous two weeks. Items are scored on a 5-point scale, ranging from 0 (=not at all) to 4 (=a whole lot). A total score is calculated by summing all 35 individual items and higher scores reflect a higher intensity of somatic complaints experienced by the child. A separate CSI-score for non-gastrointestinal (GI) symptoms can be calculated by leaving out 7 items on GI-complaints: nausea, constipation, diarrhea, epigastric and abdominal pain, vomiting and bloating. To assess GI-complaints other than abdominal pain, items on all GI-symptoms but abdominal pain are summed.

6. Health related quality of life

The KIDSCREEN-52 questionnaire is a frequently used and reliable instrument to measure health related Qol in children and adolescents and has been validated in Dutch pediatric patient groups [36,37]. It contains items on ten dimensions of health related QoL: physical well-being, psychological well-being, moods and emotions, self-perception, autonomy, relations with parents and home life, social support and peers, school environment, social acceptance (bullying) and financial resources. A 5-point Likert scale is used to score each item. Rasch scores for each individual dimension are computed from the individual items and these are transformed into T-values. Higher T-values indicate a better health related QoL and well-being.

7. Pain beliefs

Negative and positive beliefs that children have about their abdominal pain are assessed using the Pain Beliefs Questionnaire (PBQ). A Dutch translation of the PBQ, which is reliable and validated in children and adolescents is used [38,39]. The PBQ consists of 32 items scored on a 5-point Likert scale. Negative beliefs can be divided into five subscales, namely condition frequency, condition duration, condition seriousness, episode specific intensity and episode specific duration. The negative beliefs scale is calculated by summing all 20 items on negative beliefs. The other 12 items assess problem focused coping potential (PFCP) and emotion focused coping potential (EFCP). The PFCP and EFCP scales are computed by averaging the 6 items belonging to both scales. Higher scores on a scale indicate that a child has such thoughts more frequently.

8. Coping strategies

The Dutch version of the Children's Coping Strategies Checklist-revision 1 (CCSC-R1) is used to measure strategies for coping with everyday problems [40,41]. The CCSC-R1 includes 54 items, all starting with the same phrase 'if I have a problem...' and all items are scored on a 4-point Likert-scale (1 = never; 4 = always). This questionnaire has sound psychometric properties and comprises five dimensions: problem focused coping, positive cognitive reframing, distraction strategies, avoidance strategies and support seeking strategies. Scale scores on all five dimensions are calculated by averaging the individual items belonging to the five scales.

9. Cost-effectiveness/cost-utility

The Health Utility Index Mark 3 (HUI-3) is applied as a multi-attribute utility measure of health status and will be used in the cost-effectiveness and cost-utility analysis. It is suitable for assessing children, but because children may be too young to provide reliable and valid information about their own health status, proxy measurements are taken from parents [42-45]. The health utilities derived from the HUI-3 have been anchored with 1 indicating perfect health and 0 indicating death. Quality adjusted life years (QALY) will be calculated by taking the sum of the utility of health states over time by the time in between successive measurements.

In addition to the HUI-3, the Dutch Health and Labor Questionnaire (HLQ) has been adapted to the study setting to measure the direct and indirect costs of health care utilization, work absenteeism by parents, and school absenteeism by children.

10. Adequate relief

Adequate relief has been shown to be a well validated outcome measurement in trials on treatment for IBS [46]. Parents are asked whether their child has adequate relief of IBS-related abdominal pain or discomfort, using a dichotomous scale (yes/no).

Statistical analysis

Two hundred and sixty children diagnosed with IBS or FAP(S) will be included. The data will be analyzed following the intention to treat principle. The primary analyses will focus on the proportion of patients in both treatment arms in which treatment was successful (>50% reduction abdominal pain frequency and intensity) at T1 and the proportion of patients in which treatment was successful at T3. In addition, abdominal pain levels will be compared in its continuous form using all five moments of measurement during follow-up (after 4 and 8 weeks of treatment, at T1, T2 and T3). These data will be analyzed using linear mixed models to account for correlations of measurements within the same individual. Similar longitudinal, repeated measurement analyses will be performed for the secondary outcomes including depression and anxiety, somatization, health related Qol, pain beliefs, coping strategies and adequate relief. Baseline values will be incorporated in these analyses to adjust for any imbalance at baseline despite randomization and to increase precision by removing between-person variability.

Two explanatory subgroup analyses are planned to evaluate whether there are indications that treatment effects differ between clinical subgroups. Children diagnosed with IBS will be compared to children with FAP(S). Additionally, children in pre-puberty age (13 years or younger) will be compared to older children, since our previous RCT showed that younger children showed a better treatment response up till 6 months after treatment [24].

Economic evaluation will be performed from a societal perspective. Cost-effectiveness and cost-utility ratios will be calculated for the additional costs per extra patient with at least 50% reduction of abdominal pain scores and the additional costs per extra QALY.

Power

The primary analysis focuses on the proportion of patients with at least 50% reduction in abdominal pain levels compared to baseline at the end of therapy and after one year of follow up. Based on previous trials, we made a conservative estimate of this percentage being around 75% in the group receiving HT performed by a therapist. In the group assigned to self-hypnosis with CD, we anticipated this percentage to be marginally lower at 65%. In order to be a reasonable alternative treatment, this percentage should not become lower than 50% in the CD group. This non-inferiority margin should be viewed in relation to success rated with standard medical care of around 30-40% in previous trails [23,24,28]. Based on these expected proportions and a non-inferiority margin at 50%, a total of 115 patients per group are needed to achieve a power of 80% with a one-sided significance level of 5%. Since we expect less than 10% drop-out, our aim is to include 130 patients per group.

Discussion

To our knowledge, this is the first RCT comparing the effectiveness of gut-directed HT performed by a qualified therapist to home-based HT with self exercises in CD in children with IBS or FAP(S). It has been designed according to methodological recommendations on the design of treatment trials for gastrointestinal disorders and has several strengths [29]. A total of 260 children with a Rome III diagnosis of IBS or FAP(S) are included in this RCT, while previous pediatric trials on HT had sample sizes up to 52 patients [23-25,28]. Generalizability of the results of this trial will be increased, because we include both younger children and adolescents, patients from urban and rural areas in the Netherlands and recruit children from both academic centers and teaching hospitals. In addition, children are followed for a period of 1 year after the end of therapy, to evaluate whether initial effects are sustained over time. In contrast with our earlier HT trial, in which all children were treated by the same hypnotherapist [24], in this study eleven different hypnotherapists are involved in the treatment of children with abdominal pain. This will shed light on the influence of the therapist with regards to efficacy. By assessing secondary outcomes, such as depression, anxiety and somatization, it may become possible to predict response to HT, thereby allowing clinicians to select children that are likely to benefit from HT. A possible limitation of this study may be the fact that children and parents are not blinded for the received treatment, which is not possible due to the nature of HT. Recording of outcome measures by children and parents themselves at home, instead of recording of outcomes by a health care professional during a visit to the hospital, however, reduces the risk of detection bias. In addition, the fact that symptoms of abdominal pain are recorded for seven consecutive days has the benefit that it corrects for individual variability of symptoms over time. Response expectancies are known to (partly) mediate effects of psychological treatments, such as HT [47]. We therefore record expectancies about HT from the child and both parents separately to assess the magnitude of expectation bias. Another possible limitation of the design of this RCT may be the fact that we did not include a third treatment arm with children receiving standard medical care. This third treatment group however was waived, since reviewers considered it being not ethical to abstain children from treatment with HT, because previous studies have shown HT to be superior to standard medical care in this group of patients [23,24,28].

If this RCT will show that the effectiveness of home-based HT with CD is comparable to or only slightly lower than HT by a therapist, this treatment may become an attractive first line of treatment in children with IBS or FAP(S). Since it presumably is less costly and less time-consuming, it will benefit children, parents and society. In addition, the large number of children with IBS and FAP(S) combined with a shortage of qualified therapists, causes long waiting lists nowadays. Home-based HT can be started as soon as the diagnosis of IBS or FAP(S) has been made, without dealing with these long waiting lists. A potential scenario after this RCT might be that a significant proportion of children with IBS or FAP(S) can get this home-based treatment, prescribed by their general practitioner. This may subsequently lead to fewer referrals to pediatricians and/or pediatric gastroenterologists, which would lead to an additional decrease in health care costs. If this RCT indeed shows these results, the next step will be implementation of home-based HT into clinical care for children with IBS or FAP(S).

Abbreviations

CD: Compact disc; FAP: Functional abdominal pain; FAPS: Functional abdominal pain syndrome; GI: Gastrointestinal; HT: Hypnotherapy; IBS: Irritable bowel syndrome; PFS: Pain frequency score; PIS: Pain intensity score; QALY: Quality adjusted life years; QoL: Quality of life; RCT: Randomized controlled trial.

Authors' contributions

JR is primary investigator and responsible for data collection, analysis and drafting the manuscript. Participated in the design of the study and contributed to developing of the research protocols. AV supervises the study and participated in the design of the study and contributed to developing of the research protocols. Supervised drafting of the manuscript and critically reviewed it. CF participated in the design of the study, contributed to developing of the research protocols en critically reviewed the manuscript. EG participated in the design of the study, contributed to developing of the research protocols en critically reviewed the manuscript. MG participated in the design of the study, contributed to developing of the research protocols en critically reviewed the manuscript. ON participated in the design of the study, contributed to developing of the research protocols en critically reviewed the manuscript. WT participated in the design of the study, contributed to developing of the research protocols en critically reviewed the manuscript. HW participated in the design of the study, contributed to developing of the research protocols en critically reviewed the manuscript. MD participated in the design of the study, contributed to developing of the research protocols en critically reviewed the manuscript. MM participated in the design of the study, contributed to developing of the research protocols en critically reviewed the manuscript. MB supervises the study, participated in the design of the study and contributed to developing of the research protocols. Supervised drafting of the manuscript and critically reviewed it. All authors read and approved the final manuscript as submitted.

Acknowledgements

Our study is granted by the Netherlands Organization for Health Research and Development, ZonMW (ZonMW project number 171102013).

Author details

[1]Department of Pediatric Gastroenterology, Emma Children's Hospital/Academic Medical Center, PO Box 22700, 1100 DD Amsterdam, The Netherlands. [2]Department of Pediatrics, St. Antonius Hospital, Nieuwegein, The Netherlands. [3]Department of Pediatrics, Medical Center Alkmaar, Alkmaar, The Netherlands. [4]Department of Pediatrics, Maasstad Hospital, Rotterdam, The Netherlands. [5]Department of Pediatrics, Isala Clinics, Zwolle, The Netherlands. [6]Department of Pediatrics, Maxima Medical Center, Veldhoven, The Netherlands. [7]Department of Pediatrics, Amphia Hospital, Breda, The Netherlands. [8]Clinical Research Unit, Academic Medical Center, Amsterdam, The Netherlands.

References

1. Rasquin A, Di Lorenzo C, Forbes D, Guiraldes E, Hyams JS, Staiano A, Walker LS: **Childhood functional gastrointestinal disorders: child/adolescent.** *Gastroenterology* 2006, **130**:1527–1537.
2. Chitkara DK, Rawat DJ, Talley NJ: **The epidemiology of childhood recurrent abdominal pain in Western countries: a systematic review.** *Am J Gastroenterol* 2005, **100**:1868–1875.
3. Devanarayana NM, Mettananda S, Liyanarachchi C, Nanayakkara N, Mendis N, Perera N, Rajindrajith S: **Abdominal pain-predominant functional gastrointestinal diseases in children and adolescents: prevalence, symptomatology, and association with emotional stress.** *J Pediatr Gastroenterol Nutr* 2011, **53**:659–665.
4. Zhou H, Yao M, Cheng G-Y, Chen Y-P, Li D-G: **Prevalence and associated factors of functional gastrointestinal disorders and bowel habits in Chinese adolescents: a school-based study.** *J Pediatr Gastroenterol Nutr* 2011, **53**:168–173.
5. Youssef NN, Murphy TG, Langseder AL, Rosh JR: **Quality of life for children with functional abdominal pain: a comparison study of patients' and parents' perceptions.** *Pediatrics* 2006, **117**:54–59.
6. Youssef NN, Atienza K, Langseder AL, Strauss RS: **Chronic abdominal pain and depressive symptoms: analysis of the national longitudinal study of adolescent health.** *Clin Gastroenterol Hepatol* 2008, **6**:329–332.
7. Shelby GD, Shirkey KC, Sherman AL, Beck JE, Haman K, Shears AR, Horst SN, Smith CA, Garber J, Walker LS: **Functional abdominal pain in childhood and long-term vulnerability to anxiety disorders.** *Pediatrics* 2013, **132**:475–482.
8. Dhroove G, Chogle A, Saps M: **A million-dollar work-up for abdominal pain: is it worth it?** *J Pediatr Gastroenterol Nutr* 2010, **51**:579–583.
9. American College of Gastroenterology Task Force on Irritable Bowel Syndrome, Brandt LJ, Chey WD, Foxx-Orenstein AE, Schiller LR, Schoenfeld PS, Spiegel BM, Talley NJ, Quigley EM: **An evidence-based position statement on the management of irritable bowel syndrome.** *Am J Gastroenterol* 2009, **104**(Suppl 1):S1–S35.

10. Drossman DA: **The functional gastrointestinal disorders and the Rome III process.** *Gastroenterology* 2006, **130:**1377–1390.
11. Di Lorenzo C, Colletti RB, Lehmann HP, Boyle JT, Gerson WT, Hyams JS, Squires RH jr, Walker LS, Kanda PT: **Chronic abdominal pain in children: a technical report of the American academy of pediatrics and the North American society for pediatric gastroenterology, hepatology and nutrition AAP subcommittee and NASPGHAN committee on chronic abdominal pain.** *J Pediatr Gastroenterol Nutr* 2005, **40:**249–261.
12. Weydert JA, Ball TM, Davis MF: **Systematic review of treatments for recurrent abdominal pain.** *Pediatrics* 2003, **111:**e1–e11.
13. Campo JV, Di Lorenzo C, Chiappetta L, Bridge J, Colborn DK, Gartner JC Jr, Gaffney P, Kocoshis S, Brent D: **Adult outcomes of pediatric recurrent abdominal pain: do they just grow out of it?** *Pediatrics* 2001, **108:**E1.
14. Whorwell PJ, Prior A, Faragher EB: **Controlled trial of hypnotherapy in the treatment of severe refractory irritable-bowel syndrome.** *Lancet* 1984, **1:**1232–1234.
15. Palsson OS, Turner MJ, Johnson DA, Burnett CK, Whitehead WE: **Hypnosis treatment for severe irritable bowel syndrome: investigation of mechanism and effects on symptoms.** *Dig Dis Sci* 2002, **47:**2605–2614.
16. Galovski TA, Blanchard EB: **The treatment of irritable bowel syndrome with hypnotherapy.** *Appl Psychophysiol Biofeedback* 1998, **23:**219–232.
17. Forbes A, MacAuley S, Chiotakakou-Faliakou E: **Hypnotherapy and therapeutic audiotape: effective in previously unsuccessfully treated irritable bowel syndrome?** *Int J Colorectal Dis* 2000, **15:**328–334.
18. Lindfors P, Unge P, Arvidsson P, Nyhlin H, Björnsson E, Abrahamsson H, Simrén M: **Effects of gut-directed hypnotherapy on IBS in different clinical settings-results from two randomized, controlled trials.** *Am J Gastroenterol* 2012, **107:**276–285.
19. Roberts L, Wilson S, Singh S, Roalfe A, Greenfield S: **Gut-directed hypnotherapy for irritable bowel syndrome: piloting a primary care-based randomised controlled trial.** *Br J Gen Pract* 2006, **56:**115–121.
20. Gonsalkorale WM, Miller V, Afzal A, Whorwell PJ: **Long term benefits of hypnotherapy for irritable bowel syndrome.** *Gut* 2003, **52:**1623–1629.
21. Lindfors P, Unge P, Nyhlin H, Ljótsson B, Björnsson ES, Abrahamsson H, Simrén M: **Long-term effects of hypnotherapy in patients with refractory irritable bowel syndrome.** *Scand J Gastroenterol* 2012, **47:**413–420.
22. Moser G, Trägner S, Gajowniczek EE, Mikulits A, Michalski M, Kazemi-Shirazi L, Kulnigg-Dabsch S, Führer M, Ponocny-Seliger E, Dejaco C, Miehsler W: **Long-term success of GUT-directed group hypnosis for patients with refractory irritable bowel syndrome: a randomized controlled trial.** *Am J Gastroenterol* 2013, **108:**602–609.
23. Weydert JA, Shapiro DE, Acra SA, Monheim CJ, Chambers AS, Ball TM: **Evaluation of guided imagery as treatment for recurrent abdominal pain in children: a randomized controlled trial.** *BMC Pediatr* 2006, **6:**29.
24. Vlieger AM, Menko-Frankenhuis C, Wolfkamp SCS, Tromp E, Benninga MA: **Hypnotherapy for children with functional abdominal pain or irritable bowel syndrome: a randomized controlled trial.** *Gastroenterology* 2007, **133:**1430–1436.
25. Gulewitsch MD, Müller J, Hautzinger M, Schlarb AA: **Brief hypnotherapeutic-behavioral intervention for functional abdominal pain and irritable bowel syndrome in childhood: a randomized controlled trial.** *Eur J Pediatr* 2013, **172:**1043–1051.
26. Green JP, Barabasz AF, Barrett D, Montgomery GH: **Forging Ahead: the 2003 APA Division 30 definition of hypnosis.** *Int J Clin Exp Hypn* 2005, **53:**259–264.
27. Vlieger AM, Rutten JMTM, Govers AMAP, Frankenhuis C, Benninga MA: **Long-term follow-up of gut-directed hypnotherapy vs. standard care in children with functional abdominal pain or irritable bowel syndrome.** *Am J Gastroenterol* 2012, **107:**627–631.
28. Van Tilburg MAL, Chitkara DK, Palsson OS, Turner M, Blois-Martin N, Ulshen M, Whitehead WE: **Audio-recorded guided imagery treatment reduces functional abdominal pain in children: a pilot study.** *Pediatrics* 2009, **124:**e890–e897.
29. Zanten Van Veldhuyzen SJ, Talley NJ, Bytzer P, Klein KB, Whorwell PJ, Zinsmeister AR: **Design of treatment trials for functional gastrointestinal disorders.** *Gut* 1999, **45**(Suppl 2):ii69–ii77.
30. Gonsalkorale WM: **Gut-directed hypnotherapy: the Manchester approach for treatment of irritable bowel syndrome.** *Int J Clin Exp Hypn* 2006, **54:**27–50.
31. See MC, Birnbaum AH, Schechter CB, Goldenberg MM, Benkov KJ: **Double-blind, placebo-controlled trial of famotidine in children with abdominal pain and dyspepsia: global and quantitative assessment.** *Dig Dis Sci* 2001, **46:**985–992.
32. Gur RC: **Measuring hypnotic susceptibility: a guest editorial.** *Am J Clin Hypn* 1978-1979, **21:**64–67.
33. Morgan AH, Hilgard JR: **The Stanford hypnotic clinical scale for children.** *Am J Clin Hypn* 1978-1979, **21:**148–169.
34. Muris P, Meesters C, Schouten E: **A brief questionnaire of DSM-IV-defined anxiety and depression symptoms among children.** *Clin Psychol Psychoth* 2002, **9:**430–442.
35. Meesters C, Muris P, Ghys A, Reumerman T, Rooijmans M: **The Children's Somatization Inventory: further evidence for its reliability and validity in a pediatric and a community sample of Dutch children and adolescents.** *J Pediatr Psychol* 2003, **28:**413–422.
36. Ravens-Sieberer U, Gosch A, Rajmil L, Erhart M, Bruil J, Power M, Duer W, Auquier P, Cloetta B, Czemy L, Mazur J, Czimbalmos A, Tountas Y, Hagquist C, Kilroe J, the KIDSCREEN Group: **The KIDSCREEN-52 quality of life measure for children and adolescents: psychometric results from a cross-cultural survey in 13 European countries.** *Value Health* 2008, **11:**645–658.
37. The KIDSCREEN group: *The KIDSCREEN Questionnaires-Quality of Life Questoinnaires for Children and Adolescents Handbook.* Lengerich: Pabst Science Publishers; 2006.
38. Van der Veek SMC, De Haan E, Derkx HHF, Benninga MA, Lindauer RJL, Boer F: **The Relative Contribution of Parental and children's Cognitive and Behavioral Reactions to Pediatric Functional Abdominal Pain.** In *PhD Thesis: A Psychosocial Perspective on Pediatric Functional Abdominal Pain: Risk Factors and Treatment.* Academic Medical Center, University of Amsterdam; 2012:80–94.
39. Walker L, Smith C, Garber J, Claar R: **Testing a model of pain appraisal and coping in children with recurrent abdominal pain.** *Health Psychol* 2005, **24:**364–374.
40. Ayers TA, Sandler IN: **Manual for the Children's Coping Strategies Checklist & How I Coped Under Pressure Scale.** [http://prc.asu.edu/docs/CCSC-HICUPS%20%20Manual2.pdf retrieved June 2010]
41. De Boo GM, Wicherts J: **Assessing cognitive and behavioral coping strategies in children.** *Cognit Ther Res* 2007, **33:**1–20.
42. Feeny D, Furlong W, Torrance GW, Goldsmith CH, Zhu Z, DePauw S, Denton M, Boyle M: **Multiattribute and single-attribute utility functions for the health utilities index mark 3 system.** *Med Care* 2002, **40:**113–128.
43. Hille ET, Weisglas-Kuperus N, Van Goudoever JB, Jacobusse GW, Ens-Dokkum MB, De Groot L, Wit JM, Geven WB, Kok JH, De Kleine MJ, Kollée LA, Mulder AL, Van Straaten HL, De Vries LS, Van Weissenbruch MM, Verloove-Vanhorick SP, Dutch Collaborative POPS 19 study group: **Functional outcomes and participation in young adulthood for very preterm and very low birth weight infants: the Dutch Project on Preterm and Small for Gestational Age Infants at 19 years of age.** *Pediatrics* 2007, **120:**e587–e595.
44. Eiser C, Morse R: **The measurement of quality of life in children: past and future perspectives.** *J Dev Behav Pediatr* 2001, **22:**248–256.
45. Tarride J-E, Burke N, Bischof M, Hopkins RB, Goeree L, Campbell K, Xie F, O'Reilly D, Goeree R: **A review of health utilities across conditions common in paediatric and adult populations.** *Health Qual Life Outcomes* 2010, **8:**12.
46. Mangel AW, Hahn BA, Heath AT, Northcutt AR, Kong S, Dukes GE, McSorley D: **Adequate relief as an endpoint in clinical trials in irritable bowel syndrome.** *J Int Med Res* 1998, **26:**76–81.
47. Milling LS, Reardon JM, Carosella GM: **Mediation and moderation of psychological pain treatments: response expectancies and hypnotic suggestibility.** *J Consult Clin Psychol* 2006, **74:**253–262.

25

Gastrointestinal specific anxiety in irritable bowel syndrome: Validation of the Japanese version of the visceral sensitivity index for university students

Tatsuo Saigo[1,2], Jun Tayama[1], Toyohiro Hamaguchi[3], Naoki Nakaya[4], Tadaaki Tomiie[5], Peter J Bernick[1], Motoyori Kanazawa[6], Jennifer S Labus[7], Bruce D Naliboff[7], Susumu Shirabe[1] and Shin Fukudo[6*]

Abstract

Objective: The visceral sensitivity index (VSI) is a useful self-report measure of the gastrointestinal symptom-specific anxiety (GSA) of patients with irritable bowel syndrome (IBS). Previous research has shown that worsening GSA in IBS patients is related to the severity of GI symptoms, suggesting that GSA is an important endpoint for intervention. However, there is currently no Japanese version of the VSI. We therefore translated the VSI into Japanese (VSI-J) and verified its reliability and validity.

Material and methods: Participants were 349 university students aged 18 and 19 years and recruited from an academic class. We analyzed data from the VSI-J, Anxiety Sensitivity Index (ASI), Hospital Anxiety and Depression scale (HAD), and Irritable Bowel Syndrome Severity Index (IBS-SI). The internal consistency, stability, and factor structure of the VSI-J and its associations with anxiety, depression and severity measures were investigated.

Results: The factor structure of the VSI-J is unidimensional and similar to that of the original VSI (Cronbach's $\alpha = 0.93$). Construct validity was demonstrated by significant correlations with ASI ($r = 0.43$, $p < 0.0001$), HAD-ANX ($r = 0.19$, $p = 0.0003$), and IBS-SI scores ($r = 0.45$, $p < 0.0001$). Furthermore, the VSI-J was a significant predictor of severity scores on the IBS-SI and demonstrated good discriminant ($p < 0.0001$) and incremental ($p < 0.0001$) validity.

Conclusion: These findings suggest that the VSI-J is a reliable and valid measure of visceral sensitivity.

Keywords: Gastrointestinal-specific anxiety, Irritable Bowel Syndrome (IBS), Motility, Psychosomatics, Validation, Visceral Sensitivity Index (VSI)

Introduction

Irritable bowel syndrome (IBS) is a functional gastrointestinal disorder not associated with organic disease that consists of chronic abdominal discomfort associated with abnormal bowel habits [1,2]. The prevalence of IBS has been reported at approximately 5–11% in industrialized countries [3]. Patients with IBS have been shown to have poor health-related quality of life (QOL) when compared with healthy individuals [4] and often experience a significant financial burden—indeed, their economic impact factor increases from 1.1 to 6.0 when compared with non-IBS individuals [5]. The characteristic pathophysiological features of IBS are dysmotility [6,7], visceral sensitivity [8,9], and psychological disturbances [10,11]. The GI symptoms of IBS may aggravate depression and anxiety and be associated with psychosocial stress; indeed, patients with IBS symptoms improve with recovery from psychological disturbances [12-14]. At least two studies have shown that patients with IBS report a high frequency of comorbid anxiety disorders such as panic disorder, agoraphobia, generalized anxiety disorder, and post-traumatic stress disorder [14,15].

Anxiety symptoms play a major role in the onset of IBS and in the maintenance and aggravation of GI symptoms

* Correspondence: sfukudo@med.tohoku.ac.jp
[6]Department of Behavioral Medicine, Tohoku University Graduate School of Medicine, 2-1 Seiryo, Aoba, Sendai, Miyagi 980-8575, Japan
Full list of author information is available at the end of the article

[15]. Further, in IBS, the maintenance and aggravation of GI symptoms and pain is related to brain function through the emotional motor system (EMS) and responses of the neuroendocrine and autonomic nervous systems [16]. For example, in studies that used colonic barostats, the thalamus, insular cortex, anterior cingulate gyrus, and prefrontal cortex were activated; these activations were associated with abdominal pain and psychological abnormalities such as anxiety and depression [12,17-19]. Patients with IBS show greater activation of the prefrontal cortex and anterior cingulate gyrus than do healthy individuals, and also perceive more abdominal pain [12,16-18]. Patients with IBS also demonstrate enhanced pathological vigilance and selective attention for their GI symptoms [20,21]. Thus, the association of brain function with pathological vigilance and selective attention for GI symptoms suggests a neurophysiological foundation for visceral sensitivity [22-24]. GI symptoms are not only external stressors but also act as internal stressors by causing and aggravating anxiety (gastrointestinal-specific anxiety: GSA) [25]. Excessive activity of the amygdala can activate the insular cortex [26], prefrontal cortex, and the anterior cingulate gyrus, which ultimately may lead to GSA and aggravated GI symptoms [4,27]. Interventions aimed at reducing GSA associated with IBS should therefore contribute to an improvement in the QOL of patients with IBS [27,28].

GSA is defined as "the cognitive, affective, and behavioral response stemming from fear of GI sensations, symptoms, and the context in which these visceral sensations and symptoms occur" (28, p.89). For example, the fear of visceral sensations and GI symptoms is related to situations involving restaurants, parties, or first-time visits to locations where bathroom facilities are unknown or difficult to reach; such experiences may cause particular cognitive or behavioral responses. IBS patients may engage in avoidance behaviors that cause GSA, increase vigilance or attention to visceral sensations, and show excessive reactions to low-level visceral sensation [29]. Labus et al. [27] have developed the Visceral Sensitivity Index (VSI) to assess specific GSA seen in patients with IBS.

The validity and reliability of the VSI have been confirmed in several studies (27 28, 30). In studies with both university students and IBS patients, the VSI has been shown to have a unidimensional factor structure [27,28]. A high level of internal consistency has been demonstrated in a combined group of younger healthy participants, IBS patients (Cronbach's α ranging from 0.90 to 0.92), and adults with IBS (Cronbach's $\alpha = 0.93$) [27,28]. Test-retest reliability estimates showed that, four weeks after testing, the inter-class coefficient was 0.86 [30]. Further, the construct validity has been extensively studied; results for the original VSI show moderate to strong positive correlations with measures of anxiety sensitivity (AS), state anxiety, and severity of GI symptoms [27,28,30]. The original VSI also showed a strong positive correlation with the depressive symptoms of IBS patients, but there was no significant correlation with the depressive symptoms of university students with IBS [28]. In addition, the Norwegian version of the VSI showed no correlation with the depressive symptoms or indicators of food sensitivity of IBS patients [30].

There is currently no Japanese version of the VSI; however, there is a clear need for such an instrument because it could be useful for verifying treatment effects in IBS patients and may therefore be indispensable for the future development of IBS treatments [27]. In the present study, we report our newly developed Japanese version of the VSI and test its validity and reliability. Reliability and validity have been confirmed in a previous analog study of university students [28]. As a large sample was necessary to develop the Japanese version of the VSI, the present study was conducted with a sample of university students, including those with symptoms of IBS. We then tested the following hypotheses.

1. The Japanese version of the VSI will exhibit a unidimensional factor structure.
2. The Japanese version of the VSI will show moderate positive correlations with measures of AS, state anxiety, and the severity of IBS symptoms; furthermore, it will show weak positive correlations with measures of depressive symptoms.
3. The Japanese version of the VSI will predict the severity of IBS symptoms after controlling for AS and state anxiety.

Methods

Participants

We recruited 875 undergraduate student participants from Nagasaki University in Japan; Figure 1 shows the selection process. For the present study, we were interested in younger participants (less than 20 years old). After screening for age, the data of 349 students (male = 207, female = 142, mean age = 19 years) was available for analysis. The participants answered all items on the VSI questionnaire.

Japanese Version of the Visceral Sensitivity Index (VSI-J)

The VSI was translated into Japanese using a standardized procedure. Two researchers, one a clinical psychologist knowledgeable in psychosomatic medicine, translated the original version. A medical doctor who specializes in psychosomatic medicine then confirmed the consistency of the translated Japanese version. A bilingual researcher (native English speaker) back-translated the Japanese VSI into English. The VSI-J was established after comparing

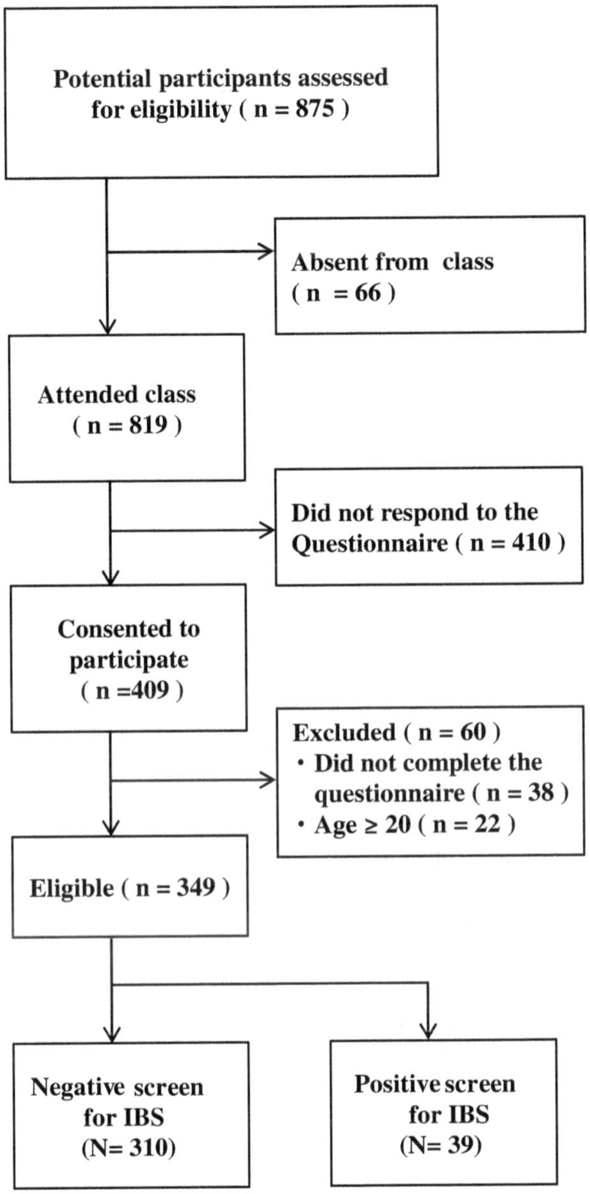

Figure 1 Flow chart showing the selection of the participants. Of 875 possible participants, 66 were absent from class, 410 did not respond to the questionnaire, 38 did not fully complete the questionnaire, and 22 were excluded because they were 20 years of age or older. We analyzed the data of the remaining 349 persons who answered all of the items on the questionnaire.

the results of the back translation to the original, and there was agreement among the researchers about the nuances (Tables 1 and 2).

The VSI measures gastrointestinal specific anxiety using 15 questionnaire items, with responses ranging from 1 (*strongly agree*) to 6 (*strongly disagree*). The VSI was "reverse scored" according to previously established methods [27], with scores ranging from 0 to 5. Total scores ranged from 0 (*no GI-specific anxiety*) to 75 (*severe GI-specific anxiety*).

Rome III diagnostic questionnaire

Rome III criteria are widely used for the diagnosis of IBS. These criteria include recurrent abdominal pain or discomfort (on at least 3 days/month in the last 3 months) associated with two or more of the following: [1] improved by defecation, [2] onset associated with a change in frequency of stool, and [3] onset associated with a change in form (appearance) of stool. The Rome III diagnostic questionnaire has been confirmed as a reliable and valid self-administered questionnaire for the purpose of diagnosing IBS (Drs. Kanazawa & Fukudo, personal communication). The questionnaire determines whether a person is IBS-positive or non-IBS.

The IBS Severity Index (IBS-SI)

In the present study, the IBS-SI was used to assess the severity of GI symptoms [31]. The IBS-SI consists of five items with total scores ranging from 0 to 500. Mild, moderate and severe symptoms of IBS are indicated by scores of 75 to 174, 175 to 299, and 300 or over, respectively [31]. The VSI has shown strong positive correlations with the severity of the GI symptoms of both healthy (non-IBS) individuals and individuals with IBS (IBS-positive) [28]. Therefore, the IBS-SI measure of symptom severity was used to examine the construct validity of the VSI-J.

The Hospital Anxiety and Depression scale (HAD)

The HAD is a 14-item self-administered anxiety and depression scale specifically designed for use in non-psychiatric settings [32]. Seven of the items relate to anxiety (HAD-ANX) and seven to depression (HAD-DEP). Participants rate each item on a scale from 0 to 3. Higher ratings indicate a greater number of symptoms of anxiety or depression. Two scores (one each for the HAD-ANX and the HAD-DEP) are calculated, each ranging from 0 to 21. Scores of 0 to 7 on the respective subscales are considered normal, with 8 to 10 being borderline and scores of 11 to 21 indicating probable clinical cases [32]. Our scoring methods conformed to those of the original version of the scale [32]. Scores on the original VSI were significantly and moderately correlated with scores on the HAD-ANX but showed a weak correlation with HAD-DEP scores [28]. Therefore, the HAD was used to examine the construct validity of the VSI-J.

The Anxiety Sensitivity Index (ASI)

The ASI is a 16-item self-administered questionnaire about anxiety sensitivity designed to assess fear of bodily sensations associated with arousal [33,34]. Items are rated on 5-point Likert scales ranging from 0 (*very little*) to 4 (*very much*). Previous research has shown that the original VSI is significantly and strongly correlated with measures of AS among both IBS patients and healthy individuals [28]. AS was related to an understanding of GSA constructed

Table 1 Original version of the VSI [27]

Visceral Sensitivity Index (VSI)

	Item	Strongly agree	Moderately agree	Mildly agree	Mildly disagree	Moderately disagree	Strongly disagree
1	I worry that whenever I eat during the day, bloating and distension in my belly will get worse.	1	2	3	4	5	6
2	I get anxious when I go to a new restaurant.	1	2	3	4	5	6
3	I often worry about problems in my belly.	1	2	3	4	5	6
4	I have a difficult time enjoying myself because I cannot get my mind off of discomfort in my belly.	1	2	3	4	5	6
5	I often fear that I won't be able to have a normal bowel movement.	1	2	3	4	5	6
6	Because of fear of developing abdominal discomfort, I seldom try new foods.	1	2	3	4	5	6
7	No matter what I eat, I will probably feel uncomfortable.	1	2	3	4	5	6
8	As soon as I feel abdominal discomfort I begin to worry and feel anxious.	1	2	3	4	5	6
9	When I enter a place I haven't been before, one of the first things I do is to look for a bathroom.	1	2	3	4	5	6
10	I am constantly aware of the feelings I have in my belly.	1	2	3	4	5	6
11	I often feel discomfort in my belly could be a sign of a serious illness.	1	2	3	4	5	6
12	As soon as I awake, I worry that I will have discomfort in my belly during the day.	1	2	3	4	5	6
13	When I feel discomfort in my belly, it frightens me.	1	2	3	4	5	6
14	In stressful situations, my belly bothers me a lot.	1	2	3	4	5	6
15	I constantly think about what is happening inside my belly.	1	2	3	4	5	6

through introspection and resulting in worry, fear, and vigilance [27,28]. Therefore, the ASI was used to examine the construct validity of the VSI-J.

Procedure

The questionnaire survey was presented in the classroom during an academic session. We explained the research procedures and general purpose, and provided both a written and verbal explanation of the intended use of the data. In addition, we explained that persons who did not consent to participate in the study would be placed at no disadvantage whatsoever. We only analyzed the data of those students who agreed to participate.

Statistical analysis

Analyses were carried out using IBM SPSS Statistics 20.0 (SPSS, Inc., Chicago, IL, USA) Descriptive statistics are presented as means ± standard deviations (SD), along with 95% confidence intervals. We used unpaired *t*-tests to compare IBS-positive and non-IBS groups. The factor structure of the VSI-J was confirmed by exploratory factor analysis (EFA). The internal consistency reliability of the VSI-J was determined using Cronbach's α. The construct validity was measured using Pearson's correlation coefficients between the VSI-J and scores on the ASI, HAD-ANX, HAD-DEP, and IBS-SI. The discriminant validity of the VSI-J was measured using the partial correlation coefficient between the VSI-J and the IBS-SI while controlling for HAD-ANX and ASI scores. Hierarchical multiple regression analyses were conducted to examine the incremental validity of the VSI-J; IBS-SI scores were the dependent variable and the scores on the VSI-J, ASI, and HAD-ANX were independent variables. For all tests, a *p*-value of .05 (two-tailed) was regarded as the cutoff for statistical significance.

Results

Demographics

Table 3 shows the demographic data for the present study participants, and reference data for university students obtained in a previous study [28]. The prevalence of IBS in the study sample was 11%; the overall gender distribution of the sample was 59% male and 41% female. However, within the IBS-positive group, 67% were female and 33% were male. The scores were significantly higher for the IBS-positive group than for the non-IBS group on the VSI-J (total; $t = 4.96$, $p < 0.0001$), the ASI ($t = 2.86$, $p = 0.0044$), and the IBS-SI

Table 2 Japanese version of the VSI

Visceral Sensitivity Index Japanese version (VSI-J)

項目		とてもあてはまる	まあまああてはまる	どちらかといえばあてはまる	どちらかといえばあてはまらない	あまりあてはまらない	まったくあてはまらない
1	何かを食べるときは、いつもおなかの膨れる感じや張る感じが悪化することを心配する	1	2	3	4	5	6
2	新しいレストランに行くときは不安になる	1	2	3	4	5	6
3	私はおなかの問題についてよく心配する	1	2	3	4	5	6
4	おなかの不快感が頭から離れないために、楽しく時間を過ごすことが難しい	1	2	3	4	5	6
5	私は排便が正常にならないのではないかとよく恐れている	1	2	3	4	5	6
6	おなかに不快感が生じることを恐れて、新しい食べ物を食べることはほとんどない	1	2	3	4	5	6
7	たとえ何を食べても、おそらく落ち着かない気持ちになる	1	2	3	4	5	6
8	おなかに不快感が生じるとすぐに悩んだり 不安になったりする	1	2	3	4	5	6
9	今まで行ったことがない場所に入った時、まず最初にトイレを探す	1	2	3	4	5	6
10	私はおなかの感覚をいつも意識している	1	2	3	4	5	6
11	おなかの不快感は深刻な病気の兆候ではないかとよく考えてしまう	1	2	3	4	5	6
12	朝起きるとすぐにその日おなかに不快感が生じることを心配する	1	2	3	4	5	6
13	おなかに不快感が生じると怖くなる	1	2	3	4	5	6
14	ストレスの多い状況では、おなかの不快感が増す	1	2	3	4	5	6
15	私は自分のおなかの中で何が起きているかをいつも考える	1	2	3	4	5	6

Table 3 Age, sex, and inventory scores

Variables	All participants	Non-IBS	IBS+	Reference value [28]	
	(*N* = 349)	(*N* = 310)	(*N* = 39)	Non-IBS	IBS+
Age	18.8 ± 0.5 [18.7–18.8]	18.8 ± 0.6 [18.7–18.9]	18.8 ± 0.6 (18.6–18.8)	19	19
Sex (% male)	59 [54–64]	63 [57–68]	33 [21–49]	-	-
IBS + (%)	11 [8–15]	-	-	-	-
VSI	15.2 ± 13.6 [13.8–16.6]	14.0 ± 12.9 [12.5–15.4]	25.1 ± 15.3 [20.2–30.1]**	8.2 [7.2–9.2]	28.0 [22.1–33.9]
ASI	16.6 ± 9.7 [15.7–17.6]	16.1 ± 9.2 [15.0–17.1]	20.8 ± 12.4 [16.7–24.8]**	18.6 [18.5–18.7]	23.2 [19.5–26.9]
HAD-ANX	8.5 ± 4.0 [8.1–8.9]	8.4 ± 4.0 [8.0–8.9]	9.3 ± 4.5 [7.8–10.7]	6.5 [6.1–6.9]	8.5 [7.7–9.3]
HAD-DEP	7.6 ± 3.1 [7.3–7.9]	7.6 ± 3.1 [7.3–8.0]	7.5 ± 2.9 [6.5–8.4]	3.1 [2.7–3.5]	5.4 [5.0–5.8]
IBS-SI	103.8 ± 86.7 [96.1–114.0]	90.9 ± 77.3 [82.3–99.6]	206.2 ± 91.0 [176.7–225.7]**	-	-

Data are expressed as: mean ± standard deviation [95% confidence interval].

Abbreviations: *VSI* Visceral Sensitivity Index, *ASI* Anxiety Sensitivity Index, *HAD-ANX* and *HAD-DEP* subscales of the Hospital Anxiety and Depression Scale, *IBS-SI* Irritable Bowel Syndrome Severity Index, *IBS* + positive diagnosis of Irritable Bowel Syndrome, *Non-IBS* no presence of Irritable Bowel Syndrome.

**$p < 0.01$ for IBS + vs. Non-IBS.

($t = 8.59$, $p < 0.0001$). However, there was no significant difference in the total HAD-ANX ($t = 1.20$, $p = 0.2305$) and total HAD-DEP ($t = 0.26$, $p = 0.7931$) scores.

Factor structure

To examine the factor structure of the VSI-J, we conducted an EFA (using maximum likelihood estimation and promax rotation) without assigning the number of factors (Table 4). There are four criteria for estimating factor structure: [1] initial eigenvalues greater than one, [2] shape of the scree plot, [3] interpretations of factor structure, and [4] factor loadings greater than 0.40. Initial eigenvalues greater than one were observed for two factors (first factor eigenvalue = 8.18, second factor eigenvalue = 1.17). However, the shape of the scree plot suggested a unidimensional factor structure. Accordingly, we then analyzed the factor structure by conducting exploratory analyses and assigning either one or two factors. The results confirmed a unidimensional factor structure. That is, a single factor accounted for 54% of the total variance. This was consistent with findings for the original VSI [27,28].

Reliability

To examine reliability, we calculated Cronbach's α for all scale measures. All measures demonstrated high internal consistency and were therefore considered reliable (VSI-J, $\alpha = 0.93$; ASI, $\alpha = 0.88$; total HAD, $\alpha = 0.73$; HAD-ANX, $\alpha = 0.66$; HAD-DEP, $\alpha = 0.50$; IBS-SI; $\alpha = 0.74$).

Validity

Construct validity

Table 5 gives Pearson's correlation coefficients among the VSI-J, ASI, HAD-ANX, HAD-DEP and IBS-SI. Overall, scores on the VSI-J were significantly correlated with scores on the ASI ($r = 0.46$, $p < 0.0001$), HAD-ANX ($r = 0.19$, $p = 0.0003$), and IBS-SI ($r = 0.43$, $p < 0.0001$). However, there was no significant correlation with the HAD-DEP ($r = 0.10$, $p = 0.0511$). For the IBS-positive group (n = 39), there was a significant correlation between scores on the VSI-J and scores on the ASI ($r = 0.44$, $p = 0.0048$), HAD-ANX ($r = 0.32$, $p = 0.0445$), and IBS-SI ($r = 0.65$, $p < 0.0001$). However, there was no significant correlation between VSI-J and HAD-DEP scores ($r = 0.27$, $p = 0.0976$). For the non-IBS group (n = 310), there was a significant correlation between scores on the VSI-J and scores on the ASI ($r = 0.41$, $p < 0.0001$), HAD-ANX ($r = 0.16$, $p = 0.0051$), and IBS-SI ($r = 0.36$, $p < 0.0001$). However, there was no significant correlation between VSI-J and HAD-DEP scores ($r = 0.09$, $p = 0.1096$).

Discriminant validity

To examine the discriminant validity of the VSI-J, we calculated the partial correlation coefficient (for the whole sample, $N = 349$) between the VSI-J and IBS-SI while controlling for scores on the HAD-ANX and ASI. The result was a significant correlation between scores on the VSI-J and the IBS-SI ($r = 0.45$, $p < 0.0001$).

Table 4 Factor analysis of the Japanese version of the Visceral Sensitivity Index

Item	Statement	Factor loadings	Item-total correlation
1	I worry that whenever I eat during the day, bloating and distension in my belly will get worse.	0.53	0.61
2	I get anxious when I go to a new restaurant.	0.42	0.52
3	I often worry about problems in my belly.	0.72	0.78
4	I have a difficult time enjoying myself because I cannot get my mind off of discomfort in my belly.	0.74	0.79
5	I often fear that I won't be able to have a normal bowel movement.	0.77	0.79
6	Because of fear of developing abdominal discomfort, I seldom try new foods.	0.56	0.62
7	No matter what I eat, I will probably feel uncomfortable.	0.62	0.66
8	As soon as I feel abdominal discomfort I begin to worry and feel anxious.	0.82	0.82
9	When I enter a place I haven't been before, one of the first things I do is to look for a bathroom.	0.58	0.62
10	I am constantly aware of the feelings I have in my belly.	0.83	0.82
11	I often feel discomfort in my belly could be a sign of a serious illness.	0.81	0.80
12	As soon as I awake, I worry that I will have discomfort in my belly during the day.	0.82	0.81
13	When I feel discomfort in my belly, it frightens me.	0.82	0.82
14	In stressful situations, my belly bothers me a lot.	0.68	0.72
15	I constantly think about what is happening inside my belly.	0.81	0.80
Eigenvalue		8.18	
Variance (%)		54.56	

Note. While factor analysis was performed with the Japanese version of the VSI, the original English items are given here for ease of reference.

Table 5 Correlation matrices for the construct validation of the Japanese version of the VSI

	VSI	ASI	HAD-ANX	HAD-DEP
All (N = 349)				
ASI	0.46**	-	-	-
HAD-ANX	0.19**	0.30**	-	-
HAD-DEP	0.10	0.17**	0.53**	-
IBS-SI	0.43**	0.24*	0.09	0.09
IBS + (N = 39)				
ASI	0.44**	-	-	-
HAD-ANX	0.32*	0.57**	-	-
HAD-DEP	0.27	0.47**	0.60**	-
IBS-SI	0.65**	0.50**	0.30	0.24
Non-IBS (N = 310)				
ASI	0.41**	-	-	-
HAD-ANX	0.16**	0.24**	-	-
HAD-DEP	0.09	0.13*	0.52**	-
IBS-SI	0.36**	0.14*	0.04	0.09

Abbreviations: *VSI* Visceral Sensitivity Index, *ASI* Anxiety Sensitivity Index, *HAD-ANX* and *HAD-DEP* subscales of the Hospital Anxiety and Depression scale, *IBS-SI* Irritable Bowel Syndrome Severity Index.
*$p < 0.05$, **$p < 0.01$.

Furthermore, there was a significant correlation between VSI-J and IBS-SI scores when controlling for only the ASI ($r = 0.40$, $p < 0.0001$).

Incremental validity

To examine the ability of the VSI-J to predict GI symptoms, we conducted a hierarchical multiple regression analysis (for the whole sample, $N = 349$) with the IBS-SI score as the dependent variable and the VSI-J, ASI, and HAD-ANX scores as independent variables (Table 6). For the first step, independent variables were the ASI and HAD-ANX scores; for the second step, the independent variable was the VSI-J score. The adjusted multiple correlation coefficient for the IBS-SI increased significantly from the first to the second step (5.2% to 20.5%). These findings suggest that the VSI-J contributed unique effects to the IBS-SI.

Table 6 Hierarchical multiple regression analysis with IBS-SI as the dependent variable

Variable	Step 1				Step 2			
	B	SE B	β	t value	B	SE B	β	t value
Step 1								
HAD-ANX	0.52	1.16	0.02	0.44	−0.13	1.16	0.01	0.12
ASI	2.06	0.49	0.23	4.22**	0.45	0.49	0.05	0.93
Step 2								
VSI					2.78	0.33	0.43	8.23**
F value	10.51**				30.94**			
Adj R^2	0.052				0.205			
ΔR^2	0.06**				0.16**			

Note. N = 349.
Abbreviations: *IBS-SI* Irritable Bowel Syndrome Severity Index, *B* regression coefficients, *SE B* standard errors for regression coefficients, β standard regression coefficient, *Adj R^2* adjusted multiple correlation coefficient, ΔR^2 changes in the multiple squared correlation coefficient, VSI = Visceral Sensitivity Index, *ASI* Anxiety Sensitivity Index, *HAD-ANX* subscale of the Hospital Anxiety and Depression scale.
**$p < 0.01$.

Discussion

Our hypotheses were mainly supported by the findings of the present study. As expected, the VSI-J exhibited a unidimensional factor structure (Hypothesis 1). Further, VSI-J scores were significantly and moderately correlated with scores on the ASI, HAD-ANX, and IBS-SI (Hypothesis 2); however, there was no significant correlation between the VSI-J scores and those of the HAD-DEP. As anticipated, when we controlled for ASI (anxiety sensitivity) and HAD-ANX (anxiety) scores, scores on the VSI-J predicted IBS-SI (GI symptom severity; Hypothesis 3).

Our study was able to demonstrate that the VSI-J is a sufficiently reliable measure of anxiety about GI symptoms. We demonstrated (using EFA) that the index has a unidimensional factor structure similar to that of the original VSI. Cronbach's α was similar to that found in previous studies [27,28] with the original VSI ($\alpha = 0.93$ vs. $\alpha = 0.90–0.93$, respectively), indicating that the VSI-J also has high levels of internal consistency.

We were also able to verify the construct validity of the VSI-J. Correlational analyses showed that scores on the VSI-J were related to scores on measures of anxiety sensitivity (ASI), anxiety (HAD-ANX), and the severity of symptoms (IBS-SI). This is consistent with previous research with the original VSI [27,28]. We found a significant correlation between measures of anxiety sensitivity and gastrointestinal specific anxiety as measured by the VSI-J, confirming previous studies showing that individuals with high trait anxiety and high anxiety sensitivity are more likely to report feeling anxious about their gastrointestinal symptoms [27,28].

Generally, in IBS, a correlation is seen between depression and anxiety [11]. It has also been reported that as GI symptoms increase in severity, psychological distress also increases [12-14]. A previous study has reported that scores on the VSI and the HAD-DEP are significantly correlated in patients with a clinical diagnosis of IBS, although this correlation was not observed in university students with symptoms of IBS [28]. Given previously reported findings regarding the correlation between depression and anxiety in individuals diagnosed with IBS, we expected to see at least a weak correlation between the VSI-J scores and the scores on the depression measure (HAD-DEP). However, we did not find such a correlation. This may be due to the fact that, of participants in this study, those with IBS symptoms only experienced moderately severe GI symptoms, as measured by the IBS-SI.

Our analyses revealed two findings important for understanding the relationship between anxiety and gastrointestinal symptoms. The results of the partial correlation analysis showed that the VSI-J has discriminant validity, as shown by a significant correlation between the VSI-J and the severity measure (IBS-SI) independent of the effects of anxiety and anxiety sensitivity. Further, the results of the hierarchical multiple regression analysis showed that the VSI-J has incremental validity that uniquely affects the IBS-SI. Therefore, it may be appropriate to assess the symptoms of the IBS patient by treating GSA rather than anxiety or AS. Together, these results suggest two intriguing possibilities. First, AS is highly relevant in cases of respiratory and cardiac sensation [35]. It is therefore possible that the VSI-J measures fear responses to GI symptoms and GI sensations, and that it is possible to predict the severity of IBS-SI scores. Second, hyperactivity in the hypothalamic-pituitary-adrenal axis and prefrontal cortex is associated with increased levels of visceral sensitivity, which may exacerbate GI symptoms [36]. Consequently, it is possible that GSA is associated with symptom severity because of the direct path of the efferent nerve originating in the brain and projecting to the gastrointestinal tract.

It is desirable to conduct additional studies to further confirm the reliability and validity of the VSI-J, and to address the following points.

First, this study included only students attending a university located in a medium-sized city on the island of Kyushu in western Japan. Additionally, the present study was based solely on results from a screening questionnaire; it did not include diagnosis or evaluation of symptom severity by a physician. Therefore, it is not known whether these results can be extended to clinical samples in the general population. It will be important to replicate our findings with a general population of patients diagnosed with IBS. At the same time, however, the prevalence of IBS in this study (14%) was similar to that reported for the general population in Japan [37]. It has also been reported that individuals who had never sought treatment for IBS symptoms had higher state anxiety compared with healthy subjects, which matches the pattern usually seen in IBS patients [37]. Thus, we believe sampling bias was unlikely to have affected the conclusions of the present study.

Additionally, at this time, the total VSI-J score does not distinguish between minor and severe symptoms. In the future, it will be necessary to set guidelines and cut-off points so that the scale may be used in clinical settings.

Finally, attention to the GI symptoms of IBS patients may be related to activity in the anterior cingulate and prefrontal cortex [38]. It is important to further study the relationship between executive functioning and GSA, so that eventually the VSI may be used as a measure of brain-gut interaction.

In terms of clinical application, reductions in visceral sensitivity (as measured by the VSI-J) are anticipated as a possible endpoint for IBS interventions, which incorporate pharmacotherapy, exercise therapy, psychotherapy, and nutritional therapy. In recent years, the VSI has been used in Western countries when implementing cognitive behavioral therapy to reduce anxiety associated with IBS symptoms [29,39,40]. Cognitive behavioral therapy is used with the goal of changing individuals' evaluations of threat in situations that cause symptom anxiety and to reduce avoidance behavior. This approach has been shown to significantly improve GI symptoms and GSA [29].

In conclusion, the present study examined the reliability and validity of the newly developed VSI-J in a sample of university students. The scale was found to be reliable and valid in a manner consistent with the original VSI. The VSI-J may now be used to better assess the impact of interventions targeting the reduction of GSA in Japanese patients with IBS. Furthermore, the results of this study may aid in efforts to use the VSI to compare psychological aspects of IBS patients across cultures.

Authors' contributions

TS and JT participated in the design of this study, carried out data collection, translated VSI into Japanese, analyzed the data and drafted the manuscript. TH, NN and TT provided the information about the psychological variables. PB carried out back translation into English, and confirmed phrasing nuances with JL and BN. MK, SS and SF evaluated the results of the study and reviewed the manuscript. All authors read and approved the final manuscript.

Acknowledgments

We would like to express our gratitude to the participants in the present study. This study was supported by the Center for Health and Community Medicine at Nagasaki University and Japan Society for the Promotion of Science KAKENHI Grant Number 24530876.

Author details

[1]Center for Health and Community Medicine, Nagasaki University, Nagasaki, Japan. [2]Department of Preventive Medicine, Graduate School of Biomedical Sciences, Nagasaki University, Nagasaki, Japan. [3]Department of Occupational Therapy, School of Health and Social Services, Saitama Prefectural University, Saitama, Japan. [4]Tohoku Medical Megabank Organization, Tohoku University, Miyagi, Japan. [5]Department of Clinical Psychology, School of Psychological Science, Health Sciences University of Hokkaido, Hokkaido, Japan. [6]Department of Behavioral Medicine, Tohoku University Graduate School of Medicine, 2-1 Seiryo, Aoba, Sendai, Miyagi 980-8575, Japan. [7]Department of Medicine, Center for Neurobiology of Stress, David Geffen School of Medicine, University of California Los Angeles, Los Angeles, CA, USA.

References

1. Drossman DA: **The functional gastrointestinal disorders and the Rome III process.** *Gastroenterology* 2006, **130:**1377–1390.

2. Longstreth GF, Thompson WG, Chey WD, Houghton LA, Mearin F, Spiller RC: **Functional bowel disorders.** *Gastroenterology* 2006, **130:**1480–1491.
3. Spiller R, Aziz Q, Creed F, Emmanuel A, Houghton L, Hungin P, Jones R, Kumar D, Rubin G, Trudgill N, Whorwell P: **Guidelines on the irritable bowel syndrome: mechanisms and practical management.** *Gut* 2007, **56:**1770–1798.
4. Jerndal P, Ringström G, Agerforz P, Karpefors M, Akkermans LM, Bayati A, Simrén M: **Gastrointestinal-specific anxiety: an important factor for severity of GI symptoms and quality of life in IBS.** *Neurogastroenterol Motil* 2010, **22:**646–e179.
5. Maxion-Bergemann S, Thielecke F, Abel F, Bergemann R: **Costs of irritable bowel syndrome in the UK and US.** *Pharmacoeconomics* 2006, **24:**21–37.
6. Kellow JE, Phillips SF: **Altered small bowel motility in irritable bowel syndrome is correlated with symptoms.** *Gastroenterology* 1987, **92:**1885–1893.
7. Drossman DA, Sandler RS, McKee DC, Levity AJ: **Bowel patterns among subjects not seeking health care.** *Gastroenterology* 1982, **83:**529–532.
8. Mayer EA, Raybould HE: **Role of visceral afferent mechanism in functional bowel disorders.** *Gastroenterology* 1987, **99:**1688–1704.
9. Fukudo S, Kanazawa M, Kano M, Sagami Y, Endo Y, Utsumi A, Nomura T, Hongo M: **Exaggerated motility of the descending colon with repetitive distention of the sigmoid colon in patients with irritable bowel syndrome.** *J Gastroenterol* 2002, **37**(suppl 14):145–150.
10. Drossman DA, McKee DC, Sandler RS, Mitchell CM, Cramer EM, Lowman BC, Burger AL: **Psychosocial factors in the irritable bowel syndrome: a multivariate study of patients and nonpatients with irritable bowel syndrome.** *Gastroenterology* 1988, **95:**701–708.
11. Whitehead WE, Bosmajian L, Zonderman AB, Costa PT, Schuster MM: **Symptoms of psychologic distress associated with irritable bowel syndrome: comparison of community and medical clinic samples.** *Gastroenterology* 1988, **95:**709–714.
12. Mertz H, Morgan V, Tanner G, Pickens D, Price R, Shyr Y, Kessler R: **Regional cerebral activation in irritable bowel syndrome and control subjects with painful and nonpainful rectal distention.** *Gastroenterology* 2000, **118:**842–848.
13. Fukudo S, Nomura T, Muranaka M, Taguchi F: **Brain-gut response to stress and cholinergic stimulation in irritable bowel syndrome: a preliminary study.** *J Clin Gastroenterol* 1993, **17:**133–141.
14. Lydiard RB: **Irritable bowel syndrome, anxiety, and depression: what are the links?** *J Clin Psychiatry* 2001, **62:**38–47.
15. Sykes MA, Blanchard EB, Lackner J, Keefer L, Krasner S: **Psychopathology in irritable bowel syndrome: support for a psychophysiological model.** *J Behav Med* 2003, **26:**361–372.
16. Mayer EA: **The neurobiology of stress and gastrointestinal disease.** *Gut* 2000, **47:**861–869.
17. Drossman DA, Ringel Y, Vogt BA, Leserman J, Lin W, Smith JK, Whitehead W: **Alterations of brain activity associated with resolution of emotional distress and pain in a case of severe irritable bowel syndrome.** *Gastroenterology* 2003, **124:**754–761.
18. Silverman DH, Munakata JA, Ennes H, Mandelkern MA, Hoh CK, Mayer EA: **Regional cerebral activity in normal and pathological perception of visceral pain.** *Gastroenterology* 1997, **112:**64–72.
19. Naliboff BD, Derbyshire SW, Munakata J, Berman S, Mandelkern M, Chang L, Mayer EA: **Cerebral activation in patients with irritable bowel syndrome and control subjects during rectosigmoid stimulation.** *Psychosom Med* 2001, **63:**365–375.
20. Munakata J, Naliboff BD, Harraf F, Kodner A, Lembo T, Chang L, Silverman DH, Mayer EA: **Repetitive sigmoid stimulation induces rectal hyperalgesia in patients with irritable bowel syndrome.** *Gastroenterology* 1997, **112:**55–63.
21. Keough ME, Timpano KR, Zawilinski LL, Schmidt NB: **The association between irritable bowel syndrome and the anxiety vulnerability factors: body vigilance and discomfort intolerance.** *J Health Psychol* 2011, **16:**91–98.
22. Yágüez L, Coen S, Gregory LJ, Amaro E, Altman C, Brammer MJ, Bullmore ET, Williams SC, Aziz Q: **Brain response to visceral aversive conditioning: a functional magnetic resonance imaging study.** *Gastroenterology* 2006, **128:**1819–1829.
23. Kanazawa M, Endo M, Yamaguchi K, Hamaguchi T, Whitehead WE, Itoh M, Fukudo S: **Classical conditioned response of rectosigmoid motility and regional cerebral activity in humans.** *Neurogastroenterol Motil* 2005, **17:**705–713.
24. Labus JS, Naliboff BD, Berman SM, Suyenobu B, Vianna EP, Tillisch K, Mayer EA: **Brain networks underlying perceptual habituation to repeated aversive visceral stimuli in patients with irritable bowel syndrome.** *Neuroimage* 2009, **47:**952–960.
25. Mayer EA, Naliboff BD, Chang L, Coutinho SV: **Stress and the gastrointestinal tract: V. stress and irritable bowel syndrome.** *Am J Physiol Gastrointest Liver Physiol* 2001, **280:**G519–G524.
26. Wilder-Smith CH, Schindler D, Lovblad K, Redmond SM, Nirkko A: **Brain functional magnetic resonance imaging of rectal pain and activation of endogenous inhibitory mechanisms in irritable bowel syndrome patient subgroups and healthy controls.** *Gut* 2004, **53:**1595–1601.
27. Labus JS, Bolus R, Chang L, Wiklund I, Naesdal J, Mayer EA, Naliboff BD: **The visceral sensitivity index: development and validation of a gastrointestinal symptom-specific anxiety scale.** *Aliment Pharmacol Ther* 2004, **20:**89–97.
28. Labus JS, Mayer EA, Chang L, Bolus R, Naliboff BD: **The central role of gastrointestinal-specific anxiety in irritable bowel syndrome: further validation of the visceral sensitivity index.** *Psychosom Med* 2007, **69:**89–98.
29. Craske MG, Wolitzky-Taylor KB, Labus J, Wu S, Frese M, Mayer EA, Naliboff BD: **A cognitive-behavioral treatment for irritable bowel syndrome using interoceptive exposure to visceral sensations.** *Behav Res Ther* 2011, **49:**413–421.
30. Lind R, Lied GA, Lillestøl K, Valeur J, Berstad A: **Do psychological factors predict symptom severity in patients with subjective food hypersensitivity?** *Scand J Gastroenterol* 2010, **45:**835–843.
31. Shinozaki M, Kanazawa M, Sagami Y, Endo Y, Hongo M, Drossman DA, Whitehead WE, Fukudo S: **Validation of the Japanese version of the Rome II modular questionnaire and irritable bowel syndrome severity index.** *J Gastroenterol* 2006, **41:**491–494.
32. Zigmond AS, Snaith PP: **The hospital anxiety and depression scale.** *Acta Psychiatr Scand* 1983, **67:**361–370.
33. Reiss S, Peterson RA, Taylor S, Schmidt N, Weems CF: *Anxiety sensitivity index consolidated user manual: ASI, ASI-3, and CASI.* Ohio: IDS Publishing Corporation; 2008.
34. Reiss S, Peterson RA, Gursky DM, Mcnally RJ: **Anxiety sensitivity, anxiety frequency and the prediction of fearfulness.** *Behav Res Ther* 1986, **24:**1–8.
35. Domschke K, Stevens S, Pfleiderer B, Gerlach AL: **Interoceptive sensitivity in anxiety and anxiety disorders: an overview and integration of neurobiological findings.** *Clin Psychol Rev* 2010, **30:**1–11.
36. Fukudo S, Saito K, Sagami Y, Kanazawa M: **Can modulating corticotropin releasing hormone receptors alter visceral sensitivity?** *Gut* 2006, **55:**146–148.
37. Kanazawa M, Endo Y, Whitehead WE, Kano M, Hongo M, Fukudo S: **Patients and nonconsulters with irritable bowel syndrome reporting a parental history of bowel problems have more impaired psychological distress.** *Dig Dis Sci* 2004, **49:**1046–1053.
38. Tillisch K, Mayer EA: **Pain perception in irritable bowel syndrome.** *CNS Spectr* 2005, **10:**877–882.
39. Gaylord SA, Palsson OS, Garland EL, Faurot KR, Coble RS, Mann JD, Frey W, Leniek K, Whitehead WE: **Mindfulness training reduces the severity of irritable bowel syndrome in women: results of a randomized controlled trial.** *Am J Gastroenterol* 2011, **106:**1677–1688.
40. Ljótsson B, Falk L, Vesterlund AW, Hedman E, Lindfors P, Rück C, Hursti T, Andréewitch S, Jansson L, Lindefors N, Andersson G: **Internet-delivered exposure and mindfulness based therapy for irritable bowel syndrome: a randomized controlled trial.** *Behav Res Ther* 2010, **48:**531–539.

26

Luminal and mucosal-associated intestinal microbiota in patients with diarrhea-predominant irritable bowel syndrome

Ian M Carroll[1], Young-Hyo Chang[2], Jiwon Park[1], R Balfour Sartor[1], Yehuda Ringel[1*]

Abstract

Background: Recent studies have suggested a role for an altered intestinal microbiota in the pathophysiology of irritable bowel syndrome (IBS). However, no consensus has been reached regarding the association between specific enteric bacterial groups and IBS. The aim of this study was to investigate the fecal and mucosal-associated microbiota using two independent techniques in intestinal samples from diarrhea-predominant IBS (D-IBS) and healthy controls.

Methods: Fecal and colonic mucosal biopsy samples were obtained from 10 D-IBS patients and 10 healthy controls. Colonic tissue was collected during a un-sedated un-prepped flexible sigmoidoscopy. Fecal and tissue samples were processed immediately upon collection for culture under aerobic and anaerobic conditions or frozen for further molecular analysis. DNA was extracted from all frozen samples and used to enumerate specific bacterial groups using quantitative real-time PCR (qPCR).

Results: Culture analysis of intestinal samples demonstrated a significant reduction in the concentration of aerobic bacteria in fecal samples from D-IBS patients when compared to healthy controls (1.4×10^7 vs. 8.4×10^8 CFUs/g feces, $P = 0.002$). qPCR analysis demonstrated a significant 3.6 fold increase ($P = 0.02$) in concentrations of fecal *Lactobacillus* species between D-IBS patients and healthy controls.

Conclusions: Our culture and molecular data indicate that quantitative differences exist in specific bacterial groups in the microbiota between D-IBS and healthy subjects.

Background

Functional gastrointestinal disorders (FGID) are highly prevalent in Western countries with Irritable Bowel Syndrome (IBS) being the most common (affecting 10-20% of adults and adolescents) [1] and best studied condition. IBS is a heterogeneous disorder that can present as diarrhea-predominant IBS (D-IBS), constipation-predominant IBS (C-IBS), or mixed bowel habit IBS (M-IBS) subsets. Traditionally IBS has been considered a disorder that arises from an altered brain-gut axis that can be associated with gastrointestinal (GI) hypersensitivity and GI motor dysfunction[2,3]. Despite intensive research, the pathophysiology of this disorder is still unclear and no single etiological factor with a defined pathogenic mechanism has been identified. However, studies have implicated new theories that associate specific etiological factors in the pathogenesis of this disorder. These factors include alterations in the normal intestinal microbiota, genetic pre-determinants, pathogenic bacterial infection, food allergy, and an altered gut immune function and inflammation[4-6].

The intestinal microbiota is a complex community of bacteria, archaea, and eukarya. Indirect evidence that the intestinal microbiota plays a role in IBS comes from epidemiologic studies identifying acute GI infection (e.g., acute gastroenteritis) as a strong predictor for the development of IBS[7,8]. Additionally, antibiotic treatment of small intestinal bacterial overgrowth (SIBO) is associated with a resolution of IBS symptoms[9-11]. To further understand the role of the intestinal microbiota in the pathophysiology of IBS several studies have characterized

* Correspondence: yehuda_ringel@med.unc.edu
[1]Division of Gastroenterology and Hepatology, Center for Gastrointestinal Biology and Disease, University of North Carolina at Chapel Hill, Chapel Hill, North Carolina, USA
Full list of author information is available at the end of the article

this complex microbial community in IBS patients. Early studies using selective and non-selective culture techniques demonstrated differing viable levels of coliforms, *Lactobacillus, Bifidobacteria* and *Enterobacteriaceae* species in fecal samples from IBS patients[12,13]. More recent studies have used molecular methods to characterize an abnormality or dysbiosis in the intestinal microbiota of IBS subjects and demonstrated variations in the levels of the *Eubacterium-Clostridium coccoides* group and *Lactobacillus, Veillonella, Coprococcus, Collinsella, Coprobacillus* species in individuals with this disorder [14-21]. However, the majority of these studies used different, often mixed, patient populations and focused their analysis on one specific intestinal niche (fecal [12,16,17,20,21] or mucosal-associated[18] microbiota) with only one study investigating both niches[14]. As the luminal and mucosal-associated microbiota differs in composition[22], it is important to investigate and compare the microbiota of both of these niches.

In the present study we used two independent techniques to quantify and compare specific bacterial groups in fecal and colonic mucosal biopsy samples (collected in a manner that accurately maintained the composition of the microbiota) from patients with D-IBS and healthy controls.

Results

I. Study Population

A total of 20 subjects (10 D-IBS and 10 healthy controls) were investigated. All subjects provided fecal and colonic mucosal samples. The study population consisted of 70% females and had a mean age of 32 years. Demographics and body mass index (BMI) were similar in the two study groups (Table 1).

II. Analysis of the fecal microbiota

The levels of aerobic bacteria in fecal samples from D-IBS patients were significantly lower compared to those from healthy controls (1.4×10^7 vs. 8.4×10^8 CFUs/g feces, $P = 0.002$) (Table 2). No significant differences were observed in the levels of anaerobic bacteria in fecal samples from D-IBS patients and healthy controls (6.24×10^9 vs. 3.12×10^9 CFUs/g feces, $P = 0.3$) (Table 2). Additionally, no significant differences between D-IBS patients and healthy controls were detected using selective media for *Bacteroides, Clostridium, Bifidobacteria, Lactobacillus* species and *Escherichia coli* concentrations in fecal samples (Table 2).

Table 1 Characteristics of D-IBS patients and Healthy Controls

	D-IBS patients	Healthy Controls
Number of subjects	10	10
Age (yr): mean (range)	31.9 (23-50)	32.4 (21-54)
Gender: F/M	8/2	6/4
BMI (kg/m^2): mean (range)	28.5 (23.1-40.6)	27.2 (19.9-36.3)

qPCR analysis detected the concentration of *Clostridium, Bacteroides, Bifidobacterium, Lactobacillus* species, and *E. coli* in all fecal DNA samples with the exception of 1 D-IBS samples that failed to amplify *Lactobacillus* species sequences. A significant 3.6 fold increase in the concentration of *Lactobacillus* species in fecal samples from D-IBS patients was observed when compared to healthy controls (HC = 10; D-IBS = 9, P = 0.02) (Figure 1E). No significant differences between groups were observed for concentrations of *Clostridium, Bacteroides, Bifidobacterium* species, and *E. coli* (Figure 1A-D). Investigation of bacterial groups using additional fecal samples from an on-going study (HC = 7, D-IBS = 6) using the same collection methods but alternative fecal DNA isolation and qPCR methods demonstrated similar results with a significant 2.7 fold increase in *Lactobacillus* species in D-IBS fecal samples compared to healthy controls (HC = 17; D-IBS = 15, P = 0.02) (Figure 2). Similarly, no significant differences between the groups in *Clostridium, Bacteroides, Bifidobacterium* species, and *E. coli* concentrations were detected between healthy controls and D-IBS patients.

III. Analysis of the mucosal-associated intestinal microbiota

No significant differences were observed in the levels of aerobic or anaerobic bacteria in colonic mucosal samples between D-IBS patients and healthy controls (Table 2). Additionally, no significant differences between D-IBS and healthy controls were detected using culture on selective media for *Bacteroides, Clostridium, Bifidobacteria, Lactobacillus* species and *Escherichia coli* (Table 2).

qPCR analysis of colonic mucosal DNA did not reveal any significant differences between groups for *Clostridium, Bacteroides, Bifidobacterium,* and *Lactobacillus* species and *Escherichia coli* (Figure 3A-E).

IV. Comparison of the fecal and mucosal-associated microbiota

Comparison of the fecal and mucosal-associated microbiota in healthy control and D-IBS groups revealed a significantly lower level of cultivable aerobic bacteria in colonic mucosal samples compared to fecal samples in both groups. However, the differences in cultivable aerobic bacteria observed between colonic mucosal and fecal samples from D-IBS patients was less obvious (Table 3). Both healthy control and D-IBS groups displayed a significant difference in cultivable anaerobes, *Bacteroides, Clostridium, Bifidobacteria* species and *E. coli* between mucosal and fecal niches (Table 3). These analyses could not be carried out on *Lactobacillus* species as the levels of these organisms were below detection limits in mucosal samples.

Table 2 Culture analysis of fecal and colonic mucosal samples from D-IBS patients and healthy controls

	Aerobic*	Anaerobic*	*Clostridium* spp.*	*Bacteroides* spp.*	*Lactobacillus* spp.*	*Bifidobacterium* spp.*	*E. coli**
Fecal samples:							
D-IBS patients	1.4×10^7	6.2×10^9	2.0×10^9	8.6×10^8	8.7×10^5	1.1×10^9	7.4×10^6
Healthy controls	8.4×10^8	3.1×10^9	6.0×10^8	3.5×10^8	8.7×10^7	6.4×10^8	1.4×10^8
P value¥	**0.002**	0.14	0.11	0.07	0.08	0.43	0.13
Mucosal samples:							
D-IBS patients	2.2×10^6	9.3×10^6	9.7×10^5	4.6×10^6	-§	1.3×10^6	1.1×10^6
Healthy controls	4.8×10^5	6.5×10^6	1.9×10^6	1.4×10^6	-§	5.9×10^5	7.5×10^3
P value¥	0.96	0.85	0.36	0.78	-	0.68	0.44

*Concentrations expressed in CFUs/g of sample.

§ Below detection levels.

¥ P value calculated using the non-parametric Mann-Whitney test.

Discussion

Recent studies have highlighted the importance of the intestinal microbiota in the well-being of the host. This diverse microbial community has been demonstrated as a critical factor for normal GI function[3,23,24]. As altered intestinal function is associated with IBS it is possible that an intestinal dysbiosis plays a role in the pathophysiology of the disorder. However, the investigation of the intestinal microbiota in IBS is difficult due to the heterogeneity of this condition, and the effects of an altered intestinal microbiota may not be consistent across all subtypes of IBS (D-IBS, C-IBS and M-IBS). In addition, the relative importance of the luminal versus the mucosal-associated niches in this disorder is not yet clear. Nevertheless, many of the studies that sought to characterize the intestinal microbiota in IBS investigated mixed populations of IBS patients[12,13,18], or focused on a single intestinal niche[12,13,15-21]. Thus, the aim of

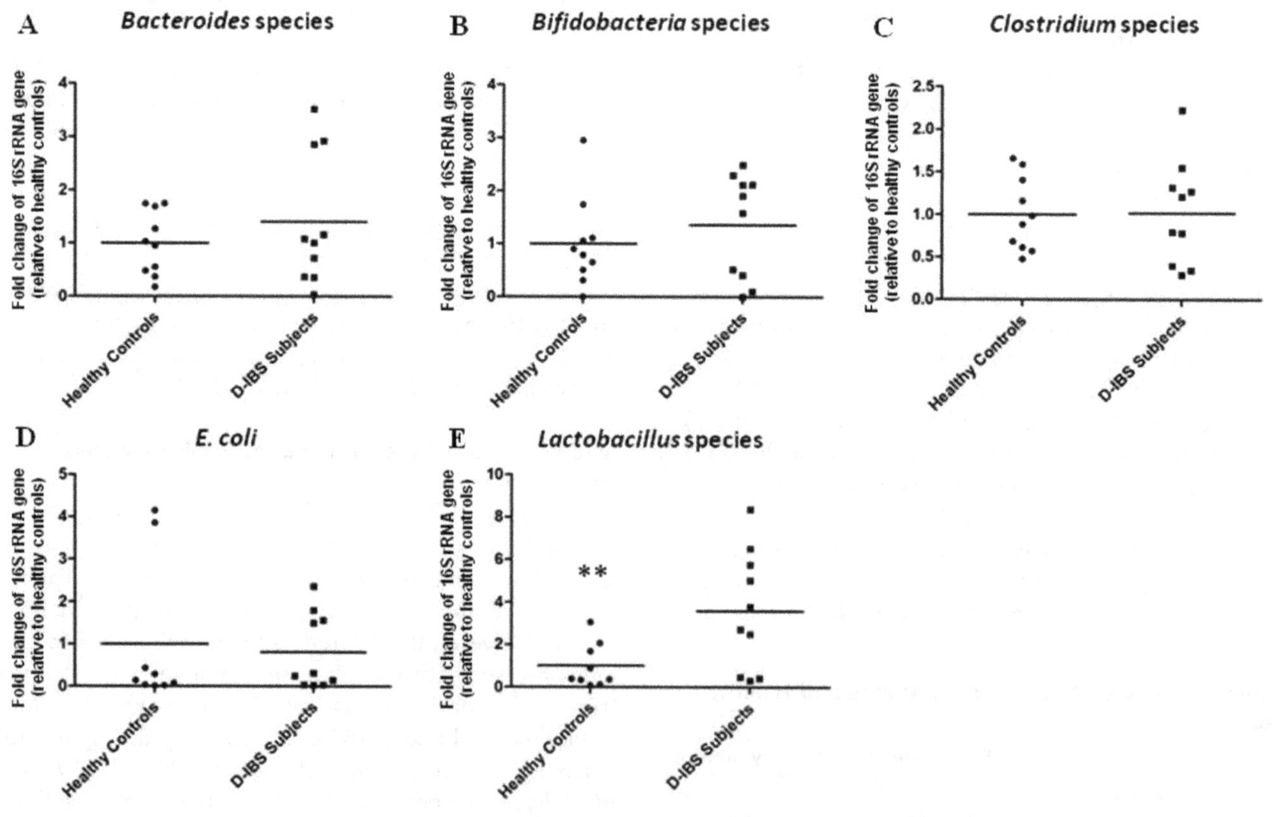

Figure 1 Fold change in concentrations of (A) *Bacteroides* species, (B) *Bifidobacterium* species, (C) *Clostridium* species, (D) *E. coli*, and (E) *Lactobacillus* species in fecal samples from D-IBS patients and healthy controls using qPCR. A significant increase in the levels of *Lactobacillus* species was detected in fecal samples from D-IBS patients (** *P* = 0.02).

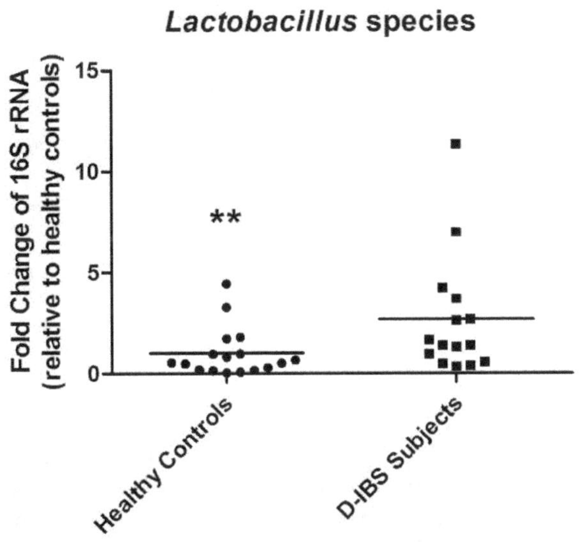

Figure 2 Fold change in concentrations of *Lactobacillus* species in fecal samples from D-IBS patients and healthy controls using a larger sample number and alternative DNA isolation and qPCR methods. A significant increase in the levels of *Lactobacillus* species was detected in fecal samples from D-IBS patients (** $P = 0.02$).

our study was to quantify and compare specific bacterial groups in both the luminal and mucosal-associated intestinal microbiota in a well-defined subgroup of patients with IBS and healthy controls. To achieve this we took the following measures; (a) we investigated a defined IBS subgroup population (D-IBS) to avoid variation in the microbiota compositions between different subtypes of IBS, (b) we used two independent techniques; culture on selective and non-selective media and qPCR, and (c) to avoid possible effects of time between delivery and analysis on the luminal microbiota, fresh fecal samples were collected from study subjects on site. These samples were immediately analyzed by culture or frozen for molecular analysis. To avoid the effect of bowel preparation on the mucosal-associated microbiota, colonic mucosal samples were collected from patients that did not receive a bowel preparation prior to the procedure.

The meticulous measures used in our study may explain some of the differences between our study results and previously reported studies investigating the intestinal microbiota in patients with IBS. For example, using non-selective culturing methods we found a decrease in concentrations of aerobic bacteria in D-IBS patients when compared to healthy controls. Additionally, using selective culture media we found no significant differences in

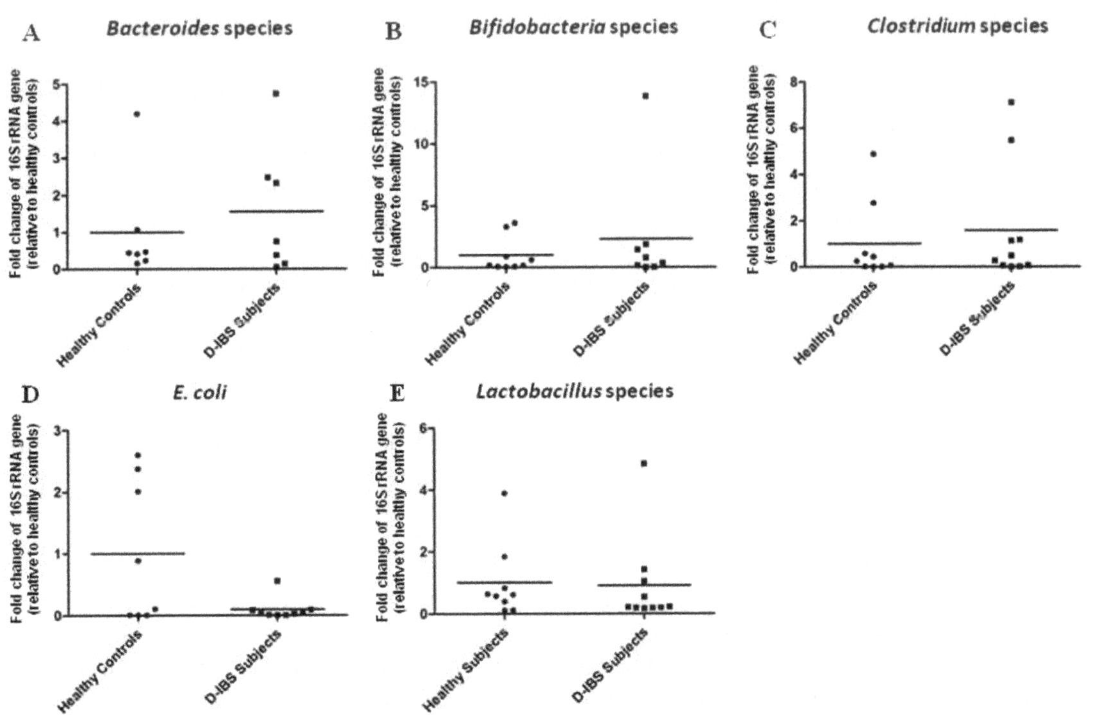

Figure 3 Fold change in concentrations of (A) *Bacteroides* species, (B) *Bifidobacterium* species, (C) *Clostridium* species, (D) *E. coli*, and (E) *Lactobacillus* species in colonic mucosal samples from D-IBS patients and healthy controls using qPCR.

Table 3 Comparison of viable bacterial groups between fecal and colonic mucosal samples

	Aerobic*	Anaerobic*	*Clostridium* spp.*	*Bacteroides* spp.*	*Lactobacillus* spp.*	*Bifidobacterium* spp.*	*E. coli**
Healthy controls:							
Feces	8.4×10^8	3.1×10^9	6.0×10^8	3.5×10^8	8.7×10^7	6.4×10^8	1.4×10^8
Mucosa	4.8×10^5	6.5×10^6	1.9×10^6	1.4×10^6	-§	5.9×10^5	7.5×10^3
P value¥	**0.0003**	**0.0001**	**0.02**	**0.004**	-	**0.04**	**0.019**
D-IBS patients:							
Feces	1.4×10^7	6.2×10^9	2.0×10^9	8.6×10^8	8.7×10^5	1.1×10^9	7.4×10^6
Mucosa	2.2×10^6	9.3×10^6	9.7×10^5	4.6×10^6	-§	1.3×10^6	1.1×10^6
P value¥	**0.05**	**0.0001**	**0.0001**	**0.0001**	-	**0.0001**	**0.01**

*Concentrations expressed in CFUs/g of sample.

§Below detection levels.

¥*P* value calculated using the non-parametric Mann-Whitney test.

concentrations of *Clostridium, Bacteroides, Bifidobacterium,* and *Lactobacillus* species or *E. coli* between D-IBS patients and healthy controls. These observations differ from those of previous studies that used culture techniques, where an increase in the total number of aerobic bacteria and a decrease in coliforms, *Lactobacillus* and *Bifidobacterium* species between IBS patients and healthy controls was reported[12,13,17]. However, these studies investigated a mixed population of IBS patients. In addition, one report investigated a population that included more than 50% of hospitalized patients[12], which may be a completely different population than the IBS population investigated in our study. It is appreciated that enumeration of specific bacterial groups using selective culture can be inaccurate and allow for organisms other than the species of interest to grow on a selective agar plate. Thus, the alternative and more accurate method of qPCR was used to enumerate different bacterial species in our samples.

Using qPCR our investigation demonstrated a significant increase in the levels of *Lactobacillus* species in fecal samples from D-IBS patients. As this finding was not *a priori* anticipated and contradict a previous study that reported a decrease in *Lactobacillus* species in D-IBS patients[16], we validated our results by reanalyzing our samples using alternate DNA extraction and qPCR methods on a larger set of fecal samples. Repeating the analysis using larger numbers and different methods yielded similar results of a significant increase in *Lactobacillus* species in the fecal samples from patients with D-IBS. Furthermore, our findings are supported by a study that demonstrated an increase in *Lactobacillus* species in IBS subjects (a mixed subtype population) using selective culturing techniques[19]. The differing reported results may be a reflection of the different ways of collecting samples as well as the alternate fecal DNA extraction and qPCR methods used. In our study we initially used a method that solely relied upon a high temperature to lyse bacterial cells. As this method may have a bias for bacteria with weaker cell walls (e.g. Gram negative bacteria) we utilized an independent method that ensures complete lysis of bacterial cells with enzymatic (lysozyme and proteinase K), chemical (sodium dodecyl sulfate), and physical disruption (bead-beating) steps. Additionally, we incorporated a universal bacterial primer set in our qPCR assay. The advantage of using this approach is that the bacterial group under investigation is determined as a percentage of total 16S rRNA genes in a sample. In addition, the differences in the reported results may relate to the differences in the study population since the reported decrease in *Lactobacillus species* was observed when comparing D-IBS and C-IBS, but not compared to healthy controls[16].

Our analysis also compared different bacterial groups harbored within fecal and mucosal niches of the intestine. We observed that in healthy individuals and D-IBS subjects the total number of cultivatable aerobic bacteria significantly differed between the microbiota located at these two intestinal sites. However, in D-IBS patients the difference in the levels of aerobic bacteria found between fecal and mucosal niches was less evident. Interestingly, an opposite trend was observed in cultivable *Bacteroides* species, where a significant decrease in the levels of this bacterial group was more obvious between mucosal and fecal niches in D-IBS patients than healthy controls. The remaining bacterial groups investigated showed similar trends between mucosal and fecal niches in both D-IBS patients and healthy controls. At this point it is not known which anaerobic bacteria or *Bacteroides* species are associated with these differences in intestinal niches between healthy individuals and D-IBS patients. However, these observations warrant further examination.

To date two studies have investigated the microbiota of luminal and mucosal niches within the intestine of IBS subjects[14,25]. However, the first of these studies did not collect mucosal samples from healthy controls[14]. In the second study, fecal and duodenal mucosa brush samples were collected from IBS subjects and healthy controls[25]. Our study differed to these previous reports as we collected fecal and colonic mucosal samples from D-IBS subjects and healthy controls. Together our study and these previous reports highlight the importance of investigating both luminal and mucosal niches in the intestine of IBS subjects and healthy controls.

Conclusions

Our data demonstrate differences in both the luminal and mucosal-associated intestinal microbiota between patients with D-IBS and healthy controls. These data suggest that both fecal and mucosal intestinal niches may independently have an important association with D-IBS. The clinical relevance of these observations still need to be addressed as it is difficult to establish whether differences in the intestinal microbiota between D-IBS patients and healthy controls are a cause of the disorder or an effect of the altered intestinal function or luminal environment in these patients. It is also appreciated that this study focused on a limited number of clinically relevant bacterial species in a small sample of patients and does not provide a generalized view of the diverse intestinal microbiota. However, our study presents interesting new findings that substantiates further in depth investigation of the fecal and mucosal-associated intestinal microbiota in IBS and sub-types of IBS using methods that characterize the composition of the intestinal microbiota in greater details.

Methods

Study Population

We studied 10 patients that met the Rome III criteria for D-IBS and 10 healthy controls[1]. Subjects were recruited from the Chapel Hill general population by advertising and from the University of North Carolina (UNC) at Chapel Hill outpatient clinics.

Inclusion criteria comprised of subjects at least 18 years of age and of any gender, race, or ethnicity. All subjects were evaluated by a physician to exclude an alternative diagnosis to IBS. D-IBS subjects had active GI symptoms at the time of sample collection. Healthy controls had no significant recurring GI symptoms. Subjects with a history of GI tract surgery other than appendectomy or cholecystectomy, a history of inflammatory bowel diseases (IBD), celiac disease, lactose malabsorption, or any other diagnosis that could explain chronic or recurring bowel symptoms were excluded from the study. In addition, participants were excluded if they had a history of antibiotic treatment or intentional probiotic consumption two months prior to the beginning of the study.

The extra subjects used to validate qPCR analysis (HC = 7, D-IBS = 6) were recruited in the same manner. The study was approved by the UNC Internal Review Board (IRB) and all subjects signed a consent form prior to participation in the study.

Sample Collection and Preparation

Fresh stool samples were collected from all 20 subjects on site during the study visit at UNC. Each fecal sample was immediately placed in an anaerobic pouch system (AnaeroPack® System, Misubishi Gas Chemical America, Inc.) and transferred on ice to the laboratory. In the laboratory, each stool sample was homogenized and divided into aliquots. Samples were immediately used for culture of viable bacteria and the remaining aliquots were stored at -80°C for DNA extraction and qPCR analysis. The extra 13 subjects included to validate our analyses (HC = 7, D-IBS = 6) provided a fecal sample which processed in the same manner for DNA extraction and qPCR analysis.

Three colonic mucosal biopsies were collected from each subject during an un-sedated flexible sigmoidoscopy. To avoid possible effects of colonic preparation on the intestinal microbiota all the procedures were carried out on un-prepped colons. Colonic mucosal biopsies were taken from the distal colon just above the rectosigmoid junction using cold forceps. Once removed from the colon each biopsy was washed in 1 ml of sterile PBS to remove non-adherent bacteria. The biopsies were then weighed and used immediately for culture of viable bacteria while other samples were flash-frozen in liquid nitrogen for further DNA extraction and qPCR analysis.

Culture of Fecal and Mucosal Microorganisms

An aliquot of a fresh fecal sample or colonic biopsy was aseptically added to sterile phosphate buffer saline (PBS) to obtain a final volume of 1 ml. Fecal samples were vortexed until a homogenous suspension was obtained and colonic biopsies were vortexed for 2 min to ensure the release of all adherent bacteria. The mixture was then serially diluted and spread onto appropriate selective and non-selective agar plates for the detection of specific bacterial groups by aerobic and anaerobic culture. The concentrations of each bacterial group were expressed as the number of colony forming units (CFUs) per gram of sample. The following types of micro-organisms were enumerated:

Total Bacterial Counts

Total aerobic and anaerobic numbers were determined by culturing diluted samples on Brain Heart Infusion (BHI) agar plates (Difico™, Franklin Lakes, NJ) supplemented with L-cystine (0.05%) and hemin (5 mg L^{-1}). Agar plates were incubated aerobically at 37°C for 24 hr to enumerate total aerobic bacteria or anaerobically (10% H_2, 80% N_2, and 10% CO_2) for 48 hr to enumerate total anaerobic bacteria. All colonies encompassing different morphologies were counted on these plates.

Bifidobacteria species

Columbia agar base plates (Difico™, Franklin Lakes, NJ) supplemented with L-cystine (0.05%), hemin (5 mg L^{-1}), horse blood (5%), and a bile salt solution (bile salts: Sodium propionate - 4.5 g L^{-1}, paromonycin sulphate - 15 g L^{-1}, Neomycin sulfate - 60 g $L^{-1}$and Lithium chloride - 900 mg g L^{-1}) were used to culture and enumerate *Bifidobacteria* species. All incubations were carried out anaerobically at 37°C.

Lactobacillus species

Man, Rogosa, and Sharpe (MRS) agar plates (Difico™, Franklin Lakes, NJ) supplemented with L-cystine (0.05%) and hemin (5 mg L^{-1}) were used to enumerate *Lactobacillus* species. All incubations were carried out anaerobically at 37°C.

Escherichia coli

McConkey agar (Difico™, Franklin Lakes, NJ) was used to enumerate *E. coli*. All incubations were carried out aerobically at 37°C.

Clostridium species

McClung Toabe agar plates (Difico™, Franklin Lakes, NJ) were used to enumerate total *Clostridium* species. All incubations were carried out anaerobically at 37°C.

Bacteroides species

Bacteroides Bile Esculin agar plates (Difico™, Franklin Lakes, NJ) were used to enumerate *Bacteroides* species. All plates were incubated anaerobically at 37°C.

Extraction of Fecal DNA

Fecal Samples

Fecal DNA was extracted using the QIAamp® DNA stool mini kit (Qiagen, Valencia, CA). Briefly, 200 mg was taken from each frozen stool sample and placed immediately into ASL buffer. Each fecal sample was homogenized by vortexing. The mixture was then heated to 95°C for 5 min to obtain bacterial lysis. Fecal DNA was further extracted and purified as per the manufacturer's instructions. DNA concentrations were determined using a NanoDrop™ (Thermo Scientific, Wilmington, DE). All fecal DNA samples were adjusted to equal concentrations for subsequent qPCR analysis.

To validate our molecular observations an alternate DNA extraction method was applied to all fecal samples with the addition of 13 extra stool specimens (HC = 7, D-IBS = 6) from an ongoing study (total sample number, HC = 17, D-IBS = 16). This method used more rigorous steps to lyse bacterial cell walls. Briefly, DNA from fecal samples was extracted using a phenol/chloroform extraction method combined with physical disruption of bacterial cells and a DNA clean-up kit (Qiagen DNeasy® Blood and Tissue extraction kit). 100 mg of frozen feces was suspended in 750 μl of sterile bacterial lysis buffer (200 mM NaCl, 100 mM Tris [pH 8.0], 20 mM EDTA, 20 mg/ml lysozyme [Sigma-Aldrich, St. Louis, MO]) and incubated at 37°C for 30 min. Next, 40 μl of proteinase K (20 mg/ml) and 85 μl of 10% SDS was added to the mixture and incubated at 65°C for 30 min. 300 mg of 0.1 mm zirconium beads (BioSpec Products, Bartlesville, OK) was then added and the mixture and homogenized in a bead beater (BioSpec Products, Bartlesville, OK) for 2 min. The homogenized mixture was cooled on ice and then centrifuged at 14,000 rpm for 5 min. The supernatant was transferred to a new 1.5 ml microfuge tube and fecal DNA was further extracted by phenol/chloroform/iso-amyl alcohol (25:24:1) and then chloroform/iso-amyl alcohol (24:1). The supernatant after extraction was precipitated by absolute ethanol at -20°C for 1 hour. The precipitated DNA was suspended in DNase free H2O and then cleaned using the DNeasy® Blood and Tissue extraction kit (Qiagen) from step 3 as per the manufacturer's instructions.

Table 4 Quantitative polymerase chain reaction (qPCR) primes used in this study to enumerate specific bacterial species

Bacterial species		Primer Sequence 5′-3′	Annealing temperature (°C)	PCR Product size (bp)
Bacteroides spp.[a]	F-	ATAGCCTTTCGAAAGRAAGAT	50	495
	R-	CCAGTATCAACTGCAATTTTA		
Clostridium spp.[b]	F-	CGGTACCTGACTAAGAAGC	50	429
	R-	AGTTTYATTCTTGCGAACG		
Escherichia coli[c]	F-	GTTAATACCTTTGCTCATTGA	52	340
	R-	ACCAGGGTATCTAATCCTGTT		
Bifidobacterium spp.[d]	F-	GGGTGGTAATGCCGGATG	55	442
	R-	TAAGCGATGGACTTTCACACC		
Lactobacillus spp.[e]	F-	AGCAGTAGGGAATCTTCCA	50	341
	R-	CACCGCTACACATGGAG		

[a]primers from Matsuki *et al.*,[26]
[b]primers from Rinttila *et al.*,[27]
[c]primers from Malinen *et al.*,[28]
[d]primers from Bartoch *et al.*,[29]
[e]primers from Maeda *et al.*,[30]

Mucosal Samples

DNA from colonic mucosal biopsies was extracted using the Qiagen Allprep DNA/RNA kit™ (Qiagen, Valencia, CA) with the addition of a lysozyme and bead-beating step. Briefly, each biopsy was incubated in 300 μl of a lysozyme solution (30 mg/ml) for 30 min at 37°C. Next, 600 μl of RLT buffer (containing β-mercaptoethanol) and 300 mg of 0.1 mm zirconium beads (BioSpec Products, Bartlesville, OK) were added and the solution was homogenized in a bead beater (BioSpec Products, Bartlesville, OK) for 2 min. The solution was centrifuged for 5 min at 14,000 rpm and DNA was further extracted from the supernatant as per the manufacturer's instructions.

Quantitative PCR

Quantitative PCR (qPCR) was performed using the QuantiTect SYBR® Green PCR kit (Qiagen, Valencia, CA) with primers that amplify the genes encoding 16S rRNA from specific bacterial groups. The primers used to amplify specific groups of are listed in Table 4. qPCR assays were conducted in 96-well plates on a real-time MX 3000*P* thermocycler (Stratagene, La Jolla, CA). Each PCR was carried out in a final volume of 25 μl and contained the following: 1 × SYBR green qPCR Master Mix (Qiagen), 0.5 μM of each primer and 50 ng of purified fecal or colonic mucosal DNA. PCR conditions were as follows: 15 min at 95°C, followed by 40 cycles of 95°C for 1 min, 30 s at the appropriate annealing temperature (Table 4), and 72°C for 1 min. Each plate included duplicate reactions per DNA sample and the appropriate set of standards. qPCR standards were generated by PCR amplifying and cloning the target 16S rRNA genes from an appropriate positive control strain. Melting curve analysis of the PCR products was conducted following each assay to confirm that the fluorescence signal originated from specific PCR products and not from primer-dimers or other artifacts. All qPCR plates included a 'no template' negative control for each primer set. The concentrations of each bacterial group in D-IBS patients were expressed as a 'fold change' with respect to the control group. All microbiology analyses of fecal and colonic mucosal samples were performed blindly, without knowledge of the subjects' clinical data.

To validate our qPCR findings an alternate qPCR method was applied to our larger number of fecal DNA samples (HC = 17, D-IBS = 16). Briefly, qPCR was performed using ABI SYBR® Green PCR Mastermix (Applied Biosystems, Carlsbad, CA) with primers that amplify the genes encoding 16S rRNA from *Lactobacillus* species (Table 4) or all bacteria (total bacterial 16S rRNA in each sample was determined using universal 16S rRNA primers; forward, 5'-GTGSTGCAYG GYTGTCGTCA-3'; reverse, 5'-ACGTCRTCCMCACCT TCCTC-3') in fecal DNA from D-IBS patients and healthy controls. qPCR assays were conducted in 96-well plates on an Eppendorf Realplex^2 mastercycler thermocycler (Eppendorf, Hauppauge, NY). Each PCR was carried out in a final volume of 12 μl and contained the following: 1 × SYBR green mastermix, 0.5 μM of each primer and approximately 50 ng of purified fecal DNA. PCR conditions were as follows: 15 min at 95°C, followed by 40 cycles of 95°C for 15 s, 30 s at the appropriate annealing temperature (Table 4), and 72°C for 45 s. Each plate included duplicate reactions per DNA sample and the appropriate set of standards. The concentration of *Lactobacillus* species were expressed as a percentage of total 16S rRNA sequences in a given sample. Analysis of melting curves confirmed that the fluorescence signal originated from specific PCR products and not from primer-dimers or other artifacts. All qPCR plates included a 'no template' negative control for each primer set. The concentrations of each bacterial group in D-IBS patients were expressed as a 'fold change' with respect to the control group.

Statistical Analysis

For culture analysis the total number of CFUs per gram of feces for aerobic, anaerobic, and each specific bacterial species investigated was determined for each sample. Mean total aerobic, anaerobic and species specific CFUs were compared between D-IBS patients and healthy controls using the non-parametric Mann-Whitney test. Similarly, for qPCR assays the concentration of each bacterium/bacterial group was determined for each sample. Mean number of 16S rRNA sequences per μg of sample DNA was compared between D-IBS patients and healthy controls using the non-parametric Mann-Whitney test. Statistical analysis was carried out using GraphPad software (v4.0a; Prism, San Diego, CA).

List of Abbreviations

IBS: irritable bowel syndrome; D/C/M-IBS: diarrhea/constipation/mixed bowel habit-predominant IBS; HC: healthy controls; CFU: colony forming units; qPCR: quantitative real-time PCR; FGID: functional gastrointestinal disorders; SIBO: small intestinal bacterial overgrowth.

Acknowledgements and Funding

The authors would like to acknowledge Sarah Van Heusen and Sarah Yeskel for their valuable contributions to this study. This study was funded by a DK067674 seed grant from the UNC Center for Functional GI Disorders awarded to YR.

Author details

[1]Division of Gastroenterology and Hepatology, Center for Gastrointestinal Biology and Disease, University of North Carolina at Chapel Hill, Chapel Hill, North Carolina, USA. [2]Korea Research Institute of Bioscience and Biotechnology (KRIBB), Dagjon, Korea.

Authors' contributions

IMC - molecular techniques, statistical analysis, and scribe of manuscript.
YHC - collection of biological samples and culture techniques.

JP - culture techniques.
RBS - study design.
YR - study design, study execution, recruitment of subjects, IRB application scribe, and recipient of funding for study.
All authors read and approved the final draft.

References

1. Longstreth GF, Thompson WG, Chey WD, Houghton LA, Mearin F, Spiller RC: **Functional bowel disorders.** *Gastroenterology* 2006, **130(5)**:1480-1491.
2. Drossman DA: **The functional gastrointestinal disorders and the Rome III process.** *Gastroenterology* 2006, **130(5)**:1377-1390.
3. Ringel Y, Carroll IM: **Alterations in the intestinal microbiota and functional bowel symptoms.** *Gastrointest Endosc Clin N Am* 2009, **19(1)**:141-150, vii.
4. Ringel Y, Sperber AD, Drossman DA: **Irritable bowel syndrome.** *Annu Rev Med* 2001, **52**:319-338.
5. Azpiroz F, Bouin M, Camilleri M, Mayer EA, Poitras P, Serra J, Spiller RC: **Mechanisms of hypersensitivity in IBS and functional disorders.** *Neurogastroenterol Motil* 2007, **19(1 Suppl)**:62-88.
6. Scanu AM, Bull TJ, Cannas S, Sanderson JD, Sechi LA, Dettori G, Zanetti S, Hermon-Taylor J: **Mycobacterium avium subspecies paratuberculosis infection in cases of irritable bowel syndrome and comparison with Crohn's disease and Johne's disease: common neural and immune pathogenicities.** *J Clin Microbiol* 2007, **45(12)**:3883-3890.
7. Rodriguez LA, Ruigomez A: **Increased risk of irritable bowel syndrome after bacterial gastroenteritis: cohort study.** *Bmj* 1999, **318(7183)**:565-566.
8. Spiller RC: **Is IBS caused by infectious diarrhea?** ***Nat Clin Pract Gastroenterol Hepatol.*** 2007, **4**(12):642-643.
9. Pimentel M, Chow EJ, Lin HC: **Normalization of lactulose breath testing correlates with symptom improvement in irritable bowel syndrome. a double-blind, randomized, placebo-controlled study.** *Am J Gastroenterol* 2003, **98(2)**:412-419.
10. Pimentel M: **Review of rifaximin as treatment for SIBO and IBS.** *Expert Opin Investig Drugs* 2009, **18(3)**:349-358.
11. Pimentel M, Chow EJ, Lin HC: **Eradication of small intestinal bacterial overgrowth reduces symptoms of irritable bowel syndrome.** *Am J Gastroenterol* 2000, **95(12)**:3503-3506.
12. Balsari A, Ceccarelli A, Dubini F, Fesce E, Poli G: **The fecal microbial population in the irritable bowel syndrome.** *Microbiologica* 1982, **5(3)**:185-194.
13. Si JM, Yu YC, Fan YJ, Chen SJ: **Intestinal microecology and quality of life in irritable bowel syndrome patients.** *World J Gastroenterol* 2004, **10(12)**:1802-1805.
14. Codling C, O'Mahony L, Shanahan F, Quigley EM, Marchesi JR: **A Molecular Analysis of Fecal and Mucosal Bacterial Communities in Irritable Bowel Syndrome.** *Dig Dis Sci* 2010, **55(2)**:392-397.
15. Kassinen A, Krogius-Kurikka L, Makivuokko H, Rinttila T, Paulin L, Corander J, Malinen E, Apajalahti J, Palva A: **The fecal microbiota of irritable bowel syndrome patients differs significantly from that of healthy subjects.** *Gastroenterology* 2007, **133(1)**:24-33.
16. Malinen E, Rinttila T, Kajander K, Matto J, Kassinen A, Krogius L, Saarela M, Korpela R, Palva A: **Analysis of the fecal microbiota of irritable bowel syndrome patients and healthy controls with real-time PCR.** *Am J Gastroenterol* 2005, **100(2)**:373-382.
17. Matto J, Maunuksela L, Kajander K, Palva A, Korpela R, Kassinen A, Saarela M: **Composition and temporal stability of gastrointestinal microbiota in irritable bowel syndrome–a longitudinal study in IBS and control subjects.** *FEMS Immunol Med Microbiol* 2005, **43(2)**:213-222.
18. Swidsinski A, Weber J, Loening-Baucke V, Hale LP, Lochs H: **Spatial organization and composition of the mucosal flora in patients with inflammatory bowel disease.** *J Clin Microbiol* 2005, **43(7)**:3380-3389.
19. Tana C, Umesaki Y, Imaoka A, Handa T, Kanazawa M, Fukudo S: **Altered profiles of intestinal microbiota and organic acids may be the origin of symptoms in irritable bowel syndrome.** *Neurogastroenterol Motil* 2010, **22(55)**:512-519.
20. Krogius-Kurikka L, Lyra A, Malinen E, Aarnikunnas J, Tuimala J, Paulin L, Makivuokko H, Kajander K, Palva A: **Microbial community analysis reveals high level phylogenetic alterations in the overall gastrointestinal microbiota of diarrhoea-predominant irritable bowel syndrome sufferers.** *BMC Gastroenterol* 2009, **9**:95.
21. Lyra A, Rinttila T, Nikkila J, Krogius-Kurikka L, Kajander K, Malinen E, Matto J, Makela L, Palva A: **Diarrhoea-predominant irritable bowel syndrome distinguishable by 16S rRNA gene phylotype quantification.** *World J Gastroenterol* 2009, **15(47)**:5936-5945.
22. Zoetendal EG, von Wright A, Vilpponen-Salmela T, Ben-Amor K, Akkermans AD, de Vos WM: **Mucosa-associated bacteria in the human gastrointestinal tract are uniformly distributed along the colon and differ from the community recovered from feces.** *Appl Environ Microbiol* 2002, **68(7)**:3401-3407.
23. Caenepeel P, Janssens J, Vantrappen G, Eyssen H, Coremans G: **Interdigestive myoelectric complex in germ-free rats.** *Dig Dis Sci* 1989, **34(8)**:1180-1184.
24. Husebye E, Hellstrom PM, Sundler F, Chen J, Midtvedt T: **Influence of microbial species on small intestinal myoelectric activity and transit in germ-free rats.** *Am J Physiol Gastrointest Liver Physiol* 2001, **280(3)**:G368-380.
25. Kerckhoffs AP, Samsom M, van der Rest ME, de Vogel J, Knol J, Ben-Amor K, Akkermans LM: **Lower Bifidobacteria counts in both duodenal mucosa-associated and fecal microbiota in irritable bowel syndrome patients.** *World J Gastroenterol* 2009, **15(23)**:2887-2892.
26. Matsuki T, Watanabe K, Fujimoto J, Takada T, Tanaka R: **Use of 16S rRNA gene-targeted group-specific primers for real-time PCR analysis of predominant bacteria in human feces.** *Appl Environ Microbiol* 2004, **70(12)**:7220-7228.
27. Rinttila T, Kassinen A, Malinen E, Krogius L, Palva A: **Development of an extensive set of 16S rDNA-targeted primers for quantification of pathogenic and indigenous bacteria in faecal samples by real-time PCR.** *J Appl Microbiol* 2004, **97(6)**:1166-1177.
28. Malinen E, Kassinen A, Rinttila T, Palva A: **Comparison of real-time PCR with SYBR Green I or 5'-nuclease assays and dot-blot hybridization with rDNA-targeted oligonucleotide probes in quantification of selected faecal bacteria.** *Microbiology* 2003, **149(Pt 1)**:269-277.
29. Bartosch S, Fite A, Macfarlane GT, McMurdo ME: **Characterization of bacterial communities in feces from healthy elderly volunteers and hospitalized elderly patients by using real-time PCR and effects of antibiotic treatment on the fecal microbiota.** *Appl Environ Microbiol* 2004, **70(6)**:3575-3581.
30. Maeda H, Fujimoto C, Haruki Y, Maeda T, Kokeguchi S, Petelin M, Arai H, Tanimoto I, Nishimura F, Takashiba S: **Quantitative real-time PCR using TaqMan and SYBR Green for Actinobacillus actinomycetemcomitans, Porphyromonas gingivalis, Prevotella intermedia, tetQ gene and total bacteria.** *FEMS Immunol Med Microbiol* 2003, **39(1)**:81-86.

Permissions

All chapters in this book were first published by BioMed Central; hereby published with permission under the Creative Commons Attribution License or equivalent. Every chapter published in this book has been scrutinized by our experts. Their significance has been extensively debated. The topics covered herein carry significant findings which will fuel the growth of the discipline. They may even be implemented as practical applications or may be referred to as a beginning point for another development.

The contributors of this book come from diverse backgrounds, making this book a truly international effort. This book will bring forth new frontiers with its revolutionizing research information and detailed analysis of the nascent developments around the world.

We would like to thank all the contributing authors for lending their expertise to make the book truly unique. They have played a crucial role in the development of this book. Without their invaluable contributions this book wouldn't have been possible. They have made vital efforts to compile up to date information on the varied aspects of this subject to make this book a valuable addition to the collection of many professionals and students.

This book was conceptualized with the vision of imparting up-to-date information and advanced data in this field. To ensure the same, a matchless editorial board was set up. Every individual on the board went through rigorous rounds of assessment to prove their worth. After which they invested a large part of their time researching and compiling the most relevant data for our readers.

The editorial board has been involved in producing this book since its inception. They have spent rigorous hours researching and exploring the diverse topics which have resulted in the successful publishing of this book. They have passed on their knowledge of decades through this book. To expedite this challenging task, the publisher supported the team at every step. A small team of assistant editors was also appointed to further simplify the editing procedure and attain best results for the readers.

Apart from the editorial board, the designing team has also invested a significant amount of their time in understanding the subject and creating the most relevant covers. They scrutinized every image to scout for the most suitable representation of the subject and create an appropriate cover for the book.

The publishing team has been an ardent support to the editorial, designing and production team. Their endless efforts to recruit the best for this project, has resulted in the accomplishment of this book. They are a veteran in the field of academics and their pool of knowledge is as vast as their experience in printing. Their expertise and guidance has proved useful at every step. Their uncompromising quality standards have made this book an exceptional effort. Their encouragement from time to time has been an inspiration for everyone.

The publisher and the editorial board hope that this book will prove to be a valuable piece of knowledge for researchers, students, practitioners and scholars across the globe.

List of Contributors

Hassan KH. Rajab
University of Tikrit, college of medicine, Department of clinical pharmacology, College of medicine, University of Tikrit, Iraq

Dharati Rami, Nehal Shah and Pinak Patel
Indubhai Patel College of Pharmacy and Research Centre, Dharmaj, Gujarat-388430, India

Vivek Rami
Internal Medicine Resident, Sheth Vadilal Sarabhai General Hospital, Ahmedabad-380006, Gujarat, India

Keyur Sheth
Department of Gastroenterology, Hepatology and Interventional Endoscopy, Chembur, Mumbai, Maharashtra, India

Khushi Bruta, Vanshika, Kishnoor Bhasin and Bhawana
Department of Biochemistry, Shaheed Rajguru College of Applied Sciences for Women, University of Delhi, Vasundhara Enclave, New Delhi 110096, India

Motoko Ida
Japan-Asia Planning & Administration, Medical & Development, Astellas Pharma Inc, 2-5-1 Nihonbashi -Honcho, Chuo-ku, Tokyo 103-8411, Japan

Akito Nishida
Development Project Management, Astellas Pharma Inc, Tokyo, Japan

Hiraku Akiho
Japan-Asia Clinical Development 2, Development, Astellas Pharma Inc, Tokyo, Japan

Yoshihiro Nakashima
Japan-Asia Data Science, Development, Astellas Pharma Inc, Tokyo, Japan

Kei Matsueda
Sakura Life Clinic, Tokyo, Japan

Shin Fukudo
Department of Behavioral Medicine, Tohoku University Graduate School of Medicine, Sendai, Japan

Nagisa Sugaya
Unit of Public Health and Preventive Medicine, School of Medicine, Yokohama City University, 3-9 Fukuura, Kanazawa-ku, Yokohama City 236-0004, Japan

Kentaro Shirotsuki
Graduate School of Human and Social Sciences, Musashino University, Tokyo, Japan
Faculty of Human Sciences, Musashino University, 3-3-3 Ariake, Koto-ku, Tokyo 135-8181, Japan

Mutsuhiro Nakao
Department of Psychosomatic Medicine, School of Medicine, International University of Health and Welfare, Chiba, Japan

Yoshitoshi Tomita
Department of Psychosomatic Medicine, National Center Hospital, National Center of Neurology and Psychiatry, 4-1-1 Ogawahigashi, Kodaira, Tokyo 187-8553, Japan

Misako Funaba
Department of Behavioral Medicine, National Institute of Mental Health, National Center of Neurology and Psychiatry, 4-1-1 Ogawahigashi, Kodaira, Tokyo 187-8553, Japan

Hiroshi Iida and Masahiko Inamori
Department of Medical Education, School of Medicine, Yokohama City University, 3-9 Fukuura, Kanazawa-ku, Yokohama 236-0004, Japan

Fumiyuki Chin Gardner
Department of Pediatrics, The Pennsylvania State University, 500 University Drive, Hershey, PA 17033, USA

Toshinari Odawara
Health Management Center, Yokohama City University, 22-2 Seto, Kanazawa-ku, Yokohama 236-0027, Japan

Tetsuya Ando
Department of Behavioral Medicine, National Institute of Mental Health, National Center of Neurology and Psychiatry, 4-1-1 Ogawahigashi, Kodaira, Tokyo 187-8553, Japan

Department of Psychosomatic Medicine, Narita Hospital, International University of Health and Welfare, 852 Hatakeda, Narita, Chiba 286-8686, Japan

Qiang Wang and Zeinab Charmchi
Department of Neurology, Kings County Hospital Center, SUNY Downstate Medical Center and Maimonides Medical Center, SUNY Downstate Health Sciences University, Brooklyn, NY, USA

Ilena C. George
Department of Neurology, Massachusetts General Hospital, 55 Fruit St, Boston, MA 02114, USA

Mei Luo, Xiaojun Zhuang, Zhenyi Tian and Lishou Xiong
Department of Gastroenterology and Hepatology, the First Affiliated Hospital of Sun Yat-Sen University, Guangzhou, China

Jiawei Zhu, Zhiying Dong and Lianna Sun
School of Pharmacy, Shanghai University of Traditional Chinese Medicine, Shanghai 201203, People's Republic of China

Jiani Chen, Zhipeng Wang and Xia Tao
Department of Pharmacy, Second Affiliated Hospital of Naval Medical University, Shanghai 200003, China

Mingming Li
School of Pharmacy, Shanghai University of Traditional Chinese Medicine, Shanghai 201203, People's Republic of China
Department of Pharmacy, Second Affiliated Hospital of Naval Medical University, Shanghai 200003, China

Xuan Liu, Jigui Tang, Cian Zhang, Jianpeng Jiao and Xiaoqiang Yue
Department of Traditional Chinese Medicine, Second Affiliated Hospital of Naval Medical University, Shanghai 200003, China

Fenghao Yin
Department of Pharmacy, 905 Hospital of People's Liberation Army Navy, Shanghai 200050, China

Shi Qiu
Traditional Chinese Medicine Resource and Technology Center, Shanghai University of Traditional Chinese Medicine, Shanghai 201203, China

Feng Zhang and Shouhong Gao
Department of Pharmacy, Second Affiliated Hospital of Naval Medical University, Shanghai 200003, China
Shanghai Key Laboratory for Pharmaceutical Metabolite Research, Shanghai 200433, China

Wansheng Chen
School of Pharmacy, Shanghai University of Traditional Chinese Medicine, Shanghai 201203, People's Republic of China
Department of Pharmacy, Second Affiliated Hospital of Naval Medical University, Shanghai 200003, China
Traditional Chinese Medicine Resource and Technology Center, Shanghai University of Traditional Chinese Medicine, Shanghai 201203, China
Shanghai Key Laboratory for Pharmaceutical Metabolite Research, Shanghai 200433, China

Qin Liu, Lin Xiao and Li-Shou Xiong
Department of Gastroenterology and Hepatology, The First Affiliated Hospital of Sun Yat-Sen University, Guangzhou 510080, China

Shima Kumei
Department of General Medicine, Asahikawa Medical University, Asahikawa, Japan

Masatomo Ishioh, Yuki Murakami and Katsuyoshi Ando
Division of Metabolism, Systemic Bioscience, Gastroenterology and Hematology/Oncology, Department of Medicine, Asahikawa Medical University, Asahikawa, Japan

Tsukasa Nozu
Department of Regional Medicine and Education, Asahikawa Medical University, Asahikawa, Japan

Toshikatsu Okumura
Department of General Medicine, Asahikawa Medical University, Asahikawa, Japan
Division of Metabolism, Systemic Bioscience, Gastroenterology and Hematology/Oncology, Department of Medicine, Asahikawa Medical University, Asahikawa, Japan

Emin Gemcioglu and Nuray Yılmaz Cakmak
Department of Internal Medicine, Ankara City Hospital, Ankara 06100, Turkey

Salih Baser
Department of Internal Medicine, Yıldırım Beyazıt University School of Medicine, Ankara, Turkey

Servet Kocaoz
Department of General Surgery, Ankara City Hospital, Ankara, Turkey

Osman Ersoy
Department of Gastroenterology, Yıldırım Beyazıt University School of Medicine, Ankara, Turkey

Ioannis D Komninos
Neapoli Primary Health Care Centre, Neapoli, Crete, Greece

Ioanna G Tsiligianni
Agia Barbara Primary Health Care Centre, Agia Barbara, Heraklion, Crete, Greece

Hugh MacPherson, Helen Tilbrook, J Martin Bland, Karen Bloor, Sally Brabyn, Helen Cox, Arthur Ricky Kang'ombe, Mei-See Man, Tracy Stuardi, David Torgerson and Ian Watt and Peter
Department of Health Sciences, University of York, York, UK

Whorwell
Wythenshawe Hospital, Manchester, UK

Elaine F Harkness and Laura Grant
Institute of Inflammation and Repair, Stopford Building, University of Manchester, Oxford Road, Manchester M13 9PL, UK

Sarah J O'Brien
Institute of Infection and Global Health, Leahurst Campus, University of Liverpool, Chester High Road, Neston, South Wirral CH64 7TE, UK

Carolyn A Chew-Graham
Research Institute, Primary Care and Health Sciences, Keele University, Keele, Staffordshire ST5 5BG, UK

David G Thompson
Gastrointestinal Centre, Institute of Inflammation & Repair, University of Manchester, Clinical Sciences Building, Salford Royal NHS Foundation Trust, Stott Lane, Salford M6 8HD, UK

Katsumi Murakami and Naohiko Moriguchi
1Department of Pediatrics, Kinki University Sakai Hospital, 2-7-1 Harayamadai, Minami-ku, Sakai, Osaka 590-0132, Japan

Chizu Habukawa
Department of Pediatrics, Minami Wakayama Medical Center, 27-1 Takinai-machi, Tanabe-shi, Wakayama 646-0015, Japan

Yukihiro Nobuta
Probiotics Research Group, Nature-Wellness research Department, Research Institute, KAGOME Co, LTD. 17Nishitomiyama, Nasushiobara, Tochigi 329-2762, Japan

Tsukasa Takemura
Department of Pediatrics, Kinki University Faculty of Medicine, 377-2, Onohigashi, Osakasayama-shi, Osaka 589-8511, Japan

David A Andrae and Paul S Covington
Furiex Pharmaceuticals, Inc, 3900 Paramount Parkway, Suite 150, Morrisville, NC 27560, USA

Donald L Patrick
Department of Health Services, University of Washington School of Public Health, Seattle, WA, USA

Douglas A Drossman
Drossman Center for the Education and Practice of Biopsychosocial Care LLC, and UNC Center for Functional GI and Motility Disorders, Chapel Hill, NC, USA

Lesley M Roberts, Deborah McCahon, Roger Holder and Sue Wilson
Primary Care Clinical Sciences, School of Health and Population Sciences, University of Birmingham, Edgbaston, Birmingham B15 2TT, UK

FD Richard Hobbs
Department of Primary Care Health Sciences, Oxford University, 2nd Floor, 23-38 Hythe Bridge Street, Oxford OX1 2ET, UK

Maria Elena Ramirez-Miranda, Rosaura Hernandez-Castellanos, Eduardo Lopez-Escamilla, David Moncada, Alberto Gonzalez-Angulo, Simon Kawa-Karasik and Pablo Maravilla
Dr. Manuel Gea Gonzalez General Hospital, Mexico, DF 14080, Mexico

Alfredo Rodriguez-Magallan and Carlos Pagaza-Melero
Hospital Juarez de Mexico, Mexico, DF 07760, Mexico

Ana Flisser
Departamento de Microbiologia y Parasitologia, Facultad de Medicina, Universidad Nacional Autonoma de Mexico, Mexico DF 04510, Mexico

Fatemeh Bazarganipour
Social Determinants of Health Research Center, Yasuj University of Medical Sciences, Yasuj, Iran

Seyed-Abdolvahab Taghavi
Medicinal Plants Research Center, Yasuj University of Medical Sciences, Yasuj, Iran

Zatollah Asemi
Research Center for Biochemistry and Nutrition in Metabolic Diseases, Institute for Basic Sciences, Kashan University of Medical Sciences, Kashan, IR, Iran

Helen Allan
Centre for Critical Research in Nursing & Midwifery, School of Health & Education, Middlesex University, London, UK

Zahra Khashavi
Infertility Clinic, Omeleila Hospital, Bandar Abbas, Hormozgan, Iran

Tahereh Safarzadeh, Shamsi Pourchangiz, Fatemeh Zare, Samaneh Ghasemi and Zivar Karimi
Student Research Committee, Hormozgan University of Medical Sciences, Bandar Abbas, Iran

Maryam Azizi Kutenaee
Fertility and Infertility Research Center, Hormozgan University of Medical Sciences, Bandar Abbas, Iran

Venu Lagishetty and Megan C. Hauer
Vatche and Tamar Manoukian Division of Digestive Diseases, Department of Medicine, David Geffen School of Medicine, University of California Los Angeles, Los Angeles, CA, USA

Jennifer S. Labus, Emeran A. Mayer, Arpana Gupta and Bruce D. Naliboff
Vatche and Tamar Manoukian Division of Digestive Diseases, Department of Medicine, David Geffen School of Medicine, University of California Los Angeles, Los Angeles, CA, USA
G. Oppenheimer Center for Neurobiology of Stress and Resilience, David Geffen School of Medicine, University of California Los Angeles, Los Angeles, CA, USA

Jonathan P. Jacobs
Vatche and Tamar Manoukian Division of Digestive Diseases, Department of Medicine, David Geffen School of Medicine, University of California Los Angeles, Los Angeles, CA, USA
G. Oppenheimer Center for Neurobiology of Stress and Resilience, David Geffen School of Medicine, University of California Los Angeles, Los Angeles, CA, USA
Division of Gastroenterology, Hepatology and Parenteral Nutrition, VA Greater Los Angeles Healthcare System, Los Angeles, CA, USA

Tien S. Dong
Vatche and Tamar Manoukian Division of Digestive Diseases, Department of Medicine, David Geffen School of Medicine, University of California Los Angeles, Los Angeles, CA, USA
Division of Gastroenterology, Hepatology and Parenteral Nutrition, VA Greater Los Angeles Healthcare System, Los Angeles, CA, USA

Ryan Toma and Momchilo Vuyisich
Viome Life Sciences, Bellevue, WA, USA

Jeffrey M. Lackner
Division of Behavioral Medicine, Department of Medicine, Jacobs School of Medicine, University at Buffalo, SUNY, Buffalo, NY, USA

Kirsten Tillisch
Vatche and Tamar Manoukian Division of Digestive Diseases, Department of Medicine, David Geffen School of Medicine, University of California Los Angeles, Los Angeles, CA, USA
G. Oppenheimer Center for Neurobiology of Stress and Resilience, David Geffen School of Medicine, University of California Los Angeles, Los Angeles, CA, USA
Integrative Medicine, VA Greater Los Angeles Healthcare System, Los Angeles, CA, USA

Tatsuo Saigo and Susumu Shirabe
Center for Health and Community Medicine, Nagasaki University, Nagasaki, Japan

Naoki Nakaya
Department of Preventive Medicine and Epidemiology, Tohoku Medical Megabank Organization, Tohoku University, Tohoku, Japan
Tohoku Medical Megabank Organization, Tohoku University, Miyagi, Japan

Masae Shinozaki and Shin Fukudo
Department of Behavioral Medicine, Tohoku University Graduate School of Medicine, Tohoku, Japan

Juliette MTM Rutten, Carla Frankenhuis and Marc A Benninga
Department of Pediatric Gastroenterology, Emma Children's Hospital/Academic Medical Center, 1100 DD Amsterdam, The Netherlands

Arine M Vlieger
Department of Pediatrics, St. Antonius Hospital, Nieuwegein, The Netherlands

Elvira K George
Department of Pediatrics, Medical Center Alkmaar, Alkmaar, The Netherlands

Michael Groeneweg
Department of Pediatrics, Maasstad Hospital, Rotterdam, The Netherlands

Obbe F Norbruis
Department of Pediatrics, Isala Clinics, Zwolle, The Netherlands

Walther Tjon a Ten
Department of Pediatrics, Maxima Medical Center, Veldhoven, The Netherlands

Herbert Van Wering
Department of Pediatrics, Amphia Hospital, Breda, The Netherlands

Marcel GW Dijkgraaf and Maruschka P Merkus
Clinical Research Unit, Academic Medical Center, Amsterdam, The Netherlands

Jun Tayama, Peter J Bernick and Susumu Shirabe
Center for Health and Community Medicine, Nagasaki University, Nagasaki, Japan

Tatsuo Saigo
Center for Health and Community Medicine, Nagasaki University, Nagasaki, Japan
Department of Preventive Medicine, Graduate School of Biomedical Sciences, Nagasaki University, Nagasaki, Japan

Toyohiro Hamaguchi
Department of Occupational Therapy, School of Health and Social Services, Saitama Prefectural University, Saitama, Japan

Tadaaki Tomiie
Department of Clinical Psychology, School of Psychological Science, Health Sciences University of Hokkaido, Hokkaido, Japan
School of Psychological Science, Health Sciences University of Hokkaido, Hokkaido, Japan

Motoyori Kanazawa and Shin Fukudo
Department of Behavioral Medicine, Tohoku University Graduate School of Medicine, 2-1 Seiryo, Aoba, Sendai, Miyagi 980-8575, Japan

Jennifer S Labus and Bruce D Naliboff
Department of Medicine, Center for Neurobiology of Stress, David Geffen School of Medicine, University of California Los Angeles, Los Angeles, CA, USA

Ian M Carroll, Jiwon Park, R Balfour Sartor and Yehuda Ringel
Division of Gastroenterology and Hepatology, Center for Gastrointestinal Biology and Disease, University of North Carolina at Chapel Hill, Chapel Hill, North Carolina, USA

Young-Hyo Chang
Korea Research Institute of Bioscience and Biotechnology (KRIBB), Dagjon, Korea

Index

www.ingramcontent.com/pod-product-compliance
Lightning Source LLC
LaVergne TN
LVHW082130200926
848484LV00008B/2037
* 9 7 9 8 8 8 7 4 0 6 4 5 9 *